NOT SURE WHAT TO CHOOSE
TO HELP YOU
OR YOUR LOVED ONES
FEEL BETTER?

THE
PILL BOOK GUIDE TO
OVER-THE-COUNTER MEDICATIONS
GIVES YOU ALL THE FACTS:

- Which leading pain reliever should be avoided if you have kidney or liver problems
- Which pain reliever is best for menstrual cramps
- How to reduce a fever without using drugs
- Why some brand-name cough products may in fact be counterproductive
- Which prescription drugs are most likely to become available over the counter and why
- Why some decongestant nose drops can make your congestion even worse
- Why using certain antihistamine creams can actually give you a rash

LET THE
PILL BOOK GUIDE TO
OVER-THE-COUNTER MEDICATIONS
BE YOUR
HOME HEALTH RESOURCE!

THE PILL BOOK
GUIDE TO OVER-THE-COUNTER MEDICATIONS
1st EDITION

Production
CMD PUBLISHING
A division of Current Medical Directions

Editor-in-Chief
ROBERT P. RAPP, Pharm. D.
Professor and Director
Division of Pharmacy Practice and Science
College of Pharmacy
University of Kentucky

Digital Photography and Color Separations
WACE, NEW YORK

BANTAM BOOKS
NEW YORK • TORONTO • LONDON • SYDNEY • AUCKLAND

THE PILL BOOK GUIDE TO OVER-THE-COUNTER MEDICATIONS

A Bantam Book / July 1997

ISBN: 0-553-57729-8

Published simultaneously in the United States and Canada

Bantam Books are published by Bantam Books, a division of Bantam Doubleday Dell Publishing Group, Inc. Its trademark, consisting of the words "Bantam Books" and the portrayal of a rooster, is Registered in U.S. Patent and Trademark Office and in other countries. Marca Registrada, Bantam Books, 1540 Broadway, New York, New York 10036.

PRINTED IN THE UNITED STATES OF AMERICA

OPM 0 9 8 7 6 5 4 3 2 1

Contents

The purpose of this book is to provide educational information to the public concerning the majority of the various types of drugs that are presently available over the counter. It is not intended to be complete or exhaustive or in any respect a substitute for personal medical care.

While every effort has been made to reproduce products on the cover and in the insert of this book in an exact fashion, certain variations in size or color may be expected as a result of the printing process. The reader should not rely solely on the photographic image to identify any pills depicted here.

The reader should regularly consult a physician in matters relating to his or her health and particularly in respect to any symptoms that may require diagnosis or medical attention.

INTRODUCTION: The Role of OTC Drug Treatment

At least once each month, 9 out of 10 Americans experience a health problem that makes them feel uncomfortable, out of sorts, or "under the weather." These problems include headaches, the common cold, allergies, muscle aches and pains, skin conditions ranging from dandruff to athlete's foot, minor wounds, upset stomach, and sleep disturbance.

Most of the time, these complaints are not serious enough to require the attention of a physician, and eventually clear up on their own. In many cases, though, they can reduce productivity, disrupt attendance at school or work, interfere with social activities, or just make life generally miserable for a few days.

For most people, the first and most sensible step in treating everyday health complaints is to use a medication available without a prescription. Nonprescription drugs—also called over-the-counter (OTC) drugs—can be purchased in pharmacies, supermarkets, and convenience stores. Many were previously available only with a doctor's prescription.

There are more than 400 medical conditions that can be treated with OTC drugs, either as the first choice of therapy or in addition to prescription treatment. And the choices are many: Thousands of OTC items crowd store shelves. At any given time, the average American medicine cabinet is stocked with about 16 different OTC medications.

OTC products are an essential part of health care today. It is not always possible, convenient, or necessary to make an appointment with a physician. Even with good health insurance, the out-of-pocket costs of doctor visits and prescriptions can mount up. OTC drugs, by contrast, are very inexpensive; on average, they cost only pennies per dose. Only 2 cents of every dollar spent on health care goes toward OTC drugs.

But the most important reason for choosing OTC products is the simple fact that they work. Used as directed for the conditions they are intended to treat, OTC drugs ease aches and pains, help wounds heal, prevent or clear up infections, and relieve the symptoms of colds, allergies, flu, and asthma.

How an OTC Drug Becomes Available

Pharmaceutical companies spend millions of dollars each year trying to discover new drugs to treat a range of illnesses. If a promising chemical is found, the company obtains a patent, which gives them the exclusive right to develop that drug into a product for sale on the market. Once a patent has been secured, the company subjects the drug to a series of tests, first in animals, then in healthy human volunteers, and finally in patients who have the illness that the medication is intended to treat.

The company then submits the results of these studies to the U.S. Food and Drug Administration (FDA). The FDA uses this information to answer 2 important questions:

- Is the drug safe—that is, do the benefits it provides outweigh any risks of side effects or adverse reactions?
- Is it effective—does it produce the results the manufacturer claims?

If the drug passes both these tests, it earns the FDA's approval and can appear for sale on the market.

Usually a new drug is available through prescription only. This means that the FDA has decided that the drug is safe and effective only if the person taking it is under the care of a licensed health care professional.

A patent on a drug is good for 17 years from the date it is first issued. After the patent expires, the chemical becomes generic. In other words, any other company that wants to make and sell the chemical may do so, provided the company submits its product for FDA review. In most cases, the generic form of the drug is still available only with a prescription. Generic drugs are cheaper than the brand-name products because the companies selling them did not have to pay for years of development and testing.

The manufacturer of a prescription drug may decide that it wants to sell its drug in OTC form. It can do so by applying to the FDA to reclassify the drug (see chapter 14).

In 1972 the FDA initiated an ongoing review of the active ingredients in OTC products to determine whether they were safe and effective and had the proper labeling. This process, known as the over-the-counter drug review, has led to the switching (reclassification of drugs from prescription to OTC status) of almost 40 prescription drugs to

OTC status. Prior to 1972, 25 drugs had already been switched, including the antifungal drug tolnaftate (Tinactin), when the FDA determined that a prescription limitation was unnecessary. See table for examples of reclassified drugs.

Selected Former Prescription Ingredients Now Available OTC

Ingredient	For Treatment of ...	Common Brand Name
cimetidine	heartburn	Tagamet HB
diphenhydramine	allergies	Benadryl
hydrocortisone	inflammation	Cortizone
ibuprofen	pain, fever	Advil
loperamide	diarrhea	Imodium A-D
miconazole	vaginal yeast infection	Monistat
minoxidil	baldness	Rogaine
nicotine polacrilex	smoking	Nicorette
permethrin	head lice	Nix
pseudoephedrine	nasal congestion	Sudafed
tolnaftate	athlete's foot	Tinactin

The Need for Information

Today, vast amounts of health care information are available from a variety of sources. Television, magazines, newspapers, the radio, and the Internet all provide a constant stream of news about medical breakthroughs, tips for staying well, and advice about diet and nutrition. People are becoming educated health care consumers, aware of their options and more forthright about asking their caregivers to provide the kind of treatment they want.

Despite—or perhaps because of—this flow of knowledge, it is easy to become confused about how to provide the best self-treatment for yourself and your family. Studies show that medicines are often used incorrectly. Perhaps 3 to 5 of every 10 doses of prescription medications are taken in the wrong amounts, at the wrong time, or under the wrong conditions. OTC drugs are just as likely to be misused. While the consequences of misusing an OTC drug as opposed to a prescription drug are generally less serious, it is possible to take too much of *any* drug and experience unpleasant, perhaps even life-threatening, side effects.

For example, ordinary aspirin is a very effective drug for reducing pain and fever, and is recommended by many physicians as a way of preventing serious illnesses such as heart conditions and colon cancer. For some people, however, aspirin can cause bleeding stomach ulcers. In children, it is associated with a serious nerve disorder called Reye's syndrome. Aspirin can also be fatal if taken in large amounts.

When taking any medication, it is important to read the package directions, follow instructions carefully, and heed any warnings. The FDA requires OTC products to provide clear, easy-to-read labels and instructions. Still, the information available with a product may not be as complete or as comprehensible as you might want. Your local pharmacist is an excellent source of information about drugs. Whenever you begin using a medication, whether prescription or OTC, ask your pharmacist to explain how the product should be taken, what results to expect, and what to do if problems arise (see box).

How to Use This Book

This book will provide you with the facts about the role of OTC drugs in helping you and your family stay healthy. You'll find overviews of the most common everyday health complaints, from hay fever to fungal infections. There are complete descriptions of hundreds of OTC products—including their active ingredients, intended uses, and possible side effects. Detailed tables allow you to compare the doses of various brand-name medications and choose the product that offers the best combination of features to treat your particular condition. You'll also find advice on when to call a physician.

Each drug profile in *The Pill Book Guide to Over-the-Counter Medications* contains the following information when applicable:

Questions to Ask Your Pharmacist

- What is the name of this drug?
- What does this drug do?
- Is a generic version of this product available?
- What dose should I take?
- At what time of day do I take this drug?
- How many times a day do I take it?
- How many days or weeks should I take it?
- Is it okay to drink alcohol while I'm taking this drug?
- Should I take the drug with food or on an empty stomach?
- How long will it take for me to notice results?
- What should I do if I skip a dose?
- What side effects might occur with this drug?
- What should I do if I notice side effects?
- Will this drug cause any problems with other prescription (or OTC) medications I am taking?
- Are there any activities I should avoid while taking this drug?
- How long does this medication stay effective—is there an expiration date on the product?
- How and where should I store the drug?
- Is it okay to keep the unused portion of the drug in the house, or should I throw it away?
- Can anyone else in my family use this drug?

Generic Name/Ingredient(s) and/or Brand Name(s)

The generic name is the name of the active chemical contained in the product while the brand name is a manufacturer's name for the drug. Many people are not aware that several different brand names can contain the same ingredient. Knowing the generic name of any OTC medication you take is the only way to ensure you are not taking the same drug under different brand names.

Type of Drug

The general classification of the chemical. For example, drugs that relieve pain are classified as analgesics; those that relieve itch are called antipruritics. Knowing what type of drug you are using helps you compare a particular product with others in the same class.

Used for
The condition(s) for which the drug is usually taken.

General Information
How the drug works, how it is similar to or different from other drugs, and how it may affect your body.

Cautions and Warnings
People with medical conditions such as heart disease or liver problems might experience adverse reactions if they take certain medications. This section alerts you to possible dangerous reactions that might arise when using the drug.

Possible Side Effects
Side effects are generally divided into 3 categories: those that are most common, those that are less common, and those that occur only rarely. For each OTC medication, a list of potential side effects is provided to help you understand what to expect from your medication. If you experience side effects that make you uncomfortable enough to want to stop taking the medication, or if you experience problems that do not appear on the list of side effects, talk to your doctor.

Drug Interactions
Sometimes the presence of 2 or more drugs in your body can cause unexpected problems. Either the 2 drugs cancel each other out, and thus make it hard to get the expected benefits, or they can cause each other to have stronger effects (including side effects) than expected. This section lists which drugs should not be taken if you are using a particular OTC product. Some interactions with other pills, alcohol, or other substances can be deadly. If you are taking another prescription or OTC medication, always ask your doctor or pharmacist about possible interactions. Your pharmacist should have a record of all medications you are currently taking. You should also keep your own record and bring it along when making a drug purchase or filling a prescription.

Food Interactions
The presence of food in your stomach might interfere with your body's ability to absorb a drug. On the other hand, food can actually help with the absorption of some drugs, or can

help minimize any potential side effects. This section lists foods to avoid while taking your medication, whether to take your medication with meals, and other related information.

Usual Dose

This section summarizes the largest and smallest doses that are typically taken. Not all products containing the same generic ingredient are taken in the same doses. Also, adult doses are usually different from those recommended for children. Your doctor may want you to take a different dose of the product than the amounts listed here. If you are uncertain about when or how often to take a pill, check with your doctor or pharmacist. Do not change the dose of any medication you take without first calling your doctor.

Overdosage

This section describes the symptoms of overdose, when applicable, and tells you what to do in an emergency.

Special Information

This section highlights important information about the specific generic ingredient or brand-name product.

Storage Instructions

Store your medicines in their original containers or in a sealed, light-resistant container to maintain maximum potency. In general medications should be stored at room temperature, away from excessive humidity. Although bathroom medicine cabinets are a common storage location for medications, they are generally inappropriate because of their high humidity. If storage instructions differ, they will be listed in this section.

How to Find Your Drug

- Start with the brand name. *The Pill Book Guide to Over-the-Counter Medications* features information on the top 200 brand-name products, which can be found at the end of each chapter. For example, Advil will be found at the end of chapter 1: Pain and Fever Relief, and Pepcid AC will be found at the end of chapter 3: Diet and Stomach Medicines. Most of the brand-name products featured can be found in the color plates.

How to Find Your Drug *(continued)*

- If you do not find your product by using the brand name, your product will be found under its generic name. The chemical that produces a drug's desired effect is known as the active ingredient. These ingredients each have a specific generic name. Many products with different brand names can contain the same generic ingredient. For example, ibuprofen is the generic name for a certain pain-relieving ingredient. Ibuprofen can be found in such brand-name products as Advil, Motrin, and Nuprin, but it is also widely available in inexpensive products sold under its generic name. *The Pill Book Guide to Over-the-Counter Medications* provides tables that show which products contain the various generic ingredients. To learn more about the drug, turn to the page describing that particular generic ingredient. By using both brand names and generic names, it is easier for you to locate information about a drug you are taking.
- All brand and generic names are cross-referenced in the index.
- The symbols A, C, and S indicate which products are alcohol-free, caffeine-free, and sugar-free.
- You can also find out about related products by turning to the pertinent chapters and their subdivisions. For example, information about all the various products available for vaginal yeast infections is presented in chapter 10: Sex.

Special Populations

Here you'll find advice relevant to people with special needs when it is applicable.

- Besides having allergies to specific drugs, people may also be allergic to other ingredients in brand-name drugs, such as sweeteners or coloring agents.
- Pregnant women need to know whether the drug might affect their fetus, while breast-feeding mothers must be aware if there is a chance the drug can be passed to the infant in breast milk.

- Infants and children are very susceptible to drug effects. No OTC medication should be given to a child under age 2 without specific approval from your physician.
- Seniors may become more susceptible to the effects of various drugs because of the age-related changes to their bodies. Because older people tend to take more prescription and OTC drugs at the same time, they should be especially aware of the possible interactions among these various medications.

Reading Labels

You must read the directions and the ingredients listed on the labels of OTC medications. This is the best way to ensure you are taking correct doses and not duplicating ingredients. For example, people with colds or flu may take acetaminophen (Tylenol), which is also found in many OTC combination products for colds and flu at regular doses. If both a combination product and acetaminophen alone are taken, an overdose can occur.

The Pill Book Guide to Over-the-Counter Medications is a unique reference tool. It amplifies the information available from your health care professionals, helps make sense of a product's labeling, and allows you to compare the various products available that contain the same generic ingredients.

This book, like medications themselves, should be handled with caution. Used properly, *The Pill Book Guide to Over-the-Counter Medications* can save you money by helping you avoid medications that are ineffective for your needs. It can help you get the most benefit from an OTC drug with the lowest risk of unwanted side effects. While every effort has been made to provide complete and accurate information, you should not use this book as a substitute for medical advice. If you are uncertain about the reason for taking a drug or how to use it, or if you read something in the book that does not agree with instructions you have received, ask your doctor or pharmacist for more information.

Points for Safe Drug Use

- Check packages before buying an OTC drug. Do not purchase a product if seals have been broken or the product appears to have been tampered with.

- Tell your doctor about all the medical problems you are currently having. Only when they know the full picture can caregivers treat you with the right medication or combination of medications.
- Tell each doctor you see about all the medications you use regularly, including both prescription and OTC drugs.
- Record any bad reactions you have had to a medication.
- Don't take more than the recommended dose without consulting your doctor or pharmacist.
- If you use an OTC cold or cough preparation, be sure to choose one that contains only the ingredients you need for your condition. Many of these products have 2 or more active ingredients; be sure you know what each of these are to avoid any possible interactions with other drugs.
- Getting all your prescriptions filled at the same pharmacy is usually the best way to centralize your records and ensure their completeness. This will avoid drug interactions and prevent taking 2 drugs of the same therapeutic class.
- Consult your pharmacist for guidance on the use of OTC drugs.
- Before taking your medicine, always read the label and follow the instructions exactly. Don't trust your memory.
- Make sure you have adequate light when taking a medication so that you can see what you're doing. If you have any questions, call your doctor or pharmacist.
- Report any unusual symptoms that you develop after taking any medicine.
- Store medications out of the sight and reach of children.
- Note the expiration date when purchasing or using a medication.
- Dispose of medicine that has passed its expiration date by flushing it down the toilet.
- Be sure the label stays on the container until the medicine is used or destroyed.
- Keep the label facing up when pouring liquid medicine from the bottle; this prevents drips and spills that can make the label hard to read.
- Use only the dropper or applicator that is packaged with the product, because different products require different dosing.

- When you travel, carry medication in its original container.
- Do not mix medications by putting 2 or more into 1 bottle.
- If you move to another city, ask your pharmacist to forward your patient records to your new pharmacy.
- Carry important medical facts about yourself in your wallet or purse. Information about drug allergies, chronic diseases such as diabetes, and so on is necessary in emergencies.

In an Emergency!

Each year, over 70,000 people experience drug-related poisoning; about 10% of those cases result in death. While OTC medications are generally safe, taken in large enough quantities they can cause serious illness or may even be fatal. Here are some general rules for dealing with drug-related poisoning.

1. Make sure the victim is breathing and call for medical help immediately.
2. Learn the phone number for your local poison control center and post it near the phone. Call the center in an emergency. When you call, be prepared to explain:
   - What drug was taken and how much.
   - What the victim is doing (is he or she conscious, sleeping, vomiting, having convulsions, etc.).
   - The age and weight of the victim.
   - Any chronic medical problems the victim has, such as diabetes, heart disease, high blood pressure, or epilepsy.
   - What other medications the victim is currently taking.
3. Remove anything that might interfere with breathing. A person who is not getting enough oxygen will turn blue (the fingernails, lips, or tongue will change color first). In such cases, lay the victim on his or her back; open the collar; place one hand under the neck; and lift, pull, or push the victim's jaw so that it juts outward. This opens the airway between the mouth and the lungs as wide as possible. Begin mouth-to-mouth resuscitation if the victim is not breathing.
4. If the victim is unconscious or is having convulsions, call for medical help immediately. While waiting for the

ambulance, lay the victim on his or her side and turn the head to one side. If the person throws up, this precaution will prevent him or her from inhaling the vomit. Do not give an unconscious person anything to eat or drink. Keep the victim warm.

5. If the victim is conscious, call for medical help and give him or her an 8-oz. glass of water to drink to dilute the poison.

Only a small number of poisoning victims require hospitalization. Most can be treated with simple steps, either at home or in the emergency room.

The poison control center may suggest inducing vomiting. The best way to do this is with ipecac syrup, which is available without a prescription at any pharmacy. Follow the directions on the label and as given by the poison control center. DO NOT induce vomiting unless specifically instructed to do so; sometimes vomiting up a poison can pose a serious risk to health. Never induce vomiting if the victim is unconscious, is having a convulsion, or has a burning feeling in the mouth or throat.

Be Prepared

The best way to deal with a poisoning is to be prepared for it. Do the following now:

1. Write the telephone number of your local poison control center next to your other emergency phone numbers.
2. Decide which hospital you will go to, if necessary, and how you will get there.
3. Buy a bottle of ipecac syrup from your pharmacy and ask your pharmacist how to use it. Remember: This is a potent drug to be used only if directed.

Reduce the Risk of Drug-Related Poisoning

1. Keep all medicines in a locked place out of the reach of young children.
2. Do not store drugs in containers that once held food.
3. Do not remove the labels from bottles so that the contents are unknown.
4. Discard all medicines when you no longer need them or when their expiration dates have passed.

Drugs and...

Drugs and Alcohol

Alcohol depresses the body's central nervous system and can either increase or decrease the effect of a drug on the nervous system. In some drug-alcohol interactions, the amount of alcohol consumed may not be as important as the chemical reaction it causes in your body. Small amounts of alcohol can cause excess stomach secretions, whereas larger amounts can inhibit stomach secretions, eroding the stomach's lining. For seniors, the use of OTC alcohol-based products is especially dangerous, since their systems may be more sensitive to alcohol. People with stomach disorders, such as peptic or gastric ulcer disease, should be fully aware of the alcohol levels in products they use.

Some OTC liquid medicines, such as decongestant cold-suppressing mixtures, contain alcohol. This ingredient may be used to dissolve the active drugs, to enhance or provide a sedative effect, or to act as a preservative. Alcohol is itself a powerful drug, and it has the potential to interact with prescription drugs. Your pharmacist can tell you which liquid medicines contain alcohol and which are alcohol-free, and *The Pill Book Guide to Over-the-Counter Medications* uses the symbol A to tell you which medicines are alcohol-free.

Alcohol does not interact with every medicine. Any potential effects of alcohol on an OTC medication can be found in the *Drug Interactions* section of each drug profile.

Drugs and Food

Foods can interfere with the ability of drugs to be absorbed into the blood through the gastrointestinal system. For this reason, most medications are best taken at least 1 hour before or 2 hours after meals, unless specific characteristics of the drug dictate otherwise. For example, some drugs (such as aspirin) can be taken with meals because food reduces the potential for drug-related stomach irritation. However, milk or milk products (such as cheese or ice cream) can interfere with the absorption of other drugs because they bind with the drug and prevent it from being absorbed into the blood.

Drugs can also affect your appetite, either by increasing it or decreasing it. For example, OTC stimulants such as phenylpropanolamine are sold as appetite suppressants. Many drugs, including antacids and laxatives, can interfere with the normal absorption of one or more body nutrients, thus posing a risk of nutritional problems.

Each drug profile in this book contains a *Food Interactions* section (if applicable) that tells you the best time to take your medicine and what foods to avoid while taking it. Check with your doctor or pharmacist if you are unsure about how best to take your medicine.

Drugs and Sexual Activity

Sexual activity is usually not affected by the use of OTC drugs, but in some instances, sex drive can be affected. In men, some drugs can cause impotence (difficulty in getting or keeping an erection). If you notice any such effects, you should discuss the problem with your doctor. A simple reduction in dosage or change to another drug in the same class may help you to deal with the problem. Each drug profile in this book will alert you to potential sexual side effects of the medicine, when they exist.

Drugs and Pregnancy

There is a risk that drug use by expectant mothers may damage a developing fetus. Some drugs can cross from the mother's bloodstream through the placenta and into the fetal blood circulation, where it may affect the normal fetal growth and development processes. Because a fetus grows much more rapidly than a fully developed human, the effects of any drug on these processes are magnified. The results can range from mild physical changes to death. Drugs can also be passed to nursing infants through breast milk.

The chances of damage to a fetus are usually greatest during the first 3 months of pregnancy, when a woman may not be aware that she is pregnant. Most doctors advise pregnant and nursing women to avoid all medicines. They suggest that pregnant women use only vitamins or iron supplements and that they limit or stop tobacco, alcohol, and caffeine intake.

If you are considering becoming pregnant, curtail drug use immediately and discuss the situation fully with your doctor. Drinking alcoholic beverages during pregnancy is associated with fetal alcohol syndrome, which causes physical deformations and mental retardation. Nobody knows how much alcohol a woman must drink before these problems will develop. To be safe, don't drink at all during pregnancy. Remember, nicotine is also a drug, and smoking may seriously complicate your pregnancy. If you plan to become pregnant and you smoke, stop!

The FDA has classified all drugs according to their safety for use during pregnancy. Every profile in this book contains information on drug safety for pregnant and nursing women.

Drugs and Children

Medicine should be given to children only on direct advice from a pediatrician, doctor, or pharmacist. Parents should be aware of all the ingredients in OTC products (including alcohol) and any possible side effects associated with use. Because their body systems are not fully developed, infants and young children are at greater risk for experiencing drug side effects and interactions. It's wise to ask your doctor whether side effects, such as fever or rash, are to be expected when a drug is given to a child.

Drug doses for children are usually lower and are often determined by body weight or by surface area. The FDA has recently encouraged drug manufacturers to study the effects of their medicines on children and submit their research for government evaluation. As a result, many more medicines are being officially approved for children's use, even though they have been widely used in children for years. Find out all there is to know about a drug before you give it to your child. Check with your doctor or pharmacist to make sure OTC medicines will not interact with any other drugs your child is taking.

Drugs and Seniors

Two-thirds of people over age 65 take medications regularly. Senior citizens make up only about 13% of the population, but they consume 25% of all prescription drugs and 33% of all OTC drugs sold.

Studies show that 70% to 90% of seniors take pills and OTC medicines with little knowledge of their dangerous effects. Bodily changes caused by age or disease make older adults 3 times more likely than younger persons to suffer an adverse drug reaction. Since many older adults take more than 1 medicine, their potential for drug interactions is much greater. Older adults often suffer from undetected reactions caused by slowly rising amounts of drugs that are not being properly metabolized by their bodies, which work less efficiently as they age. In some cases older adults may develop speech or hearing problems, become absentminded, or experience symptoms that are assumed to be part of the aging process, when in fact they are symptoms of drug reactions. Adjustment of dosage often causes these symptoms to vanish.

Seniors are often victims of overdose. Body weight fluctuations and normal changes in body functions lead to overdose unless the dosage of a drug is altered accordingly.

It's important to make sure that older adults understand their drugs as completely as possible. Develop a simple recording system that lists the pills being taken, the sequence in which they should be taken, the time of day and how they should be taken, and a line to check off what was taken. Every drug profile in this book contains special drug information for seniors, if applicable.

Part I

Chapter 1: Pain and Fever Relief

Pain begins when cells and tissues are damaged by inflammation or injury. The damaged cells release chemicals that trigger pain receptors, which send messages to the brain that an injury has occurred. Drugs used to treat pain either block the transmission of the message to the brain or blunt the brain's perception of the pain signals. Hence, although there is still tissue damage, the pain signal sent to the brain is temporarily blocked, and the pain is relieved.

Terms That Describe Pain

Acute pain occurs suddenly and is typically the result of a specific event; it may last minutes to hours. Example: burns.

Chronic pain is long-term pain (lasting more than 3 months) that may, from time to time, flare up into acute pain. Example: arthritis.

Localized pain is confined to a specific area of the body. Example: calf muscle pull.

Generalized pain is spread over a large area of the body. Example: body aches caused by the flu.

Medically based (or somatic) pain results from a specific injury; most pain is somatic. Example: a knife cut.

Psychologically based pain is influenced by the mind. Example: a backache or headache caused by severe stress. However, medically based pain is also usually affected by the mind.

Referred pain comes from one area of the body but is felt in another. Example: the pain of a heart attack, which originates in the heart but may be felt in the neck, jaw, or left arm.

Common Types of Pain

Headache

Headache is perhaps the most common pain. Most headaches are minor and are easily treated. Others, such as migraines, are severe and require medical attention. Infrequently, head pain can signal a serious, life-threatening condition.

Headaches are divided into 3 major types based on their cause. It's important to know which type of headache you suffer from, because the treatment may be different for different types.

Tension headaches are caused by muscle contractions in the back, neck, and scalp. They are characterized by:
- a steady, nonpulsing ache
- tightness at the temples or back of the head
- bandlike pain around the head
- occurrence in the morning or evening
- difficulty falling asleep
- association with depression, stress, or fatigue
- cramping sensations in the neck and upper back
- pain on one or both sides of the head

Migraine headaches and *cluster headaches* are caused by the abnormal dilation (widening) of blood vessels in the head. Although the brain itself actually has no pain receptors, the pressure against the walls of the blood vessels in the head causes the pain associated with migraines. People who are prone to tension headaches often suffer from migraine headaches, and vice versa; features of both may appear at the same time.

Migraine headaches are characterized by:
- feelings of pulsating or throbbing
- pain on one or both sides of the head, especially in the temples
- pain above the eyebrows
- nausea, vomiting, and sensitivity to light
- several days' duration
- an aura or sensation of light before the headache begins

Cluster headaches are characterized by:
- excruciating, burning, one-sided pain
- pain mostly around the eye
- flushing, tearing, or runny nose on the affected side
- frequent occurrence at night during sleep
- 10 to 60 minutes' duration
- attacks occurring in groups (especially nightly) over a period of several weeks

Organic disease may cause headaches that occur because of infection, for example an infection of the sinuses or meningitis (inflammation of the membranes of the brain), or because of a brain tumor or aneurysm (dilated blood vessel). These types of headaches always require immediate medical attention.

Headaches due to organic disease are characterized by:
- severe headache accompanied by fever, vomiting, confusion, drowsiness, or stiff neck
- deterioration in speech, vision, or sensation
- sudden weakness in arms or legs

Seek medical attention if any of the following applies to you

- Sudden onset of headaches
- More frequent and more severe headaches
- Headache after physical exercise
- Headache for more than 3 days
- Headache stopping you from daily activities
- Feelings of an explosion in your head
- Stiff neck or fever
- Vomiting without nausea, especially on first awakening
- Vision difficulties
- Cognitive difficulties (problems thinking)
- Speech difficulties
- Poor coordination
- Weak arms or legs

Reducing stress and fatigue are important in reducing headache pain. Tension headaches are easily treated with OTC analgesic (pain-relieving) preparations. Of the available medications, aspirin and ibuprofen may be the most effective because they lower the levels of the body's prostaglandins, chemicals that mediate pain. Because caffeine speeds the absorption of aspirin and also constricts the dilated, painful arteries that cause head pain, taking a headache preparation that contains aspirin, ibuprofen, or acetaminophen combined with caffeine may help. However, taking caffeine close to bedtime can interfere with sleep.

OTC Treatment for Headaches

Acetaminophen
Aspirin
Caffeine
Ibuprofen
Naproxen sodium
Ketoprofen
Salicylates (choline salicylate, magnesium salicylate, sodium salicylate)

Muscle Pain

Muscle pain, usually the result of overworked muscles, is a warning to slow down and take it easy. When a muscle is overused, the tiny fibers that make up the muscle begin to tear, and the muscle contracts to allow the fibers to heal. Hence, your muscle feels tight and sore. Occasionally, the muscle is overworked due to stress. Muscles, especially in the head, neck, and back, respond to stress by staying tense, causing a vicious cycle of tension and pain. If this condition affects several areas of the body, it is called fibromyalgia. Most muscle pain responds to RICE treatment (see box); however, the pain of fibromyalgia is often difficult to relieve completely. Muscle pain also responds well to aspirin and ibuprofen.

RICE Treatment

Rest—To allow the injury to heal, avoid unnecessary movement
Ice—Apply an ice pack to decrease pain, muscle spasm, and swelling
Compression—Use an elastic bandage or other wrap to help bring swelling down
Elevation—Raise the injured arm or leg above the level of your heart

Related types of pain include the following:

Chest wall pain is common and harmless. It is usually centered on the front of the chest and is a result of injury to the muscles and cartilage that connect your ribs to your breastbone. Pain and tenderness may be felt in small areas around the breastbone, or may be more diffuse. This type of pain is usually caused by overexertion, whether from rigorous sports or too much coughing during a bout with the flu. Chest wall pain can also result from trauma, such as a blow to the chest or a fall, or even from chronic overwork and stress. Aspirin or another analgesic and heat will relieve symptoms.

Arm/leg pain caused by common muscle pulls, strains, and contusions (injury to tissue, such as a bruise) can generally be self-diagnosed and treated with RICE treatment and OTC pain medications.

Joint pain is generally caused by inflammation or wear and tear of cartilage. It may be the result of injury, overuse, or repetitive movements, or of conditions such as arthritis or rheumatism. Symptoms include pain and stiffness in one or more joints. The area may be warm, red, and inflamed. Treatment with ice or heat and OTC pain relievers, rest, and gentle exercise may be recommended.

Seek medical attention if any of the following applies to you

- Inability to use the affected muscle
- Intolerable pain
- Muscle pain accompanied by fever
- Severe or unexplained joint pain
- Pain lasting more than a week
- Joint injured by a sharp blow
- Pain not reduced by OTC pain relievers and ice or heat
- Hot, red or swollen, and painful joint

OTC Treatment for Muscle Pain

Acetaminophen
Aspirin
Ibuprofen
Naproxen sodium
Ketoprofen
Salicylates (choline salicylate, magnesium salicylate, sodium salicylate)

Menstrual Pain

Menstrual cramps are a common symptom accompanying a woman's monthly period. Cramps are a result of the uterus contracting while it expels the uterine lining. Cramping and other pain associated with menstruation (in the abdomen and lower back, for example) have been linked to the increased production of prostaglandins in the uterus, which is at its peak during the first 2 to 3 days of a woman's period. Severe cramping may also indicate a medical condition such as endometriosis, when bits of the tissue that normally lines the uterus become attached to other pelvic organs. Other conditions that can cause uterine cramping are fibroids (noncancerous growths in the uterus) or miscarriage of an undiagnosed pregnancy. Most cramps are relieved with OTC preparations, especially ibuprofen, ketoprofen, and naproxen sodium. Ibuprofen in particular has been proven in many studies to be effective against menstrual pain and cramping. Exercise, relaxation, heat, ice, and dietary changes can also help relieve menstrual cramps. Mild diuretics may alleviate the swelling in the hands and feet experienced by some women during their periods.

Seek medical attention if any of the following applies to you

- Severe pain with your first or second period (if you have just started menstruating)
- Severe cramps that keep you home from school or work
- Nausea, headaches, diarrhea, and vomiting with your cramps
- Very heavy bleeding or clots for more than 1 day
- Cramps associated with fever
- Severe cramps while taking birth control pills
- Painful cramps that began suddenly
- Menstrual pain not helped by OTC pain relievers

OTC Treatment for Menstrual Pain

Acetaminophen
Aspirin
Caffeine
Ibuprofen
Naproxen sodium
Ketoprofen
Salicylates (choline salicylate, magnesium salicylate, sodium salicylate)

Backache

Backaches most often occur in the lower back and neck. The majority of backaches are due to overexertion, poor posture, and stress. Many of us are out of shape, so when the time comes to play or shovel snow, our muscles are weak. It's important to gradually get into shape and keep muscles limber and toned by stretching and using them every day. Many backaches are caused by weak stomach muscles, the opposing muscle group. Strengthening the stomach and abdominal muscles will help prevent low back pain. Acute low back pain can be treated with a variety of OTC pain preparations, particularly a nonsteroidal anti-inflammatory drug (NSAID) such as aspirin, ibuprofen, naproxen sodium, or ketoprofen, which helps reduce inflammation. Chiropractic work may alleviate some cases of chronic low back pain. Surgery is usually reserved for severe disk problems, which cause only a small number of back pain cases.

Seek medical attention if any of the following applies to you

- Severe back pain lasting for more than 3 days
- Difficulty working because of intense pain
- Pain radiating to your legs, feet, or toes
- Numbness or weakness in one leg
- Difficulty with bowel or urine control

OTC Treatment for Backache

Acetaminophen
Aspirin
Ibuprofen
Naproxen sodium
Ketoprofen
Salicylates (choline salicylate, magnesium salicylate, sodium salicylate)

Treatment for Pain

Early treatment helps prevent the cycle of pain and lessens its severity. It also helps relieve the anxiety surrounding pain, which contributes to the emotional experience of pain.

The commonly available OTC analgesics include aspirin and the other salicylates (choline salicylate, magnesium salicylate, sodium salicylate), acetaminophen, ibuprofen, naproxen sodium, and ketoprofen. All of these, with the exception of acetaminophen, are NSAIDs. NSAIDs reduce inflammation by inhibiting the production of prostaglandins, hormonelike substances that make nerves more sensitive to pain. Acetaminophen, in contrast, relieves pain but does not reduce inflammation.

Your choice of pain reliever should depend primarily on the type of pain you are experiencing. For example, because the cramping associated with menstrual pain is caused by the production of prostaglandins, an NSAID such as ibuprofen or naproxen sodium is a good choice. Acetaminophen may be a better choice for pain accompanied by fever, which may occur with the common cold, flu, or viral infections. Acetaminophen is also free of many of the side effects associated with aspirin and can be taken by people who are allergic to aspirin. However, too much acetaminophen (more than 3000 to 4000 mg/day) may cause liver damage, especially in people who drink alcohol regularly. Finally, choline salicylate, magnesium salicylate, and sodium salicylate are no more effective as pain relievers than aspirin and share its potential for drug interactions. However, because they are easier on the stomach, these other salicylates may be taken by those who cannot tolerate aspirin's gastrointestinal effects.

Fever

The average adult temperature is 98.6°, although variations in either direction are normal. Healthy body temperature can vary throughout the day between 97° and 99°. Generally it is lowest in the morning and highest in the evening. Low-grade adult fever is present at temperatures 1 to 2 degrees above your normal temperature.

Fever is part of the body's natural defenses and can accompany many minor ailments. Viral and bacterial infections are a common cause of fever. Fever below 103°, a mild sore throat, aches and pains, headache, runny nose, and sneezing are symptoms of the common cold or flu.

Fever can be caused by any infection, as well as a wide range of conditions and diseases, some of which can be serious. Cold symptoms along with shortness of breath or coughing-up discolored sputum can indicate pneumonia or bronchitis. Kidney, urinary tract, and female reproductive infections can cause a sudden high fever (usually over 102°) with shaking and chills. Frequent urination, blood or vaginal discharge, lower back pain, and nausea are further symptoms of kidney, urinary tract, and female reproductive infections. Fever right after childbirth or pain in the lower abdomen accompanied by smelly or heavy vaginal discharge can signal a serious infection and should be treated immediately. Fevers can also be caused by sore throat, sinusitis, hepatitis, diarrhea, cholecystitis, allergies, sunstroke and heat exhaustion, mononucleosis, and meningitis.

Treatment for Fever

High fevers (103°F and higher) require medical attention. Any fever in a child less than 3 months old should be treated by a doctor immediately. Most low-grade fevers will go away within 1 or 2 days without treatment. Soaking in a bath of tepid water while sponging the skin will help lower a fever. The water should be about 70°; it does not have to be extremely cold to be effective at reducing fever. If necessary repeat the bath every two hours. Although "feed a fever" is traditional advice, eat only if you are hungry. It is much more important to drink plenty of fluids. Because fever dehydrates the body, drink plenty of water. Juices, sports drinks, and chicken and beef broth are also recommended to restore minerals. Aspirin, acetaminophen, and ibuprofen are OTCs that reduce fever.

Seek medical attention if any of the following applies to you

- You have a fever of 103 °F or more
- You have a fever that persists for more than 3 days
- You have a fever and a history of heart disease, diabetes, or any chronic illness
- You have a fever accompanied by any of the following:
  - Recurrent shaking or chills
  - Pain while urinating
  - Cough with discolored phlegm
  - Shortness of breath
  - Convulsions
  - Severe headache
  - Stiff neck
  - Nausea or vomiting
  - Change in alertness
  - Hypersensitivity to light

Aspirin and Reye's Syndrome

Aspirin—even so-called children's aspirin—should not be taken by anyone under age 16 unless recommended by a doctor, because of the risk of a rare complication called Reye's syndrome. This disease, occurring mainly in children, causes damage to nerves, brain, and liver; in about 30% of cases, it is fatal.

OTC Treatment for Fever

Acetaminophen
Aspirin
Ibuprofen

Analgesics

BRAND NAME	acetaminophen	aspirin	caffeine	ibuprofen	other analgesic
Acephen	120mg; 325mg; 650mg				
Aceta [A] [C]	160mg/5ml				
Acetaminophen Uniserts [C]	120mg; 325mg; 650mg				
Actamin [C]	325mg				
Actamin Extra [C]	500mg				
Actamin Super	500mg		65mg		
Actron					ketoprofen 12.5mg
Addaprin [C]				200mg	
Adprin B [C]		325mg			
Adprin B Extra Strength [C]		500mg			
Advil [C]				200mg	
Aleve [C]					naproxen 200mg
Alka-Seltzer	500mg				
Alka-Seltzer Extra Strength [C]		500mg			
Alka-Seltzer Original/Lemon-Lime [C]		325mg			
Aminofen	324mg				
Aminofen Max [S]	500mg				
Anacin		400mg	32mg		
Anacin Aspirin Free Maximum Strength	500mg				
Anacin Maximum Strength		500mg	32mg		
Anodynos		410mg	60mg		salicylamide 30mg
APAP (suppository)	650mg				
APAP (tablet)	325mg				
APAP Extra Strength	500mg				
APAP, Children's (elixir) [A]	80mg/2.5ml				

BRAND NAME	acetaminophen	aspirin	caffeine	ibuprofen	other analgesic
APAP, Children's (suspension) [A] [C]	80mg/2.5ml				
APAP, Children's (tablet)	80mg				
APAP, Infants' [A]	80mg/0.8ml				
APAP, Infants' Suspension [A] [C]	80.0/8ml				
APAP, Pediatric	120mg				
Arthriten [S]	250mg				magnesium salicylate, 250mg
Arthritis Foundation Aspirin Free	500mg				
Arthritis Foundation Ibuprofen				200mg	
Arthritis Foundation Safety Coated Aspirin		500mg			
Arthritis Pain Formula [C]		500mg			
Arthropan					choline salicylate 174mg/ml
Ascriptin Arthritis Pain [C]		325mg			
Ascriptin Maximum Strength [C]		500mg			
Ascriptin Regular Strength [C]		325mg			
Aspercin [C]		324mg			
Aspercin Extra [C]		500mg			
Aspergum [C]		227mg			
Aspermin [C]		324mg			
Aspermin Extra [C]		500mg			
Aspirin Free Pain Relief [C]	325mg; 500mg				
Aspirin Free, Children's [A]	80mg/2.5ml				
Aspirin Free, Infants' [A] [C]	80mg/0.8ml				
Aspirtab [C]		324mg			
Aspirtab Max [C]		500mg			
Azo-Dine					phenazopyridine HCl 97.2mg
Azo-Standard					phenazopyridine HCl 95mg

Back-Quell [C]		425mg			
Backache from the Makers of Nuprin [C]					magnesium salicylate 580mg
Baridium [C]					phenazopyridine HCl 95mg
Bayer 8-Hour Aspirin Extended-Release [C]		650mg			
Bayer Arthritis Pain Regimen Extra Strength [C]		500mg			
Bayer Aspirin Extra Strength [C]		500mg			
Bayer Aspirin Regimen Adult Low Strength [C]		81mg			
Bayer Aspirin Regimen Regular Strength [C]		325mg			
Bayer Aspirin, Genuine [C]		325mg			
Bayer Children's Aspirin [C]		81mg			
Bayer Plus Extra Strength [C]		500mg			
Bayer Select Aspirin-Free Headache	500mg		65mg		
Bayer Select Ibuprofen Pain Relief [C]				200mg	
BC (powder)		650mg	32mg		salicylamide 195mg
BC (tablet)		325mg	16mg		salicylamide 95mg
BC Arthritis Strength		742mg	36mg		salicylamide 222mg
Bromo-Seltzer	325mg/capful				
Buffaprin [C]		325mg			
Buffaprin Extra [C]		500mg			
Buffasal [C]		324mg			
Buffasal Max [C]		500mg			
Bufferin Arthritis Strength, Tri-Buffered [C]		500mg			
Bufferin Extra Strength, Tri-Buffered [C]		500mg			
Bufferin, Tri-Buffered [C]		325mg			
Buffets II	162mg	226.8mg	32.4mg		
Buffinol [C]		325mg			

BRAND NAME	acetaminophen	aspirin	caffeine	ibuprofen	other analgesic
Buffinol Extra [C]		500mg			
Cope		421mg	32mg		
Cystex					sodium salicylate 162.5mg
Doan's Extra Strength [C]					magnesium salicylate 580mg
Doan's Regular Strength [C]					magnesium salicylate 377mg
Dyspel	325mg				
Ecotrin Adult Low Strength		81mg			
Ecotrin Maximum Strength		500mg			
Ecotrin Regular Strength		325mg			
Ed-APAP Liquid [A] [C]	80mg/2.5ml				
Emagrin		410mg	30mg		salicylamide 60mg
Empirin [C]		325mg			
Excedrin Aspirin Free	500mg		65mg		
Excedrin Extra Strength	250mg	250mg	65mg		
Feverall Adult Strength [C]	650mg				
Feverall Junior Strength [C]	325mg				
Feverall Sprinkle Caps Powder, Children's Strength [C]	80mg				
Feverall Sprinkle Caps, Junior Strength [C]	160mg				
Feverall, Children's [C]	120mg				
Feverall, Infants' [C]	80mg				
Genapap Extra Strength	500mg				
Genapap, Children's (elixir) [A]	80mg/2.5ml				
Genapap, Children's (suspension) [A] [C]	80mg/2.5ml				
Genapap, Children's (tablet)	80mg				
Genapap, Infants'	80mg/0.8ml				
Genebs	325mg				

Genebs Extra Strength	500mg			
Genpril			200mg	
Genprin		325mg		
Gensan		400mg	32mg	
Goody's Extra Strength	130mg	260mg	16.25mg	
Goody's Extra Strength Headache	260mg	520mg	32.5mg	
Halfprin Low Strength Enteric Coated		81mg; 162mg		
Haltran			200mg	
Heartline		81mg		
Liquiprin for Children [A] [C]	48mg/ml			
Midol IB Cramp Relief Formula [C]			200mg	
Midol Menstrual Regular Strength Multisymptom Formula [C]	325mg			
Mobigesic [S]				magnesium salicylate 325mg
Momentum [C]				magnesium salicylate 580mg
Motrin IB [C]			200mg	
Motrin, Children's			100mg/5ml	
Neopap	125mg			
Norwich Aspirin (caplet) [C]		500mg		
Norwich Aspirin (tablet) [C]		325mg		
Norwich Aspirin, Enteric Coated [C]		325mg; 500mg		
Nuprin [C]			200mg	
Orudis KT [C]				ketoprofen 12.5mg
P-A-C		400mg	32mg	
Panadol Junior Strength [C]	160mg			
Panadol Maximum Strength [C]	500mg			
Panadol, Children's (liquid) [A] [C]	32mg/ml			

BRAND NAME	acetaminophen	aspirin	caffeine	ibuprofen	other analgesic
Panadol, Children's (tablet) C	80mg				
Panadol, Infants' A C	80mg/0.8ml				
PediApap A C	160mg				
Percogesic Coated C	325mg				
Prodium C					phenazopyridine HCl 95mg
Re-Azo					phenazopyridine HCl 97.5mg
Regipren Enteric Coated		81mg			
Rid-a-Pain Compound	226.8mg		32.4mg		salicylamide 97.2mg
Rid-a-Pain with Codeine	97.2mg	226.8mg	32.4mg		salicylamide 32.4mg; codeine phosphate, 1mg
St. Joseph Low Dose Adult Aspirin		81mg			
Stanback AF Extra-Strength C	950mg				
Stanback, Original Formula		650mg	32mg		salicylamide 200mg
Supac S	160mg	230mg	33mg		
Tapanol Extra Strength	500mg				
Tempra 1 A C	80mg/0.8ml				
Tempra 2 A C	160mg/5ml				
Tempra 3 C	80mg				
Tempra 3, Double Strength C	160mg				
Tycolene C	325mg				
Tycolene Extra Strength C	500mg				
Tylenol Extended Relief C	650mg				
Tylenol Extra Strength C	500mg				
Tylenol Extra Strength Adult C	166.7mg/5ml				
Tylenol Extra Strength Headache Plus C	500mg				
Tylenol Junior Strength C	160mg				
Tylenol Regular Strength C	325mg				

Tylenol, Children's (elixir, liquid) [A] [C]	80mg/2.5ml			
Tylenol, Children's (tablet) [C]	80mg			
Tylenol, Infants' [A] [C]	80mg/0.8ml			
Tylenol, Infants' Suspension [A] [C]	80mg/0.8ml			
Ultraprin [C]				200mg
Valorin [C]	325mg			
Valorin Extra [C]	500mg			
Valorin Super	500mg			
Valprin [C]				200mg
Vanquish	194mg	227mg	33mg	

External Analgesics

BRAND NAME	COUNTERIRRITANT							
	camphor	capsaicin	eucalyptol	menthol	methyl nicotinate	methyl salicylate	phenol	other
Absorbine Jr.	3.1%			1.27%				
Absorbine Jr. Extra Strength				4%				
Absorbine Jr. Power Gel				4%				
Arthricare Double Ice Pain Relieving Rub (cream)				4%				
Arthricare Double Ice Pain Relieving Rub (gel)				1.25%	0.25%			
Arthricare Triple Medicated Pain Relieving Rub				1.25%	0.25%	30%		
Arthritis Hot				10%		15%		
Arthritis Rub Extra Strength				8%		30%		

BRAND NAME	COUNTERIRRITANT							
	camphor	capsaicin	eucalyptol	menthol	methyl nicotinate	methyl salicylate	phenol	other
Aspercreme								trolamine salicylate 10%
Banalg Muscle Pain Reliever	2%			1%		4.9%		
Ben-Gay Arthritis Formula				8%		30%		
Ben-Gay Greaseless Formula				10%		15%		
Ben-Gay Original Formula				16%		18.3%		
Ben-Gay Ultra Strength	4%			10%		30%		
Ben-Gay Vanishing Scent				2.5%				
Betuline	x			x		x		
Campho-phenique Pain Relieving Antiseptic	10.8%						4.7%	
Capzasin-P		0.025%						
Cool Heat				2%				
Deep-Down	0.5%			5%		15%		
Dencorub (cream)	3.1%			1.25%		15%		
Dencorub (liquid)		0.025%						
Epiderm Balm				x		x		
Eucalyptamint Arthritis Pain Reliever				16%				
Eucalyptamint Muscle Pain Relief				8%				
Exocaine Medicated Rub						25%		
Exocaine Odor Free								trolamine salicylate 10%
Exocaine Plus Rub						30%		
First Aid Medicated Powder			x	x		x		
Flex-All				7%		x		
Flex-All 454 Maximum Strength				16%		x		

Gold Bond Medicated			x	x		
Gold Bond Medicated Anti-Itch			x	x		
Gordogesic				10%		
Heet	3.6%	0.025%		15%		
Icy Hot			10%	30%		
Icy Hot Chill Stick			10%	30%		
Icy Hot Extra Strength			7.6%	29%		
Menthacin		0.025%	0.4%			
Mentholatum	9%		1.3%			
Mentholatum Deep Heating			6%	20%		
Mentholatum Deep Heating Arthritis Formula			8%	30%		
Mentholatum Deep Heating Rub			5.8%	12.7%		
Methagual			8%			guaiacol 2%
Minit-Rub	2.3%		3.5%	15%		
Mobisyl						trolamine salicylate 10%
Muscle Rub			16%	18.3%		
Myoflex						trolamine salicylate 10%
Noxzema Original	x		x		x	
Numol	9.6%		3.1%	9.7%		mustard oil
Pain Doctor		0.025%	10%	25%		
Pain Gel Plus			4%			
Pain Patch			154mg			
Pain Relief			7%			
PainBreak			5%	x		
Rid-a-Pain (cream)		0.025%				
Rid-a-Pain (ointment)			15%			

BRAND NAME	COUNTERIRRITANT							
	camphor	capsaicin	eucalyptol	menthol	methyl nicotinate	methyl salicylate	phenol	other
Rid-a-Pain HP		0.075%						
Sarna	0.5%			0.5%				
Sloan's		0.025%						turpentine oil 47%
Soltice Quick Rub	5.1%			5.1%				
Sports Spray Extra Strength	5%			10%		35%		
Sportscreme								trolamine salicylate 10%
Thera-Gesic				x		15%		
Therapeutic Blue Ice				2.5%				
Therapeutic Mineral Ice				2%				
Therapeutic Mineral Ice Exercise Formula				4%				
Vicks VapoRub (cream)	5.2%			2.8%				spirits of turpentine
Vicks VapoRub (ointment)	4.8%			2.6%				
Vicks VapoSteam	6.2%			3.2%				
Wonder Ice				x				
Zostrix		0.025%						
Zostrix-HP		0.075%						
Zostrix Sports		0.075%						

Advil (ADD-VIL)

*see **Ibuprofen,** page 845*

Brand Name

Aleve (uh-LEAVE)

Generic Ingredient

Naproxen sodium

Type of Drug

Nonsteroidal anti-inflammatory drug (NSAID), analgesic (pain reliever), and antipyretic (fever reducer).

Used for

Temporary relief of mild to moderate pain associated with headache, colds, toothache, muscle ache, backache, arthritis, menstrual cramps and menstrual pain, and reduction of fever.

General Information

NSAID is the general term used for a group of drugs that are effective in reducing inflammation and pain. Other OTC drugs in this group are aspirin, ibuprofen, and ketoprofen. It is not known exactly how NSAIDs work. However, part of their action may be due to an ability to inhibit the body's production of a hormone called prostaglandin, as well as other body chemicals (e.g., cyclooxygenase, lipoxygenase, leukotrienes, lysosomal enzymes) that sensitize pain receptors and stimulate the inflammatory response. NSAIDs are generally quickly absorbed into the bloodstream, and pain and fever relief usually occurs within 1 hour of taking the first dose and can last up to 6 hours. The anti-inflammatory effect of these agents generally takes longer to work (several days to 2 weeks) and may take a month or more to reach maximum effect.

Naproxen sodium was approved for sale OTC in 1994. It works in much the same way and is as effective as ibuprofen. Naproxen sodium may work for a longer period of time than ibuprofen, but the significance of this is not clear. A difference between the drugs may be seen only at the higher doses sometimes needed by people with arthritis.

Aleve is available in tablet and caplet forms.

Cautions and Warnings

Do not take Aleve for more than 10 consecutive days or, in the presence of fever, for more than 3 days, unless directed by your doctor. Notify your doctor if Aleve does not relieve your symptoms in that time.

Do not exceed the recommended daily dosage of Aleve.

Naproxen sodium, the active ingredient in Aleve, can cause gastrointestinal (GI) bleeding, ulcers, and stomach perforation. This can occur at any time, with or without warning, in anyone who takes this drug for a long period of time. People with a history of active GI bleeding should avoid taking any NSAID without checking with the physician. Minor stomach upset, distress, or gas is common during the first few days of use. If you develop bleeding or ulcers, stop taking Aleve and contact your doctor.

Sodium and water retention leading to peripheral edema (swelling in the arms, legs, or feet) may occur in some persons using Aleve. Therefore, people with heart failure, high blood pressure, or other conditions that are worsened with fluid and sodium retention should avoid taking Aleve without checking with their physician.

People with a history of asthma attacks brought on by an NSAID, iodides, or aspirin should not take Aleve.

Do not take acetaminophen, aspirin, another NSAID, or any product containing them, while taking Aleve.

Aleve can make you drowsy. Be careful when driving a motor vehicle or operating heavy machinery.

To avoid stomach irritation, don't lie down for at least 15 to 30 minutes after you have taken Aleve.

If you develop any severe GI effects, blurred vision, or a rash while you are taking Aleve, consult your doctor.

Naproxen sodium, the active ingredient in Aleve, can have damaging effects on the kidneys. It may increase blood levels of urea nitrogen and serum creatinine. These effects are especially dangerous in patients with kidney damage or congestive heart failure. This may be more likely to occur in older people, those who use diuretics, and in those with hypertension (abnormally high blood pressure), diabetes, and/or atherosclerotic heart disease. If any of the above applies to you, do not take Aleve without first consulting your doctor.

Aleve can affect platelets and blood clotting at high doses, and should therefore be avoided by people with bleeding disorders and by those taking warfarin, an anticoagulant (blood-thinning) drug.

Aleve should be taken at a lower dose by people with severe liver disease.

If you generally have 3 or more alcoholic drinks per day, consult your doctor before taking Aleve to determine proper dosage.

Possible Side Effects

- ▼ Most common: GI problems (e.g., constipation, indigestion, heartburn, nausea, diarrhea, and stomach irritation).
- ▼ Less common: stomach ulcers, GI bleeding, loss of appetite, hepatitis, gallbladder problems, painful urination, poor kidney function, kidney inflammation, blood in the urine, dizziness, fainting, and nervousness.
- ▼ Rare: severe allergic reactions, including closing of the throat; fever and chills; changes in liver function; jaundice; kidney failure; ringing in the ears; and blurred vision.

Drug Interactions

• If you are currently taking an anticoagulant (blood-thinning) drug, such as warfarin, you should not take Aleve without first consulting your doctor (see "Cautions and Warnings"). Aleve can increase risk of bleeding if taken with an anticoagulant.

• Aleve may work against the effects of drugs taken to lower blood pressure, including diuretics, angiotensin-converting enzyme (ACE) inhibitors, and beta blockers. If you are taking any of these drugs along with Aleve, the dose of your blood-pressure-lowering drug may need to be changed or the Aleve discontinued.

• Aleve interferes with the action of methotrexate, which is used to treat cancer, severe psoriasis, severe rheumatoid arthritis, and to induce abortion, and can increase methotrexate's toxicity.

• Taking Aleve with aspirin, other salicylates, acetaminophen, or other NSAIDs (e.g., ibuprofen, ketoprofen) is not necessary and carries an increased risk of side effects.

Food Interactions

If Aleve upsets your stomach, take it with meals or milk.

Usual Dose

Each tablet or caplet contains 220 mg of naproxen sodium.

Pain Relief

Adult and Child (age 12–64): 1–2 tablets/caplets every 8–12 hours (no more than 3 tablets/caplets in 24 hours).

Adult (age 65 and over): 1 tablet/caplet every 12 hours (no more than 2 tablets/caplets in 24 hours).

Child (under age 12): Consult your doctor.

Drink 8 oz. of fluid with each dose of Aleve.

Overdosage

Symptoms of overdose include drowsiness, nausea, vomiting, diarrhea, abdominal pain, rapid breathing, rapid heartbeat, sweating, ringing or buzzing in the ears, confusion, disorientation, stupor, and coma. Severe metabolic acidosis and movement disorders have also been reported.

Even if the victim is not displaying any of the symptoms listed above, do the following in case of accidental overdose: If the victim is unconscious or having convulsions, call for an ambulance immediately. If you take the victim to an emergency room, be sure to bring the bottle or container with you. If the victim is conscious, call your local poison control center or a health care professional. The poison control center may suggest inducing vomiting with ipecac syrup (available without a prescription at any pharmacy). DO NOT induce vomiting unless specifically instructed to do so.

Special Populations

Allergies

People who are allergic to aspirin or to any other NSAID should not take Aleve.

Pregnancy/Breast-feeding

It is not generally recommended that pregnant women take any drugs, particularly during the first 3 months after conception.

If you are or might be pregnant, consult your doctor before using Aleve. It is especially important not to use naproxen sodium during the last 3 months of pregnancy; if naproxen sodium is taken during this time it can cause problems in the unborn child or complications in delivery.

Naproxen sodium has been shown to pass into breast milk. If you must take Aleve, bottle-feed your baby with formula.

Infants/Children

Do not give Aleve to children under age 12 without consulting your doctor.

Seniors

Seniors may be more likely to experience side effects when taking Aleve, and should take lower doses (see "Usual Dose").

Brand Names

Alka-Seltzer Original Effervescent Antacid Pain Reliever

(AL-kuh-SELTZ-er)

Alka-Seltzer Extra Strength Effervescent Antacid Pain Reliever

(AL-kuh-SELTZ-er)

Generic Ingredients

Aspirin
Sodium bicarbonate

Type of Drug

Nonsterodial anti-inflammatory drug (NSAID), analgesic (pain reliever), and antacid.

Used for

Temporary relief of body aches and pains, sour stomach with headache, acid indigestion, and heartburn.

General Information

NSAID is the general term used for a group of drugs that is effective in reducing pain. Aspirin, one of the active ingredients in Alka-Seltzer Original Effervescent and Extra Strength Effervescent, and other NSAIDs are generally quickly absorbed into the bloodstream. Pain relief usually occurs within 1 hour of taking the first dose and lasts for 4 to 6 hours. Aspirin is also a member of the group of drugs called salicylates.

Aspirin's effect on pain is thought to be related to its ability to prevent the manufacture of complex body hormones called prostaglandins, which sensitize pain receptors.

Aspirin presents risks to certain populations: Aspirin is associated with gastrointestinal (GI) irritation, erosion, and bleeding, and should not be used by individuals with a GI bleeding disorder or a history of peptic ulcers. Because it has been shown to be harmful to the developing fetus, aspirin should not be taken by pregnant women. Finally, aspirin should not be used by children under age 16 because of the risk of Reye's syndrome (see "Cautions and Warnings").

Sodium bicarbonate (also known as baking soda) is the antacid ingredient in these products. All antacids neutralize stomach acid but vary in their adverse effects and in their interactions with other drugs, as well as in their speed of onset and duration of action. Sodium bicarbonate dissolves quickly in stomach acid and provides a rapid effect, but has the shortest duration of action of any antacid.

In general, an antacid taken on an empty stomach leaves the stomach rapidly, and works for only 20 to 40 minutes. However, when taken after a meal, it leaves the stomach more slowly. When taken 1 hour after a meal, an antacid can work for up to 3 hours.

Cautions and Warnings

Do not use Alka-Seltzer Original Effervescent or Extra Strength Effervescent for more than 10 days, or if fever is present, for more than 3 days, without consulting your doctor. If your condition worsens or persists, if new symptoms occur, or if there is redness or swelling, consult your doctor.

Do not exceed the recommended daily dosage of these products.

People with liver damage or severe kidney failure should avoid these products.

These products should not be used by patients with a history of bleeding disorders or by patients taking drugs for anticoagulation (blood thinning) without checking with your doctor.

These products should be avoided prior to surgery to reduce the risk of bleeding. Check with your physician regarding the duration of time to avoid use of these products prior to a surgical procedure.

Alcohol can aggravate the stomach irritation caused by these products. The risk of aspirin-related ulcers is increased by alcohol.

These products should not be used by patients with a history of ulcer disease.

If you develop continuous stomach pain, dizziness, hearing loss, or ringing or buzzing in the ears, stop using these products and consult your doctor.

If you have a history of asthma, do not use these products without consulting your doctor.

Children with the flu or chicken pox who are given these products may develop Reye's syndrome, a life-threatening condition characterized by vomiting, progressive damage to the central nervous system (CNS), liver injury, and abnormally low blood sugar. Up to 30% of those who develop Reye's syndrome die and permanent brain damage is possible in those who survive. Because of the risk of Reye's syndrome, do not give these products to children under age 16.

Patients with AIDS and AIDS-related complex who take zidovudine (AZT) should avoid using these products because they increase their risk of bleeding.

These products are very high in sodium, which can lead to fluid retention. If you must restrict your sodium intake because of hypertension (high blood pressure), heart failure, kidney failure, or cirrhosis, avoid these products.

Antacids like sodium bicarbonate may relieve symptoms of a serious condition such as peptic ulcer disease. If you take these products for a prolonged period, you run the risk of unknowingly masking the symptoms of a serious GI disease and delaying diagnosis.

Call your doctor if you have severe stomach pains after taking these products.

Call your doctor if your stool is black or tarry or looks like coffee grounds, which indicates bleeding in the intestines or stomach. These may be signs of a serious GI disorder that cannot and should not be treated with an OTC product without your doctor's supervision.

Sodium bicarbonate is completely absorbed into the blood stream. When taken in large doses or by people with impaired kidney function, it can cause systemic metabolic alkalosis (a condition in which the blood becomes low in acidity, affecting the kidney, blood, and salt balance).

Large doses of these products, when combined with milk or calcium, can cause milk-alkali syndrome, which occurs when there is a high intake of calcium combined with anything producing alkalosis (imbalance of acid and base in body fluids). Symptoms include headache, nausea, irritability, vertigo (dizziness), and vomiting. Left unchecked, the syndrome can cause irreversible kidney damage.

Do not take these products if you are overfull from eating or drinking.

Possible Side Effects

- ▼ Most common: gastric distension (swelling), flatulence (gas), nausea, upset stomach, heartburn, and loss of appetite, and appearance of small amounts of blood in the stool.
- ▼ Less common: fluid retention and weight gain.
- ▼ Rare: hives, rashes, liver damage, fever, thirst, and difficulties with vision. Alka-Seltzer Original Effervescent and Extra Strength Effervescent may contribute to the formation of stomach ulcers and bleeding. People who are allergic to aspirin and those with a history of nasal polyps, asthma, or rhinitis may experience breathing difficulty and a stuffy nose.

Drug Interactions

• Do not take Alka-Seltzer Original Effervescent and Extra Strength Effervescent if you are currently taking methotrexate, which is used to treat cancer, severe psoriasis, severe rheumatoid arthritis, and to induce abortion; or valproic acid, an anticonvulsant. These products increase the toxicity of methotrexate and valproic acid.

• These products should also not be taken with anticoagulant (blood-thinning) drugs, such as warfarin and dicumarol. The effects of warfarin and dicumarol will be intensified by these products and increase the risk of abnormal bleeding.

• The possibility of a stomach ulcer is increased if either of these products is taken together with an adrenal corticosteroid such as hydrocortisone, another NSAID such as phenylbutazone, or alcoholic beverages. Taking these products with another NSAID has no benefit and carries a greatly increased risk of side effects.

• These products will counteract the effects of the antigout medications probenecid and sulfinpyrazone and may counteract the effects of angiotensin-converting enzyme (ACE) inhibitors and beta blockers, which work to lower blood pressure. These products may also counteract the effects of some diuretics in people with severe liver disease.

• Combining nitroglycerin tablets and either of these products may lead to a drop in blood pressure.

• These products decrease the absorption of iron and ketoconazole, (an antifungal agent), reducing their effects. If you are taking either of these products at the same time as iron or ketoconazole, separate your dose of each drug by at least 2 hours.

• These products decrease the elimination of amphetamine, (used to treat narcolepsy and obesity); and quinidine (an antiarrhythmic), leading to possible retention of these drugs and intoxication. Do not use either of these products at the same time as amphetamine or quinidine.

Food Interactions

Take Alka-Seltzer Original Effervescent and Extra Strength Effervescent with food, milk, or water to reduce the chance of upset stomach or bleeding.

Usual Dose

Each tablet of Alka-Seltzer Original Effervescent contains 325 mg of aspirin and 1916 mg of sodium bicarbonate.

Each tablet of Extra Strength Effervescent contains 500 mg of aspirin and 1985 mg of sodium bicarbonate.

Alka-Seltzer Original Effervescent

Adult (age 60 and older): Dissolve 2 tablets in 4 oz. of water every 4 hours, not to exceed 4 tablets in 24 hours.

Adult (age 16–59): Dissolve 2 tablets in 4 oz. of water every 4 hours, not to exceed 8 tablets in 24 hours.

Child (under age 16): not recommended.

Extra Strength Effervescent

Adult (age 60 and older): Dissolve 2 tablets in 4 oz. of water every 6 hours, not to exceed 4 tablets in 24 hours.

Adult (age 16–59): Dissolve 2 tablets in 4 oz. of water every 6 hours, not to exceed 7 tablets in 24 hours.

Child (under age 16): not recommended.

Overdosage

Symptoms of overdosage include rapid or deep breathing, nausea, vomiting, dizziness, ringing or buzzing in the ears, flushing, sweating, thirst, headache, drowsiness, diarrhea, rapid heartbeat, fever, excitement, low blood sugar, confusion, convulsions, liver or kidney failure, coma, and bleeding.

Even if the victim is not displaying any of the symptoms listed above, do the following in case of accidental overdose: If the victim is unconscious or having convulsions, call for an ambulance immediately. If you take the victim to an emergency room, be sure to bring the bottle or container with you. If the victim is conscious, call your local poison control center or a health care professional. The poison control center may suggest inducing vomiting with ipecac syrup (available without a prescription at any pharmacy). DO NOT induce vomiting unless specifically instructed to do so.

Special Information

A strong vinegary smell means that Alka-Seltzer Original Effervescent or Extra Strength Effervescent has started to break down in the bottle and should be discarded.

Special Populations

Allergies

If you are allergic to indomethacin, sulindac, ibuprofen, ketoprofen, fenoprofen, naproxen, tolmetin, or meclofenamate sodium, or to products containing tartrazine (a commonly used orange dye and food coloring), you may also be allergic to Alka-Seltzer Original Effervescent and Extra Strength Effervescent.

People with asthma and/or nasal polyps are more likely to be allergic to these products.

Pregnancy/Breast-feeding

Do not take these products if you are pregnant. Aspirin can cause bleeding problems in the developing fetus and can lead to a low-birth-weight infant; it can also cause bleeding problems in the mother before, during, or after pregnancy.

These products pass into breast milk. Check with your doctor before self-medicating with these products if you are breast-feeding.

Infants/Children

These products should not be taken by children under age 16 unless directed by a doctor, due to the risk of Reye's syndrome (see "Cautions and Warnings").

Seniors

Seniors may find the aspirin in these products irritating to the stomach, especially in larger doses. Older adults with liver disease or severe kidney impairment should not use these products.

Be advised that many older patients are at high risk for complications from ulcers, yet often do not show classic ulcer symptoms. Discuss the possible causes of your gastric discomfort with your pharmacist before self-medicating with these products, and possibly delaying diagnosis of an ulcer. Be aware of possible interactions between these products and other medications you may be taking.

Many seniors are on low-sodium diets because of high blood pressure or congestive heart failure. Do not take these products if your sodium intake is restricted.

Brand Name

Arthropan (ar-THROE-pan)

Generic Ingredient

Choline salicylate (KOE-leen SAL-ih-SILL-ate)

Type of Drug

Analgesic (pain reliever) and antipyretic (fever reducer).

Used for

Temporary relief of mild to moderate pain and fever associated with the common cold, flu, viral infections, or other disorders (neuritis, neuralgia, bursitis, arthritis, rheumatism, simple headache, menstrual cramps, tooth and periodontic pain, sprains, and minor muscular aches). It may also be taken to relieve arthritis or inflammation of bones, joints, or body tissues.

General Information

Choline salicylate is a member of the group of drugs called salicylates. Other members of this group include aspirin, sodium salicylate, and magnesium salicylate. Choline salicylate reduces fever by causing the blood vessels in the skin to open, allowing heat to leave the body more rapidly. Choline salicylate's effects on pain and inflammation are thought to be related to its ability to prevent the manufacture of complex body hormones called prostaglandins.

Although choline salicylate is absorbed more quickly from the stomach than aspirin, this does not mean that it is a more effective pain reliever or fever reducer. However, there are other differences between these pain relievers that should be considered when choosing which one to take. Because aspirin has the greatest effect on prostaglandin production of the salicylates, it causes the strongest gastrointestinal effects; choline salicylate may be less irritating to the stomach. Choline salicylate can also be used by people who cannot tolerate the side effects associated with aspirin or who are allergic to aspirin. However, unlike aspirin, choline salicylate does not inhibit platelet aggregation and therefore cannot be substituted for aspirin in the prevention of heart attack or stroke. Choline salicylate is also more expensive than aspirin.

Arthropan is available in an oral liquid form.

Cautions and Warnings

Do not take Arthropan for more than 10 consecutive days or, in the presence of fever, 3 days, unless directed by your doctor. Notify your doctor if this product does not relieve your symptoms in that time.

Do not exceed the recommended daily dosage of Arthropan.

Do not take Arthropan if you have gout.

Stop taking this product and notify your doctor if you develop ringing in the ears or hearing loss.

Children with the flu or chicken pox who are given salicylates may develop Reye's syndrome, a life-threatening condition characterized by vomiting, progressive damage to the central nervous system, liver injury, and abnormally low blood sugar. Up to 30% of those who develop Reye's syndrome die and permanent brain damage is possible in those who survive. Because of the risk of Reye's syndrome, do not give Arthropan to children under age 16. Acetaminophen can usually be substituted.

Possible Side Effects

- ▼ Most common: nausea, upset stomach, heartburn, loss of appetite, and loss of small amounts of blood in the stool.
- ▼ Rare: hives, rashes, liver damage, fever, thirst, and difficulties with vision.

Drug Interactions

- Arthropan should not be used by individuals currently taking methotrexate, which is used to treat cancer, severe psoriasis, severe rheumatoid arthritis, and to induce abortion; or valproic acid, an anticonvulsant. It can increase the toxicity of these drugs.

• Arthropan should also not be taken with anticoagulant (blood-thinning) drugs, such as warfarin and dicumarol. It will exaggerate the effects of these drugs and increase the risk of abnormal bleeding.

• The possibility of stomach ulcer is increased if Arthropan is taken together with an adrenal corticosteroid, such as hydrocortisone; phenylbutazone, a nonsteroidal anti-inflammatory drug (NSAID); or alcoholic beverages.

• Arthropan will counteract the effects of the antigout medications probenecid and sulfinpyrazone and may counteract the effects of angiotensin-converting enzyme (ACE) inhibitors and beta blockers, which work to lower blood pressure.

• Arthropan can lower blood sugar, which can combine with the effects of oral sulfonylurea antidiabetes drugs, such as chlorpropamide or tolbutamide, and further suppress blood sugar levels in people with diabetes.

• Taking Arthropan with an NSAID has no benefit and carries a greatly increased risk of side effects, especially stomach irritation.

• Never mix Arthropan with any alkaline solution (including antacids) because this will make its characteristically "fishy" odor stronger.

Food Interactions

If you dislike the odor of Arthropan, you can mix it with fruit juice, a carbonated beverage, or water just before you take it. Even if you decide not to mix it, you should take Arthropan with food, milk, or water to reduce the risk of stomach irritation.

Usual Dose

Analgesic or Antipyretic:

Adult (age 16 and over): 435–870 mg every 4 hours, as needed. Do not take more than 6 daily doses. Try to take the smallest possible dose that works for you.

Child (under age 16): not recommended because of the risk of Reye's syndrome (see "Cautions and Warnings").

Arthritis or Inflammation:

Adult (age 16 and over): 4.8–7.2 g daily, given in divided doses. Try to take the smallest possible dose that works for you.

Child (under age 16): not recommended because of the risk of Reye's syndrome (see "Cautions and Warnings").

Overdosage

Do the following in case of accidental overdose: If the victim is unconscious or having convulsions, call for an ambulance immediately. If you take the victim to an emergency room, be sure to bring the bottle or container with you. If the victim is conscious, call your local poison control center or a health care professional. The poison control center may suggest inducing vomiting with ipecac syrup (available without a prescription at any pharmacy). DO NOT induce vomiting unless specifically instructed to do so.

Special Populations

Allergies

You may be able to take Arthropan if you are allergic to aspirin, but check with your doctor first.

Pregnancy/Breast-feeding

It is not generally recommended that pregnant women take any drugs, particularly during the first 3 months after conception.

Choline salicylate can cause bleeding problems in the developing fetus and can lead to a low-birth-weight infant; it can also cause bleeding problems in the mother before, during, or after pregnancy. Avoid Arthropan if you are or might be pregnant.

Although choline salicylate passes into breast milk, no adverse effects have been shown to occur in the nursing infant if the drug is taken only occasionally, in low doses. Do not take Arthropan on a regular basis unless it is approved by your physician. Acetaminophen may be a better choice if you are nursing.

Infants/Children

Arthropan is not recommended for use in children under age 16 because of the risk of Reye's syndrome.

Seniors

Seniors should exercise the same caution as younger adults when using Arthropan.

Brand Name

Aspercreme (ASS-per-kreem)

Generic Ingredients

Trolamine salicylate
Triethanolamine

Type of Drug

Topical analgesic.

Used for

Relief of soreness, stiffness, and pain in muscles, joints, and tendons.

General Information

Topical analgesics are one of the most popular types of OTC drugs, and the number of these drugs sold continues to increase year after year. Many of the people using these products are over age 50; in fact, 40% of individuals in this age group use topical analgesics on a regular basis. Younger people may use topical analgesics to relieve pain and soreness brought on by exercising or playing sports.

Salicylates (e.g., aspirin, sodium salicylate, magnesium aslicylate) are thought to relieve pain by affecting the body's production of complex hormones known as prostaglandins. However, it has not been proven that trolamine salicylate, a topical member of the group, works in this way when applied to the skin, nor does it work as a counterirritant to relieve pain. Although there have been some published reports indicating that trolamine salicylate, the active ingredient in Aspercreme, may be effective in relieving pain and soreness caused by exercise and weight training, the FDA does not recognize trolamine salicylate as an effective OTC analgesic.

Cautions and Warnings

Do not use Aspercreme for longer than 10 consective days.

If redness is present or your condition worsens, or if the pain persists for more than 7 days or is recurrent, stop using Aspercreme and consult your doctor.

Do not exceed the recommended daily dosage of Aspercreme.

If you have experienced an allergic reaction to aspirin or salicylates, consult your doctor before using Aspercreme.

Do not use Aspercreme on children under the age of 12.

Aspercreme should be used only on the skin. Don't apply it near your eyes or to mucous membranes (i.e., inside the mouth, nose, rectum, or vagina).

Do not use Aspercreme on red or irritated skin. Stop using it if irritation develops, and call your doctor.

To avoid the risk of irritation, redness, or blistering, don't use a tight bandage or dressing over the skin where you apply Aspercreme.

Do not use Aspercreme on broken or sunburned skin, or on an open wound.

If you wear contact lenses, don't take them out or put them in your eyes after you use Aspercreme without first washing your hands.

Possible Side Effect

▼ When used extensively, Aspercreme may cause mild to moderate peeling of the skin. This does not necessarily require that you discontinue using Aspercreme unless the peeling worsens or becomes infected.

Drug Interactions

• Some people taking the anticoagulant (blood-thinning) drug warfarin who also used a topical analgesic containing a salicylate, such as trolamine salicylate, the active ingredient in Aspercreme, have experienced an increase in the effect of warfarin. If you take warfarin, talk to your doctor or pharmacist before you self-medicate with Aspercreme.

Usual Dose

Aspercreme contains trolamine salicylate 10%.

Adult and Child (age 12 and over): Apply generously to the affected area, massaging the medication into the skin, up to 4 times a day. Be sure to wash your hands thoroughly afterward. If you are treating pain in your hands, wait 30 minutes before washing.

Child (under age 12): Consult your doctor.

Overdosage

Do the following in case of accidental ingestion: If the victim is unconscious or having convulsions, call for an ambulance immediately. If you take the victim to an emergency room, be sure to bring the bottle or container with you. If the victim is conscious, call your local poison control center or a health care professional. The poison control center may suggest inducing vomiting with ipecac syrup (available without a prescription at any pharmacy). DO NOT induce vomiting unless specifically instructed to do so.

Special Information

Besides using a topical preparation, there are also physical methods of easing the pain of an overworked muscle, such as by gently massaging the injured area. In fact, some of the benefit gained from using topical medications may simply be due to the fact that they are applied by being rubbed and massaged into the skin. Another way to ease pain is to apply heat to the skin with a hot water bottle or heating pad; in addition to reducing pain, heat helps the collagen in your skin regain its elasticity and lose its stiffness after a stretching injury.

Special Populations

Allergies

If you are allergic to aspirin or to other salicylates, check with your doctor before using Aspercreme.

Pregnancy/Breast Feeding

It is not generally recommended that pregnant women take any drugs, particularly during the first 3 months after conception. Check with your doctor if you are or might be pregnant, or if you are breast-feeding.

Infants/Children

Aspercreme should not be used on children under age 12, unless directed by a doctor.

Seniors

Seniors should exercise the same caution as younger adults when using Aspercreme.

Bayer (BAY-er)

*see **Aspirin,** page 672*

Brand Name

Doan's Ⓒ (Dohnz)

Gereric Ingredient

Magnesium salicylate

Type of Drug

Analgesic (pain reliever) and antipyretic (fever reducer).

Used for

Temporary relief of minor backache pain.

General Information

Magnesium salicylate's effects on pain and inflammation are thought to be related to its ability to prevent the manufacture of complex body hormones called prostaglandins.

Although magnesium salicylate has not been proven to be more effective than aspirin, it has some advantages that should be considered when choosing which pain reliever to take. Because aspirin has the greatest effect on prostaglandin production of the salicylates, it causes the strongest gastrointestinal effects; magnesium salicylate may be less irritating to the stomach. Magnesium salicylate can also be used by people who cannot tolerate the side effects associated with aspirin or who are allergic to aspirin.

Cautions and Warnings

Do not take Doan's for more than 5 consecutive days or, in the presence of fever, 3 days, unless directed by your doctor. Notify your doctor if Doan's does not relieve your symptoms in that time.

Do not exceed the recommended daily dosage of Doan's.

Do not take Doan's if you have asthma.

People with chronically impaired kidney function should not use Doan's because of the risk of magnesium buildup in the body.

Stop taking Doan's and notify your doctor if you develop ringing in the ears or hearing loss.

Children with the flu or chicken pox who are given salicylates may develop Reye's syndrome, a life-threatening condition characterized by vomiting, progressive damage to the central nervous system, liver injury, and abnormally low blood sugar. Up to 30% of those who develop Reye's syndrome die and permanent brain damage is possible in those who survive. Because of the risk of Reye's syndrome, do not give Doan's to children under age 16. Acetaminophen can usually be substituted.

Possible Side Effects

- ▼ Most common: nausea, upset stomach, heartburn, loss of appetite, and appearance of small amounts of blood in the stool.
- ▼ Less common: hives, rashes, liver damage, fever, thirst, and difficulties with vision.

Drug Interactions

• Doan's should not be used by individuals currently taking methotrexate, which is used to treat cancer, severe psoriasis, severe rheumatoid arthritis, and to induce abortion; or valproic acid, an anticonvulsant. It can increase the toxicity of these drugs.

• Doan's should not be taken with anticoagulant (blood-thinning) drugs, such as warfarin and dicumarol. It will exaggerate the effects of these drugs and increase the risk of abnormal bleeding.

• The possibility of stomach ulcer is increased if Doan's is taken together with an adrenal corticosteroid such as hydrocortisone; phenylbutazone, a nonsteroidal anti-inflammatory drug (NSAID); or alcoholic beverages.

• Doan's will counteract the effects of the antigout medications probenicid and sulfinpyrazone and may counteract the effects of angiotensin-converting enzyme (ACE) inhibitors and beta blockers, which work to lower blood pressure.

• Taking Doan's with an NSAID has no benefit and carries a greatly increased risk of side effects, especially stomach irritation.

Food Interactions

Take Doan's with food, milk, or water to reduce the chance of upset stomach or bleeding.

Usual Dose

Each caplet of Doan's Regular Strength contains 377 mg of magnesium salicylate. Each caplet of Doan's Extra Strength contains 580 mg of magnesium salicylate.

Regular Strength

Adult (age 16 and over): 2 caplets every 4 hours, not to exceed 12 caplets in 24 hours.

Child (under age 16): not recommended because of the risk of Reye's syndrome (see "Cautions and Warnings").

Extra Strength

Adult (age 16 and over): 2 caplets every 6 hours, not to exceed 8 caplets in 24 hours.

Child (under age 16) : not recommended because of the risk of Reye's syndrome (see "Cautions and Warnings").

Overdosage

Do the following in case of accidental overdose: If the victim is unconscious or having convulsions, call for an ambulance immediately. If you take the victim to an emergency room, be sure to bring the bottle or container with you. If the victim is conscious, call your local poison control center or a health care professional. The poison control center may suggest inducing vomiting with ipecac syrup (available without a prescription at any pharmacy). DO NOT induce vomiting unless specifically instructed to do so.

Special Populations

Allergies

You may be able to take Doan's if you are allergic to aspirin, but check with your doctor first.

Pregnancy/Breast-feeding

Magnesium salicylate can cause bleeding problems in the developing fetus and can lead to a low-birth-weight infant; it can also cause bleeding problems in the mother before, during, or after pregnancy. Avoid Doan's if you are or might be pregnant.

Although magnesium salicylate passes into breast milk, no adverse effects have been shown to occur in the nursing infant if the drug is taken only occasionally, in low doses. Do not take Doan's on a regular basis unless it is approved by your physician. Acetaminophen may be a better choice if you are nursing.

Infants/Children

Doan's is not recommended for use in children under age 16 because of the risk of Reye's syndrome.

Seniors

Seniors should exercise the same caution as younger adults when using Doan's.

Ecotrin

*see **Aspirin,** page 672*

Brand Name

Excedrin Aspirin-Free Analgesic Caplets (ex-SED-rin)

Generic Ingredients

Acetaminophen
Caffeine

Type of Drug

Analgesic (pain reliever), mild diuretic, and central nervous system (CNS) stimulant.

Used for

Temporary relief of the pain of headache, sinusitis, colds, muscular aches, menstrual discomfort, toothaches, and minor arthritis pain.

General Information

The acetaminophen in Excedrin Aspirin-Free Analgesic Caplets is used to relieve pain associated with the common cold, flu, viral infections, or other disorders (neuritis, neuralgia, bursitis, arthritis, rheumatism, simple headache, menstrual cramps, tooth and periodontic pain, sprains, and minor muscular aches).

Caffeine, a diuretic and CNS stimulant, is used in OTC medications to help fight off sleep, increase mental alertness, and improve coordination. In Excedrin Aspirin-Free it is combined with acetaminophen and aspirin to treat headache or the fluid retention, tension, and fatigue that can accompany menstruation.

Cautions and Warnings

Do not take Excedrin Aspirin-Free for pain for more than 10 days, or in the presence of fever, for more than 3 days, unless directed by your doctor.

Do not exceed the recommended daily dosage of Excedrin Aspirin-Free.

If pain or fever persists or worsens, if new symptoms occur, or if there is redness or swelling, consult your doctor.

In doses of more than 4 grams per day, the acetaminophen ingredient in Excedrin Aspirin-Free is potentially toxic to the liver. Use Excedrin Aspirin-Free with caution if you have kidney or liver disease or viral infections of the liver. Studies have shown that the risk of liver damage with acetaminophen is associated with fasting and alcohol use. People with pre-existing liver disease who are taking other drugs that are potentially damaging to the liver, who do not eat regularly, or who drink alcohol (even moderately) are especially at risk. Alcohol can also lead to adverse gastrointestinal (GI) effects if taken with Excedrin Aspirin-Free. If you take Excedrin Aspirin-Free regularly, avoid drinking alcoholic beverages and/or fasting.

The effectiveness of Excedrin Aspirin-Free may be decreased if you smoke, and you may need a higher dose to achieve the desired effect.

Excedrin Aspirin-Free should be used with caution by individuals with a history of peptic ulcer because it may lead to GI irritation.

The caffeine in Excedrin Aspirin-Free may have the potential to cause cardiac arrhythmia (irregular heartbeats), although this effect is still under investigation. As a precaution, individuals should avoid Excedrin Aspirin-Free if they have symptomatic cardiac arrhythmias and/or palpitations and if they are in the first several days or weeks of recovery after a heart attack.

Excedrin Aspirin-Free may increase aggressive behavior, worsen symptoms in people with anxiety or panic disorder, or worsen symptoms in women with moderate to severe premenstrual syndrome (PMS).

Excedrin Aspirin-Free may have adverse effects on the quality of your sleep. You may wake up more frequently during the night or be awakened more easily by noises or other disturbances.

Possible Side Effects

▼ Most common: lightheadedness, insomnia, restlessness, nervousness, headache, irritability, nausea, vomiting, and upset stomach.

▼ Less common: trembling and pain in lower back or side.

▼ Rare: extreme fatigue, rash, itching, or hives; sore throat or fever; unexplained bleeding or bruising; anemia; yellowing of the skin or eyes; blood in urine; painful or frequent urination; and decreased output of urine volume; excitability; agitation; shakiness; anxiety; scintillating scotoma (a sensation of light before the eyes); hyperesthesia (unusual sensitivity of the skin or of a particular sense); ringing in the ears; and rapid or premature heartbeat or other cardiac arrhythmias.

Drug Interactions

• The effects of Excedrin Aspirin-Free may be reduced by long-term use or large doses of barbiturate drugs; the anticonvulsants carbamazepine and phenytoin (and other similar drugs); rifampin, used to treat tuberculosis (TB); and sulfinpyrazone, used to treat gout. These drugs may also increase the chances of liver toxicity if taken with Excedrin Aspirin-Free.

• Taking chronic, large doses of Excedrin Aspirin-Free with isoniazid (used to treat TB) may also increase the risk of liver damage.

• If Excedrin Aspirin-Free is taken with an anticoagulant such as warfarin, it may increase the blood-thinning effect of the anti-coagulant agent. This does not occur with occasional use.

• Alcohol increases the liver toxicity caused by large doses of Excedrin Aspirin-Free (see "Cautions and Warnings"). Alcohol, can also increase the adverse GI effects of Excedrin Aspirin-Free. If you take Excedrin Aspirin-Free regularly, avoid alcohol.

• Nonsteroidal anti-inflammatory drugs (NSAIDs) and corticosteroids may increase the risk of adverse GI effects in people taking Excedrin Aspirin-Free.

• It has been reported that patients with AIDS and AIDS-related complex taking zidovudine (AZT) with acetaminophen, one of the active ingredients in Excedrin Aspirin-Free, have an increased incidence of bone marrow suppression. However, studies performed to try to determine if a harmful interaction exists have not shown that short-term use of acetaminophen (less than 7 days) increases the risk of bone marrow suppression or causes a decrease in white blood cells in AIDS patients taking AZT. Acetaminophen, when taken on a short-term basis or only as needed, is the recommended OTC pain-relieving drug for these patients.

• The body's metabolism of caffeine, the other active ingredient in Excedrin Aspirin-Free, is inhibited by the following drugs: mexiletine, an antiarrhythmic; cimetidine, used to treat peptic ulcers, heartburn, and acid indigestion; the fluoroquinolone anti-infectives norfloxacin, enoxacin, and ciprofloxacin; and oral contraceptives containing estrogen. This effect is also seen when caffeine is ingested with alcohol or the drug disulfiram, which is used in the treatment of chronic alcoholism.

• Because Excedrin Aspirin-Free may decrease the body's absorption of iron, iron supplements should be taken 1 hour before or 2 hours after the dose of Excedrin Aspirin-Free.

• Taken together, Excedrin Aspirin-Free and the decongestant phenylpropanolamine may increase blood pressure.

• Excedrin Aspirin-Free may interfere with the therapeutic benefit of drugs given to regulate heart rhythm, such as quinidine, and propranolol. It may also increase the breakdown of phenobarbitol or aspirin, thus decreasing the beneficial effects of these drugs.

• The effects of both the benzodiazepine tranquilizer, diazepam, and Excedrin Aspirin-Free may either be increased or decreased (depending on dose and specific behavioral tests used) when these drugs are taken together.

• Excedrin Aspirin-Free may cause false-positive results in tests performed to diagnose pheochromocytoma (tumor of the adrenal gland) or neuroblastoma (tumor of the nervous system), and may also affect readings of uric acid concentrations.

Food Interactions

To avoid the potential danger of caffeine overdose, be aware of your consumption of coffee, tea, cola drinks, chocolate, and other caffeine-containing foods if you are taking Excedrin Aspirin-Free. Check with your doctor about a safe level of caffeine intake for you.

Usual Dose

Each caplet contains 500 mg of acetaminophen and 65 mg of caffeine.

Adult and Child (age 12 and over): 2 caplets every 6 hours, not to exceed 8 caplets in 24 hours.

Child (under age 12): Consult your doctor.

Overdosage

Symptoms of overdose include nausea, vomiting, drowsiness, confusion, abdominal pain, low blood pressure, yellowing of the skin and eyes, liver damage, restlessness, excitability, increased heart rate, sleeplessness, frequent urination, flushing, muscle twitching, and disordered thoughts and speech.

Even if the victim is not displaying any of the symptoms listed above, do the following in case of accidental overdose: If the victim is unconscious or having convulsions, call for an ambulance immediately. If you take the victim to an emergency room, be sure to bring the bottle or container with you. If the victim is conscious, call your local poison control center or a health care professional. The poison control center may suggest inducing vomiting with ipecac syrup (available without a prescription at any pharmacy). DO NOT induce vomiting unless specifically instructed to do so.

Special Populations:

Pregnancy/Breast-feeding

It is not generally recommended that pregnant women take any drugs, particularly during the first 3 months after conception. Although taking normal dosages of acetaminophen is considered relatively safe for the expectant mother and her baby, taking continual high doses may cause birth defects or interfere with the baby's development.

Caffeine has been shown to cross the placenta in pregnant women, which means that it passes from the mother to the fetus. The FDA recommends that women should limit their caffeine intake or avoid caffeine entirely during pregnancy. Studies in humans suggest that adverse effects of caffeine during pregnancy are related to the amount ingested; doses of more than 300 mg per day have been linked to slowed growth and low birth weight of the infant.

Acetaminophen is considered acceptable for use during breast-feeding by the American Academy of Pediatrics. Although acetaminophen does pass into breast milk when taken by nursing mothers, the only side effect reported in infants is a rash that goes away when the mother stops taking the drug.

Caffeine passes into breast milk and may cause wakefulness and irritability in nursing infants of mothers taking high doses (600 mg per day). Because the highest concentrations of caffeine in breast milk occur within 1 hour of caffeine intake, you may want to avoid caffeine until just after you nurse. Keep your caffeine intake at moderate levels, especially if your child is under 4 months old. Another alternative is simply to avoid caffeine entirely until your child is weaned.

Check with your doctor before using acetaminophen or caffeine if you are or might be pregnant, or if you are breast-feeding.

Infants/Children

Children may be more susceptible to the CNS effects of Excedrin Aspirin-Free. Don't give Excedrin Aspirin-Free to children under age 12 without consulting your doctor.

Seniors

Because acetaminophen may clear the body more slowly in older adults, the side effects of Excedrin Aspirin-Free may be more noticeable.

Older people may be more sensitive to the stimulant effects of Excedrin Aspirin-Free and may be more liable to have nervousness, anxiety, sleeplessness, and irritability. Be especially cautious about your caffeine intake if you are taking other drugs that stimulate the CNS, such as theophylline, amantadine (used to treat Parkison's disease), tricyclic antidepressants, or appetite suppressants.

Brand Name

Excedrin Extra Strength (ex-SED-rin)

Generic Ingredients

Aspirin
Acetaminophen
Caffeine

Type of Drug

Nonsteroidal anti-inflammatory drug (NSAID), analgesic (pain reliever), and central nervous system (CNS) stimulant, and diuretic.

Used for

Temporary relief of headache, body aches, minor arthritis pain, toothache, and pain associated with nasal congestion, colds, and menstrual discomfort.

General Information

Some OTC products use a combination of drugs to relieve aches and pains. Excedrin Extra Strength contains an NSAID, a second pain reliever, and a mild CNS stimulant/diuretic.

Excedrin Extra Strength contains aspirin, which is an NSAID. NSAID is the general term for a group of drugs that reduce inflammation and pain. Aspirin is also a member of the group of drugs called salicylates, which are also pain relievers. Aspirin's effects on pain and inflammation are thought to be related to its ability to prevent the manufacture of complex hormones called prostaglandins, which sensitize pain receptors and stimulate the inflammatory response. Of all the salicylates, aspirin has the greatest effect on prostaglandin production.

The second pain reliever in Excedrin Extra Strength is acetaminophen, whose action is similar to aspirin's. Acetaminophen and aspirin have been shown to be equally effective in reducing most types of pain.

Excedrin Extra Strength also contains caffeine. Caffeine has been reported to increase the pain-relieving effects of both aspirin and acetaminophen, and caffeine alone may relieve certain types of headaches. Caffeine also has diuretic properties, and is used with aspirin and acetaminophen to treat the fluid retention, tension, and fatigue that may accompany menstruation.

Cautions and Warnings

Unless directed by your doctor, do not take Excedrin Extra Strength for more than 10 days continuously, or in the presence of fever, for more than 3 days continuously.

Do not exceed the recommended daily dosage of Excedrin Extra Strength.

If dizziness, hearing loss, ringing or buzzing in the ears, or continuous stomach pain occur while using Excedrin Extra Strength or any other aspirin product, stop taking the drug immediately and call your doctor.

Children with the flu or chicken pox who are given aspirin or other salicylates may develop Reye's syndrome, a life-threatening condition characterized by vomiting, progressive damage to the central nervous system, liver injury, and abnormally low blood sugar. Up to 30% of children who develop Reye's syndrome die, and permanent brain damage is possible in those who survive. Because of the risk of Reye's syndrome, do not give Excedrin Extra Strength to children under age 16. A product that contains only acetaminophen can usually be substituted for aspirin or an aspirin combination.

Aspirin is associated with gastrointestinal (GI) irritation, erosion, and bleeding. Unless directed by a doctor, people with GI bleeding or a history of peptic ulcers should not take Excedrin Extra Strength. Be aware that the risk of aspirin-related ulcers is increased by alcohol.

People with liver or kidney damage should avoid aspirin.

People with a history of asthma, nasal polyps, or rhinitis should not use aspirin without checking with a doctor.

To reduce the risk of bleeding, aspirin should be avoided prior to surgery. Ask your doctor how long before surgery you should avoid taking Excedrin Extra Strength and any other aspirin product.

In doses of more than 4 grams per day, acetaminophen is potentially toxic to the liver. Use Excedrin Extra Strength with caution if you have kidney or liver disease or viral infections of the liver. Studies have shown that the risk of liver damage with acetaminophen is associated with fasting and alcohol use. People with liver disease who are taking other drugs that are potentially damaging to the liver, people who do not eat regularly, or who drink alcohol (even moderately) are especially at risk. If you take Excedrin Extra Strength regularly, avoid drinking alcohol and/or fasting.

The caffeine in Excedrin Extra Strength may cause cardiac arrhythmia (irregular heart beat), although this effect is still under investigation. As a precaution, it is recommended that caffeine be avoided by people with a history of irregular heart beat and/or heart palpitations, and during the first several days to weeks after a heart attack.

Caffeine may lead to certain side effects involving mood, including a decrease in aggressive behavior, a worsening of anxiety or panic disorder, and worsening of moderate to severe premenstrual syndrome.

Over the long term, high caffeine intake can lead to tolerance of, and physical and psychological dependence on the drug. If caffeine is stopped abruptly, physical signs of withdrawal may occur. The most common symptoms of caffeine withdrawal are fatigue and a throbbing headache, followed by vomiting, impaired physical coordination, irritability, restlessness, drowsiness, and sometimes yawning and a runny nose. These symptoms usually begin 12 to 24 hours after caffeine is stopped and reach their maximum in 20 to 48 hours; they may last for as long as 7 days.

Caffeine may have adverse effects on the quality of your sleep. You may wake up more frequently during the night or may be awakened more easily by noises or other disturbances.

Possible Side Effects

▼ Most common: nausea, upset stomach, vomiting, heartburn, loss of appetite; small amounts of blood in the stool, lightheadedness, restlessness, nervousness, sleeplessness, irritability, tremors, and headache.

Possible Side Effects *(continued)*

- ▼ Less common: excitability, anxiety, tremors, scintillating scotoma (a sensation of light before the eyes), hyperesthesia (unusual sensitivity of one of the senses), ringing in the ears, increased urination, and rapid or irregular heat beat.
- ▼ Rare: rashes, hives, liver damage, fever, thirst, and difficulty breathing.

Drug Interactions

• Excedrin Extra Strength should not be taken by individuals currently taking methotrexate, used to treat cancer, severe psoriasis, severe rheumatoid arthritis, and to induce abortion; or valproic acid, an anticonvulsant. The aspirin in Excedrin Extra Strength can increase the toxicity of these drugs.

• The possibility of a stomach ulcer is increased if aspirin is taken together with alcoholic beverages; an adrenal corticosteroid, such as hydrocortisone; or phenylbutazone, another NSAID. Taking Excedrin Extra Strength with another NSAID has no benefit and carries a greatly increased risk of side effects.

• The aspirin in Excedrin Extra Strength will counteract the effects of the antigout medications probenecid and sulfinpyrazone, and may counteract the effects of angiotensin-converting enzyme (ACE) inhibitors and beta blockers, which work to lower blood pressure. Aspirin may also counteract the effects of some diuretics in people with severe liver disease.

• Combining nitroglycerin tablets and aspirin may lead to an unexpected drop in blood pressure.

• People with AIDS and AIDS-related complex who take zidovudine (AZT) should avoid using Excedrin Extra Strength because the aspirin in it may increase the risk of bleeding. For people taking AZT, the recommended alternative to aspirin is acetaminophen alone—but only taken as needed or for no longer than 7 consecutive days, unless directed otherwise by your doctor. (If acetaminophen is taken at the same time as AZT for anything other than short periods, people with AIDS may experience increased suppression of bone marrow production.)

• Excedrin Extra Strength should also not be taken with

anticoagulant (blood-thinning) drugs, such as warfarin and dicumarol. Both aspirin and acetaminophen may exaggerate the effects of these drugs and increase the risk of abnormal bleeding.

• The effect of the acetaminophen in Excedrin Extra Strength may be reduced by long-term use or large doses of barbiturate drugs; the anticonvulsants carbamazepine and phenytoin (and other similar drugs); rifampin, used to treat tuberculosis (TB) and sulfinpyrazone, used to treat gout. These drugs may also increase the chances of liver toxicity if taken with acetaminophen. Taking chronic, large doses of acetaminophen with isoniazid (used to treat TB) may also increase the risk of liver damage.

• Because of its caffeine content, Excedrin Extra Strength should not be used at the same time as a monoamine oxidase inhibitor (MAOI) or within 2 weeks of stopping treatment with an MAOI. MAOIs are used to treat depression, other psychiatric or emotional conditions, and Parkinson's disease. If you are not sure whether you are or have been taking an MAOI, check with your doctor or pharmacist before you use Excedrin Extra Strength.

• Because caffeine may decrease the body's absorption of iron, iron supplements should be taken 1 hour before or 2 hours after Excedrin Extra Strength is taken.

• Caffeine may interact adversely with other CNS stimulants, including theophylline, a bronchodilator; amanatadine, used to treat Parkinson's disease; tricyclic antidepressants; appetite suppressants, decongestants, and additional caffeine. These combinations can cause disorientation, delirium, and other side effects.

• The body's metabolism of caffeine is inhibited by the following drugs: mexiletine, an antiarrhythmic; cimetidine, used to treat peptic ulcers, heartburn, and acid indigestion; the fluoroquinolone anti-infectives norfloxacin, enoxacin, and ciprofloxacin; and oral contraceptives containing estrogen. This effect is also seen when caffeine is ingested with alcohol or the drug disulfiram, which is used in the treatment of chronic alcoholism.

• The effects of both caffeine and the benzodiazepine tranquilizer diazepam may either be increased or decreased (depending on dose and specific behavioral tests used) when these drugs are taken together.

• Caffeine may cause false-positive results in tests performed to diagnose pheochromocytoma (tumor of the adrenal gland) or neuroblastoma (tumor of the nervous system), and may also affect readings of uric acid concentrations.

• Avoid alcohol when you are taking Excedrin Extra Strength. (Be aware that alcohol is present in many OTC preparations). Alcohol aggravates the stomach irritation associated with both aspirin and caffeine, and increases the risk of aspirin-related ulcers. Alcohol also increases the risk of liver damage associated with acetaminophen (see "Cautions and Warnings").

Food Interactions

Taking Excedrin Extra Strength along with food, milk, or water reduces the risk of upset stomach or GI bleeding from aspirin.

The caffeine in Excedrin Extra Strength can interact adversely with additional caffeine (see "Drug Interactions"). Be aware that caffeine is found in many popular beverages, including coffee, tea, and cola, and in chocolate. Check with your doctor regarding your safe level of caffeine intake.

Usual Dose

Each tablet or caplet of Excedrin Extra Strength contains 250 mg of aspirin, 250 mg of acetaminophen, and 65 mg of caffeine.

Adult (age 16 and over): 2 tablets or caplets every 6 hours. Do not exceed 8 tablets or caplets in a 24-hour period.

Child (under age 16): Consult your doctor.

Overdosage

Symptoms of overdose include ringing or buzzing in the ears, rapid and deep breathing, rapid or irregular heartbeat, sweating, flushed face, thirst, headache, drowsiness, dizziness, muscle twitches, abdominal pain, nausea, vomiting, diarrhea, fever, nervousness, restlessness, sleeplessness, excitability, confusion, low blood sugar, convulsions, yellowing of the skin and eyes, liver or kidney failure, and bleeding. Symptoms may develop within 30 minutes, or may not be seen for as long as 2 days after the overdose.

Even if the victim is not displaying any of the symptoms listed above, do the following in case of accidental overdose: If the victim is unconscious or having convulsions, call for an ambulance immediately. If you take the victim to an

emergency room, be sure to bring the bottle or container with you. If the victim is conscious, call your local poison control center or a health care professional. The poison control center may suggest inducing vomiting with ipecac syrup (available without a prescription at any pharmacy). DO NOT induce vomiting unless specifically instructed to do so.

Special Populations

Pregnancy/Breast-feeding

Do not take Excedrin Extra Strength if you are or might be pregnant.

Aspirin, acetaminophen, and caffeine are known to pass into the breast milk of nursing mothers and may cause side effects in infants. Check with your doctor before taking Excedrin Extra Strength if you are breast-feeding.

Infants/Children

Aspirin should not be used by children under 16 unless directed by your doctor because of the risk of Reye's syndrome (see "Cautions and Warnings"). Do not give Excedrin Extra Strength to a child under age 16 unless directed by your doctor.

Seniors

Older individuals may find the aspirin in Excedrin Extra Strength irritating to the stomach, especially in large doses. Older adults with liver disease or severe kidney impairment should not use aspirin.

Older people may also be more sensitive to the caffeine in Excedrin Extra Strength and may experience nervousness, anxiety, sleeplessness, and irritability. Seniors should also be especially aware that caffeine may interact with other drugs that stimulate the CNS (see "Drug Interactions").

Brand Name

Mobigesic (moe-bi-JEE-zik)

Generic Ingredients

Magnesium salicylate
Phenyltoloxamine citrate

Type of Drug

Analgesic (pain reliever).

Used for

Temporary relief of mild to moderate pain and fever associated with the common cold, flu, viral infections, or other disorders (neuritis, neuralgia, bursitis, arthritis, rheumatism, simple headache, menstrual cramps, tooth and periodontic pain, sprains, and minor muscular aches). It may also be taken to relieve arthritis or inflammation of bones, joints, or other body tissues.

General Information

Magnesium salicylate is a member of the group of drugs called salicylates. Other members of this group include aspirin, sodium salicylate, and choline salicylate. Magnesium salicylate reduces fever by causing the blood vessels in the skin to open, allowing heat to leave the body more rapidly. Magnesium salicylate's effects on pain and inflammation are thought to be related to its ability to prevent the manufacture of complex body hormones called prostaglandins.

Although magnesium salicylate has not been proven to be more effective than aspirin, it has some advantages that should be considered when choosing which pain reliever to take. Of the salicylates, aspirin has the greatest effect on prostaglandin production causes and the strongest gastrointestinal effects; magnesium salicylate may be less irritating to the stomach. Magnesium salicylate can also be used by people who cannot tolerate the side effects associated with aspirin or who are allergic to aspirin. However, unlike aspirin, magnesium salicylate does not inhibit platelet aggregation, and therefore cannot be substituted for aspirin in the prevention of heart attack or stroke.

Phenyltoloxamine citrate is an antihistamine that is sometimes combined with an analgesic (pain reliever), such as magnesium salicylate to enhance the effectiveness of the analgesic.

Cautions and Warnings

Do not take Mobigesic for more than 5 consecutive days or, in the presence of fever, 3 days, unless directed by your doctor. Notify your doctor if Mobigesic does not relieve your symptoms in that time.

Do not exceed the recommended daily dosage of Mobigesic.

Do not take Mobigesic if you have asthma.

People with chronically impaired kidney function should not use products containing magnesium salicylate, because of the risk of magnesium buildup in the body.

Stop taking Mobigesic and notify your doctor if you develop ringing in the ears or hearing loss.

Children with the flu or chicken pox who are given salicylates may develop Reye's syndrome, a life-threatening condition characterized by vomiting, progressive damage to the central nervous system, liver injury, and abnormally low blood sugar. Up to 30% of those who develop Reye's syndrome can die, and permanent brain damage is possible in those who survive. Because of the risk of Reye's syndrome, do not give salicylates to children under age 16.

Possible Side Effects

▼ Most common: nausea, upset stomach, heartburn, loss of appetite, and loss of small amounts of blood in the stool.

▼ Less common: hives, rashes, liver damage, fever, thirst, and difficulties with vision.

Drug Interactions

• Mobigesic should not be taken by individuals currently taking methotrexate, which is used to treat cancer, severe psoriasis, and severe rheumatoid arthritis and to induce abortion; or valproic acid, an anticonvulsant. The magnesium salicylate in mobigesic can increase the toxicity of these drugs.

• Mobigesic should also not be taken with anticoagulant (blood-thinning) drugs, such as warfarin and dicumarol. The magnesium salicylate in mobigesic will exaggerate the effects of these drugs and increase the risk of abnormal bleeding.

• The possibility of stomach ulcer is increased if magnesium salicylate is taken together with an adrenal corticosteroid such as hydrocortisone; phenylbutazone, a nonsteroidal anti-inflammatory drug (NSAID); or alcoholic beverages.

• Magnesium salicylate will counteract the effects of the antigout medications probenecid and sulfinpyrazone and may counteract the effects of angiotesin-converting enzyme (ACE) inhibitors and beta blockers, which work to lower blood pressure.

• Magnesium salicylate can lower blood sugar, which can combine with the effects of oral sulfonylurea antidiabetes drugs, such as chlorpropamide or tolbutamide, and further suppress blood sugar levels in people with diabetes.

• Taking Mobigesic with an NSAID has no benefit and carries a greatly increased risk of side effects, especially stomach irritation.

Food Interactions

Take Mobigesic with food, milk, or water to reduce the chance of upset stomach or bleeding.

Usual Dose

Each tablet contains 325 mg of magnesium salicylate and 30 mg of phenyltoloxamine citrate.

Analgesic or Antipyretic

Adult (age 16 and over): initial dose 500 mg–1 g, followed by 500 mg every 4 hours, as needed. Do not take more than 3.5 g in 24 hours. Try to take the smallest possible dose that works for you.

Child (under age 16): not recommended because of the risk of Reye's syndrome (see "Cautions and Warnings").

Arthritis or Inflammation

Adult (age 16 and over): 545mg–1.2g, 3 or 4 times a day. Try to take the smallest possible dose that works for you.

Child (under age 16) : not recommended because of the risk of Reye's syndrome (see "Cautions and Warnings").

Overdosage

Do the following in case of accidental overdose: If the victim is unconscious or having convulsions, call for an ambulance immediately. If you take the victim to an emergency room, be sure to bring the bottle or container with you. If the victim is conscious, call your local poison control center or a health care professional. The poison control center may suggest inducing vomiting with ipecac syrup (available without a prescription at any pharmacy). DO NOT induce vomiting unless specifically instructed to do so.

Special Populations

Allergies
If you are allergic to aspirin you may be able to take mobigesic, but check with your doctor first.

Pregnancy/Breast-feeding
It is not generally recommended that pregnant women take any drugs, particularly during the first 3 month after conception. Magnesium salicylate can cause bleeding problems in the developing fetus and can lead to a low-birth-weight infant; it can also cause bleeding problems in the mother before, during, or after pregnancy. Avoid magnesium salicylate if you are pregnant, especially during the last 3 months.

Magnesium salicylate passes into breast milk, although no adverse effects have been shown to occur in the nursing infant (when the drug is taken occasionally in low doses). If you must take Mobigesic, bottle-feed your baby with formula.

Infants/Children
Magnesium salicylate is not recommended for use in children under age 16 because of the risk of Reye's syndrome.

Seniors
Seniors should exercise the same caution as younger adults when taking Mobigesic.

Motrin

*see **Ibuprofen,** page 845*

Nuprin

*see **Ibuprofen,** page 845*

Orudis KT ¢ (uh-ROOD-iss)

*see **Ketoprofen,** page 862*

Tylenol (TYE-leh-nol)

*see **Acetaminophen,** page 659*

Chapter 2: Cough, Cold, Flu, and Asthma Treatment

Colds and Coughs

No human ailment is so widespread, or causes so much general misery, as the common cold. This nagging, persistent disease has become a symbol of frustration with the medical profession, as heard in the lament: "They can put a man on the moon; why can't they come up with a cure for the common cold?"

Symptoms from allergies (e.g., allergic rhinitis) resemble those of colds, and they are often treated with some of the same medications, but allergies arise from very different causes (see chapter 7).

A cold—also known as acute infectious rhinitis or an upper respiratory tract infection—is caused by one of dozens of viruses. You can contract a virus by touching something (such as a glass) that has also been touched by someone with a cold and then rubbing your eyes or putting your fingers in your mouth, or (less commonly) by inhaling droplets of moisture that have been expelled into the air during a sneeze or a cough. When the virus enters your body, it produces inflammation of the membranes that line the nose, mouth, throat, and sinuses.

Colds are hardly life-or-death emergencies, but they cause a great deal of discomfort and days lost from school and work. In severe cases, colds can lead to secondary bacterial ear or sinus infections, and they increase the risk of lower respiratory tract infections such as bronchitis and pneumonia. They can also trigger asthma symptoms.

Preventing a cold is largely a matter of common sense: wash your hands frequently and avoid contact with people who have colds. There is no vaccine against colds. Despite the widespread belief, vitamin C, even in huge doses, will not prevent colds. People who smoke or who experience a great deal of stress are more susceptible to viral infections.

Sore throat is usually the first sign of a cold, followed by nasal symptoms such as stuffiness, runny nose, and postnasal drip (mucus dripping from the back of the nose into the throat). Other typical symptoms include watery eyes, sneezing, and cough (see box). In the first days of a cold, mucus from the nose is typically thin and watery, but over time the discharge usually thickens and becomes green or yellow. Cough can also be a symptom of other diseases, including allergies, acute bronchitis, a chronic obstructive pulmonary disease (such as emphysema or chronic bronchitis), pneumonia, cancer, and congestive heart failure. People with these conditions should be treated by a physician.

Symptoms of the Common Cold

Frequent
- Runny nose
- Nasal congestion
- Sneezing
- Sore throat
- Watery eyes

Less frequent
- Headache
- Body aches and pains
- Fatigue and weakness
- Cough (usually one that does not produce mucus)
- Laryngitis

Infrequent
- Fever

A Sore Subject

The sore throat that comes with a cold is caused by viruses, but bacterial infections can also cause sore throat. Here are some ways to tell the difference.

Characteristic	Viral Sore Throat	Bacterial Sore Throat
Onset	Slow	Rapid
Soreness	Moderate	Severe
Respiratory symptoms	Usually present	Not usually present
Glands	Slight enlargement, not tender	Enlarged, tender
Fever	Uncommon	Common

Seek medical attention if any of the following applies to you

- Persistent cough
- Sore throat or nasal congestion that lasts more than 7 days
- Symptoms that spread beyond the nose or throat
- Ear or chest infection made worse by the cold

Treatment for Colds and Coughs

There is no medication that will cure your cold; the most you can hope for is some relief of symptoms. Usually the cold will disappear on its own within 5 to 10 days whether you treat it or not. Sensible strategies include getting as much rest as possible and drinking plenty of fluids (but not caffeinated beverages or alcohol, which act as diuretics to remove water from the body). If you feel well enough to go to work or school, reduce the risk of spreading the infection by limiting your contact with other people.

If you opt to use an OTC medication, choose a product (or products) that contains only the ingredients you need to address your specific symptoms. There is no reason to take a cough suppressant, for example, if you do not have a cough.

Sore throat can be treated with lozenges or hard candy, which stimulates the flow of saliva and soothes irritated membranes. Lozenges that contain zinc may actually lessen the severity of cold symptoms if used soon after the symptoms appear. Gargling with warm salt water (1 to 3 teaspoons of salt dissolved in 8 to 12 ounces of water) can help, as can drinking fruit juice. Products containing local anesthetics such as menthol, benzocaine, or dyclonine hydrochloride are available as lozenges or sprays. The anesthetic ingredient deadens the nerve endings and relieves pain. Pain relievers such as aspirin or acetaminophen may also be effective for some people. Some cough and cold products also contain ingredients to fight bacterial infection, but these do not work against viruses, which are the cause of colds.

Nasal symptoms are treated with decongestants. The active ingredients in these products are vasoconstrictors, which cause blood vessels to contract, thus reducing swelling, leakage of fluid, and pressure. Examples include ephedrine, naphazoline, oxymetazoline, phenylephrine, propylhexedrine, tetrahydrozoline, and xylometazoline. Decongestants are available in topical form (applied directly to the nasal membranes through drops or sprays) or as oral products that act systemically (tablets or liquids). The topical forms should be used for no more than 3 to 5 days, while the oral products are generally safe for longer-term use. Be aware that using topical decongestants for too long a period can make your nasal symptoms worse.

Guidelines for Use of Decongestants

- Always check the expiration date before using.
- Discard the product if it is discolored or cloudy.
- Do not use for more than 5 days.
- Do not share spray bottles or droppers with another person.
- Blow your nose before using the product, and wait a few minutes after use before blowing your nose again.
- Do not shake the bottle before use.
- Keep your head upright and sniff deeply while spraying.
- If using drops, tilt your head gently from side to side to allow medication to reach the entire area.
- Repeat in both nostrils if necessary.
- Rinse the bottle tip with hot water (but do not let water get into the bottle) and let it air-dry.

Antitussives (cough suppressants) work best against a dry, hacking cough. As a rule, they should not be used for productive coughs (those that produce mucus), because such coughs are the body's way of removing the excess sputum (fluid). However, if a productive cough is preventing you from sleeping, use of a cough suppressant at night may be a good idea.

The most powerful cough suppressant is codeine, which is available without a prescription in some states. This drug is also used as an analgesic (pain reliever), but the dose of codeine in cough products is lower than that used for pain relief. There is a small risk that people using a codeine product will become dependent on it (that is, they will continue to take the medication after the need for it has stopped). Other common cough suppressants are dextromethorphan and diphenhydramine. Unlike codeine, dextromethorphan is not a pain reliever and poses little risk of dependency. Some experts believe it is just as effective as codeine. Diphenhydramine works to reduce the activity of nerves that trigger cough, but it also acts as an antihistamine, which means it can be sedating. Generally, antihistamines are not as effective as decongestants in treating symptoms of the common cold.

In addition to an antitussive, some OTC cough products contain an expectorant called guaifenesin, which loosens mucus secretions and makes them easier to expel. However, it doesn't make sense to take a cough medicine that simultaneously suppresses the cough and increases mucus flow, since you'll be less able to cough up secretions. Drinking 6 to 8 glasses (a glass equals 8 ounces) of water a day also makes mucus thinner and less sticky, and thus easier to expel through coughing. Breathing humidified air also helps. Other cough products contain camphor or menthol, which can be applied to the skin as an ointment or cream, or inhaled in steam. Menthol is also found in lozenges and tablets. The efficacy of these products is marginal, but using them seems to make many people feel better.

As a rule, the common cold does not produce fever, although in some cases body temperature may rise slightly to a little over 100°F. OTC pain and fever relievers, including aspirin and acetaminophen, are usually effective. Children and adolescents should avoid products containing aspirin.

Influenza (Flu)

Like the common cold, the flu is caused by a virus (the influenza virus) and is spread hand to mouth or through droplets sneezed or coughed into the air. Most outbreaks of flu tend to occur in the winter, because people spend more time indoors during that season and are therefore more likely to make contact with an infected person. There are several kinds of flu virus, and headlines seem to report the appearance of yet another new strain each year. This is of concern to doctors and patients alike, because vaccinations that protect against one type of flu may be ineffective against next year's virus; hence the need for annual immunization against flu (especially in seniors and those with chronic diseases).

Flu symptoms resemble those of the common cold, but they are generally more severe and appear in a different pattern. The first sign of flu is usually a sudden fever, accompanied by chills, fatigue, headache, and intense general body aches. After the second day these symptoms start to diminish, but respiratory symptoms and weakness persist. Typically the disease clears up after a week to 10 days. The stress of fighting off flu can weaken the body's immune defense system and make it vulnerable to other bacterial infections, especially pneumonia. This is a special concern in children, seniors, and those with chronic diseases, such as heart or lung disease or diabetes mellitus.

Symptoms of Flu

Frequent/severe

- Fever
- Chills
- Fatigue, weakness, exhaustion
- Sore throat
- Cough (nonproductive)
- Headache
- Body aches and pains

Less frequent

- Runny nose
- Nasal congestion
- Sore throat
- Soreness or burning sensation in the eyes

Treatment of Flu

Vaccines can reduce the risk of contracting flu. Many physicians recommend that older people and those (including children) with respiratory or heart diseases receive vaccinations each year at the start of flu season. Most experts today believe that flu vaccinations can be beneficial to almost everyone. However, vaccines are not foolproof; they work in only about 6 or 7 of every 10 people who receive them.

If flu strikes, treatment is aimed at relieving symptoms, since there is no medication that will eradicate the virus (if started very early, there are medicines that may shorten the duration of certain strains of flu; e.g., amantidine, which is available by prescription only). Bed rest is essential, especially until the fever diminishes. Analgesics (aspirin or nonaspirin products such as acetaminophen and ibuprofen) will ease the aches and fever. As with colds, drinking extra fluids and inhaling humidified air or steam will soothe sore throats and irritated lungs.

The medicines to relieve cold symptoms described above will also ease common flu symptoms such as cough, congestion, and sore throat. Eyedrops containing saline (salt water) or other active ingredients (such as tetrahydrozaline) may alleviate soreness in the eyes.

Seek medical attention if any of the following applies to you

- Symptoms (fever, pain, fatigue) persisting longer than 7 to 10 days
- Heart disease, a respiratory condition, or a pre-existing infection
- Age 60 or over
- Progressively worse, productive cough

OTC Treatment for Colds, Coughs, and Flu

Symptom	Treatment
Sore throat	Local anesthetic Lozenges, especially those containing zinc Pain relievers Salt-water gargles
Nasal symptoms	Oral decongestant Decongestant nasal spray (short-term use only)
Cough	Cough suppressant Expectorant Lozenges
Fever, headache	Pain relievers

Asthma

Asthma is a chronic respiratory disease that causes attacks of breathlessness, coughing, and wheezing during exhalation. Symptoms caused by mild attacks can sometimes be relieved through the use of OTC medications. Avoiding substances or activities that can bring on attacks and reducing the presence of potential triggers in the home environment can reduce the risk of asthma attacks (see Box).

There is no cure for asthma, but treatment can reduce the number and severity of asthma episodes. If you have moderate or severe asthma, you need careful management by a physician, including prescription medications. Hospitalization may be needed in the case of serious attacks.

Typically, asthma first arises during childhood, usually before the age of 5, although it can develop in adulthood. Childhood asthma often becomes less severe over the years. About 1 in 10 children have asthma; the rate among adults is about 1 in 20. During the past decade, the number of people with asthma has increased, possibly due to rising levels of environmental pollution.

Common Asthma Triggers

Air pollution
Bronchial infections
Chemicals
Cockroach particles (feces)
Cold weather
Dander from warm-blooded animals (cats, dogs, birds, rodents)
Dust mites
Emotional excitement
Exercise
Feathers
Fumes (paint, solvents, cleaning products)
Other infections (ear infections, sinus infections, etc.)
Medications
Mold
Perfume
Pollen
Smoke (tobacco, wood)

In recent years, doctors have learned a great deal about the nature of asthma. These new discoveries have changed the way the disease is treated. The most important discovery is that asthma results from chronic inflammation of the airways, the passages from the mouth to the lungs through which air moves when we breathe. The passages into the lungs are also called the bronchial tubes, or trachea. The cells that make up the bronchial tubes can become irritated if they are exposed to allergens (allergy-triggering substances) such as pollen, animal dander, or pollution. People with asthma are especially sensitive to allergens; doctors describe these people as having hyper-reactive airways.

When the cells in the air passages become irritated, they release histamine (and other chemicals) that produce symptoms of inflammation, including itching, redness, and swelling. In the airways, histamine also stimulates the production of the thick, sticky fluid called mucus. During an asthma attack, the airways narrow; this is known as bronchoconstriction.

The symptoms of asthma, then, result from a complicated process. First something happens to trigger a reaction in a person with hyper-reactive bronchial passages—either exposure to an allergen or to a stress factor such as exercise, cold air, or a respiratory infection. In response, the airways become constricted and inflamed. At the same time, they become clogged with mucus. As a result, the person experiences the symptoms of asthma: difficulty breathing, coughing, and wheezing.

Episodes of asthma can last anywhere from a few minutes to several days. Usually people with asthma do not experience symptoms between episodes. However, prompt treatment of an episode is needed, because if the attack continues it can progressively worsen, requiring hospitalization and occasionally intubation for assisted breathing.

Seek medical attention if any of the following applies to you

- Persistent or worsening cough
- Wheezing (especially when exhaling)
- Difficulty breathing
- Chest tightness

Treatment for Asthma

Bronchodilators

It's important to understand the role of inflammation in asthma because it has a direct impact on treatment. The only OTC asthma treatments available are bronchodilators. As the name indicates, these medications work by dilating (widening) the bronchial passages. Bronchodilators provide rapid relief of mild asthma symptoms, but *they do not address the underlying inflammation that is causing the symptoms.* For this reason, people with asthma, especially asthma that is moderate or severe, need to be under the care of a physician who can prescribe additional medications that are unavailable in OTC form.

Bronchodilators are available in oral or inhaled forms. One of the 2 OTC bronchodilators is ephedrine, which is available only in oral form. It can take up to an hour for ephedrine's maximum effect to be felt, and the effects may last up to 5 hours. Unfortunately, because ephedrine can be used to make illegal drugs such as methamphetamine, the FDA may restrict its availability in the near future.

The other available bronchodilator is epinephrine, which is available as an inhalant and a solution (liquid). The inhalant comes in canisters (also called metered-dose inhalers) that deliver the correct dose of medication in an aerosol spray. When the medication is inhaled, it enters the air passages and widens the bronchial tubes. Epinephrine solution is delivered via a special machine called a nebulizer. The liquid is placed in a container connected to a tube, which is attached to a mask that fits over the nose and mouth. The nebulizer pumps air into the container, turning the solution into a spray that is then inhaled through the mask. This form of delivery is used primarily for young children who cannot yet learn to use inhalers properly or for people who are unable to use inhalers. Epinephrine is not available in oral form, because the medication does not survive the process of digestion well enough to provide any benefits.

One key to effective asthma management is knowing when to take these medications. The OTC inhaled bronchodilators are short-acting medications—relief occurs within minutes, but the effects last only about 3 hours or less. If you have mild asthma, and suffer from asthma symptoms only occasionally (less than once a week), it is not a good idea to use a bronchodilator on a regular basis (for example, every morning) as a way to prevent attacks. Instead, these medications should be used only as needed, when symptoms develop. However, if you know that exercise or exposure to cold air is likely to trigger an attack, or that you have trouble breathing whenever you visit the house of someone who owns a cat or smokes cigarettes, it is a good idea to use the bronchodilator 10 or 15 minutes ahead of time as a preventative measure. If symptoms break through despite your use of the medication, additional doses can be taken.

The other important aspect of asthma treatment is knowing how to use the inhaler properly (see box). Some people find it hard to release the spray and inhale in the correct way to get the proper dose of medication. If you use an inhaler, be sure and ask your doctor, nurse, or pharmacist to teach you the right method. Some people, including most children, find it easier to use an inhaler to which a special chamber, called a spacing device, is attached. This chamber holds the medication for a few seconds so that it can be inhaled effectively.

Proper Use of a Metered-Dose Inhaler

1. Remove the cap; check the mouthpiece and remove any foreign objects. Hold the inhaler upright with the mouthpiece at the bottom, and shake the container well to mix the medication.
2. Tilt your head back slightly.
3. Position the inhaler 1½ to 2 inches in front of your mouth.
4. Open your mouth wide and breathe out normally.
5. Press down once on the inhaler to release the medication. At the same time, begin a slow deep breath.
6. Inhale slowly for 3 to 5 seconds.
7. Hold your breath for 10 seconds to allow the medication to penetrate the lungs.
8. Resume normal breathing.
9. If you do not experience adequate relief, or if instructed to do so by your physician, wait 1 minute and repeat the process.
10. Do not take more than 2 puffs of medication at a time, and do not take more than 2 puffs every 3 to 4 hours.

Antihistamines

Medications containing an antihistamine block the effects of histamine, which, as described earlier, causes the inflammation, swelling, and bronchial constriction experienced during an asthma attack. However, most of the antihistamines available in OTC products cause unwanted side effects and should not be used for relief of asthma. Prescription medications such as cetirizine (Zyrtec) and loratidine (Claritin) contain newer antihistamines that pose a lower risk of side effects. These may be of some benefit to people with mild asthma if their symptoms are triggered by an allergic reaction such as hay fever. In such cases, the antihistamine should not be thought of as a treatment for asthma per se but as a treatment for the hay fever; as a bonus, treating the hay fever reduces the risk of triggering asthma symptoms.

Expectorants

Most oral bronchodilators contain the expectorant guaifenesin. Removing mucus helps clear air passages, but it is probably not necessary to take an additional medication specifically for this purpose. Instead, drinking plenty of fluids is a safe strategy that is just as helpful.

Cough Medications

Cough is a common symptom of asthma; in fact, persistent cough is often the main symptom that leads to the doctor visit during which asthma is first diagnosed. Coughing is the body's way of removing mucus from the airways; taking a medication to suppress cough is counterproductive. Use of an inhaled bronchodilator is usually sufficient to relieve coughing caused by asthma.

OTC Treatment for Asthma

Ephedrine
Epinephrine

Cough, Cold, and Flu Products

Analgesics
Acet = acetaminophen
Asp = aspirin
Ibu = ibuprofen
Sali = salicylamide
Sod-Sali = sodium salicylate

Antihistamines
Brom = brompheniramine maleate
Chlor = chlorpheniramine maleate
ClemF = clemastine fumarate
Diph = diphenhydramine HCl
Dox = doxylamine succinate
PhenylT = phenyltoloxamine citrate
Pyril = pyrilamine maleate
Trip = triprolidine HCl

Antitussives
Cam = camphor
Cod-Phos = codeine phosphate
Dex-Hydro = dextromethorphan hydrobromide
Euc = eucalyptol
Euc-Oil = eucalyptus oil
Menth = menthol
Pepp = peppermint oil
Thym = thymol
Turp = spirits of turpentine

Decongestants
Eph = ephedrine
Phen-Eph = phenylephrine
Phenyl = phenylpropanolamine HCl
Prop = phenylpropanolamine bitartrate
Pseudo = pseudoephedrine HCl
Pseudo-Sulf = pseudoephedrine sulfate

Expectorants
Amm-Chlor = ammonium chloride
Guai = guaifenesin
Ipecac = ipecac fluid/extract
Sod-cit = sodium citrate

BRAND NAME	Analgesic	Antihistamine	Antitussive	Decongestant	Expectorant
A.R.M.		Chlor 4mg		Phenyl 25mg	
Actifed		Trip 2.5mg		Pseudo 60mg	
Actifed Allergy Daytime				Pseudo 30mg	
Actified Allergy Nightime		Diph 25mg		Pseudo 30mg	
Actifed Cold & Sinus	Acet 500mg	Trip 1.25mg		Pseudo 30mg	
Actifed Sinus Daytime/Nighttime	Acet 500mg	Diph 25mg		Pseudo 30mg	
Advil Cold & Sinus	Ibu 200mg			Pseudo 30mg	
Alka-Seltzer Plus Cold & Cough Medicine	Asp 500 mg	Chlor 2mg	Dex-Hydro 10mg	Prop 24.08mg	
Alka-Seltzer Plus Cold & Cough Medicine Liqui-Gels	Acet 250mg	Chlor 2mg	Dex-Hydro 10mg	Pseudo 30mg	
Alka-Seltzer Plus Cold Medicine	Asp 325mg	Chlor 2mg		Prop 24mg	
Alka-Seltzer Plus Cold Medicine Liqui-Gels	Acet 250mg	Chlor 2mg		Pseudo 30mg	
Alka-Seltzer Plus Flu & Body Aches	Acet 325mg	Chlor 2mg	Dex-Hydro 10mg	Prop 20mg	
Alka-Seltzer Plus Flu & Body Aches Liqui-Gels	Acet 250mg		Dex-Hydro 10mg	Pseudo 30mg	
Alka-Seltzer Plus Maximum Strength Sinus Medicine	Asp 500mg	Brom 2mg		Prop 24.08mg	
Alka-Seltzer Plus Night-Time Cold Medicine	Asp 500 mg	Brom 2mg	Dex-Hydro 10mg	Prop 20mg	

BRAND NAME	Analgesic	Antihistamine	Antitussive	Decongestant	Expectorant
Alka-Seltzer Plus Night-Time Cold Medicine Liqui-Gels	Acet 250mg	Dox 6.25mg	Dex-Hydro 10mg	Pseudo 30mg	
Alka-Seltzer Plus Sinus Medicine			Dex-Hydro 10mg		
Aller-med		Diph 25mg			
Allerest Maximum Strength		Chlor 2mg		Pseudo 30mg	
Allerest No Drowsiness	Acet 325mg			Pseudo 30mg	
Allerest Sinus Pain Formula	Acet 500mg	Chlor 2mg		Pseudo 30mg	
Allergy Relief		Chlor 4mg			
AllerMax Caplet		Diph 50mg			
AllerMax Syrup		Diph 12.5mg/5ml	*Menth*		
Anti-Tuss					Guai 100mg/5ml
Anti-Tuss DM			Dex-Hydro 15mg/5ml		Guai 100mg/5ml
Anti-Tuss DM					Guai 100mg/5ml
Antihist-1		ClemF 1.34mg			
Babee Cof [A]			Dex-Hydro 7.5mg/5ml		
Bayer Select Aspirin-Free Sinus Pain Relief	Acet 500mg			Pseudo 30mg	
BC Allergy-Sinus-Cold	Asp 650mg	Chlor 4mg		Phenyl 25mg	
BC Sinus-Cold	Asp 650mg			Phenyl 25mg	
Benadryl Allergy Capsule		Diph 25mg			
Benadryl Allergy Chewable Tablet		Diph 12.5mg			
Benadryl Allergy Liquid [A]		Diph 12.5mg/5ml			
Benadryl Allergy Tablet		Diph 25mg			
Benadryl Allergy Decongestant Liquid [A]		Diph 12.5mg/5ml		Pseudo 30mg/5ml	
Benadryl Allergy Decongestant Tablet		Diph 25mg		Pseudo 60mg	
Benadryl Allergy Dye-Free [A]		Diph 6.25mg/5ml			
Benadryl Allergy Dye-Free Liqui-Gels		Diph 25mg			
Benadryl Allergy Cold	Acet 500mg	Diph 12.5mg		Pseudo 30mg	
Benadryl Allergy Sinus Headache Formula	Acet 500mg	Diph 12.5mg		Pseudo 30mg	

Benylin Adult Cough Formula [A]			Dex-Hydro 15mg/5ml		
Benylin Cough Suppressant Expectorant [A]			Dex-Hydro 5mg/5ml		Guai 100mg/5ml
Benylin Multi-Symptom Formula [A]			Dex-Hydro 5mg/5ml	Pseudo 15mg/5ml	Guai 100mg/5ml
Benylin Pediatric Cough Formula [A]			Dex-Hydro 7.5mg/5ml		
Bromatapp Extended Release		*Brom*		*Phenyl*	
Bromfed [A]		Brom 2mg/5ml		Pseudo 30mg/5ml	
Bromotap		Brom 2mg/5ml		Phenyl 12.5mg/5ml	
Cenafed Syrup [A]				Pseudo 30mg/5ml	
Cenafed Tablet				Pseudo 30mg	
Cenafed Tablet				Pseudo 60mg	
Cenafed Plus Tablet		Trip 2.5mg		Pseudo 60mg	
Cepacol Maximum Strength			Menth 2mg		
Cepacol Sore Throat, Cherry			Menth 3.6mg		
Cepacol Sore Throat, Mint			Menth 2mg		
Cepacol, Cherry or Honey-Lemon			Menth 3.6mg		
Cepacol, Menthol-Eucalyptus			Menth 5mg *Euc*		
Cerose-DM		Chlor 4mg	Dex-Hydro 15mg/5ml	Phen-Eph 10mg/5ml	
Cheracol D			Dex-Hydro 10mg		Guai 100mg
Cheracol Plus		Chlor 4mg	Dex-Hydro 20mg	Phenyl 25mg	
Chlor-Trimeton 12-Hour Allergy		Chlor 12mg			
Chlor-Trimeton 12-Hour Allergy Decongestant		Chlor 8mg		Pseudo-Sulf 120mg	
Chlor-Trimeton 4-Hour Allergy		Chlor 4mg			
Chlor-Trimeton 4-Hour Allergy Decongestant		Chlor 4mg		Pseudo-Sulf 60mg	
Chlor-Trimeton 8-Hour Allergy		Chlor 8mg			
Chlor-Trimeton Allergy [A]		Chlor 2mg/5ml			
Chlor-Trimeton Allergy, Sinus, Headache	Acet 500mg	Chlor 2mg		Phenyl 12.5mg	
Chlor-Trimeton Non-Drowsy 4-Hour				Pseudo-Sulf 60mg	

BRAND NAME	Analgesic	Antihistamine	Antitussive	Decongestant	Expectorant
Clear Cough DM [A]			Dex-Hydro 15mg/5ml		Guai 100mg/5ml
Clear Cough Night Time	Acet 166.67mg/5ml	Dox 2.08mg/5ml	Dex-Hydro 5mg/5ml		
Clear Tussin 30 [A]			Dex-Hydro 15mg/5ml		Guai 100mg/5ml
Codimal Capsule [A]	Acet 325mg	Chlor 2mg		Pseudo 30mg	
Codimal Tablet	Acet 325mg	Chlor 2mg		Pseudo 30mg	
Codimal DM [A]		Pyril 8.3mg/5ml	Dex-Hydro 10mg/5ml	Phen-Eph 5mg/5ml	
Codimal PH [A]		Pyril 8.3mg/5ml	Cod-Phos 10mg/5ml	Phen-Eph 5mg/5ml	
Cold and Allergy Extended-Release		Brom 12mg		Phenyl 75mg	
Cold and Allergy Maximum Strength 4-Hour Liquid Gelcaps		Brom 4mg		Phenyl 25mg	
Coldonyl	Acet 325mg			Phen-Eph 5mg	
Comtrex Allergy-Sinus	Acet 500mg	Chlor 2mg		Pseudo 30mg	
Comtrex Maximum Strength (caplet, tablet)	Acet 500mg	Chlor 2mg	Dex-Hydro 15mg	Pseudo 30mg	
Comtrex Maximum Strength Liqui-Gel	Acet 500mg	Chlor 2mg	Dex-Hydro 15mg	Phenyl 12.5mg	
Comtrex Maximum Strength Liquid	Acet 1000mg/30ml	Chlor 4mg/30ml	Dex-Hydro 30mg/30ml	Pseudo 60mg/30ml	
Comtrex Maximum Strength Day Caplet	Acet 500mg		Dex-Hydro day=15mg	Pseudo day=30mg	
Comtrex Maximum Strength Night Liquid	Acet 1000mg/30ml	Chlor 4mg/30ml	Dex-Hydro 30mg/30ml	Pseudo 60mg/30ml	
Comtrex Maximum Strength Day & Night Tablet	Acet 500mg	Chlor 2mg	Dex-Hydro 15mg	Pseudo 30mg	
Comtrex Maximum Strength Non-Drowsy Caplet	Acet 500mg		Dex-Hydro 15mg	Pseudo 30mg	
Comtrex Maximum Strength Non-Drowsy Liqui-gel	Acet 500mg		Dex-Hydro 15mg	Phenyl 12.5mg	
Congestac				Pseudo 60mg	Guai 400mg
Congestion Relief				Pseudo 60mg	
Contac 12-Hour Allergy		ClemF 1.34mg			
Contac 12-Hour Cold		Chlor 8mg		Phenyl 75mg	
Contac 12-Hour Maximum Strength		Chlor 12mg		Phenyl 75mg	
Contac Day Allergy/Sinus	Acet 650mg			Pseudo 60mg	
Contac Night Allergy/Sinus	Acet 650mg	Diph 50mg		Pseudo 60mg	
Contac Day & Night Cold/Flu	Acet 650mg			Pseudo 60mg	

Contac Non-Drowsy	Acet 325mg			Pseudo 30mg	
Contac Severe Cold & Flu Maximum Strength	Acet 500mg	Chlor 2mg	Dex-Hydro 15mg	Phenyl 12.5mg	
Coricidin Cold & Flu	Acet 325mg	Chlor 2mg			
Coricidin Cough & Cold		Chlor 4mg	Dex-Hydro 30mg		
Coricidin D	Acet 325mg	Chlor 2mg		Phenyl 12.5mg	
Cough-X			Dex-Hydro 5mg		
Creomulsion Complete [A]			Dex-Hydro 6mg/5ml	Pseudo 20mg/5ml	
Creomulsion Cough Medicine [A]			Dex-Hydro 6.67mg/5ml		
Creomulsion for Children [A]			Dex-Hydro 5mg/5ml		
Creomulsion Pediatric [A]			Dex-Hydro 5mg/5ml	Pseudo 1mg/5ml	
Dallergy-D [A]				Phen-Eph 5mg/5ml	
DayGel	Acet 250mg		Dex-Hydro 10mg	Pseudo 30mg	Guai 100mg
Decongestant Cough Formula D			Dex-Hydro 10mg/5ml	Pseudo 20mg/5ml	
Delsym Extended Release [A]			Dex-Hydro 30mg/5ml		
Demazin Syrup [A]				Phenyl 12.5mg/5ml	
Demazin Timed Release Tablet				Phenyl 25mg	
Diabe-tuss DM [A]			Dex-Hydro 15mg/5ml		
Diabetic Tussin Cough Drops, Cherry			*Euc Oil* Menth 5mg		
Diabetic Tussin Cough Drops, Menthol-Eucalyptus			*Euc Oil* Menth 6mg		
Diabetic Tussin DM [A]			Dex-Hydro 10mg/5ml		Guai 100mg/5ml
Diabetic Tussin DM Maximum Strength [A]			Dex-Hydro 10mg/5ml		Guai 200mg/5ml
Diabetic Tussin EX [A]			*Menth*		Guai 100mg/5ml
Diabetic Tussin, Children's [A]			Dex-Hydro 10mg/5ml *Menth*		Guai 100mg/5ml
Dimacol			Dex-Hydro 10mg	Pseudo 30mg	Guai 100mg
Dimetane Allergy Extentabs		Brom 12mg			
Dimetapp [A]		Brom 2mg/5ml		Pseudo 12.5mg/5ml	
Dimetapp 12-Hour Maximum Strength Extentabs		Brom 12mg		Phenyl 75mg	

BRAND NAME	Analgesic	Antihistamine	Antitussive	Decongestant	Expectorant
Dimetapp 4-Hour Maximum Strength		Brom 4mg		Phenyl 25mg	
Dimetapp 4-Hour Maximum Strength Liqui-Gels		Brom 4mg		Phenyl 25mg	
Dimetapp Allergy		Brom 4mg			
Dimetapp Allergy Liqui-Gels		Brom 4mg			
Dimetapp Allergy Sinus	Acet 500mg	Brom 2mg		Phenyl 12.5mg	
Dimetapp Allergy, Children's A		Brom 2mg/5ml			
Dimetapp Cold & Allergy		Brom 1mg		Phenyl 6.25mg	
Dimetapp Cold & Cough Maximum Strength		Brom 4mg	Dex-Hydro 20mg	Phenyl 25mg	
Dimetapp Cold & Fever, Children's A	Acet 160mg/5ml	Brom 1mg/5ml		Pseudo 15mg/5ml	
Dimetapp Decongestant Non-Drowsy Liqui-Gels				Pseudo 30mg	
Dimetapp Decongestant, Pediatric A				Pseudo 7.5mg/0.8ml	
Dimetapp DM A		Brom 2mg/5ml	Dex-Hydro 10mg/5ml	Phenyl 12.5mg/5ml	
Diphenadryl		Diph 12.5mg/5ml			
Diphenadryl Cough		Diph 12.5mg/5ml	*Menth*		
Disophrol Chronotabs Sustained Action		Dexbrom 6mg		Pseudo-Sulf 120mg	
DM Cough & Cold		Brom 2mg/5ml	Dex-Hydro 10mg/5ml	Phenyl 12.5mg/5ml	
Dorcol Children's Cough A			Dex-Hydro 5mg/5ml	Pseudo 15mg/5ml	Guai 50mg/5ml
Dristan Cold & Cough Liqui-Gels	Acet 250mg		Dex-Hydro 10mg	Pseudo 30mg	Guai 100mg
Dristan Cold Maximum Strength No Drowsiness Caplet	Acet 500mg			Pseudo 30mg	
Dristan Cold Maximum Strength No Drowsiness Gel Caplet	Acet 500mg			Pseudo 30mg	
Dristan Cold Multi-Symptom	Acet 325mg	Chlor 2mg		Phen-Eph 5mg	
Dristan Cold Multi-Symptom Maximum Strength	Acet 500mg	Brom 2mg		Pseudo 30mg	
Dristan Sinus	Ibu 200mg			Pseudo 30mg	
Drixoral Allergy Sinus Extended Release	Acet 500mg	Dexbrom 3mg		Pseudo-Sulf 60mg	
Drixoral Cold & Allergy Sustained Action		Dexbrom 6mg		Pseudo-Sulf 120mg	
Drixoral Cold & Flu	Acet 500mg	Dexbrom 3mg		Pseudo-Sulf 60mg	
Drixoral Cough & Congestion Liquid Caps			Dex-Hydro 30mg	Pseudo 60mg	

Drixoral Cough & Sore Throat Liquid Caps	Acet 325mg		Dex-Hydro 15mg		
Drixoral Cough Liquid Caps			Dex-Hydro 30mg		
Drixoral Non-Drowsy Extended Release				Pseudo-Sulf 120mg	
Duadacin	Acet 325mg	Chlor 2mg		Phenyl 12.5mg	
Dynafed Jr.	Acet 325mg			Pseudo 30mg	
Dynafed Plus	Acet 500mg			Pseudo 30mg	
Dynafed Pseudo				Pseudo 60mg	
Efidac 24 Chlorpheniramine		Chlor 16mg			
Efidac/24				Pseudo 240mg	
Emagrin Forte	Acet 260mg			Phen-Eph 5mg	Guai 101mg
Excedrin Sinus	Acet 500mg			Pseudo 30mg	
Fedahist		Chlor 4mg		Pseudo 60mg	
Fendol	Acet 354mg Sali 65mg			Phen-Eph 5mg	Guai 101mg
Fisherman's Friend, Extra Strong, Sugar Free S			*Euc Oil* Menth 10mg		
Fisherman's Friend, Licorice Strong			Menth 6mg		
Fisherman's Friend, Original Extra Strong			*Euc Oil* Menth 10mg		
Fisherman's Friend, Refreshing Mint, Sugar Free S			Menth 3mg *Pepp*		
Flu, Cold, and Cough Medicine	Acet 500mg	Chlor 4mg	Dex-Hydro 20mg	Pseudo 60mg	
Flu-Relief	Acet 325mg	Chlor 2mg		Pseudo 30mg	
Genac		Trip 2.5mg		Pseudo 60mg	
Genahist Capsule		Diph 25mg			
Genahist Elixir		Diph 12.5mg/5ml			
Genamin		Chlor 2mg/5ml		Phenyl 12.5mg/5ml	
Genapap Maximum Strength Sinus	Acet 500mg			Pseudo 30mg	
Genaphed				Pseudo 30mg	
Genatap		Brom 2mg/5ml		Phenyl 12.5mg/5ml	
Genatuss					Guai 100mg/5ml
Genatuss DM			Dex-Hydro 15mg/5ml		Guai 100mg/5ml

BRAND NAME	Analgesic	Antihistamine	Antitussive	Decongestant	Expectorant
Gencold		Chlor 8mg		Phenyl 75mg	
Gendecon	Acet 325mg	Chlor 2mg		Phen-Eph 5mg	
Genite	Acet 167mg/5ml	Dox 1.25mg/5ml	Dex-Hydro 5mg/5ml	Pseudo 10mg/5ml	
GG-Cen					Guai 200mg
Guaifed [A]			*Menth*	Pseudo 30mg/5ml	Guai 200mg/5ml
GuiaCough			*Menth*		Guai 100mg/5ml
GuiaCough CF			Dex-Hydro 10mg/5ml *Menth*	Phenyl 12.5mg/ml	Guai 100mg/5ml
GuiaCough PE				Pseudo 30mg/5ml	Guai 100mg/5ml
Guiatuss CF [A]			Dex-Hydro 10mg/5ml	Phenyl 12.5mg/ml	Guai 100mg/5ml
Guiatuss Cough & Cold			Dex-Hydro 10mg	Pseudo 30mg	Guai 200mg/5ml
Halls Juniors Sugar Free Cough Drops, Grape/Orange [S]			*Euc Oil* Menth 2.5mg		
Halls Mentho-Lyptus Cough Drops, Cherry/Menthol-L.			*Euc Oil* Menth 6.1mg		
Halls Mentho-Lyptus Cough Drops, Honey-Lemon			*Euc Oil* Menth 8.4mg		
Halls Mentho-Lyptus Cough Drops, Spearmint			*Euc Oil* Menth 5mg		
Halls Mentho-Lyptus Ex. Strength Cough Drops, Ice Blue			*Euc Oil* Menth 12mg		
Halls Mentho-Lyptus Sugar Free Cough Drops, Bl. Cherry [S]			*Euc Oil* Menth 5mg		
Halls Mentho-Lyptus Sugar Free Cough Drops, Citrus [S]			*Euc Oil* Menth 5mg		
Halls Mentho-Lyptus Sugar Free Cough Drops, Menthol [S]			*Euc Oil* Menth 6mg		
Halls Plus Max. Strength; Cherry, Honey-Lemon Mentho-Lyptus			*Euc Oil* Menth 10mg		
Hay Fever & Allergy Relief		Chlor 2mg		Phenyl 18.7mg	
Hayfebrol [A] [S]		Chlor 2mg/5ml	*Menth*	Pseudo 30mg/5ml	
Herbal-Menthol [S]			*Euc Oil* Menth 6mg *Pepp*		
Histatab Plus		Chlor 2mg Phen/Eph 5mg			
Hold			Dex-Hydro 5mg		
Humibid GC [C] [S]			Dex-Hydro 10mg	Pseudo 30mg	Guai 200mg
Hydramine Cough		Diph 12.5mg/5ml			

Hytuss					Guai 100mg
Hytuss 2X					Guai 200mg
Ipsatol [A]			Dex-Hydro 10mg/5ml	Phenyl 9mg/5ml	Guai 100mg/5ml
Isodettes			Menth 10mg		
Kodet-SE				Pseudo 30mg	
Koldets Cough Drops			*Euc Oil* Menth 6.1mg		
Kolephrin	Acet 325mg	Chlor 2mg		Pseudo 30mg	
Kolephrin DM	Acet 325mg	Chlor 2mg	Dex-Hydro 10mg	Pseudo 30mg	
Kolephrin GG/DM [A]			Dex-Hydro 10mg/5ml		Guai 150mg/5ml
Kophane Cough and Cold Medication [A]		Chlor 2mg/5ml	Dex-Hydro 10mg/5ml *Menth*	Phenyl 12.5mg/5ml	
Luden's Maximum Strength Sugar Free, Cherry [S])			*Euc Oil* Menth 10mg		
Luden's Maximum Strength, Cherry			*Euc Oil* Menth 10mg		
Luden's Maximum Strength, Menthol Eucalyptus			*Euc Oil* Menth 10mg		
Mini Thin Pseudo				Pseudo 60mg	
Multi-Symptom Cough Formula M	Acet 125mg/5ml	Chlor 1mg/5ml	Dex-Hydro 7.5mg/5ml	Pseudo 15mg/5ml	
N'Ice 'N Clear, Cherry Eucalyptus			Menth 7mg		
N'Ice 'N Clear, Menthol Eucalyptus			Menth 5mg		
N'Ice Sore Throat & Cough, Assorted or Citrus			Menth 5mg		
Naldecon DX, Adult [A]			Dex-Hydro 10mg/5ml	Phenyl 12.5mg/5ml	Guai 200mg/5ml
Naldecon DX, Children's [A]			Dex-Hydro 5mg/5ml	Phenyl 6.25mg/5ml	Guai 100mg/5ml
Naldecon DX, Pediatric [A]			Dex-Hydro 5mg/5ml	Phenyl 6.25mg/5ml	Guai 50mg/ml
Naldecon EX, Children's [A]				Phenyl 6.25mg/5ml	Guai 100mg/ml
Naldecon EX, Pediatric [A]				Phenyl 6.25mg/5ml	Guai 50mg/ml
Naldecon Senior DX [A]			Dex-Hydro 10mg/5ml		Guai 200mg/5ml
Naldecon Senior EX [A]					Guai 200mg/5ml
Napril		Chlor 4mg		Pseudo 60mg	
Nasal-D [S]				Pseudo 60mg	

BRAND NAME	Analgesic	Antihistamine	Antitussive	Decongestant	Expectorant
ND-Gesic	Acet 300mg	Pyril 12.5mg Chlor 2mg		Phen-Eph 5mg	
Night Time Cold Medicine [A]	Acet 1000mg/oz	Dox 7.5mg/oz	Dex-Hydro 30mg/oz	Pseudo 60mg/oz	
Night Time Cold Medicine Softgels	Acet 250mg	Dox 6.25mg	Dex-Hydro 10mg	Pseudo 30mg	
NiteGel	Acet 250mg	Dox 6.25mg	Dex-Hydro 10mg	Pseudo 30mg	
Nolahist		Phentart 25mg			
Novahistine		Chlor 2mg/5ml		Phen-Eph 5mg/5ml	
Novahistine DH		Chlor 2mg/5ml	Cod-Phos 10mg/5ml	Pseudo 30mg/5ml	
Novahistine DMX			Dex-Hydro 10mg/5ml	Pseudo 30mg/5ml	Guai 100mg/5ml
Novahistine Expectorant			Cod-Phos 10mg/5ml	Pseudo 30mg/5ml	Guai 100mg/5ml
Oranyl				Pseudo 30mg	
Oranyl Plus	Acet 500mg			Pseudo 30mg	
Ornex Maximum Strength	Acet 500mg			Pseudo 30mg	
Ornex Regular Strength	Acet 325mg			Pseudo 30mg	
P.C. Nasal Decongestant				Pseudo 30mg	
PediaCare Cough-Cold Formula Chewable Tablet			Dex-Hydro 5mg	Pseudo 15mg	
PediaCare Cough-Cold Formula Liquid [A]			Dex-Hydro 5mg/5ml	Pseudo 15mg/5ml	
PediaCare Infants' Decongestant [A]				Pseudo 7.5mg/0.8ml	
PediaCare Infants' Decongestant Plus Cough [A]			Dex-Hydro 2.5mg/0.8ml	Pseudo 7.5mg/0.8ml	
PediaCare Night Rest Cough-Cold Formula [A]		Chlor 1mg/5ml	Dex-Hydro 7.5mg/5ml	Pseudo 15mg/5ml	
Pediacon DX, Children's [A]			Dex-Hydro 5mg/5ml	Phenyl 6.25mg/5ml	Guai 100mg/5ml
Pediacon DX, Pediatric [A]			Dex-Hydro 5mg/1ml	Phenyl 6.25mg/1ml	Guai 50mg/1ml
Pediacon EX, Pediatric [A]				Phenyl 6.25mg/1ml	Guai 50mg/1ml
Pertussin CS			Dex-Hydro 7mg/10ml		
Pertussin ES			Dex-Hydro 10mg/10ml		
Phenylgesic	Acet 325mg	PhenylT 30mg			
Pinex			Dex-Hydro 7.5mg/5ml		
Pinex Concentrate			Dex-Hydro 7.5mg/5ml		

Prominicol Cough		Chlor 2mg	Dex-Hydro 10mg	Phenyl 12.5mg	
Propagest [S]				Phenyl 25mg	
Protac DM			Dex-Hydro 10mg		Guai 100mg
Protac SF [A]		Chlor 4mg	Dex-Hydro 15mg		
Pyrroxate	Acet 500mg	Chlor 4mg		Phenyl 25mg	
Quelidrine Cough		Chlor 2mg/5ml	Dex-Hydro 10mg/5ml	Eph 5mg/5ml Phen-Eph 5mg/5ml	Amm-Chlor 40mg/5ml Ipecac 0.005ml/5ml
REM [A]			Dex-Hydro 5mg/5ml		
Ricola Cough Drops, Original Flavor			Menth 3mg		
Ricola Sugar Free Herb Throat Drops, Alpine-Mint [S]			Menth 4.8mg		
Ricola Sugar Free Herb Throat Drops, Cherry/Lemon-Mint [S]			Menth 1mg		
Ricola Sugar Free Herb Throat Drops, Mountain Herb [S]			Menth 1.5mg		
Ricola Throat Drops, Cherry-Mint			Menth 1.5mg		
Ricola Throat Drops, Honey-Herb			Menth 2.4mg		
Ricola Throat Drops, Lemon-Mint/Orange-Mint			Menth 1.25mg		
Ricola Throat Drops, Menthol-Eucalyptus			Menth 4.5mg		
Robitussin [A]					Guai 100mg/5ml
Robitussin CF [A]			Dex-Hydro 10mg/5ml	Phenyl 12.5mg/5ml	Guai 100mg/5ml
Robitussin Cold & Cough Liqui-Gels			Dex-Hydro 10mg	Pseudo 30mg	Guai 200mg
Robitussin Cold, Cough, & Flu Liqui-Gels	Acet 250mg		Dex-Hydro 10mg	Pseudo 30mg	Guai 100mg
Robitussin Cough Calmers			Dex-Hydro 5mg		
Robitussin Cough Drops, Cherry/Menthol Eucalyptus			*Euc Oil* Menth 7.4mg		
Robitussin Cough Drops, Honey-Lemon			*Euc Oil* Menth 10mg		
Robitussin DM			Dex-Hydro 10mg/5ml		Guai 100mg/5ml
Robitussin Liquid Center Cough Drops, Cherry w/ Honey-Lemon			*Euc Oil* Menth 8mg		
Robitussin Liquid Center Cough Drops, Honey-Lemon w/ Cherry			*Euc Oil* Menth 10mg		

BRAND NAME	Analgesic	Antihistamine	Antitussive	Decongestant	Expectorant
Robitussin Liquid Center Cough Drops, Menthol Eucalyptus w/ Cherry			*Euc Oil* Menth 8mg		
Robitussin Maximum Strength Cough			Dex-Hydro 15mg/5ml		
Robitussin Maximum Strength Cough & Cold			Dex-Hydro 15mg/5ml	Pseudo 30mg/5ml	
Robitussin Night Relief [A]	Acet 108.33mg/5ml	Pyril 8.33mg/5ml	Dex-Hydro 5mg/5ml	Pseudo 10mg/5ml	
Robitussin Night-Time Cold Formula	Acet 325mg	Dox 6.25mg	Dex-Hydro 15mg	Pseudo 30mg	
Robitussin PE [A]				Pseudo 30mg/5ml	Guai 100mg/5ml
Robitussin Pediatric [A]			Dex-Hydro 5mg/2.5ml	Pseudo 15mg/2.5ml	Guai 100mg/2.5ml
Robitussin Pediatric Cough [A]			Dex-Hydro 7.5mg/5ml		
Robitussin Pediatric Cough & Cold [A]			Dex-Hydro 7.5mg/5ml	Pseudo 15mg/5ml	
Robitussin Pediatric Night Relief [A]		Chlor 1mg/5ml	Dex-Hydro 7.5mg/5ml	Pseudo 15mg/5ml	
Robitussin Severe Congestion Liqui-Gels				Pseudo 30mg	Guai 200mg
Robitussin Sugar Free Cough Drops [S]			Menth 10mg		
Safe Tussin 30 [A]			Dex-Hydro 30mg/5ml		Guai 200mg/5ml
Scot-Tussin Allergy Relief Formula [A] [S]		Diph 12.5mg/5ml	*Menth*		
Scot-Tussin DM [A] [S]		Chlor 2mg/5ml	Dex-Hydro 15mg/5ml *Menth*		
Scot-Tussin DM Cough Chasers [S]			Dex-Hydro 2.5mg *Pepp*		
Scot-Tussin Expectorant [A] [S]			*Menth*		Guai 100mg/5ml
Scot-Tussin Original [A] [S]	Sod-Sali 83.3mg/5ml	Phen 13.33mg/5ml		Phen-Eph 4.2mg/5ml	Sod-cit 83.3mg/5ml
Scot-Tussin Senior [A] [S]			Dex-Hydro 15mg/5ml		Guai 200mg/5ml
Sinapils	Acet 325mg	Chlor 2mg		Phenyl 12.5mg	
Sinarest Extra Strength	Acet 500mg	Chlor 2mg		Pseudo 30mg	
Sinarest No Drowsiness	Acet 325mg			Pseudo 30mg	
Sinarest Sinus Medicine	Acet 325mg	Chlor 2mg		Pseudo 30mg	
Sine-Aid IB	Ibu 200 mg			Pseudo 30mg	
Sine-Aid Maximum Strength Caplet	Acet 500mg			Pseudo 30mg	
Sine-Aid Maximum Strength Gelcap	Acet 500mg			Pseudo 30mg	

Sine-Aid Maximum Strength Tablet	Acet 500mg			Pseudo 30mg	
Sine-Off Maximum Strength No Drowsiness Formula	Acet 500mg			Pseudo 30mg	
Sine-Off Sinus Medicine	Acet I500mg	Chlor 2mg		Pseudo 30mg	
Singlet	Acet 650mg	Chlor 4mg		Pseudo 60mg	
Sinulin [S]	Acet 650mg	Chlor 4mg		Phenyl 25mg	
Sinus	Acet 325mg			Pseudo 30mg	
Sinus Relief Extra Strength	Acet 500mg	Chlor 2mg		Pseudo 30mg	
Sinutab Non-Drying				Pseudo 30mg	Guai 200mg
Sinutab Sinus Allergy Medication Maximum Strength	Acet 500mg	Chlor 2mg		Pseudo 30mg	
Sinutab Sinus Non-Drowsiness	Acet 325mg			Pseudo 30mg	
Sinutab Sinus without Drowsiness Maximum Strength	Acet 500mg			Pseudo 30mg	
Sinutol Maximum Strength	Acet 500mg			Pseudo 30mg	
Spec-T Sore Throat Cough Suppressant			Dex-Hydro 10mg		
Spec-T Sore Throat Decongestant				Phen-Eph 5mg Phenyl 10.5mg	
St. Joseph Cough Suppressant for Children			Dex-Hydro 7.5mg/5ml		
Sucrets 4-Hour Cough Suppressant, Cherry/Menthol			Dex-Hydro 15mg *Menth*		
Sudafed				Pseudo 60mg	
Sudafed				Pseudo 30mg	
Sudafed 12-Hour Extended Release				Pseudo 120mg	
Sudafed Children's Cold & Cough [A] [S]			Dex-Hydro 5mg/5ml	Pseudo 15mg/5ml	Guai 100mg/5ml
Sudafed Children's Nasal Decongestant [A] [S]				Pseudo 15mg/5ml	
Sudafed Cold & Allergy		Chlor 4mg		Pseudo 60mg	
Sudafed Cold & Cough	Acet 250mg		Dex-Hydro 10mg	Pseudo 30mg	Guai 100mg
Sudafed Pediatric Nasal Decongestant [A] [S]				Pseudo 7.5mg/0.8ml	
Sudafed Severe Cold Formula	Acet 500mg		Dex-Hydro 15mg	Pseudo 30mg	
Sudafed Sinus Non-Drowsy Maximum Strength	Acet 500mg			Pseudo 30mg	
Sudafed Sinus Non-Drying Non-Drowsy Maximum Strength				Pseudo 30mg	Guai 200mg

BRAND NAME	Analgesic	Antihistamine	Antitussive	Decongestant	Expectorant
Sudanyl				Pseudo 30mg	
Tavist-1 Antihistamine		ClemF 1.34mg			
Tavist-D Antihistamine/Nasal Decongestant		ClemF 1.34mg		Phenyl 75mg	
Teldrin		Chlor 8mg		Phenyl 75mg	
Tetrahist	Acet 325mg	Chlor 2mg	Dex-Hydro 15mg	Pseudo 30mg	
TheraFlu Flu and Cold Medicine	Acet 650mg	Chlor 4mg		Pseudo 60mg	
TheraFlu Flu, Cold, & Cough Medicine	Acet 650mg	Chlor 4mg	Dex-Hydro 20mg	Pseudo 60mg	
TheraFlu Max. Strength Flu & Cold Medicine for Sore Throat	Acet 1000mg	Chlor 4mg		Pseudo 60mg	
TheraFlu Max. Strength Flu, Cold & Cough Medicine NightTime	Acet 1000mg	Chlor 4mg	Dex-Hydro 30mg	Pseudo 60mg	
TheraFlu Maximum Strength Non-Drowsy	Acet 500mg		Dex-Hydro 15mg	Pseudo 30mg	
TheraFlu Maximum Strength Sinus Non-Drowsy	Acet 500mg			Pseudo 30mg	
Tolu-Sed DM			Dex-Hydro 10mg/5ml		Guai 100mg/5ml
Tri-Fed		Trip 2.5mg		Pseudo 60mg	
Tri-Nefrin Extra Strength		Chlor 4mg		Phenyl 25mg	
Triaminic AM, Non-Drowsy Cough & Decongestant Formula [A]			Dex-Hydro 7.5mg/5ml	Pseudo 15mg/5ml	
Triaminic AM, Non-Drowsy Decongestant Formula [A]				Pseudo 15mg/5ml	
Triaminic DM, Cough Relief [A]			Dex-Hydro 5mg/5ml	Phenyl 6.25/5ml	
Triaminic Expectorant, Chest & Head Congestion [A]				Phenyl 6.25/5ml	Guai 50mg/5ml
Triaminic Infant, Oral Decongestant [A]				Pseudo 7.5mg/0.8ml	
Triaminic Night Time [A]		Chlor 1mg/5ml	Dex-Hydro 7.5mg/5ml	Pseudo 15mg/5ml	
Triaminic Sore Throat, Throat Pain & Cough [A]	Acet 160mg/5ml		Dex-Hydro 7.5mg/5ml	Pseudo 15mg/5ml	
Triaminic, Cold & Allergy [A]		Chlor 1mg/5ml		Phenyl 6.25/5ml	
Triaminicin	Acet 650mg	Chlor 4mg		Phenyl 25mg	
Triaminicol Multi-Symptom Relief [A]		Chlor 1mg/5ml	Dex-Hydro 5mg/5ml	Phenyl 6.25mg/5ml	
Tricodene Forte [A]		Chlor 2mg/5ml	Dex-Hydro 10mg/5ml	Phenyl 12.5mg/5ml	

Tricodene NN Cough and Cold Medication [A]		Chlor 2mg/5ml	Dex-Hydro 10mg/5ml *Menth*	Phenyl 12.5mg/5ml	
Tricodene No. 1 [A]		Pyril 12.5mg/5ml	Cod-Phos 8.2mg/5ml *Menth*		
Tricodene Sugar Free [A] [S]		Chlor 2mg/5ml	Dex-Hydro 10mg/5ml *Menth*		
Tricodene, Pediatric [A]			Dex-Hydro 10mg/5ml	Phenyl 12.5mg/5ml	
Tuss-DM			Dex-Hydro 10mg		Guai 200mg
Tussar-2			Cod-Phos 10mg/5ml	Pseudo 30mg/5ml	Guai 100mg/5ml
Tussar-DM [A]		Chlor 2mg/5ml	Dex-Hydro 15mg/5ml	Pseudo 30mg/5ml	
Tussar-SF			Cod-Phos 10mg/5ml	Pseudo 30mg/5ml	Guai 100mg/5ml
Tylenol Allergy Sinus Maximum Strength Caplet	Acet 500mg	Chlor 2mg		Pseudo 30mg	
Tylenol Allergy Sinus Maximum Strength Gelcap	Acet 500mg	Chlor 2mg		Pseudo 30mg	
Tylenol Allergy Sinus Maximum Strength Geltab	Acet 500mg	Chlor 2mg		Pseudo 30mg	
Tylenol Allergy Sinus NightTime Maximum Strength	Acet 500mg	Diph 25mg		Pseudo 30mg	
Tylenol Children's Cold Multi-Symptom Chewable Tablet	Acet 80mg	Chlor 0.5mg		Pseudo 7.5mg	
Tylenol Children's Cold Multi-Symptom Liquid [A]	Acet 160mg/5ml	Chlor 1mg/5ml		Pseudo 15mg/5ml	
Tylenol Children's Cold Plus Cough Chewable Tablet	Acet 80mg	Chlor 0.5mg	Dex-Hydro 2.5mg	Pseudo 7.5mg	
Tylenol Children's Cold Plus Cough Liquid [A]	Acet 160mg/5ml	Chlor 1mg/5ml	Dex-Hydro 5mg/5ml	Pseudo 15mg/5ml	
Tylenol Cold Medication Multi-Symptom Formula (caplet/tablet)	Acet 325mg	Chlor 2mg	Dex-Hydro 15mg	Pseudo 30mg	
Tylenol Cold Multi-Symptom	Acet 650mg/packet	Chlor 4mg/packet	Dex-Hydro 30mg/packet	Pseudo 60mg/packet	
Tylenol Cold No Drowsiness Formula Caplet	Acet 325mg		Dex-Hydro 15mg	Pseudo 30mg	
Tylenol Cold No Drowsiness Formula Gelcap	Acet 325mg		Dex-Hydro 15mg	Pseudo 30mg	
Tylenol Cough Multi-Symptom	Acet 650mg/15ml		Dex-Hydro 30mg/15ml		
Tylenol Cough with Decongestant Multi-Symptom	Acet 650mg/15ml		Dex-Hydro 10mg/15ml	Pseudo 60mg/15ml	
Tylenol Flu Maximum Strength	Acet 500mg		Dex-Hydro 15mg	Pseudo 30mg	

BRAND NAME	Analgesic	Antihistamine	Antitussive	Decongestant	Expectorant
Tylenol Flu NightTime Maximum Strength	Acet 500mg	Diph 25mg		Pseudo 30mg	
Tylenol Flu NightTime Maximum Strength Hot Medication	Acet 1000mg/packet	Diph 50mg/packet		Pseudo 60mg/packet	
Tylenol Infants' Cold Decongestant and Fever Reducer [A]	Acet 80mg/0.8ml			Pseudo 7.5mg/0.8ml	
Tylenol Severe Allergy Maximum Strength	Acet 500mg	Diph 12.5mg			
Tylenol Sinus Maximum Strength (caplet/tablet)	Acet 500mg			Pseudo 30mg	
Tylenol Sinus Maximum Strength (gelcap/geltab)	Acet 500mg			Pseudo 30mg	
Vicks 44 LiquiCaps Cough, Cold, & Flu Relief	Acet 250mg	Chlor 2mg	Dex-Hydro 10mg	Pseudo 30mg	
Vicks 44 LiquiCaps Non-Drowsy Cough & Cold			Dex-Hydro 30mg	Pseudo 60mg	
Vicks 44 Soothing Cough Relief			Dex-Hydro 10mg/5ml		
Vicks 44d Pediatric Cough & Head Congestion Relief [A]			Dex-Hydro 15mg/15ml	Pseudo 30mg/15ml	
Vicks 44d Soothing Cough & Head Congestion Relief			Dex-Hydro 10mg/5ml	Pseudo 20mg/5ml	
Vicks 44e Pediatric Cough & Chest Congestion Relief [A]			Dex-Hydro 10mg/15ml		Guai 100mg/15ml
Vicks 44e Soothing Cough & Chest Congestion Relief			Dex-Hydro 20mg/15ml		Guai 200mg/15ml
Vicks 44m Pediatric Cough & Cold Relief [A]		Chlor 2mg/15ml	Dex-Hydro 15mg/15ml	Pseudo 30mg/15ml	
Vicks 44m Soothing Cough Cold & Flu Relief	Acet 162.5mg/5ml	Chlor 1mg/5ml	Dex-Hydro 7.5mg/5ml	Pseudo 15mg/5ml	
Vicks Chloraseptic Cough and Throat Drops			Menth 10mg		
Vicks Cough Drops, Cherry			*Euc Oil* Menth 1.7mg		
Vicks Cough Drops, Menthol			*Euc Oil* Menth 3.3mg		
Vicks DayQuil Allergy Relief 12-Hour		Brom 12mg		Phenyl 75mg	
Vicks DayQuil Children's Allergy Relief		Chlor 2mg/15ml		Pseudo 30mg/15ml	
Vicks DayQuil LiquiCaps Multi-Symptom Cold/Flu Relief	Acet 250mg		Dex-Hydro 10mg	Pseudo 30mg	Guai 100mg
Vicks DayQuil Multi-Symptom Cold/Flu Relief [A]	Acet 650mg/30ml		Dex-Hydro 20mg/30ml	Pseudo 60mg/30ml	Guai 200mg/30ml
Vicks DayQuil Sinus Pressure & Congestion Relief				Phenyl 25mg	Guai 200mg
Vicks DayQuil Sinus Pressure & Pain Relief with Ibuprofen	Ibu 200mg			Pseudo 30mg	

Vicks NyQuil Children's Cold/Cough Medicine [A]		Chlor 2mg/15ml	Dex-Hydro 15mg/15ml	Pseudo 30mg/15ml
Vicks NyQuil Hot Therapy	Acet 1000mg	Dox 12.5mg	Dex-Hydro 30mg	Pseudo 60mg
Vicks NyQuil LiquiCaps Multi-Symptom Cold/Flu Relief	Acet 250mg	Dox 6.25mg	Dex-Hydro 10mg	Pseudo 30mg
Vicks NyQuil Multi-Symptom Cold/Flu Relief, Cherry	Acet 1000mg/30ml	Dox 12.5mg/30ml	Dex-Hydro 30mg/30ml	Pseudo 60mg/30ml
Vicks NyQuil Multi-Symptom Cold/Flu Relief, Original	Acet 1000mg/30ml	Dox 12.5mg/30ml	Dex-Hydro 30mg/30ml	Pseudo 30mg/30ml
Vicks Original Cough Drops, Cherry			Menth 3.1mg	

Miscellaneous Cough Products

BRAND NAME	Camphor	Eucalyptus Oil	Menthol	Peppermint	Spirits of Turpentine	Thymol
Mentholatum	9%		1.3%			
Mentholatum Cherry Chest Rub for Kids	4.7%	1.2%	2.6%			
Vaporizer in a Bottle Air Wick Inhaler	3.6%	x	0.55%	x		
Vicks Original Cough Drops, Menthol	x	x	6.6mg			x
Vicks VapoRub (cream)	5.2%	1.2%	2.8%		x	x
Vicks VapoRub (ointment)	4.8%	1.2%	2.6%		x	x
Vicks VapoSteam	6.2%	1.5%	3.2%			

Sore Throat Products

BRAND NAME	ANESTHETIC							ANTIBACTERIAL	
	benzocaine	dyclonine HCl	eucalyptol	eucalyptus oil	menthol	phenol	alcohol	cetylpyridinium chloride	hexyl-resorcinol
Celestial Seasonings Soothers Herbal Throat Drops					x				
Cepacol Anesthetic	10mg							1.4%	
Cepacol Maximum Strength	10mg				2mg			x	
Cepacol Sore Throat, Cherry					3.6mg			x	
Cepacol Sore Throat, Mint					2mg			x	
Cepacol, Cherry or Honey-Lemon					3.6mg			x	
Cepacol, Menthol-Eucalyptus			x		5mg			x	
Cepacol, Original Flavor								1.4%	
Cepastat Extra Strength Sore Throat				x	x	29mg			
Cepastat Sore Throat (lozenge)					x	14.5mg			
Cepastat Sore Throat (spray)						1.4%	12.5%		
Fisherman's Friend, Extra Strong, Sugar Free S				x	10mg				
Fisherman's Friend, Licorice Strong					6mg				
Fisherman's Friend, Original Extra Strong				x	10mg				
Fisherman's Friend, Refreshing Mint, Sugar Free S					3mg				
Halls Juniors Sugar Free Cough Drops S				x	2.5mg				
Halls Mentho-Lyptus Cough Suppressant Drops, Cherry or Mentho-Lyptus				x	6.1mg				
Halls Mentho-Lyptus Cough Suppressant Drops, Honey-Lemon				x	8.4mg				
Halls Mentho-Lyptus Cough Suppressant Drops, Spearmint				x	5mg				
Halls Mentho-Lyptus Cough Suppressant Drops, Ice Blue				x	12mg				

Halls Mentho-Lyptus Sugar Free Cough Suppressant Drops, Black Cherry or Citrus [S]		x	5mg		
Halls Mentho-Lyptus Sugar Free Cough Suppressant Drops, Menthol [S]		x	6mg		
Halls Plus Maximum Strength		x	10mg		
Herbal-Menthol [S]		x	6mg		
Isodettes (lozenge)	6mg		10mg		
Isodettes (spray)				1.4%	
Koldets Cough Drops		x	6.1mg		
Luden's Maximum Strength, Sugar Free [S]		x	10mg		
Luden's Maximum Strength		x	10mg		
Luden's Original Menthol			x		
Mycinette (spray) [A]				1.4%	
Mycinettes (lozenges)	15mg		x		2.5mg
N'Ice 'N Clear, Cherry Eucalyptus			7mg		
N'Ice 'N Clear, Menthol Eucalyptus			5mg		
N'Ice Sore Throat & Cough			5mg		
Painalay Sore Throat Gargle				0.5%	
Protac	10mg				2.5mg
Ricola Cough Drops, Original Flavor			3mg		
Ricola Sugar Free Herb Throat Drops, Alpine-Mint [S]			4.8mg		
Ricola Sugar Free Herb Throat Drops, Cherry-Mint or Lemon-Mint [S]			1mg		
Ricola Sugar Free Herb Throat Drops, Mountain Herb [S]			1.5mg		
Ricola Throat Drops, Cherry-Mint			1.5mg		
Ricola Throat Drops, Honey-Herb			2.4mg		
Ricola Throat Drops, Lemon-Mint or Orange-Mint			1.25mg		

BRAND NAME	ANESTHETIC						ANTIBACTERIAL		
	benzocaine	dyclonine HCl	eucalyptol	eucalyptus oil	menthol	phenol	alcohol	cetylpyridinium chloride	hexylresorcinol
Ricola Throat Drops, Menthol-Eucalyptus					4.5mg				
Robitussin Cough Drops, Cherry or Menthol Eucalyptus				x	7.4mg				
Robitussin Cough Drops, Honey-Lemon				x	10mg				
Robitussin Liquid Center Cough Drops, Cherry with Honey-Lemon				x	8mg				
Robitussin Liquid Center Cough Drops, Honey-Lemon with Cherry				x	10mg				
Robitussin Liquid Center Cough Drops, Menthol Eucalyptus with Cherry				x	8mg				
Robitussin Sugar Free Cough Drops [S]					10mg				
Spec-T Sore Throat Anesthetic	10mg								
Spec-T Sore Throat Cough Suppressant	10mg								
Spec-T Sore Throat Decongestant	1omg								
Sucrets Children's Sore Throat		1.2mg							
Sucrets Maximum Strength Sore Throat		3mg							
Sucrets Sore Throat, Assorted Flavors		2mg							
Sucrets Sore Throat, Original Mint									2.4mg
Throat Discs									
Throtoceptic						1.4%			
Vicks Chloraseptic Sore Throat, Cherry Menthol [A]						1.4%			
Vicks Chloraseptic Sore Throat, Cherry or Menthol	6mg				10mg				
Vicks Cough Drops, Cherry				x	1.7mg				
Vicks Cough Drops, Menthol				x	3.3mg				
Vicks Original Cough Drops, Cherry					3.1mg				
Vicks Original Cough Drops, Menthol				x	6.6mg				

Inhaled Asthma Medications

BRAND NAME	epinephrine	sodium chloride
Asthma Haler [A]	0.16mg base/spray (epinephrine bitartrate, 0.3mg/spray)	
Asthma Nefrin [A]	2.25% base (racemic epinephrine HCl)	x
Breatheasy	2.2% (epinephrine HCl)	
Broncho Saline [A]		0.9%
Bronkaid Mist	0.25mg base/spray	
Bronkaid Mist Suspension	7mg/ml (epinephrine bitartrate)	
Micro NEFRIN	2.25% base (racemic epinephrine HCl)	
Primatene Mist	5.5mg/ml	

Oral Asthma Medications

BRAND NAME	ephedrine	expectorant (guaifenesin)
Bronkaid Dual Action Formula	25mg	400mg
Dynafed Two-Way	25mg	200mg
Mini Thin Two-Way	25mg	200mg
Primatene	12.5mg	200mg
Tedrigen	25mg	

Brand Name

Alka-Seltzer Plus Cold & Cough Medicine Effervescent Tablets (AL-kuh-SELTZ-er)

Generic Ingredients

Aspirin	Dextromethorphan
Chlorpheniramine maleate	Phenylpropanolamine

Type of drug

Antihistamine, decongestant, nonsteroidal anti-inflammatory drug (NSAID), analgesic (pain reliever), antipyretic (fever reducer), and antitussive (cough suppressant).

Used for

Temporary relief of runny nose, sneezing, nasal and sinus congestion, minor sore throat, headache, body aches, fever, and cough associated with colds and flu.

General Information

Some OTC products use a combination of drugs to relieve symptoms that can accompany colds and flu. Alka-Seltzer Plus Cold & Cough contains an antihistamine, a decongestant, an NSAID/analgesic/antipyretic to reduce pain and fever, and an antitussive to suppress cough.

The antihistamine ingredient in Alka-Seltzer Plus Cold & Cough is chlorpheniramine maleate. Antihistamines block the release of histamine in the body, relieving the sneezing and itching that often occurs with colds. They can also aid in stopping a runny nose by reducing the secretions caused by histamine release.

The decongestant ingredient in Alka-Seltzer Plus Cold & Cough is phenylpropanolamine, an oral decongestant. Decongestants relieve nasal congestion by narrowing or constricting blood vessels in the nose. This action reduces the blood supplied to the nose and decreases the swelling of nasal mucous membranes. Unlike topical decongestants (decongestant nasal sprays) that act on local blood vessels, oral decongestants may constrict blood vessels throughout the body.

The analgesic/antipyretic ingredient in Alka-Seltzer Plus Cold & Cough is aspirin. Aspirin is classified as an NSAID, a group of drugs that reduce inflammation and pain. Aspirin is also a member of the group of drugs called salicylates. Aspirin reduces inflammation and fever and relieves pain.

Aspirin's effects on pain and inflammation are thought to be related to its ability to prevent the manufacture of complex hormones called prostaglandins, which sensitize pain receptors and stimulate the inflammatory response. Aspirin reduces fever by acting on the heat-regulating center in the brain. This causes the blood vessels in the skin to dilate, which allows heat to leave the body more rapidly.

The cough suppressant in Alka-Seltzer Plus Cold & Cough is dextromethorphan, a common antitussive in OTC cough preparations. Dextromethorphan suppresses the cough reflex by acting directly on the cough center in the brain. Unlike some cough suppressants, dextromethorphan does not depress breathing and has a low potential for addiction.

Alka-Seltzer Plus Cold & Cough will not cure or prevent colds or flu. The best you can hope for is symptomatic relief. Colds will usually go away in 1 to 2 weeks whether they are treated or not.

Cautions and Warnings

Do not take Alka-Seltzer Plus Cold & Cough for more than 7 days continuously, or 3 days continuously in the presence of fever. If symptoms do not improve, see your doctor.

If a severe sore throat persists for longer than 2 days, or is accompanied by fever, headache, nausea, or vomiting, consult a doctor immediately.

If a cough lasts longer than 7 days, or keeps coming back, consult your doctor. A persistent cough may be the sign of a more serious condition.

Do not exceed the recommended daily dosage of Alka-Seltzer Plus Cold & Cough.

If you experience fever, rash, or persistent headache while taking Alka-Seltzer Plus Cold & Cough, stop taking it immediately and call your doctor.

If dizziness, hearing loss, ringing or buzzing in the ears, or continuous stomach pain occur while using Alka-Seltzer Plus Cold & Cough, stop taking the drug immediately and call your doctor.

Alka-Seltzer Plus Cold & Cough should be used with caution if you have a condition that causes breathing problems, such as emphysema, chronic bronchitis, asthma, nasal polyps, or rhinitis. Consult your doctor before using Alka-Seltzer Plus Cold & Cough if you have any of these conditions.

Alka-Seltzer Plus Cold & Cough should be used with caution by people with glaucoma, hyperthyroidism, heart disease, high blood pressure, diabetes, an enlarged prostate, or liver disease. If you have any of these conditions, ask your doctor before using Alka-Seltzer Plus Cold & Cough.

The antihistamine ingredient in Alka-Seltzer Plus Cold & Cough acts as a depressant on the central nervous system (CNS), and can cause sleepiness or grogginess and interfere with the ability to concentrate. Your ability to perform activities that require your full alertness and coordination, such as driving a motor vehicle or operating machinery, may be affected. Refrain from drinking alcohol while you are taking Alka-Seltzer Plus Cold & Cough, because alcohol aggravates these effects.

The aspirin ingredient in Alka-Seltzer Plus Cold & Cough is associated with gastrointestinal (GI) irritation, erosion, and bleeding. Unless directed by a doctor, people with GI bleeding or a history of peptic ulcers should not take Alka-Seltzer Plus Cold & Cough. Be aware that the risk of aspirin-related ulcers is increased by alcohol.

Children with the flu or chicken pox who are given aspirin may develop Reye's syndrome, a life-threatening condition characterized by vomiting, progressive damage to the central nervous system, liver injury, and abnormally low blood sugar. Up to 30% of children who develop Reye's syndrome die, and permanent brain damage is possible in those who survive. Because of the risk of Reye's syndrome, do not give Alka-Seltzer Plus Cold & Cough to children under age 16.

People with liver or kidney damage should avoid Alka-Seltzer Plus Cold & Cough.

To reduce the risk of bleeding, Alka-Seltzer Plus Cold & Cough should be avoided prior to surgery. Ask your doctor how long before surgery you should refrain from taking Alka-Seltzer Plus Cold & Cough.

Because productive coughing (coughing that brings up mucus) actually helps relieve the underlying condition, some doctors do not believe that suppressing a productive cough makes good sense. However, a severe cough can interfere with sleep, and loss of sleep can contribute to the severity and duration of an illness. In the balance, the most appropriate use of cough suppressants may be to relieve a dry, nonproductive cough.

Unless directed by your doctor, do not take Alka-Seltzer Plus Cold & Cough if you have a chronic cough, such as that associated with smoking, asthma, chronic bronchitis, or emphysema, or for coughs associated with excessive mucus.

Dextromethorphan, the antitussive ingredient in Alka-Seltzer Plus Cold & Cough, is not recommended for people confined to bed rest or under sedation.

Alka-Seltzer Plus Cold & Cough is high in sodium, which can lead to fluid retention. Do not take Alka-Seltzer Plus Cold & Cough if you must restrict your sodium intake because of high blood pressure, heart disease, or kidney disease.

Phenylketonurics (people who cannot digest phenylalanine) should be aware that Alka-Seltzer Plus Cold & Cough contains aspartame (NutraSweet), which breaks down in the GI tract to phenylalanine.

Possible Side Effects

▼ Most common: restlessness, nervousness, sleeplessness or drowsiness, sedation, excitability, dizziness, poor coordination, upset stomach, nausea, heartburn, loss of appetite, and small amounts of blood in the stool.

▼ Less common: dry eyes, nose, and mouth; blurred vision; difficulty urinating; irritability (at high doses); increased blood pressure; increased or irregular heart rate; and heart palpitations.

▼ Rare: severe headache, feelings of tightness in the chest, greatly elevated blood pressure, heart contractions, hives, rash, fever, thirst, and liver damage.

Drug Interactions

• The antihistamine ingredient in Alka-Seltzer Plus Cold & Cough can enhance the effect of other drugs that depress the CNS, such as barbiturates, tranquilizers, sleeping medications, and alcohol (present in many OTC preparations). If you are taking other depressant drugs, check with your doctor before taking these products. Avoid drinking alcohol if you are taking Alka-Seltzer Plus Cold & Cough.

• Antihistamines can also affect the results of skin and blood tests. Notify your health care professional before scheduling these tests if you are taking Alka-Seltzer Plus Cold & Cough.

• Alka-Seltzer Plus Cold & Cough should not be used at the same time as a monoamine oxidase inhibitor (MAOI) or within 2 weeks of stopping treatment with an MAOI. MAOIs are used to treat depression, other psychiatric or emotional conditions, and Parkinson's disease. If you are not sure whether you are or have been taking an MAOI, check with your doctor or pharmacist before using Alka-Seltzer Plus Cold & Cough.

• The effects of phenylpropanolamine, the decongestant in Alka-Seltzer Plus Cold & Cough, may combine with those of caffeine, a CNS stimulant found in many prescription and OTC drugs. This combination can cause disorientation, delirium, and other side effects.

• Taking Alka-Seltzer Plus Cold & Cough along with another decongestant can increase the risk of adverse effects and toxicity. If you are taking another decongestant, do not use Alka-Seltzer Plus Cold & Cough without first asking your doctor.

• Alka-Seltzer Plus Cold & Cough should not be taken by individuals currently taking methotrexate, used to treat cancer, severe psoriasis, severe rheumatoid arthritis, and to induce abortion; or valproic acid, an anticonvulsant.

• Alka-Seltzer Plus Cold & Cough should also not be taken with anticoagulant (blood-thinning) drugs, such as warfarin and dicumarol. It will exaggerate the effects of these drugs and increase the risk of abnormal bleeding.

• People with AIDS and AIDS-related complex who take zidovudine (AZT) should avoid using Alka-Seltzer Plus Cold & Cough because the aspirin in it may increase the risk of bleeding.

• The possibility of a stomach ulcer is increased if Alka-Seltzer Plus Cold & Cough is taken together with alcoholic beverages; an adrenal corticosteroid, such as hydrocortisone; or phenylbutazone, another NSAID. Taking Alka-Seltzer Plus Cold & Cough with another NSAID has no benefit and carries a greatly increased risk of side effects.

• The aspirin in Alka-Seltzer Plus Cold & Cough will counteract the effects of the antigout medications probenecid and sulfinpyrazone, and may counteract the effects of angiotensin-converting enzyme (ACE) inhibitors and beta blockers, which work to lower blood pressure. Alka-Seltzer Plus Cold & Cough may also counteract the effects of some diuretics in people with severe liver disease.

• Combining nitroglycerin tablets and Alka-Seltzer Plus Cold & Cough may lead to an unexpected drop in blood pressure.

Food Interactions

The decongestant in Alka-Seltzer Plus Cold & Cough interacts adversely with caffeine (see "Drug Interactions"), which is found in many popular beverages, including coffee, tea, and cola, and in chocolate.

Usual Dose

Each tablet contains 2 mg of chlorpheniramine, 20 mg of phenylpropanolamine, 325 mg of aspirin, and 10 mg of dextromethorphan.

Adult and Child (age 16 and over): 2 tablets dissolved in 4 oz. of water every 4 hours. Do not exceed 8 tablets in a 24-hour period.

Child (under age 16): not recommended because of the risk of Reye's syndrome (see "Cautions and Warnings").

Overdosage

Symptoms of overdose include nausea, vomiting, urinary retention, shallow breathing, rapid breathing, rapid heartbeat, sweating, fever, thirst, headache, diarrhea, flushed face, dry mouth, ringing or buzzing in the ears, blurred vision, dilated pupils, rapid rolling of the eyeballs, loss of muscle coordination, excitability, confusion, drowsiness, dizziness, hallucinations, seizures, liver or kidney failure, coma, and bleeding.

Even if the victim is not displaying any of the symptoms listed above, do the following in case of accidental overdose: If the victim is unconscious or having convulsions, call for an ambulance immediately. If you take the victim to an emergency room, be sure to bring the bottle or container with you. If the victim is conscious, call your local poison control center or a health care professional. The poison control center may suggest inducing vomiting with ipecac syrup (available without a prescription at any pharmacy). DO NOT induce vomiting unless specifically instructed to do so.

Special Populations

Pregnancy/Breast-feeding

Do not take Alka-Seltzer Plus Cold & Cough if you are or might be pregnant.

The active ingredients in Alka-Seltzer Plus Cold & Cough have been shown to pass into the breast milk of nursing mothers and may cause side effects in infants. Check with your doctor before taking Alka-Seltzer Plus Cold & Cough if you are breast-feeding.

Infants/Children

Alka-Seltzer Plus Cold & Cough should not be given to a child under age 16 unless directed by a doctor, due to the risk of Reye's syndrome (see "Cautions and Warnings").

Seniors

Seniors may be more sensitive to the side effects of Alka-Seltzer Plus Cold & Cough. They may experience nervousness, irritability, and restlessness. Dizziness, sedation, and low blood pressure may also occur. Older men may experience difficulty in urinating. Most mild reactions may be handled by either lowering your dose or trying another antihistamine/decongestant combination.

Seniors taking Alka-Seltzer Plus Cold & Cough should be especially cautious about the amount of caffeine they ingest (see "Drug Interactions").

Older individuals may find Alka-Seltzer Plus Cold & Cough irritating to the stomach, especially in large doses. Older adults with liver disease or severe kidney impairment should not use Alka-Seltzer Plus Cold & Cough.

Brand Names

Alka-Seltzer Plus Cold & Cough Medicine Liqui-Gels
(AL-kuh-SELTZ-er)

Children's Tylenol Cold Plus Cough (TYE-leh-nol)

Theraflu Flu, Cold & Cough Medicine, Original Formula
(THER-uh-flu)

Theraflu Flu, Cold & Cough Medicine, Maximum Strength Night Time

Tylenol Cold Multi-Symptom Hot Medication

Generic Ingredients

Acetaminophen
Chlorpheniramine maleate
Dextromethorphan
Pseudoephedrine

Type of Drug

Antihistamine, decongestant, analgesic (pain reliever), antipyretic (fever reducer), and antitussive (cough suppressant).

Used for

Temporary relief of runny nose, sneezing, nasal and sinus congestion, minor sore throat, headache, body ache, fever, and cough associated with colds and flu.

General Information

Some OTC products use a combination of drugs to relieve symptoms that can accompany colds and flu. Alka-Seltzer Plus Cold & Cough Liqui-Gels; Children's Tylenol Cold Plus

Cough; Theraflu Flu, Cold & Cough; and Tylenol Cold Multi-Symptom Hot Medication each contain an antihistamine, a decongestant, an analgesic/antipyretic to reduce pain and fever, and an antitussive to suppress cough.

The antihistamine ingredient in these products is chlorpheniramine maleate. Antihistamines block the release of histamine in the body, relieving the sneezing and itching that often occur with colds and flu. They can also aid in stopping a runny nose by reducing the secretions caused by histamine release.

The decongestant ingredient in these products is pseudoephedrine, an oral decongestant. Decongestants relieve nasal congestion by narrowing or constricting blood vessels in the nose, which reduces the blood supplied to the nose and decreases the swelling of nasal mucous membranes. Unlike topical decongestants (decongestant nasal sprays) that act on local blood vessels, oral decongestants may constrict blood vessels throughout the body.

The analgesic/antipyretic ingredient in these products is acetaminophen. Acetaminophen provides effective relief from the aches and fever associated with a cold or the flu.

The cough suppressant in these products is dextromethorphan, a common antitussive in OTC cough preparations. Dextromethorphan suppresses the cough reflex by acting directly on the cough center in the brain. However, unlike some antitussives, it does not depress breathing. It also has a low potential for addiction.

These products will not cure or prevent colds or flu. The best you can hope for is symptomatic relief. Colds will usually go away in 1 to 2 weeks whether they are treated or not.

Cautions and Warnings

Do not take Alka-Seltzer Plus Cold & Cough Liqui-Gels; Children's Tylenol Cold Plus Cough; Theraflu Flu, Cold & Cough; or Tylenol Cold Multi-Symptom Hot Medication for more than 7 days continuously. If fever is present do not take them for more than 3 days continuously. If symptoms do not improve, see your doctor.

If a severe sore throat persists for longer than 2 days, or is accompanied by fever, headache, nausea, or vomiting, consult a doctor immediately.

If a cough lasts longer than 7 days, or keeps coming back, consult your doctor. A persistent cough may be the sign of a more serious condition.

Do not exceed the recommended daily dosage of these products.

If you experience fever, rash, or persistent headache while taking these products, stop taking them immediately and call your doctor.

These products should be used with caution if you have a condition that causes breathing problems, such as emphysema, chronic bronchitis, or asthma. Consult your doctor before using them if you have any of these conditions.

These products should be used with caution by people with glaucoma, hyperthyroidism, heart disease, high blood pressure, diabetes, an enlarged prostate, or liver disease; if you have any of these conditions, ask your doctor before using them.

The antihistamine ingredient in these products acts as a depressant on the central nervous system (CNS), and can cause sleepiness or grogginess and interfere with the ability to concentrate. Your ability to perform activities that require your full alertness and coordination, such as driving a motor vehicle or operating machinery, may be affected. Refrain from drinking alcohol while you are taking these products, because alcohol aggravates these effects.

In doses of more than 4 grams per day, acetaminophen is potentially toxic to the liver. Use these products with caution if you have kidney or liver disease or viral infections of the liver. Studies have shown that the risk of liver damage with acetaminophen is associated with fasting and alcohol use. People with liver disease who are taking other drugs that are potentially damaging to the liver, people who do not eat regularly, or who drink alcohol (even moderately) are especially at risk. If you take these products regularly, avoid drinking alcohol and/or fasting.

Because productive coughing (coughing that brings up mucus) actually helps relieve the underlying condition, some doctors do not believe that suppressing a productive cough makes good sense. However, a severe cough can interfere with sleep, and loss of sleep can contribute to the severity and duration of an illness. In the balance, the most appropriate use of cough suppressants may be to relieve a dry, nonproductive cough, especially at night.

Unless directed by your doctor, do not take these products if you have a chronic cough, such as that associated with smoking, asthma, chronic bronchitis, or emphysema, or for coughs associated with excess mucus.

Dextromethorphan, the antitussive ingredient in these products, is not recommended for people confined to bed rest or under sedation.

Possible Side Effects

- ▼ Most common: lightheadedness, restlessness, nervousness, sleeplessness, sedation, excitability, dizziness, poor coordination, headache, and upset stomach.
- ▼ Less common: dry eyes, nose, and mouth; blurred vision; difficulty urinating; irritability (at high doses); increased blood pressure; and increased or irregular heart rate.
- ▼ Rare: nausea, difficulty breathing, anxiety, extreme fatigue, rashes, hives, sore throat, fever, unexplained bleeding or bruising, anemia, yellowing of the skin or eyes, blood in the urine, painful or frequent urination, decreased output of urine volume, tremor, hallucinations, seizures, and cardiovascular collapse.

Drug Interactions

• The antihistamine ingredient in Alka-Seltzer Plus Cold & Cough Liqui-Gels; Children's Tylenol Cold Plus Cough; Theraflu Flu, Cold & Cough; and Tylenol Cold Multi-Symptom Hot Medication, can enhance the effect of other drugs that depress the CNS, such as barbiturates, tranquilizers, sleeping medications, and alcohol (present in many OTC preparations). If you are taking other depressant drugs, check with your doctor before taking these products.

• Antihistamines can also affect the results of skin and blood tests. Notify your health care professional before scheduling these tests if you are taking these products.

• These products should not be used at the same time as a monoamine oxidase inhibitor (MAOI) or within 2 weeks of stopping treatment with an MAOI. MAOIs are used to treat depression, other psychiatric or emotional conditions, and Parkinson's disease. If you are not sure whether you are or have been taking an MAOI, check with your doctor or pharmacist before you use these products.

• The effects of the decongestant in these products may combine with those of caffeine, a CNS stimulant found in many prescription and OTC drugs. This combination can cause disorientation, delirium, and other side effects.

• Taking these products along with another decongestant can increase the risk of adverse effects and toxicity; if you are taking another decongestant, do not use these products without first asking your doctor.

• The effect of the acetaminophen in these products may be reduced by long-term use or large doses of barbiturate drugs; the anticonvulsants carbamazepine and phenytoin (and other similar drugs); rifampin, used to treat tuberculosis (TB); and sulfinpyrazone, used to treat gout. These drugs may also increase the chances of liver toxicity if taken with acetaminophen. Chronically taking large doses of acetaminophen with isoniazid (used to treat TB) may also increase the risk of liver damage.

• If these products are taken with an anticoagulant such as warfarin, the acetaminophen in them may increase the blood-thinning effect of the anticoagulant agent. This does not occur with occasional use.

• Avoid alcohol while taking these products. (Be aware that alcohol is found in many OTC preparations.) Alcohol may contribute to the risk of liver damage associated with acetaminophen; it also increases the sedative effects of antihistamines (see "Cautions and Warnings").

Food Interactions

The decongestant in Alka-Seltzer Plus Cold & Cough Liqui-Gels; Children's Tylenol Cold Plus Cough; Theraflu Flu, Cold & Cough; and Tylenol Cold Multi-Symptom Hot Medication interacts adversely with caffeine (see "Drug Interactions"), which is found in many popular beverages, including coffee, tea, and cola, and in chocolate.

Usual Dose

Alka-Seltzer Plus Cold & Cough Liqui-Gels
Each softgel contains 2 mg of chlorpheniramine, 30 mg of pseudoephedrine, 250 mg of acetaminophen, and 10 mg of dextromethorphan.

Adult and Child (age 12 and over): 2 softgels every 4 hours. Do not exceed 4 doses in a 24-hour period.

Child (age 6–11): 1 softgel every 4 hours. Do not exceed 4 doses in a 24-hour period.

Child (under age 6): Consult your doctor.

Children's Tylenol Cold Plus Cough
Each packet contains 0.5 mg of chlorpheniramine, 7.5 mg of pseudoephedrine, 80 mg of acetaminophen, and 2.5 mg of dextromethorphan.

Child (age 6–11): 4 tablets every 4–6 hours. Do not exceed 4 doses in a 24-hour period.

Child (under age 6): Consult your doctor.

Theraflu Flu, Cold & Cough
Each packet of Original Formula contains 4 mg of chlorpheniramine, 60 mg of pseudoephedrine, 650 mg of acetaminophen, and 20 mg of dextromethorphan. Each packet of Maximum Strength Night Time formula contains 4 mg of chlorpheniramine, 60 mg of pseudoephedrine, 1000 mg of acetaminophen, and 30 mg of dextromethorphan.

Adult and Child (age 12 and over): One packet dissolved in 6 oz. of hot water, every 4–6 hours for the Original Formula, and every 6 hours for the Maximum Strength Night Time formula. Do not exceed 4 doses in a 24-hour period.

Child (under age 12): Consult your doctor.

Tylenol Cold Multi-Symptom Hot Medication
Each packet contains 4 mg of chlorpheniramine, 60 mg of pseudoephedrine, 650 mg of acetaminophen, and 30 mg of dextromethorphan.

Adult and Child (age 12 and over): One packet dissolved in 6 oz. of hot water every 6 hours. Do not exceed 4 doses in a 24-hour period.

Child (under age 12): not recommended unless directed by your doctor.

Overdosage

Symptoms of overdose include nausea, vomiting, abdominal pain, urinary retention, low blood pressure, shallow breathing, fever, flushed face, dry mouth, dilated pupils, blurred vision, rapid rolling of the eyeballs, loss of muscle coordination, confusion, excitability, hallucinations, drowsiness, dizziness, coma, seizures, yellowing of the skin and eyes, and liver damage. Symptoms may develop within 30 minutes, but may not be seen for as long as 2 days after the overdose.

Even if the victim is not displaying any of the symptoms listed above, do the following in case of accidental overdose: If the victim is unconscious or having convulsions, call for an ambulance immediately. If you take the victim to an emergency room, be sure to bring the bottle or container with you. If the victim is conscious, call your local poison control center or a health care professional. The poison control center may suggest inducing vomiting with ipecac syrup (available without a prescription at any pharmacy). DO NOT induce vomiting unless specifically instructed to do so.

Special Populations

Pregnancy/Breast-feeding

Antihistamines are not recommended for use during pregnancy unless directed by your doctor. Antihistamines, decongestants, and acetaminophen are known to pass into the breast milk of nursing mothers and may cause side effects in infants. Check with your doctor before taking Alka-Seltzer Plus Cold & Cough Liqui-Gels; Children's Tylenol Cold Plus Cough; Theraflu Flu, Cold & Cough; or Tylenol Cold Multi-Symptom Hot Medication if you are or might be pregnant, or if you are breast-feeding.

Infants/Children

Children may be more susceptible to the side effects of these products. They are also more susceptible to accidental antihistamine overdose. Unless directed by your doctor, do not give Alka-Seltzer Plus Cold & Cough Liqui-Gels or Children's Tylenol Cold Plus Cough to a child under age 6. Do not give Theraflu Flu, Cold & Cough or Tylenol Cold Multi-Symptom Hot Medication to a child under age 12 unless directed by your doctor.

Seniors

Older persons may be more sensitive to the side effects of Alka-Seltzer Plus Cold & Cough Liqui-Gels; Theraflu Flu, Cold & Cough; and Tylenol Cold Multi-Symptom Hot Medication. They may experience nervousness, irritability, restlessness, dizziness, sedation, urinary retention, low blood pressure, hallucinations, and seizures. Most mild reactions may be handled by either lowering your dose or trying another product.

Seniors taking these products should be especially cautious about the amount of caffeine they ingest (see "Drug Interactions").

Brand Name

Alka-Seltzer Plus Cold Medicine Effervescent Tablets (AL-kuh-SELTZ-er)

Generic Ingredients

Aspirin
Chlorpheniramine maleate
Phenylpropanolamine

Type of drug

Antihistamine, decongestant, nonsteroidal anti-inflammatory drug (NSAID), analgesic (pain reliever), and antipyretic (fever reducer).

Used for

Temporary relief of runny nose, sneezing, nasal and sinus congestion, minor sore throat, headache, body aches, and fever associated with colds and flu.

General Information

Some OTC products use a combination of drugs to relieve symptoms that can accompany colds and flu. Alka-Seltzer Plus Cold Medicine contains an antihistamine, a decongestant, an NSAID/analgesic/antipyretic to reduce pain and fever, and an antitussive to suppress cough.

The antihistamine ingredient in Alka-Seltzer Plus Cold

is chlorpheniramine maleate. Antihistamines block the release of histamine in the body, relieving the sneezing and itching that often occur with colds. They can also aid in stopping a runny nose by reducing the secretions caused by histamine release.

The decongestant ingredient in Alka-Seltzer Plus Cold is phenylpropanolamine, an oral decongestant. Decongestants relieve nasal congestion by narrowing or constricting blood vessels in the nose, which reduces the blood supplied to the nose and decreases the swelling of nasal mucous membranes. Unlike topical decongestants (decongestant nasal sprays) that act on local blood vessels, oral decongestants may constrict blood vessels throughout the body.

The analgesic/antipyretic ingredient in Alka-Seltzer Plus Cold is aspirin. Aspirin is classified as an NSAID, a group of drugs that reduce inflammation and pain. Aspirin is also a member of the group of drugs called salicylates. Aspirin reduces inflammation and fever and relieves pain.

Aspirin's effects on pain and inflammation are thought to be related to its ability to prevent the manufacture of complex hormones called prostaglandins, which sensitize pain receptors and stimulate the inflammatory response. Aspirin reduces fever by acting on the heat-regulating center in the brain. This causes the blood vessels in the skin to dilate which allows heat to leave the body more rapidly.

Alka-Seltzer Plus Cold Medicine will not cure or prevent colds or flu. The best you can hope for is symptomatic relief. Colds will usually go away in 1 to 2 weeks whether they are treated or not.

Cautions and Warnings

Do not take Alka-Seltzer Plus Cold for 7 days continuously, or 3 days continuously in the presence of fever. If symptoms do not improve, see your doctor.

If a severe sore throat persists for longer than 2 days, or is accompanied by fever, headache, nausea, or vomiting, consult your doctor immediately.

Do not exceed the recommended daily dosage of Alka-Seltzer Plus Cold.

If dizziness, hearing loss, ringing or buzzing in the ears, or continuous stomach pain occur while using Alka-Seltzer

Plus Cold, stop taking the drug immediately and call your doctor.

Alka-Seltzer Plus Cold should be used with caution if you have a condition that causes breathing problems, such as emphysema, chronic bronchitis, asthma, nasal polyps, or rhinitis. Consult your doctor before using Alka-Seltzer Plus Cold if you have any of these conditions.

Alka-Seltzer Plus Cold should be used with caution by people with glaucoma, hyperthyroidism, heart disease, high blood pressure, diabetes, an enlarged prostate, or liver disease. If you have any of these conditions, ask your doctor before using Alka-Seltzer Plus Cold.

The antihistamine ingredient in Alka-Seltzer Plus Cold acts as a depressant on the central nervous system (CNS), and can cause sleepiness or grogginess and interfere with the ability to concentrate. Your ability to perform activities that require your full alertness and coordination, such as driving a motor vehicle or operating machinery, may be affected. Refrain from drinking alcohol while you are taking Alka-Seltzer Plus Cold, because alcohol aggravates these effects.

The aspirin ingredient in Alka-Seltzer Plus Cold is associated with gastrointestinal (GI) irritation, erosion and bleeding. Unless directed by a doctor, people with GI bleeding or a history of peptic ulcers should not take Alka-Seltzer Plus Cold. Be aware that the risk of aspirin-related ulcers is increased by alcohol.

Children with the flu or chicken pox who are given aspirin may develop Reye's syndrome, a life-threatening condition characterized by vomiting, progressive damage to the central nervous system, liver injury, and abnormally low blood sugar. Up to 30% of children who develop Reye's syndrome die, and permanent brain damage is possible in those who survive. Because of the risk of Reye's syndrome, do not give Alka-Seltzer Plus Cold to children under age 16.

People with liver or kidney damage should avoid Alka-Seltzer Plus Cold.

To reduce the risk of bleeding, Alka-Seltzer Plus Cold should be avoided prior to surgery. Ask your doctor how long before surgery you should refrain from taking Alka-Seltzer Plus Cold.

Alka-Seltzer Plus Cold is high in sodium, which can lead to fluid retention. Do not take Alka-Seltzer Plus Cold if you must restrict your sodium intake because of high blood pressure, heart disease, or kidney disease.

Possible Side Effects

- ▼ Most common: restlessness, nervousness, sleeplessness or drowsiness, sedation, excitability, dizziness, poor coordination, upset stomach, nausea, heartburn, loss of appetite, and small amounts of blood in the stool.
- ▼ Less common: dry eyes, nose, and mouth; blurred vision; difficulty urinating; irritability (at high doses); increased blood pressure; increased or irregular heart rate; and heart palpitations.
- ▼ Rare: severe headache, feelings of tightness in the chest, greatly elevated blood pressure, heart contractions, hives, rash, fever, thirst, and liver damage.

Drug Interactions

• The antihistamine ingredient in Alka-Seltzer Plus Cold can enhance the effect of other drugs that depress the CNS, such as barbiturates, tranquilizers, sleeping medications, and alcohol (present in many OTC preparations). If you are taking other depressant drugs, check with your doctor before taking Alka-Seltzer Plus Cold. Avoid drinking alcohol while you are taking this product because alcohol aggravates these effects.

• Antihistamines can also affect the results of skin and blood tests. Notify your health care professional before scheduling these tests if you are taking Alka-Seltzer Plus Cold.

• Alka-Seltzer Plus Cold should not be used at the same time as a monoamine oxidase inhibitor (MAOI) or within 2 weeks of stopping treatment with an MAOI. MAOIs are used to treat depression, other psychiatric or emotional conditions, and Parkinson's disease. If you are not sure whether you are or have been taking an MAOI, check with your doctor or pharmacist before using Alka-Seltzer Plus Cold.

• The effects of phenylpropanolamine, the decongestant in Alka-Seltzer Plus Cold, may combine with those of caffeine, a CNS stimulant found in many prescription and OTC drugs. This combination can cause disorientation, delirium, and other side effects.

• Taking Alka-Seltzer Plus Cold along with another decongestant can increase the risk of adverse effects and toxicity If you are taking another decongestant, do not use Alka-Seltzer Plus Cold without first asking your doctor.

• Alka-Seltzer Plus Cold should not be taken by individuals currently taking methotrexate, used to treat cancer, severe psoriasis, severe rheumatoid arthritis, and to induce abortion; or valproic acid, an anticonvulsant.

• Alka-Seltzer Plus Cold should also not be taken with anticoagulant (blood-thinning) drugs, such as warfarin and dicumarol. It will exaggerate the effects of these drugs and increase the risk of abnormal bleeding.

• People with AIDS and AIDS-related complex who take zidovudine (AZT) should avoid using Alka-Seltzer Plus Cold because the aspirin in it may increase the risk of bleeding.

• The possibility of a stomach ulcer is increased if Alka-Seltzer Plus Cold is taken together with alcoholic beverages; an adrenal corticosteroid, such as hydrocortisone; or phenylbutazone, another NSAID. Taking Alka-Seltzer Plus Cold with another NSAID has no benefit and carries a greatly increased risk of side effects.

• The aspirin in Alka-Seltzer Plus Cold will counteract the effects of the antigout medications probenecid and sulfinpyrazone, and may counteract the effects of angiotensin-converting enzyme (ACE) inhibitors and beta blockers, which work to lower blood pressure. Alka-Seltzer Plus Cold may also counteract the effects of some diuretics in people with severe liver disease.

• Combining nitroglycerin tablets and Alka-Seltzer Plus Cold may lead to an unexpected drop in blood pressure.

Food Interactions

The decongestant in Alka-Seltzer Plus Cold interacts adversely with caffeine (see "Drug Interactions"), which is found in many popular beverages, including coffee, tea, and cola, and in chocolate.

Usual Dose

Each tablet contains 2 mg of chlorpheniramine, 24.08 mg of phenylpropanolamine, and 325 mg of aspirin.

Adult and Child (age 16 and over): 2 tablets dissolved in 4 oz. of water every 4 hours. Do not exceed 8 tablets in a 24-hour period.

Child (under age 16): not recommended because of the risk of Reye's syndrome (see "Cautions and Warnings").

Overdosage

Symptoms of overdose include nausea, vomiting, rapid breathing, rapid heartbeat, sweating, fever, thirst, headache, diarrhea, flushed face, dry mouth, ringing or buzzing in the ears, dilated pupils, loss of muscle coordination, excitability, confusion, drowsiness, dizziness, hallucinations, seizures, liver or kidney failure, coma, and bleeding.

Even if the victim is not displaying any of the symptoms listed above, do the following in case of accidental overdose: If the victim is unconscious or having convulsions, call for an ambulance immediately. If you take the victim to an emergency room, be sure to bring the bottle or container with you. If the victim is conscious, call your local poison control center or a health care professional. The poison control center may suggest inducing vomiting with ipecac syrup (available without a prescription at any pharmacy). DO NOT induce vomiting unless specifically instructed to do so.

Special Populations

Pregnancy/Breast-feeding

Do not take Alka-Seltzer Plus Cold if you are or might be pregnant.

The active ingredients in Alka-Seltzer Plus Cold have been shown to pass into the breast milk of nursing mothers and may cause side effects in infants. Check with your doctor before taking Alka-Seltzer Plus Cold if you are breast-feeding.

Infants/Children

Alka-Seltzer Plus Cold should not be given to a child under age 16 unless directed by a doctor, due to the risk of Reye's syndrome (see "Cautions and Warnings").

Seniors

Seniors may be more sensitive to the side effects of Alka-Seltzer Plus Cold. They may experience nervousness, irritability, and restlessness. Dizziness, sedation, and low blood pressure may also occur. Older men may experience difficulty in urinating. Most mild reactions may be handled by either lowering your dose or trying another antihistamine/decongestant combination.

Seniors taking Alka-Seltzer Plus Cold should be especially cautious about the amount of caffeine they ingest (see "Drug Interactions").

Older individuals may find Alka-Seltzer Plus Cold irritating to the stomach, especially in large doses. Older adults with liver disease or severe kidney impairment should not use Alka-Seltzer Plus Cold.

Brand Names

Alka-Seltzer Plus Cold Medicine Liqui-Gels (AL-kuh-SELTZ-er)

Children's Tylenol Cold Multi Symptom Liquid (TYE-leh-nol)

Generic Ingredients

Acetaminophen
Chlorpheniramine maleate
Pseudoephedrine

Type of Drug

Antihistamine, decongestant, analgesic (pain reliever), and antipyretic (fever reducer).

Used for

Temporary relief of runny nose, sneezing, nasal and sinus congestion, minor sore throat, headache, body ache, and fever associated with colds and flu.

General Information

Some OTC products use a combination of drugs to relieve symptoms that can accompany colds and flu. Alka-Seltzer Plus Cold Liqui-Gels and Children's Tylenol Cold Multi Symptom Liquid contain an antihistamine, a decongestant, and an analgesic/antipyretic to reduce pain and fever.

The antihistamine ingredient in these products is chlorpheniramine maleate. Antihistamines block the release of histamine in the body, relieving the sneezing and itching that often occur with colds and flu. They can also aid in stopping a runny nose by reducing the secretions caused by histamine release.

The decongestant ingredient in these products is pseudoephedrine, an oral decongestant. Decongestants relieve nasal congestion by narrowing or constricting blood vessels in the nose, which reduces the blood supplied to the nose and decreases the swelling of nasal mucous membranes. Unlike topical decongestants (decongestant nasal sprays) that act on local blood vessels, oral decongestants may constrict blood vessels throughout the body.

The analgesic/antipyretic ingredient in these products is acetaminophen. Acetaminophen provides effective relief from the aches and fever associated with a cold or the flu.

Neither of these products will cure or prevent colds or flu. The best you can hope for is symptomatic relief. Colds will usually go away in 1 to 2 weeks whether they are treated or not.

Cautions and Warnings

Do not take Alka-Seltzer Plus Cold Liqui-Gels for more than 7 days continuously, or more than 3 days continuously in the presence of fever. Do not give a child Children's Tylenol Cold Multi Symptom Liquid for more than 5 days continuously, or more than 3 days continuously in the presence of fever. If symptoms do not improve, see your doctor.

If a severe sore throat persists for longer than 2 days, or is accompanied by fever, headache, nausea, or vomiting, consult a doctor immediately.

Do not exceed the recommended daily dosage of these products.

These products should be used with caution if you or your child has a condition that causes breathing problems, such as emphysema, chronic bronchitis, or asthma. Its antihistamine ingredient dries the mucous membranes. This in turn can inhibit the ability of the lungs to move or get rid of the excess secretions that these conditions produce.

These products should be used with caution by people with glaucoma, hyperthyroidism, heart disease, high blood pressure, diabetes, or an enlarged prostate. If you or your child has any of these conditions, ask your doctor before using these products.

The antihistamine ingredient in these products acts as a depressant on the central nervous system (CNS), and can cause sleepiness or grogginess and interfere with the ability to concentrate. Your ability to perform activities that require your full alertness and coordination, such as driving a motor vehicle or operating machinery, may be affected. Refrain from drinking alcohol while you are taking Alka-Seltzer Plus Cold Liqui-Gels.

In doses of more than 4 grams per day, acetaminophen is potentially toxic to the liver. Use these products with caution if you or your child has kidney or liver disease or viral infections of the liver. Studies have shown that the risk of liver damage with acetaminophen is associated with fasting and alcohol use. People with liver disease who are taking other drugs that are potentially damaging to the liver, people who do not eat regularly, or who drink alcohol (even moderately) are especially at risk. If you use these products regularly, avoid drinking alcohol and/or fasting.

Possible Side Effects

- ▼ Most common: lightheadedness, restlessness, nervousness, sleeplessness, sedation, excitability, dizziness, poor coordination, headache, and upset stomach.
- ▼ Less common: dry eyes, nose, and mouth; blurred vision; difficulty urinating; irritability (at high doses); increased blood pressure; and increased or irregular heart rate.
- ▼ Rare: difficulty breathing, anxiety, extreme fatigue, rashes, hives, sore throat, fever, unexplained bleeding or bruising, anemia, yellowing of the skin or eyes, blood in the urine, painful or frequent urination, decreased output of urine volume, tremor, hallucinations, seizures, and cardiovascular collapse.

Drug Interactions

• The antihistamine ingredient in Alka-Seltzer Plus Cold Liqui-Gels and Children's Tylenol Cold Multi Symptom Liquid can enhance the effect of other drugs that depress the CNS, such as barbiturates, tranquilizers, sleeping medications, and alcohol (present in many OTC preparations). If you or your child is taking other depressant drugs, check with your doctor before taking these products.

• Antihistamines can also affect the results of skin and blood tests. Notify your health care professional before scheduling these tests if you are using these products.

• These products should not be used at the same time as a monoamine oxidase inhibitor (MAOI) or within 2 weeks of stopping treatment with an MAOI. MAOIs are used to treat depression, other psychiatric or emotional conditions, and Parkinson's disease. If you are not sure whether you or your child is or has been taking an MAOI, check with your doctor or pharmacist before using these products.

• The effects of the decongestant in these products may combine with those of caffeine, a CNS stimulant found in many prescription and OTC drugs. This combination can cause disorientation, delirium, and other side effects.

• Taking these products along with another decongestant can increase the risk of adverse effects and toxicity. If you or your child is taking another decongestant, do not use these products without first asking your doctor.

• The effect of the acetaminophen in these products may be reduced by long-term use or large doses of barbiturate drugs; the anticonvulsants carbamazepine and phenytoin (and other similar drugs); rifampin, used to treat tuberculosis (TB); and sulfinpyrazone, used to treat gout. These drugs may also increase the chances of liver toxicity if taken with acetaminophen. Chronically taking large doses of acetaminophen along with isoniazid (used to treat TB) may also increase the risk of liver damage.

• If these products are taken with an anticoagulant such as warfarin, the acetaminophen in them may increase the blood-thinning effect of the anticoagulant agent. This does not occur with occasional use.

• Avoid alcohol while taking these products. (Be aware that alcohol is found in many OTC preparations.) Alcohol may contribute to the risk of liver damage associated with acetaminophen; it also increases the sedative effects of antihistamines (see "Cautions and Warnings").

Food Interactions

The decongestant in Alka-Seltzer Plus Cold Liqui-Gels and Children's Tylenol Cold Multi Symptom Liquid interacts adversely with caffeine (see "Drug Interactions"), which is found in many popular beverages, including coffee, tea, and cola, and in chocolate.

Usual Dose

Alka-Seltzer Plus Cold Liqui-Gels
Each softgel contains 2 mg of chlorpheniramine, 30 mg of pseudoephedrine, and 250 mg of acetaminophen.

Adult and Child (age 12 and over): 2 softgels every 4 hours. Do not exceed 8 softgels in a 24-hour period.

Child (age 6–11): 1 softgel every 4 hours. Do not exceed 4 softgels in a 24-hour period.

Child (under age 6): Consult your doctor.

Children's Tylenol Cold Multi Symptom Liquid
Each 5 ml (1 tsp.) contains 1 mg of chlorpheniramine, 15 mg pseudoephedrine, and 160 mg of acetaminophen.

Child (age 6–11): 2 tsp. every 4–6 hours. Do not exceed 8 tsp. in a 24-hour period.

Child (under age 6): Consult your doctor.

Overdosage

Symptoms of overdose include nausea, vomiting, abdominal pain, low blood pressure, fever, flushed face, dry mouth, dilated pupils, loss of muscle coordination, confusion, excitability, hallucinations, drowsiness, coma, seizures, yellowing of the skin and eyes, and liver damage. Symptoms may develop within 30 minutes, or may not be seen for as long as 2 days after the overdose.

Even if the victim is not displaying any of the symptoms listed above, do the following in case of accidental overdose: If the victim is unconscious or having convulsions, call for an ambulance immediately. If you take the victim to an emergency room, be sure to bring the bottle or container with you. If the victim is conscious, call your local poison control center or a health care professional. The poison control center may suggest inducing vomiting with ipecac syrup (available without a prescription at any pharmacy). DO NOT induce vomiting unless specifically instructed to do so.

Special Populations

Pregnancy/Breast-feeding

Antihistamines are not recommended for use during pregnancy unless directed by your doctor. Antihistamines, decongestants, and acetaminophen are known to pass into the breast milk of nursing mothers and may cause side effects in infants. Check with your doctor before taking Alka-Seltzer Plus Cold Liqui-Gels if you are or might be pregnant, or if you are breast-feeding.

Infants/Children

Children may be more susceptible to the side effects of these products. They are also more susceptible to accidental antihistamine overdose. Do not give Alka-Seltzer Plus Cold Liqui-Gels to a child under age 6 unless directed by your doctor. Give Children's Tylenol Cold Multi Symptom Liquid to a child under 6 according to your doctor's instructions.

Seniors

Older persons may be more sensitive to the side effects of Alka-Seltzer Plus Cold Liqui-Gels. They may experience nervousness, irritability, restlessness, dizziness, sedation, urinary retention, low blood pressure, hallucinations, and seizures. Most mild reactions may be handled by either lowering your dose or trying another product.

Seniors taking Alka-Seltzer Plus Cold Liqui-Gels should be especially cautious about the amount of caffeine they ingest (see "Drug Interactions").

Brand Name

Alka-Seltzer Plus Flu & Body Aches Formula Effervescent Tablets

(AL-kuh-SELTZ-er)

Generic Ingredients

Acetaminophen	Dextromethorphan
Chlorpheniramine maleate	Phenylpropanolamine

Type of Drug

Antihistamine, decongestant, analgesic (pain reliever), antipyretic (fever reducer), antitussive (cough suppressant).

Used for

Temporary relief of runny nose, sneezing, nasal and sinus congestion, minor sore throat, cough, headache, body aches, and fever associated with colds and flu.

General Information

Some OTC drugs use a combination of medications to relieve the many symptoms that can accompany colds and flu. Alka-Seltzer Plus Flu & Body Aches Formula contains an antihistamine, a decongestant, an analgesic/antipyretic, and a cough suppressant.

The antihistamine in Alka-Seltzer Plus Flu & Body Aches Formula is chlorpheniramine maleate. Antihistamines block the release of histamine in the body, relieving the sneezing and itching that often occur with colds and allergies. They can also aid in stopping a runny nose by reducing the secretions caused by histamine release.

Decongestants relieve nasal congestion by narrowing or constricting blood vessels in the nose, reducing the blood supplied to the nose, and decreasing the swelling of nasal mucous membranes. Unlike topical decongestants (decongestant nasal sprays), which act locally on blood vessels of the nose, oral decongestants constrict blood vessels throughout the body.

Acetaminophen, the analgesic/antipyretic ingredient, provides effective relief from the aches and fever associated with a cold or the flu.

Dextromethorphan suppresses the cough reflex by acting directly on the cough center in the brain. Unlike some antitussives, it does not depress breathing and has a low potential for addiction.

Alka-Seltzer Plus Flu & Body Aches Formula will not cure or prevent colds or flu. The best you can hope for is temporary relief of symptoms.

Cautions and Warnings

Do not take Alka-Seltzer Plus Flu & Body Aches Formula for more than 7 consecutive days, or 3 consecutive days in the presence of fever, unless under the supervision of a doctor.

Do not exceed the recommended daily dosage of Alka-Seltzer Plus Flu & Body Aches Formula.

If a severe sore throat persists for longer than 2 days, or is accompanied by fever, headache, nausea, or vomiting, consult your doctor immediately.

If your cough lasts longer than 7 days, is recurrent, or is accompanied by fever, rash, or persistent headache, call your doctor. A persistent cough may be a sign of a more serious condition.

If you experience fever, rash, or persistent headache while taking Alka-Seltzer Plus Flu & Body Aches Formula, stop taking it and call your doctor immediately.

If you have hyperthyroidism, glaucoma, heart disease, high blood pressure, an enlarged prostate, or diabetes, you should take Alka-Seltzer Plus Flu & Body Aches Formula only under the supervision of a doctor, because it can aggravate these conditions. When used by individuals with diabetes, phenylpropanolamine may increase blood sugar.

Unless directed by a doctor, Alka-Seltzer Plus Flu & Body Aches Formula should not be used by people who have asthma or a chronic breathing problem such as emphysema or bronchitis.

The effects of Alka-Seltzer Plus Flu & Body Aches Formula on the central nervous system (CNS) can make you feel sleepy or reduce your concentration. Your ability to perform activities that require your full alertness and coordination, such as driving a motor vehicle or operating machinery, may be affected. Drinking alcohol while you are taking Alka-Seltzer Plus Flu & Body Aches Formula can add to these effects.

Acetaminophen can cause liver toxicity in doses exceeding 4 grams per day. Use Alka-Seltzer Plus Flu & Body Aches Formula with caution if you have kidney or liver disease or viral infection of the liver. People with liver disease who are taking other hepatotoxic drugs, who do not eat regularly, and who drink alcohol (even moderately) are especially at risk. You should avoid alcohol and fasting if you take Alka-Seltzer Plus Flu & Body Aches Formula regularly.

Phenylketonurics (people who cannot digest the amino acid phenylalanine) should be aware that Alka-Seltzer Plus Flu & Body Aches Formula contains aspartame (NutraSweet), which breaks down in the gastrointestinal tract to phenylalanine.

Because productive coughing (coughing that brings up mucus) actually helps relieve the underlying condition, some doctors do not believe that suppressing a productive cough makes good sense. However, a severe cough can interfere with sleep, and loss of sleep can contribute to the severity and duration of an illness. For that reason, the most appropriate use of cough suppressants may be to relieve dry cough, especially at night.

Unless directed by your doctor, do not take Alka-Seltzer Plus Flu & Body Aches Formula if you have a chronic cough, such as that associated with smoking, asthma, chronic bronchitis, or emphysema, or a cough associated with excessive mucus.

Alka-Seltzer effervescent products are very high in sodium. If you must restrict your sodium intake because of high blood pressure, heart failure, or kidney failure, consider taking another medication for relief of your symptoms.

Possible Side Effects

- ▼ Most common: nervousness, restlessness, insomnia, drowsiness, dizziness, lightheadedness, poor coordination, headache, and upset stomach.
- ▼ Less common: increased blood pressure; increased or irregular heart rate; heart palpitations; dry eyes, nose, and mouth; blurred vision; difficulty urinating; irritability (at high doses); and loss of appetite.

Possible Side Effects *(continued)*

▼ Rare: nausea, extreme fatigue, rashes, hives, sore throat, fever, unexplained bleeding or bruising, anemia, yellowing of the skin or eyes, blood in the urine, painful or frequent urination, decreased output of urine volume, severe headache, feelings of tightness in the chest, greatly elevated blood pressure, and rapid heartbeat.

Drug Interactions

• The antihistamine ingredient in Alka-Seltzer Plus Flu & Body Aches Formula can enhance the effect of other drugs that depress the CNS, including barbiturates, tranquilizers, sleeping medications, and alcohol (present in many OTC preparations). If you are taking other depressant drugs, check with your doctor before you take Alka-Seltzer Plus Flu & Body Aches Formula.

• Antihistamines can affect the results of skin and blood tests. Notify your health care professional before scheduling these tests if you are taking Alka-Seltzer Plus Flu & Body Aches Formula.

• Alka-Seltzer Plus Flu & Body Aches Formula should not be used at the same time as a monoamine oxidase inhibitor (MAOI) or within 2 weeks of stopping treatment with an MAOI. MAOIs are used to treat depression, other psychiatric or emotional conditions, and Parkinson's disease. If you are not sure whether you are or have been taking an MAOI, check with your doctor or pharmacist before you use Alka-Seltzer Plus Flu & Body Aches Formula

• Taking Alka-Seltzer Plus Flu & Body Aches Formula along with another decongestant can increase the risk of adverse effects and toxicity. If you are taking another decongestant, do not take Alka-Seltzer Plus Flu & Body Aches Formula without first asking your doctor.

• The effects of the decongestant in Alka-Seltzer Plus Flu & Body Aches Formula may combine with those of caffeine, a CNS stimulant found in many prescription and OTC drugs. This combination can cause disorientation, delirium, and other side effects.

• The effects of the acetaminophen in Alka-Seltzer Plus Flu & Body Aches Formula may be reduced by long-term use or large doses of barbiturate drugs; carbamazepine, an anticonvulsant; phenytoin (and other similar drugs), used to treat epilepsy; rifampin, an antitubercular drug; and sulfinpyrazone, an antigout medication. These drugs may also increase the chances of liver toxicity if taken with acetaminophen. Taking Alka-Seltzer Plus Flu & Body Aches Formula with the antitubercular drug isoniazid may also increase the risk of liver damage.

• If Alka-Seltzer Plus Flu & Body Aches Formula is taken with an anticoagulant such as warfarin, it may increase the blood-thinning effect of the anticoagulant agent. This does not occur with occasional use.

• Avoid alcohol while taking Alka-Seltzer Plus Flu & Body Aches Formula. (Be aware that alcohol is found in many OTC preparations.) Alcohol may contribute to the risk of liver damage associated with acetominophen; alcohol also increases the sedative effects of Alka-Seltzer Plus Flu & Body Aches Formula (see "Cautions and Warnings").

Food Interactions

Decongestants interact adversely with caffeine (see "Drug Interactions"), which is found in many popular beverages, including coffee, tea, and cola, and in chocolate.

Usual Dose

Each tablet contains 325 mg of acetaminophen, 10 mg of dextromethorphan, 20 mg of phenylpropanolamine, and 2 mg of chlorpheniramine maleate.

Adult and Child (age 12 and over): Take 2 tablets dissolved in approximately 4 oz. of water every 4 hours, not to exceed 8 tablets in a 24-hour period.

Child (under age 12): not recommended unless directed by your doctor.

Overdosage

Symptoms of overdose include nausea, vomiting, abdominal pain, low blood pressure, fever, flushed face, dry mouth, dilated pupils, blurred vision, rapid rolling of the eyeballs, loss of muscle coordination, confusion, excitability, shallow breathing, hallucinations, dizziness, drowsiness, stupor, coma, toxic psychosis, seizures, urinary retention, yellowing of the skin and eyes, and liver damage. Symptoms may develop within 30 minutes, but may not be seen for as long as 2 days after the overdose.

Even if the victim is not displaying any of the symptoms listed above, do the following in case of accidental overdose: If the victim is unconscious or having convulsions, call for an ambulance immediately. If you take the victim to an emergency room, be sure to bring the bottle or container with you. If the victim is conscious, call your local poison control center or a health care professional. The poison control center may suggest inducing vomiting with ipecac syrup (available without a prescription at any pharmacy). DO NOT induce vomiting unless specifically instructed to do so.

Special Populations

Pregnancy/Breast-feeding

Antihistamines are not recommended for use during pregnancy unless directed by your doctor. Antihistamines, decongestants, and acetaminophen are known to pass into the breast milk of nursing mothers and may cause side effects in infants. Check with your doctor before taking Alka-Seltzer Plus Flu & Body Aches Formula if you are or might be pregnant, or if you are breast-feeding.

Infants/Children

Children may be more susceptible to the side effects of Alka-Seltzer Plus Flu & Body Aches Formula. They are also more susceptible to accidental antihistamine overdose. Do not give Alka-Seltzer Plus Flu & Body Aches Formula to a child under 12 unless directed by your doctor.

Seniors

Older persons may be more sensitive to the side effects of antihistamines and decongestants. They may experience nervousness, irritability, blurred vision, constipation, urinary retention, confusion, restlessness, dizziness, sedation, hallucinations, seizures, and low blood pressure. Most mild reactions may be handled by either lowering the dose or by switching to another product.

Seniors taking Alka-Seltzer Plus Flu & Body Aches Formula should be especially cautious about the amount of caffeine they ingest (see "Drug Interactions").

Brand Names

Alka-Seltzer Plus Flu & BodyAches Liqui-Gels

(AL-kuh-SELTZ-er)

Sudafed Severe Cold Formula

(SOO-dah-fed)

Tylenol Cold Non Drowsy Medication **(TYE-leh-nol)**

Tylenol Flu Maximum Strength Gelcaps

Generic Ingredients

Acetaminophen
Dextromethorphan
Pseudoephedrine

Type of Drug

Decongestant, analgesic (pain reliever), antipyretic (fever reducer), and antitussive (cough suppressant).

Used for

Temporary relief of nasal and sinus congestion, minor sore throat, headache, body aches, fever, and cough associated with colds and flu.

General Information

Some OTC products use a combination of drugs to relieve symptoms that can accompany colds and flu. Alka-Seltzer Plus Flu & BodyAches Liqui-Gels, Sudafed Severe Cold Formula, Tylenol Cold Non Drowsy Medication, and Tylenol Flu Maximum Strength Gelcaps contain a decongestant, an analgesic/antipyretic to reduce pain and fever, and an antitussive to suppress cough.

The decongestant ingredient in these products is pseudoephedrine, an oral decongestant. Decongestants relieve nasal congestion by narrowing or constricting blood vessels in the nose, which reduces the blood supplied to the nose and decreases the swelling of nasal mucous membranes. Unlike topical decongestants (decongestant nasal sprays) that act on local blood vessels, oral decongestants may constrict blood vessels throughout the body.

The analgesic/antipyretic ingredient in these products is acetaminophen. Acetaminophen provides effective relief from the aches and fever associated with a cold or the flu.

The cough suppressant in these products is dextromethorphan, a common antitussive in OTC cough preparations. Dextromethorphan suppresses the cough reflex by acting directly on the cough center in the brain. However, unlike some antitussives, it does not depress breathing. It also has a low potential for addiction.

These products will not cure or prevent colds or flu. The best you can hope for is symptomatic relief. Colds will usually go away in 1 to 2 weeks whether they are treated or not.

Cautions and Warnings

If symptoms do not improve while taking Alka-Seltzer Plus Cold Medicine Liqui-Gels, Sudafed Severe Cold Formula, Tylenol Cold Non Drowsy Medication, or Tylenol Flu Maximum Strength Gelcaps for 7 consecutive days, or 3 consecutive days in the presence of fever, see your doctor.

If a severe sore throat persists for longer than 2 days, or is accompanied by fever, headache, nausea, or vomiting, consult a doctor immediately.

If a cough lasts longer than 7 days, or keeps coming back, consult your doctor. A persistent cough may be the sign of a more serious condition.

Do not exceed the recommended daily dosage of these products.

If you experience fever, rash, or persistent headache while taking these products, stop taking them immediately and call your doctor.

These products should be used with caution by people with hyperthyroidism, heart disease, high blood pressure, diabetes, an enlarged prostate, asthma, or liver disease; if you have any of these conditions, ask your doctor before using them.

In doses of more than 4 grams per day, acetaminophen is potentially toxic to the liver. Use these products with caution if you have kidney or liver disease or viral infections of the liver. Studies have shown that the risk of liver damage with acetaminophen is associated with fasting and alcohol use. People with liver disease who are taking other drugs that are potentially damaging to the liver, people who do not eat regularly, or who drink alcohol (even moderately) are especially at risk. If you take these products regularly, avoid drinking alcohol and/or fasting.

Because productive coughing (coughing that brings up mucus) actually helps relieve the underlying condition, some doctors do not believe that suppressing a productive cough makes good sense. However, a severe cough can interfere with sleep, and loss of sleep can contribute to the severity and duration of an illness. In the balance, the most appropriate use of cough suppressants may be to relieve a dry, nonproductive cough, especially at night.

Unless directed by your doctor, do not use these products if you have a chronic cough, such as that associated with smoking, asthma, chronic bronchitis, or emphysema, or for coughs associated with excessive mucus.

Dextromethorphan, the antitussive ingredient in these products, is not recommended for people confined to bed rest or under sedation.

Possible Side Effects

▼ Most common: lightheadedness, restlessness, nervousness, excitability, sleeplessness, dizziness, weakness, drowsiness, and headache.

▼ Less common: increased blood pressure, increased or irregular heart rate, and heart palpitations.

▼ Rare: nausea, difficulty breathing, anxiety, extreme fatigue, rashes, hives, sore throat, fever, unexplained bleeding or bruising, anemia, yellowing of the skin or eyes, blood in the urine, painful or frequent urination, decreased output of urine volume, tremor, hallucinations, seizures, and cardiovascular collapse.

Drug Interactions

• Alka-Seltzer Plus Flu & BodyAches Liqui-Gels, Sudafed Severe Cold Formula, Tylenol Cold Non Drowsy Medication, or Tylenol Flu Maximum Strength Gelcaps should not be used at the same time as a monoamine oxidase inhibitor (MAOI) or within 2 weeks of stopping treatment with an MAOI. MAOIs are used to treat depression, other psychiatric or emotional conditions, and Parkinson's disease. If you are not sure whether you are or have been taking an MAOI, check with your doctor or pharmacist before you use these products.

• The effects of the decongestant in these products may combine with those of caffeine, a central nervous system stimulant found in many prescription and OTC drugs. This combination can cause disorientation, delirium, and other side effects.

• Taking these products along with another decongestant can increase the risk of adverse effects and toxicity; if you are taking another decongestant, do not use these products without first asking your doctor.

• The effect of the acetaminophen in these products may be reduced by long-term use or large doses of barbiturate drugs; the anticonvulsants carbamazepine and phenytoin (and other similar drugs); rifampin, used to treat tuberculosis (TB); and sulfinpyrazone, used to treat gout. These drugs may also increase the chances of liver toxicity if taken with acetaminophen. Chronically taking large doses of acetaminophen with isoniazid (used to treat TB) may increase the risk of liver damage.

• If these products are taken with an anticoagulant such as warfarin, the acetaminophen in them may increase the blood-thinning effect of the anticoagulant agent. This does not occur with occasional use.

• Avoid alcohol while taking these products. (Be aware that alcohol is found in many OTC preparations.) Alcohol may contribute to liver damage associated with acetaminophen (see "Cautions and Warnings").

Food Interactions

The decongestant in Alka-Seltzer Plus Flu & Body Aches Liqui-Gels, Sudafed Severe Cold Formula, Tylenol Cold Non Drowsy Medication, and Tylenol Flu Maximum Strength Gelcaps interacts adversely with caffeine (see "Drug Interactions"), which is found in many popular beverages, including coffee, tea, and cola, and in chocolate.

Usual Dose

Alka-Seltzer Plus Flu & Body Aches Liqui-Gels
Each softgel contains 30 mg of pseudoephedrine, 250 mg of acetaminophen, and 10 mg of dextromethorphan.

Adult and Child (age 12 and over): 2 softgels every 4 hours. Do not exceed 8 softgels in a 24-hour period.

Child (age 6–12): 1 softgel every 4 hours. Do not exceed 4 softgels in a 24-hour period.

Child (under age 6): Consult your doctor.

Sudafed Severe Cold Formula
Each caplet or tablet contains 30 mg of pseudoephedrine, 500 mg of acetaminophen, and 15 mg of dextromethorphan.

Adult and Child (age 12 and over): 2 caplets or tablets every 6 hours. Do not exceed 8 caplets or tablets in a 24-hour period.

Child (under age 12): not recommended unless directed by your doctor.

Tylenol Cold Non Drowsy Medication
Each caplet or gelcap contains 30 mg of pseudoephedrine, 325 mg of acetaminophen, and 15 mg of dextromethorphan.

Adult and Child (age 12 and over): 2 caplets or gelcaps every 6 hours. Do not exceed 8 caplets or gelcaps in a 24-hour period.

Child (age 6–11): 1 caplet or gelcap every 6 hours. Do not exceed 4 caplets or gelcaps in a 24-hour period.

Child (under age 6): not recommended unless directed by your doctor.

Tylenol Flu Maximum Strength Gelcaps
Each gelcap contains 30 mg of pseudoephedrine, 500 mg of acetaminophen, and 15 mg of dextromethorphan.

Adult and Child (age 12 and over): 2 gelcaps every 6 hours. Do not exceed 8 gelcaps in a 24-hour period.

Child (under age 12): not recommended unless directed by your doctor.

Overdosage

Symptoms of overdose include nausea, vomiting, abdominal pain, urinary retention, low blood pressure, shallow breathing, blurred vision, rapid rolling of the eyeballs, loss of muscle coordination, confusion, hallucinations, drowsiness, dizziness, coma, yellowing of the skin and eyes, and liver damage. Symptoms may develop within 30 minutes, or may not be seen for as long as 2 days after the overdose.

Even if the victim is not displaying any of the symptoms listed above, do the following in case of accidental overdose: If the victim is unconscious or having convulsions, call for an ambulance immediately. If you take the victim to an emergency room, be sure to bring the bottle or container with you. If the victim is conscious, call your local poison control center or a health care professional. The poison control center may suggest inducing vomiting with ipecac syrup (available without a prescription at any pharmacy). DO NOT induce vomiting unless specifically instructed to do so.

Special Populations

Pregnancy/Breast-feeding

Alka-Seltzer Plus Flu & Body Aches Liqui-Gels, Sudafed Severe Cold Formula, Tylenol Cold Non Drowsy Medication, and Tylenol Flu Maximum Strength Gelcaps are not recommended for use during pregnancy unless directed by your doctor. Decongestants and acetaminophen are known to pass into the breast milk of nursing mothers and may cause side effects in infants. Check with your doctor before taking these products if you are or might be pregnant, or if you are breast-feeding.

Infants/Children

Unless directed by your doctor, do not give Alka-Seltzer Plus Flu & Body Aches Liqui-Gels or Tylenol Cold Non Drowsy Medication to a child under age 6, and do not give Sudafed Severe Cold Formula or Tylenol Flu Maximum Strength Gelcaps to a child under age 12.

Seniors

Older persons may be more sensitive to the side effects of these products. They may experience nervousness, irritability, restlessness, dizziness, sedation, hallucinations, seizures, and low blood pressure. Most mild reactions may be handled by either lowering your dose or trying another product.

Seniors taking these products should be especially cautious about the amount of caffeine they ingest (see "Drug Interactions").

Brand Name

Alka-Seltzer Plus Night-Time Cold Medicine Effervescent Tablets

(AL-kuh-SELTZ-er)

Generic Ingredients

Aspirin
Dextromethorphan
Doxylamine succinate
Phenylpropanolamine

Type of drug

Antihistamine, decongestant, analgesic (pain reliever), antipyretic (fever reducer), and antitussive (cough suppressant).

Used for

Temporary relief of runny nose, sneezing, nasal and sinus congestion, minor sore throat, headache, body aches, fever, and cough associated with colds and flu.

General Information

Some OTC products use a combination of drugs to relieve symptoms that can accompany colds and flu. Alka-Seltzer Plus Night-Time Cold Medicine contains an antihistamine, a decongestant, an NSAID/analgesic/antipyretic to reduce pain and fever, and an antitussive to suppress cough.

The antihistamine ingredient in Alka-Seltzer Plus Night-Time Cold Medicine is doxylamine succinate. Antihistamines block the release of histamine in the body, relieving the sneezing and itching that often occurs with colds. They can also aid in stopping a runny nose by reducing the secretions caused by histamine release. Doxylamine is also used as a sleep aid in OTC preparations.

The decongestant ingredient in Alka-Seltzer Plus Night-Time Cold Medicine is phenylpropanolamine, an oral decongestant. Decongestants relieve nasal congestion by narrowing or constricting blood vessels in the nose, which reduces the blood supplied to the nose and decreases the swelling of nasal mucous membranes. Unlike topical decongestants (decongestant nasal sprays) that act on local blood vessels, oral decongestants may constrict blood vessels throughout the body.

The analgesic/antipyretic ingredient in Alka-Seltzer Plus Night-Time Cold Medicine is aspirin. Aspirin is classified as an NSAID, a group of drugs that reduce inflammation and pain. Aspirin is also a member of the group of drugs called salicylates. Aspirin reduces inflammation, relieves pain, and reduces fever.

Aspirin's effects on pain and inflammation are thought to be related to its ability to prevent the manufacture of complex hormones called prostaglandins, which sensitize pain receptors and stimulate the inflammatory response. Of all the salicylates, aspirin has the greatest effect on prostaglandin production. Aspirin reduces fever by acting on the heat-regulating center in the brain. This causes the blood vessels in the skin to dilate which allows heat to leave the body more rapidly.

The cough suppressant in Alka-Seltzer Plus Night-Time Cold Medicine is dextromethorphan. Dextromethorphan suppresses the cough reflex by acting directly on the cough center in the brain. Unlike some antitussives, it does not depress breathing and has a low potential for addiction.

Alka-Seltzer Plus Night-Time Cold Medicine will not cure or prevent colds or allergies. The best you can hope for is symptomatic relief. Colds will usually go away in 1 to 2 weeks whether they are treated or not.

Cautions and Warnings

Do not take Alka-Seltzer Plus Night-Time Cold Medicine for 7 days continuously, or 3 days continuously in the presence of fever. If symptoms do not improve, see your doctor.

If a severe sore throat persists for longer than 2 days, or is accompanied by fever, headache, nausea, or vomiting, consult a doctor immediately.

If a cough lasts longer than 7 days, or keeps coming back, consult your doctor. A persistent cough may be the sign of a more serious condition.

Do not exceed the recommended daily dosage of Alka-Seltzer Plus Night-Time Cold Medicine.

If you experience fever, rash, or persistent headache while taking Alka-Seltzer Plus Night-Time Cold Medicine, stop taking it immediately and call your doctor.

If dizziness, hearing loss, ringing or buzzing in the ears, or continuous stomach pain occur while using Alka-Seltzer Plus Night-Time Cold Medicine, stop taking the drug immediately and call your doctor.

Alka-Seltzer Plus Night-Time Cold Medicine should be used with caution if you have a condition that causes breathing problems, such as emphysema, chronic bronchitis, asthma, nasal polyps, or rhinitis. Consult your doctor before using Alka-Seltzer Plus Night-Time Cold Medicine if you have any of these conditions.

Alka-Seltzer Plus Night-Time Cold Medicine should be used with caution by people with glaucoma, hyperthyroidism, heart disease, high blood pressure, diabetes, an enlarged prostate, or liver disease. If you have any of these conditions, ask your doctor before using Alka-Seltzer Plus Night-Time Cold Medicine.

The antihistamine ingredient in Alka-Seltzer Plus Night-Time Cold Medicine acts as a depressant on the central nervous system (CNS), and can cause sleepiness or grogginess and interfere with the ability to concentrate. Your ability to perform activities that require your full alertness and coordination, such as driving a motor vehicle or operating machinery, may be affected. Refrain from drinking alcohol while you are taking Alka-Seltzer Plus Night-Time Cold Medicine, because alcohol aggravates these effects.

Children with the flu or chicken pox who are given aspirin or other salicylates may develop Reye's syndrome, a life-threatening condition characterized by vomiting, progressive damage to the central nervous system, liver injury, and abnormally low blood sugar. Up to 30% of children who develop Reye's syndrome die, and permanent brain damage is possible in those who survive. Because of the risk of Reye's syndrome, do not give Alka-Seltzer Plus Night-Time Cold Medicine to children under age 16.

Aspirin is associated with gastrointestinal (GI) irritation, erosion and bleeding. Unless directed by a doctor, people with GI bleeding or a history of peptic ulcers should not take Alka-Seltzer Plus Night-Time Cold Medicine. Be aware that the risk of aspirin-related ulcers is increased by alcohol.

People with liver or kidney damage should avoid aspirin.

To reduce the risk of bleeding, aspirin should be avoided prior to surgery. Ask your doctor how long before surgery you should refrain from taking Alka-Seltzer Plus Night-Time

Cold Medicine and any other aspirin product.

Because productive coughing (coughing that brings up mucus) actually helps relieve the underlying condition, some doctors do not believe that suppressing a productive cough makes good sense. However, a severe cough can interfere with sleep, and loss of sleep can contribute to the severity and duration of an illness. In the balance, the most appropriate use of cough suppressants may be to relieve a dry, nonproductive cough, especially at night.

Unless directed by your doctor, do not take Alka-Seltzer Plus Night-Time Cold Medicine if you have a chronic cough, such as that associated with smoking, asthma, chronic bronchitis, or emphysema, or for coughs associated with excessive mucus.

Dextromethorphan, the antitussive ingredient in Alka-Seltzer Plus Night-Time Cold Medicine, is not recommended for people confined to bed rest or under sedation.

Alka-Seltzer Plus Night-Time Cold Medicine is high in sodium, which can lead to fluid retention. Do not take Alka-Seltzer Plus Night-Time Cold Medicine if you must restrict your sodium intake because of high blood pressure, heart disease, or kidney disease.

Phenylketonurics (people who cannot digest phenylalanine) should be aware that Alka-Seltzer Plus Night-Time Cold Medicine contains aspartame (NutraSweet), which breaks down in the GI tract to phenylalanine.

Possible Side Effects

- ▼ Most common: restlessness, nervousness, sleeplessness or drowsiness, sedation, excitability, dizziness, poor coordination, upset stomach, nausea, heartburn, and small amounts of blood in the stool.
- ▼ Less common: dry eyes, nose, and mouth; blurred vision; difficulty urinating; irritability (at high doses); increased blood pressure; increased or irregular heart rate; heart palpitations, and loss of appetite.
- ▼ Rare: nausea, severe headache, feelings of tightness in the chest, greatly elevated blood pressure, heart contractions, hives, rash, fever, thirst, and liver damage.

Drug Interactions

• The antihistamine ingredient in Alka-Seltzer Plus Night-Time Cold Medicine can enhance the effect of other drugs that depress the CNS, such as barbiturates, tranquilizers, sleeping medications, and alcohol (present in many OTC preparations). If you are taking other depressant drugs, check with your doctor before taking this product. Avoid drinking alcohol if you are taking Alka-Seltzer Plus Night-Time Cold Medicine.

• Antihistamines can also affect the results of skin and blood tests. Notify your health care professional before scheduling these tests if you are taking Alka-Seltzer Plus Night-Time Cold Medicine.

• Alka-Seltzer Plus Night-Time Cold Medicine should not be used at the same time as a monoamine oxidase inhibitor (MAOI) or within 2 weeks of stopping treatment with an MAOI. MAOIs are used to treat depression, other psychiatric or emotional conditions, and Parkinson's disease. If you are not sure whether you are or have been taking an MAOI, check with your doctor or pharmacist before using Alka-Seltzer Plus Night-Time Cold Medicine.

• The effects of the decongestant in Alka-Seltzer Plus Night-Time Cold Medicine may combine with those of caffeine, a CNS stimulant found in many prescription and OTC drugs. This combination can cause disorientation, delirium, and other side effects.

• Taking Alka-Seltzer Plus Night-Time Cold Medicine along with another decongestant can increase the risk of adverse effects and toxicity; if you are taking another decongestant, do not use Alka-Seltzer Plus Night-Time Cold Medicine without first asking your doctor.

• Alka-Seltzer Plus Night-Time Cold Medicine should not be taken by individuals currently taking methotrexate, used to treat cancer, severe psoriasis, severe rheumatoid arthritis, and to induce abortion; or valproic acid, an anticonvulsant. The aspirin in Alka-Seltzer Plus Night-Time Cold Medicine can increase the toxicity of these drugs.

• Aspirin should also not be taken with anticoagulant (blood-thinning) drugs, such as warfarin and dicumarol. It will exaggerate the effects of these drugs and increase the risk of abnormal bleeding.

• People with AIDs and AIDs-related complex who take zidovudine (AZT) should avoid using Alka-Seltzer Plus Night-Time Cold Medicine because the aspirin in it may increase the risk of bleeding.

• The possibility of a stomach ulcer is increased if aspirin is taken together with alcoholic beverages; an adrenal corticosteroid, such as hydrocortisone; or phenylbutazone, another NSAID. Taking Alka-Seltzer Plus Night-Time Cold Medicine with another NSAID has no benefit and carries a greatly increased risk of side effects.

• The aspirin in Alka-Seltzer Plus Night-Time Cold Medicine will counteract the effects of the antigout medications probenecid and sulfinpyrazone, and may counteract the effects of angiotensin-converting enzyme (ACE) inhibitors and beta blockers, which work to lower blood pressure. Aspirin may also counteract the effects of some diuretics in people with severe liver disease.

• Combining nitroglycerin tablets and aspirin may lead to an unexpected drop in blood pressure.

Food Interactions

The decongestant in Alka-Seltzer Plus Night-Time Cold Medicine interacts adversely with caffeine (see "Drug Interactions"), which is found in many popular beverages, including coffee, tea, and cola, and in chocolate.

Usual Dose

Each tablet contains 6.25 mg doxylamine, 20 mg of phenylpropanolamine, 500 mg of aspirin, and 15 mg of dextromethorphan.

Adult and Child (age 16 and over): 2 tablets dissolved in 4 oz. of water every 4 hours. Do not exceed 8 tablets in a 24-hour period.

Child (under age 16): not recommended because of the risk of Reye's syndrome (see "Cautions and Warnings").

Overdosage

Symptoms of overdose include nausea, vomiting, urinary retention, shallow breathing, rapid breathing, rapid heartbeat, sweating, fever, thirst, headache, diarrhea, flushed face, dry mouth, ringing or buzzing in the ears, blurred vision, dilated pupils, rapid rolling of the eyeballs, loss of muscle coordination, excitability, confusion, drowsiness, dizziness, hallucinations, seizures, liver or kidney failure, coma, and bleeding.

Even if the victim is not displaying any of the symptoms listed above, do the following in case of accidental overdose: If the victim is unconscious or having convulsions, call for an ambulance immediately. If you take the victim to an emergency room, be sure to bring the bottle or container with you. If the victim is conscious, call your local poison control center or a health care professional. The poison control center may suggest inducing vomiting with ipecac syrup (available without a prescription at any pharmacy). DO NOT induce vomiting unless specifically instructed to do so.

Special Populations

Pregnancy/Breast-feeding

Do not take Alka-Seltzer Plus Night-Time Cold Medicine if you are or might be pregnant.

The active ingredients in Alka-Seltzer Plus Night-Time Cold Medicine have been shown to pass into the breast milk of nursing mothers and may cause side effects in infants. Check with your doctor before taking Alka-Seltzer Plus Night-Time Cold Medicine if you are breast-feeding.

Infants/Children

Aspirin should not be used by children under 16 unless directed by your doctor, because of the risk of Reye's syndrome (see "Cautions and Warnings"). Children are also more susceptible to accidental antihistamine overdose. Do not give Alka-Seltzer Plus Night-Time Cold Medicine to a child under age 16 unless directed by your doctor.

Seniors

Older persons may be more sensitive to the side effects of Alka-Seltzer Plus Night-Time Cold Medicine. They may experience nervousness, irritability, and restlessness. Dizziness, sedation, and low blood pressure may also occur. Older men may experience difficulty in urinating. Most mild reactions may be handled by either lowering your dose or trying another antihistamine/decongestant combination.

Seniors taking Alka-Seltzer Plus Night-Time Cold Medicine should be especially cautious about the amount of caffeine they ingest (see "Drug Interactions").

Older individuals may find aspirin irritating to the stomach, especially in large doses. Older adults with liver disease or severe kidney impairment should not use aspirin.

Brand Names

Alka-Seltzer Plus Night-Time Cold Medicine Liqui-Gels

(AL-kuh-SELTZ-er)

Vicks NyQuil

(VIKS NYE-kwill)

Generic Ingredients

Acetaminophen
Dextromethorphan
Doxylamine succinate
Pseudoephedrine

Type of Drug

Antihistamine, decongestant, analgesic (pain reliever), antipyretic (fever reducer), and antitussive (cough suppressant).

Used for

Temporary relief of runny nose, sneezing, nasal and sinus congestion, minor sore throat, headache, body ache, fever, and cough associated with colds and flu.

General Information

Some OTC products use a combination of drugs to relieve symptoms that can accompany colds and flu. Alka-Seltzer Plus Night-Time Cold Medicine Liqui-Gels and Vicks NyQuil contain an antihistamine, a decongestant, an analgesic/antipyretic to reduce pain and fever, and an antitussive to suppress cough.

The antihistamine ingredient in Alka-Seltzer Plus Night-Time Cold and NyQuil is doxylamine succinate. Antihistamines block the release of histamine in the body, relieving the sneezing and itching that often occurs with colds and flu. They can also aid in stopping a runny nose by reducing the secretions caused by histamine release.

The decongestant ingredient in these products is pseudoephedrine, an oral decongestant. Decongestants relieve nasal congestion by narrowing or constricting blood vessels in the nose, which reduces the blood supplied to the nose and decreases the swelling of nasal mucous membranes. Unlike topical decongestants (decongestant nasal sprays) that act on local blood vessels, oral decongestants may constrict blood vessels throughout the body.

The analgesic/antipyretic ingredient in Alka-Seltzer Plus Night-Time Cold and NyQuil is acetaminophen. Acetaminophen provides effective relief from the aches and fever associated with a cold or the flu.

The cough suppressant in these products is dextromethorphan, a common antitussive in OTC cough preparations. Dextromethorphan suppresses the cough reflex by acting directly on the cough center in the brain. However, unlike some antitussives, it does not depress breathing. It also has a low potential for addiction.

Alka-Seltzer Plus Night-Time Cold and NyQuil will not cure or prevent colds or flu. The best you can hope for is symptomatic relief. Colds will usually go away in 1 to 2 weeks whether they are treated or not.

Cautions and Warnings

Do not take Alka-Seltzer Plus Night-Time Cold or NyQuil for more than 7 days continuously. If fever is present do not take them for more than 3 days continuously. If symptoms do not improve, see your doctor.

If a severe sore throat persists for longer than 2 days, or is accompanied by fever, headache, nausea, or vomiting, consult a doctor immediately.

If a cough lasts longer than 7 days, or keeps coming back, consult your doctor. A persistent cough may be the sign of a more serious condition.

Do not exceed the recommended daily dosage of these products.

If you experience fever, rash, or persistent headache while taking these products, stop taking them immediately and call your doctor.

Alka-Seltzer Plus Night-Time Cold and NyQuil should be used with caution if you have a condition that causes breathing problems, such as emphysema, chronic bronchitis, or asthma: if you have any of these conditions, ask your doctor before using these products.

These products should be used with caution by people with glaucoma, hyperthyroidism, heart disease, high blood pressure, diabetes, an enlarged prostate, or liver disease. If you have any of these conditions, ask your doctor before using Alka-Seltzer Plus Night-Time Cold or NyQuil.

The antihistamine ingredient in these products acts as a depressant on the central nervous system (CNS), and can cause sleepiness or grogginess and interfere with the ability to concentrate. Your ability to perform activities that require your full alertness and coordination, such as driving a motor vehicle or operating machinery, may be affected. Refrain from drinking alcohol while you are taking these products because alcohol aggravates these effects.

In doses of more than 4 grams per day, acetaminophen is potentially toxic to the liver. Use these products with caution if you have kidney or liver disease or viral infections of the liver. Studies have shown that the risk of liver damage with acetaminophen is associated with fasting and alcohol use. People with liver disease who are taking other drugs that are potentially damaging to the liver, people who do not eat regularly, or who drink alcohol (even moderately) are especially at risk. If you take Alka-Seltzer Plus Night-Time Cold or NyQuil regularly, avoid drinking alcohol and/or fasting.

Because productive coughing (coughing that brings up mucus) actually helps relieve the underlying condition, some doctors do not believe that suppressing a productive cough makes good sense. However, a severe cough can interfere with sleep, and loss of sleep can contribute to the severity and duration of an illness. In the balance, the most appropriate use of cough suppressants may be to relieve a dry, nonproductive cough, especially at night.

Unless directed by your doctor, do not take these products if you have a chronic cough, such as that associated with smoking, asthma, chronic bronchitis, or emphysema, or for coughs associated with excess mucus.

Dextromethorphan, the antitussive ingredient in these products, is not recommended for people confined to bed rest or under sedation.

Possible Side Effects

- ▼ Most common: lightheadedness, restlessness, nervousness, sleeplessness, sedation, excitability, dizziness, poor coordination, headache, and upset stomach.
- ▼ Less common: dry eyes, nose, and mouth; blurred vision; difficulty urinating; irritability (at high doses); increased blood pressure; and increased or irregular heart rate.
- ▼ Rare: nausea, difficulty breathing, anxiety, extreme fatigue, rashes, hives, sore throat, fever, unexplained bleeding or bruising, anemia, yellowing of the skin or eyes, blood in the urine, painful or frequent urination, decreased output of urine volume, tremor, hallucinations, seizures, and cardiovascular collapse.

Drug Interactions

• The antihistamine ingredient in Alka Seltzer Plus Night-Time Cold and NyQuil can enhance the effect of other drugs that depress the CNS, such as barbiturates, tranquilizers, sleeping medications, and alcohol (present in many OTC preparations). If you are taking other depressant drugs, check with your doctor before taking Alka-Seltzer Plus Night-Time Cold or NyQuil.

• Antihistamines can also affect the results of skin and blood tests. Notify your health care professional before scheduling these tests if you are taking these products.

• These products should not be used at the same time as a monoamine oxidase inhibitor (MAOI) or within 2 weeks of stopping treatment with an MAOI. MAOIs are used to treat depression, other psychiatric or emotional conditions, and Parkinson's disease. If you are not sure whether you are or have been taking an MAOI, check with your doctor or pharmacist before you use Alka-Seltzer Plus Night-Time Cold or NyQuil.

• The effects of pseudoephedrine, the decongestant in these products, may combine with those of caffeine, a CNS stimulant found in many prescription and OTC drugs. This combination can cause disorientation, delirium, and other side effects.

• Taking these products along with another decongestant can increase the risk of adverse effects and toxicity. If you are taking another decongestant, do not use Alka Seltzer Plus Night-Time Cold or NyQuil without first asking your doctor.

• The effect of the acetaminophen in these products may be reduced by long-term use or large doses of barbiturate drugs; the anticonvulsants carbamazepine and phenytoin (and other similar drugs); rifampin, used to treat tuberculosis (TB); and sulfinpyrazone, used to treat gout. These drugs may also increase the chances of liver toxicity if taken with acetaminophen. Chronically taking large doses of acetaminophen with isoniazid (used to treat TB) may also increase the risk of liver damage.

• If these products are taken with an anticoagulant such as warfarin, the acetaminophen in them may increase the blood-thinning effect of the anticoagulant agent. This does not occur with occasional use.

• Avoid alcohol while taking Alka-Seltzer Plus Night-Time Cold or NyQuil. (Be aware that alcohol is found in many OTC preparations.) Alcohol may contribute to the risk of liver damage associated with acetaminophen; it also increases the sedative effects of antihistamines (see "Cautions and Warnings").

Food Interactions

The decongestant in these products interacts adversely with caffeine (see "Drug Interactions"), which is found in many popular beverages, including coffee, tea, and cola, and in chocolate.

Usual Dose

Alka-Seltzer Plus Night-Time Cold Medicine Liqui-Gels
Each softgel contains 6.25 mg of doxylamine, 30 mg of pseudoephedrine, 250 mg of acetaminophen, and 10 mg of dextromethorphan.

Adult and Child (age 12 and over): 2 softgels at bedtime. Do not exceed 2 softgels in a 24-hour period.

Child (under age 12): not recommended unless directed by your doctor.

Vicks NyQuil LiquiCaps
Each softgel contains 6.25 mg of doxylamine, 30 mg of pseudoephedrine, 250 mg of acetaminophen, and 10 mg of dextromethorphan.

Adult and Child (age 12 and over): 2 softgels every 4 hours. Do not exceed 8 softgels in a 24-hour period.

Child (under age 12): not recommended unless directed by your doctor.

Vicks NyQuil Liquid
Each 15 ml (1 tsp.) contains 6.25 mg of doxylamine, 30 mg of pseudoephedrine, 500 mg of acetaminophen, and 15 mg of dextromethorphan.

Adult and Child (age 12 and over): 30 ml every 6 hours. Do not exceed 4 doses in a 24-hour period.

Child (under age 12): not recommended unless directed by your doctor.

Overdosage

Symptoms of overdose include nausea, vomiting, abdominal pain, urinary retention, low blood pressure, shallow breathing, fever, flushed face, dry mouth, dilated pupils, blurred vision, rapid rolling of the eyeballs, loss of muscle coordination, confusion, excitability, hallucinations, drowsiness, dizziness, coma, seizures, yellowing of the skin and eyes, and liver damage. Symptoms may develop within 30 minutes, but may not be seen for as long as 2 days after the overdose.

Even if the victim is not displaying any of the symptoms listed above, do the following in case of accidental overdose: If the victim is unconscious or having convulsions, call for an ambulance immediately. If you take the victim to an emergency room, be sure to bring the bottle or container with you. If the victim is conscious, call your local poison control center or a health care professional. The poison control center may suggest inducing vomiting with ipecac syrup (available without a prescription at any pharmacy). DO NOT induce vomiting unless specifically instructed to do so.

Special Populations

Pregnancy/Breast-feeding
Antihistamines are not recommended for use during pregnancy unless directed by your doctor. Antihistamines, decongestants, and acetaminophen are known to pass into the breast milk of nursing mothers and may cause side effects in infants. Check with your doctor before taking Alka-Seltzer Plus Night-Time Cold or NyQuil if you are or might be pregnant, or if you are breast-feeding.

Infants/Children

Children may be more susceptible to the side effects of these products. They are also more susceptible to accidental antihistamine overdose. Unless directed by your doctor, do not give Alka Seltzer Plus Night-Time Cold or NyQuil to a child under age 12.

Seniors

Older persons may be more sensitive to the side effects of these products. They may experience nervousness, irritability, restlessness, dizziness, sedation, urinary retention, low blood pressure, hallucinations, and seizures. Most mild reactions may be handled by either lowering your dose or trying another product.

Seniors taking these products should be especially cautious about the amount of caffeine they ingest (see "Drug Interactions").

Children's Tylenol Cold Multi Symptom Liquid (TYE-leh-nol)

see ***Alka-Seltzer Plus Cold Medicine Liqui-Gels,*** *page 130*

Brand Name

Contac 12 Hour Cold Capsules (CON-tak)

Generic Ingredients

Chlorpheniramine maleate
Phenylpropanolamine

Type of drug

Antihistamine and decongestant.

Used for

Temporary relief of runny nose, sneezing, nasal congestion, itchy and watery eyes, and itching of the nose and throat associated with colds and allergies.

General Information

Some OTC products use a combination of drugs to relieve symptoms that can accompany colds and allergies. Contac contains an antihistamine and a decongestant.

The antihistamine ingredient in Contac is chlorpheniramine maleate. Antihistamines block the release of histamine in the body, relieving the sneezing and itching that often occurs with colds and allergies. They can also aid in stopping a runny nose by reducing the secretions caused by histamine release.

Since histamine is only one of several substances released by the body during an allergic reaction, antihistamines can only reduce about 40% to 60% of allergic symptoms.

The decongestant ingredient in Contac is phenylpropanolamine, an oral decongestant. Decongestants relieve nasal congestion by narrowing or constricting blood vessels in the nose, which reduces the blood supplied to the nose and decreases the swelling of nasal mucous membranes. Unlike topical decongestants (decongestant nasal sprays) that act on local blood vessels, oral decongestants may constrict blood vessels throughout the body.

Contac will not cure or prevent colds or allergies. The best you can hope for is symptomatic relief. Colds will usually go away in 1 to 2 weeks whether they are treated or not.

Cautions and Warnings

Do not take Contac for more than 7 days continuously. If symptoms do not improve or if fever is present, see your doctor.

Do not exceed the recommended daily dosage of Contac.

Contac should be used with caution if you have a condition that causes breathing problems, such as emphysema, chronic bronchitis, or asthma. Its antihistamine ingredient dries the mucous membranes. This in turn can inhibit the ability of the lungs to move or get rid of the excess secretions that these conditions produce.

Contac should be used with caution by people with glaucoma, hyperthyroidism, heart disease, high blood pressure, diabetes, or an enlarged prostate; if you have any of these conditions, ask your doctor before using it.

The antihistamine ingredient in Contac acts as a depressant on the central nervous system (CNS), and can cause sleepiness or grogginess and interfere with the ability to concentrate. Your ability to perform activities that require your full alertness and coordination, such as driving a motor vehicle or operating machinery, may be affected. Refrain from drinking alcohol while you are taking Contac, because alcohol aggravates these effects.

Possible Side Effects

▼ Most common: restlessness, nervousness, sleeplessness or drowsiness, sedation, excitability, dizziness, poor coordination, and upset stomach.

▼ Less common: dry eyes, nose, and mouth; blurred vision; difficulty urinating; irritability (at high doses); increased blood pressure; increased or irregular heart rate; heart palpitations, and loss of appetite.

▼ Rare: severe headache, feelings of tightness in the chest, greatly elevated blood pressure, and heart contractions.

Drug Interactions

• The antihistamine ingredient in Contac can enhance the effect of other drugs that depress the CNS, such as barbiturates, tranquilizers, sleeping medications, and alcohol (present in many OTC preparations). If you are taking other depressant drugs, check with your doctor before taking Contac. Avoid drinking alcohol if you are taking Contac.

• The antihistamine ingredient in Contac can affect the results of skin and blood tests. Notify your health care professional before scheduling these tests if you are taking Contac.

• Contac should not be used at the same time as a monoamine oxidase inhibitor (MAOI) or within 2 weeks of stopping treatment with an MAOI. MAOIs are used to treat depression, other psychiatric or emotional conditions, and Parkinson's disease. If you are not sure whether you are or have been taking an MAOI, check with your doctor or pharmacist before you use Contac.

• The effects of the decongestant in Contac may combine with those of caffeine, a CNS stimulant found in many prescription and OTC drugs. This combination can cause disorientation, delirium, and other side effects.

• Taking Contac along with another decongestant can increase the risk of adverse effects and toxicity; if you are taking another decongestant, do not use Contac without first asking your doctor.

Food Interactions

The decongestant in Contac interacts adversely with caffeine (see "Drug Interactions"), which is found in many popular beverages, including coffee, tea, and cola, and in chocolate.

Usual Dose

If you are taking Contac for allergies, it is best to take it on a schedule rather than as needed because histamine is released almost continuously.

Each Contac Capsule contains 8 mg chlorpheniramine and 75 mg of phenylpropanolamine.

Adult and Child (age 12 and over): 1 capsule every 12 hours. Do not exceed 2 capsules in a 24-hour period.

Child (under age 12): Consult your doctor.

If you forget to take a dose of Contac, do so as soon as you remember. If it is almost time for your next dose, skip the one you forgot and continue with your regular schedule. Do not take a double dose.

Overdosage

Symptoms of overdose in children include dilated pupils, flushed face, dry mouth, fever, excitability, hallucinations, loss of muscle coordination, and seizures.

In adults, severe overdose can cause drowsiness or coma, which may be followed by excitability or seizures. Eventually fluid can build up in the brain; the kidneys may fail, and the heart and lungs stop working, resulting in death. Symptoms may develop within 30 minutes to 2 hours following an overdose, and death may occur within 18 hours.

Even if the victim is not displaying any of the symptoms listed above, do the following in case of accidental overdose: If the victim is unconscious or having convulsions, call for an ambulance immediately. If you take the victim to an emergency room, be sure to bring the bottle or container with you. If the victim is conscious, call your local poison control center or a health care professional. The poison control center may suggest inducing vomiting with ipecac syrup (available without a prescription at any pharmacy). DO NOT induce vomiting unless specifically instructed to do so.

Special Populations

Pregnancy/Breast-feeding

Antihistamines are not recommended for use during pregnancy unless directed by your doctor. Antihistamines and decongestants are known to pass into the breast milk of nursing mothers and may cause side effects in infants. Check with your doctor before taking Contac if you are or might be pregnant, or if you are breast-feeding.

Infants/Children

Children may be more susceptible to the side effects of these products. They are also more susceptible to accidental antihistamine overdose. Do not give Contac to a child under age 12 unless directed by your doctor.

Seniors

Older individuals should not take Contac, which is an extended-release preparation, until they have first tried a short-acting product containing the decongestant phenylpropanolamine and experienced no ill effects.

Older persons may be more sensitive to the side effects of Contac. They may experience nervousness, irritability, and restlessness. Dizziness, sedation, and low blood pressure may also occur. Older men may experience difficulty in urinating. Most mild reactions may be handled by either lowering your dose or trying another antihistamine/decongestant combination.

Seniors taking Contac should be especially cautious about the amount of caffeine they ingest (see "Drug Interactions").

Brand Name

Coricidin D (kor-uh-SEE-din)

Generic Ingredients

Acetaminophen
Chlorpheniramine maleate
Phenylpropanolamine

Type of Drug

Antihistamine, decongestant, analgesic (pain reliever), and antipyretic (fever reducer).

Used for

Temporary relief of runny nose, sneezing, nasal and sinus congestion, headache, body ache, pains, and fever associated with colds and flu.

General Information

Some OTC products use a combination of drugs to relieve symptoms that can accompany colds and flu. Coricidin D contains an antihistamine, a decongestant, and an analgesic/antipyretic to reduce pain and fever.

The antihistamine ingredient in Coricidin is chlorpheniramine maleate. Antihistamines block the release of histamine in the body, relieving the sneezing and itching that often occurs with colds and flu. They can also aid in stopping a runny nose by reducing the secretions caused by histamine release.

The decongestant ingredient in Coricidin is phenylpropanolamine, an oral decongestant. Decongestants relieve nasal congestion by narrowing or constricting blood vessels in the nose. This action reduces the blood supplied to the nose and decreases the swelling of nasal mucous membranes. Unlike topical decongestants (decongestant nasal sprays) that act on local blood vessels, oral decongestants may constrict blood vessels throughout the body.

The analgesic/antipyretic ingredient in Coricidin is acetaminophen. Acetaminophen relieves aches and pains, and reduces fever.

Coricidin will not cure or prevent colds or flu. The best you can hope for is symptomatic relief. Colds will usually go away in 1 to 2 weeks whether they are treated or not.

Cautions and Warnings

Do not take Coricidin for more than 10 days continuously, or more than 3 days continuously in the presence of fever. Children ages 6 to 11 should not take Coricidin for more than 5 days continuously, or 3 days continuously in the presence of fever. If symptoms do not improve, or if congestion lasts longer than 7 days, see your doctor.

Do not exceed the recommended daily dosage of Coricidin.

Coricidin should be used with caution if you have a condition that causes breathing problems, such as emphysema, chronic bronchitis, or asthma. Its antihistamine ingredient dries the mucous membranes. This in turn can inhibit the ability of the lungs to move or get rid of the excess secretions that these conditions produce.

Coricidin should be used with caution by people with glaucoma, hyperthyroidism, heart disease, high blood pressure, diabetes, or an enlarged prostate. If you have any of these conditions, ask your doctor before using Coricidin.

The antihistamine ingredient in Coricidin acts as a depressant on the central nervous system (CNS), and can cause sleepiness or grogginess and interfere with the ability to concentrate. Your ability to perform activities that require your full alertness and coordination, such as driving a motor vehicle or operating machinery, may be affected. Refrain from drinking alcohol while you are taking Coricidin because alcohol aggravates these effects.

In doses of more than 4 grams per day, acetaminophen is potentially toxic to the liver. Use Coricidin with caution if you have kidney or liver disease or viral infections of the liver. Studies have shown that the risk of liver damage with acetaminophen is associated with fasting and alcohol use. People with liver disease who are taking other drugs that are potentially damaging to the liver, people who do not eat regularly, or who drink alcohol (even moderately) are especially at risk. If you take Coricidin regularly, avoid drinking alcohol and/or fasting.

Possible Side Effects

- ▼ Most common: lightheadedness, restlessness, nervousness, sleeplessness, sedation, excitability, dizziness, poor coordination, headache, and upset stomach.
- ▼ Less common: dry eyes, nose, and mouth; blurred vision; difficulty urinating; irritability (at high doses); increased blood pressure; increased or irregular heart rate; and loss of appetite.
- ▼ Rare: extreme fatigue, rashes, hives, sore throat, fever, unexplained bleeding or bruising, anemia, yellowing of the skin or eyes, blood in the urine, painful or frequent urination, decreased output of urine volume, severe headache, feelings of tightness in the chest, greatly elevated blood pressure, and heart contractions.

Drug Interactions

• The antihistamine ingredient in Coricidin can enhance the effect of other drugs that depress the CNS, such as barbiturates, tranquilizers, sleeping medications, and alcohol (present in many OTC preparations). If you are taking other depressant drugs, check with your doctor before taking Coricidin.

• Antihistamines can also affect the results of skin and blood tests. Notify your health care professional before scheduling these tests if you are taking Coricidin.

• Coricidin should not be used at the same time as a monoamine oxidase inhibitor (MAOI) or within 2 weeks of stopping treatment with an MAOI. MAOIs are used to treat depression, other psychiatric or emotional conditions, and Parkinson's disease. If you are not sure whether you are or have been taking an MAOI, check with your doctor or pharmacist before you use Coricidin.

• The effects of phenylpropanolamine, the decongestant in Coricidin may combine with those of caffeine, a CNS stimulant found in many prescription and OTC drugs. This combination can cause disorientation, delirium, and other side effects.

• Taking Coricidin along with another decongestant can increase the risk of adverse effects and toxicity. If you are taking another decongestant, do not use Coricidin without first asking your doctor.

• The effect of the acetaminophen in Coricidin may be reduced by long-term use or large doses of barbiturate drugs; the anticonvulsants carbamazepine and phenytoin (and other similar drugs); rifampin, used to treat tuberculosis (TB); and sulfinpyrazone, used to treat gout. These drugs may also increase the chances of liver toxicity if taken with acetaminophen. Taking chronic, large doses of acetaminophen with isoniazid (used to treat TB) may also increase the risk of liver damage.

• If Coricidin is taken with an anticoagulant such as warfarin, the acetaminophen in them may increase the blood-thinning effect of the anticoagulant agent. This does not occur with occasional use.

• People with AIDS and AIDS-related complex who are taking zidovudine (AZT) may experience increased suppression of bone marrow production if they also take products that contain acetaminophen, such as Coricidin. However, studies have not shown that short-term use (less than 7 days) of acetaminophen increases the risk of bone marrow suppression or causes a decrease in white blood cells in people taking AZT. Contact your doctor for proper monitoring of AZT and acetaminophen interaction.

• Avoid alcohol while taking Coricidin. (Be aware that alcohol is found in many OTC preparations.) Alcohol may contribute to the risk of liver damage associated with acetaminophen; it also increases the sedative effects of antihistamines (see "Cautions and Warnings").

Food Interactions

The decongestant in Coricidin interacts adversely with caffeine (see "Drug Interactions"), which is found in many popular beverages, including coffee, tea, and cola, and in chocolate.

Usual Dose

Each tablet contains 2 mg of chlorpheniramine, 12.5 mg of phenylpropanolamine, and 325 mg of acetaminophen.

Adult and Child (age 12 and over): 2 tablets every 4 hours. Do not exceed 12 tablets in a 24-hour period.

Child (age 6–11): 1 tablet every 4 hours. Do not exceed 5 tablets in a 24-hour period.

Child (under age 6): Consult your doctor.

Overdosage

Symptoms of overdose include nausea, vomiting, abdominal pain, low blood pressure, fever, flushed face, dry mouth, dilated pupils, loss of muscle coordination, confusion, excitability, hallucinations, drowsiness, coma, seizures, yellowing of the skin and eyes, and liver damage. Symptoms may develop within 30 minutes, or may not be seen for as long as 2 days after the overdose.

Even if the victim is not displaying any of the symptoms listed above, do the following in case of accidental overdose: If the victim is unconscious or having convulsions, call for an ambulance immediately. If you take the victim to an emergency room, be sure to bring the bottle or container with you. If the victim is conscious, call your local poison control center or a health care professional. The poison control center may suggest inducing vomiting with ipecac syrup (available without a prescription at any pharmacy). DO NOT induce vomiting unless specifically instructed to do so.

Special Populations

Pregnancy/Breast-feeding
Antihistamines are not recommended for use during pregnancy unless directed by your doctor. Antihistamines, decongestants, and acetaminophen are known to pass into the breast milk of nursing mothers and may cause side effects in infants. Check with your doctor before taking Coricidin if you are or might be pregnant, or if you are breast-feeding.

Infants/Children
Children may be more susceptible to the side effects of Coricidin. They are also more susceptible to accidental antihistamine overdose. Do not give Coricidin to a child under age 6 unless directed by your doctor.

Seniors
Seniors may be more sensitive to the side effects of Coricidin. They may experience nervousness, irritability, restlessness, dizziness, sedation, urinary retention, low blood pressure, hallucinations, and seizures. Most mild reactions may be handled by either lowering your dose or trying another product.

Seniors taking Coricidin should be especially cautious about the amount of caffeine they ingest (see "Drug Interactions").

Brand Name

Dimetapp DM A (DYE-muh-tap)

Generic Ingredients

Brompheniramine maleate
Dextromethorphan
Phenylpropanolamine

Type of Drug

Antihistamine, decongestant, and antitussive (cough suppressant).

Used for

Relief of nasal congestion, itchy and watery eyes, itching of the nose and throat, runny nose, sneezing, and cough associated with cold and allergy.

General Information

Some OTC drugs use a combination of medications to relieve the many symptoms that can accompany colds and allergies. Dimetapp DM contains an antihistamine, a decongestant, and an antitussive.

The antihistamine in Dimetapp DM is brompheniramine maleate. Antihistamines block the release of histamine in the body, relieving the sneezing and itching that often occur with colds and allergies. They can also aid in stopping a runny nose by reducing the secretions caused by histamine release. (Generally, though, a decongestant is used in combination products for that purpose.)

Since histamine is only one of several substances released by the body during an allergic reaction, antihistamines can only reduce about 40% to 60% of allergic symptoms.

The decongestant in Dimetapp DM is phenylpropanolamine, an oral decongestant. Decongestants work by narrowing or constricting the blood vessels. This relieves the puffiness and swelling of nasal and bronchial mucous membranes. Unlike topical decongestants (decongestant nasal sprays) that act on local blood vessels, oral decongestants may constrict blood vessels throughout the body.

The antitussive ingredient in Dimetapp DM is dextromethorphan. This drug is found in many OTC cough preparations. Dextromethorphan suppresses the cough reflex by acting directly on the cough center in the brain. However, unlike other cough suppressants, dextromethorphan does not have pain-relieving effects, does not depress breathing, and has a low potential for addictions.

Dimetapp DM will not cure or prevent allergies or colds. The best you can hope for is symptomatic relief. Colds will usually go away in 1 to 2 weeks whether they are treated or not.

Cautions and Warnings

Do not take Dimetapp DM for more than 7 days continuously. If symptoms do not improve, or fever is present, see a doctor.

If your cough lasts longer than 7 days or keeps coming back, contact your doctor. A persistent cough can be a sign of a more serious condition.

Do not exceed the recommended daily dosage of Dimetapp DM.

If you experience fever, rash, or persistent headache while taking Dimetapp DM, call your doctor.

Dimetapp DM should be used with caution if you have a condition that causes breathing problems, such as emphysema, chronic bronchitis, or asthma. Its antihistamine ingredient, brompheniramine, acts to dry the mucous membranes. This in turn can inhibit the ability of the lungs to move or get rid of the excess secretions that these conditions produce.

Dimetapp DM should be used with caution by people with glaucoma, hyperthyroidism, heart disease, high blood pressure, diabetes, an enlarged prostate, or liver disease. If you have any of these conditions, take Dimetapp DM only on the advice of your doctor.

Antihistamines act as a depressant on the central nervous system (CNS), which can cause sleepiness or grogginess and can interfere with the ability to concentrate. Your ability to perform activities that require your full alertness and coordination, such as driving a motor vehicle or operating machinery, may be affected. Refrain from drinking alcohol while you are taking Dimetapp DM because alcohol aggravates these effects.

Because productive coughing (coughing that brings up mucus) actually helps relieve the underlying condition, some doctors do not believe that suppressing a productive cough makes good sense. However, a severe cough can interfere with sleep, and loss of sleep can contribute to the severity and duration of an illness. In the balance, the most appropriate use of cough suppressants may be to relieve a dry, nonproductive cough, especially at night.

Unless directed by your doctor, do not take Dimetapp DM if you have a chronic cough, such as that associated with smoking, asthma, chronic bronchitis, or emphysema, or cough with excessive mucus.

Possible Side Effects

- ▼ Most common: restlessness, nervousness, sleeplessness or drowsiness, dizziness, excitability, poor muscle coordination, headache, and upset stomach.
- ▼ Less common: dry eyes, nose, and mouth; blurred vision; difficulty urinating; irritability (at high doses); increased blood pressure; increased or irregular heart rate; heart palpitations; and loss of appetite.
- ▼ Rare: nausea, severe headache, feelings of tightness in the chest, greatly elevated blood pressure, and heart contractions.

Drug Interactions

• Antihistamines can enhance the effect of other drugs that depress the CNS, such as barbiturates, tranquilizers, sleeping medications, and alcohol (present in many OTC preparations). If you are taking other depressant drugs, check with your doctor before taking Dimetapp DM. Avoid drinking alcohol while taking Dimetapp DM.

• Antihistamines can affect skin and blood tests. Notify your health care professional before scheduling these tests if you are taking Dimetapp DM.

• Dimetapp DM should not be used at the same time as a monoamine oxidase inhibitor (MAOI) or within 2 weeks of stopping treatment with an MAOI. MAOIs are used to treat depression, other psychiatric or emotional conditions, and Parkinson's disease. If you are not sure whether you are or have been taking an MAOI, check with your doctor or pharmacist before you use Dimetapp DM.

• Taking Dimetapp DM along with another decongestant can increase the risk of adverse effects and toxicity. If you are taking another decongestant do not take Dimetapp DM without first asking your doctor.

• The effects of the decongestant phenylpropanolamine may also combine with those of caffeine, a CNS stimulant found in many prescription and OTC drugs. This combination can cause disorientation, delirium, and other side effects.

Food Interactions

Decongestants interact adversely with caffeine (see "Drug Interactions"), which is found in many popular beverages, including coffee, tea, and cola, and in chocolate.

Usual Dose

If you are taking Dimetapp DM for allergies, it is best to take it on a schedule rather than as needed because histamine is released almost continuously.

Each 5 ml (1 tsp.) of Dimetapp DM contains 2 mg of brompheniramine, 12.5 mg of phenylpropanolamine, and 10 mg dextromethorphan.

Adult and Child (age 12 and over): 2 tsp. every 4 hours. Do not exceed 6 doses in a 24-hour period.

Child (age 6–11): 1 tsp. every 4 hours. Do not exceed 6 doses in a 24-hour period.

Child (under age 6): Consult your doctor.

You may minimize the inconvenience of the sedative effects of Dimetapp DM by taking a full dose at bedtime and using the smallest recommended doses during the day. You can establish the lowest dose necessary for effective relief by starting with the lowest dose when you begin taking the drug, and gradually increasing the dosage over several days, as needed.

If you forget to take a dose of Dimetapp DM, do so as soon as you remember. If it is almost time for your next dose, skip the one you forgot and continue with your regular schedule. Do not take a double dose.

Overdosage

Symptoms of overdose include nausea, vomiting, urinary retention, shallow breathing, flushed face, dry mouth, blurred vision, dilated pupils, rapid rolling of the eyeballs, loss of muscle coordination, excitability, confusion, drowsiness, dizziness, hallucinations, seizures, and coma.

Even if the victim is not displaying any of the symptoms listed above, do the following in case of accidental overdose: If the victim is unconscious or having convulsions, call for an ambulance immediately. If you take the victim to an emergency room, be sure to bring the bottle or container with you. If the victim is conscious, call your local poison control center or a health care professional. The poison control center may suggest inducing vomiting with ipecac syrup (available without a prescription at any pharmacy). DO NOT induce vomiting unless specifically instructed to do so.

Special Populations

Pregnancy/Breast-feeding

Antihistamines are not recommended for use during pregnancy unless directed by your doctor. Antihistamines and decongestants are known to pass into the breast milk of nursing mothers and may cause side effects in infants. Check with your doctor before taking Dimetapp DM if you are or might be pregnant, or if you are breast-feeding.

Infants/Children

Children may be more susceptible to the side effects of Dimetapp DM. They are also more susceptible to accidental antihistamine overdose. Do not give Dimetapp DM to a child under 6 unless directed by a doctor.

Seniors

Seniors may be more sensitive to the side effects of antihistamines and decongestants. They may experience nervousness, irritability, restlessness, dizziness, sedation, hallucinations, seizures, and low blood pressure. Most mild reactions may be handled by either lowering the dose or switching to another product.

Seniors taking Dimetapp DM should be especially cautious about the amount of caffeine they ingest (see "Drug Interactions").

Brand Name

Dimetapp Extentabs (DYE-muh-tap)

Generic Ingredients

Brompheniramine maleate
Phenylpropanolamine

Type of Drug

Antihistamine and decongestant.

Used for

Relief of runny nose, sneezing, itching of the nose or throat, nasal congestion, and itchy eyes associated with cold and allergy.

General Information

Some OTC drugs use a combination of medications to relieve the many symptoms that can accompany colds and allergies. Dimetapp Extentabs contain an antihistamine and a decongestant.

The antihistamine in Dimetapp is brompheniramine maleate. Antihistamines block the release of histamine in the body, relieving the sneezing and itching that often occurs with colds and allergies. They can also aid in stopping a runny nose by reducing the secretions caused by histamine release. (Generally, though, a decongestant is used in combination products for that purpose.)

Since histamine is only one of several substances released by the body during an allergic reaction, antihistamines can only reduce about 40% to 60% of allergic symptoms.

The decongestant in Dimetapp is phenylpropanolamine, an oral decongestant. Decongestants work by narrowing or constricting the blood vessels. This relieves the puffiness and swelling of nasal and bronchial mucous membranes. Unlike topical decongestants (decongestant nasal sprays) that act on local blood vessels, oral decongestants may constrict blood vessels throughout the body.

Dimetapp will not cure or prevent allergies or colds. The best you can hope for is symptomatic relief. Colds will usually go away in 1 to 2 weeks whether they are treated or not.

Cautions and Warnings

Do not take Dimetapp Extentabs for more than 7 days continuously. If symptoms do not improve, or fever is present, see a doctor.

Do not exceed the recommended daily dosage of Dimetapp.

Dimetapp should be used with caution if you have a condition that causes breathing problems, such as emphysema, chronic bronchitis, or asthma. Its antihistamine ingredient, brompheniramine, acts to dry the mucous membranes. This in turn can inhibit the ability of the lungs to move or get rid of the excess secretions that these conditions produce.

Dimetapp should be used with caution by people with glaucoma, hyperthyroidism, heart disease, high blood pressure, diabetes, or an enlarged prostate. If you have any of these conditions, take Dimetapp only on the advice of your doctor.

Antihistamines act as a depressant on the central nervous system (CNS), which can cause sleepiness or grogginess and can interfere with the ability to concentrate. Your ability to perform activities that require your full alertness and coordination, such as driving a motor vehicle or operating machinery, may be affected. Refrain from drinking alcohol while you are taking Dimetapp because alcohol aggravates these effects.

Possible Side Effects

- ▼ Most common: restlessness, nervousness, sleeplessness or drowsiness, dizziness, excitability, poor muscle coordination, headache, and upset stomach.
- ▼ Less common: dry eyes, nose, and mouth; blurred vision; difficulty urinating; irritability (at high doses); increased blood pressure; increased or irregular heart rate; heart palpitations; and loss of appetite.
- ▼ Rare: severe headache, feelings of tightness in the chest, greatly elevated blood pressure, and heart contractions.

Drug Interactions

• Antihistamines can enhance the effect of other drugs that depress the central nervous system, such as barbiturates, tranquilizers, sleeping medications, and alcohol (present in many OTC preparations). If you are taking other depressant drugs, check with your doctor before taking Dimetapp Extentabs. Avoid drinking alcohol while taking Dimetapp.

• Antihistamines can affect the results of skin and blood tests. Notify your health care professional before scheduling these tests if you are taking Dimetapp.

• Dimetapp should not be used at the same time as a monoamine oxidase inhibitor (MAOI) or within 2 weeks of stopping treatment with an MAOI. MAOIs are used to treat depression, other psychiatric or emotional conditions, and Parkinson's disease. If you are not sure whether you are or have been taking an MAOI, check with your doctor or pharmacist before you use Dimetapp.

• Taking Dimetapp along with another decongestant can increase the risk of adverse effects and toxicity. If you are taking another decongestant, do not take Dimetapp without first asking your doctor.

• The effects of the decongestant phenylpropanolamine may combine with caffeine, a CNS stimulant found in many prescription and OTC drugs. This combination can cause disorientation, delirium, and other side effects.

Food Interactions

Decongestants interact adversely with caffeine (see "Drug Interactions"), which is found in many popular beverages, including coffee, tea, and cola, and in chocolate.

Usual Dose

If you are taking Dimetapp Extentabs for allergies, it is better to take it on a schedule rather than as needed because histamine is released nearly continuously.

Each tablet contains 12 mg of brompheniramine and 75 mg of phenylpropanolamine.

Adult and Child (age 12 and over): One tablet every 12 hours. Do not exceed 1 tablet every 12 hours or 2 tablets in a 24-hour period.

Child (under age 12): not recommended unless directed by your doctor.

If you forget to take a dose of Dimetapp, do so as soon as you remember. If it is almost time for your next dose, skip the one you forgot and continue with your regular schedule. Do not take a double dose.

Overdosage

Symptoms of overdose in children include dilated pupils, flushed face, dry mouth, fever, excitability, hallucinations, loss of muscle coordination, and seizures.

In adults, severe overdose can cause drowsiness or coma, which may be followed by excitability or seizures. Eventually fluid can build up in the brain; the kidneys may fail, and the heart and lungs may stop working, resulting in death. Symptoms may develop within 30 minutes to 2 hours following an overdose, and death may occur within 18 hours.

Even if the victim is not displaying any of the symptoms

listed above, do the following in case of accidental overdose: If the victim is unconscious or having convulsions, call for an ambulance immediately. If you take the victim to an emergency room, be sure to bring the bottle or container with you. If the victim is conscious, call your local poison control center or a health care professional. The poison control center may suggest inducing vomiting with ipecac syrup (available without a prescription at any pharmacy). DO NOT induce vomiting unless specifically instructed to do so.

Special Populations

Pregnancy/Breast-feeding

Antihistamines are not recommended for use during pregnancy unless directed by your doctor. Antihistamines and decongestants are known to pass into the breast milk of nursing mothers and may cause side effects in infants. Check with your doctor before taking Dimetapp Extentabs if you are or might be pregnant, or if you are breast-feeding.

Infants/Children

Children may be more susceptible to the side effects of Dimetapp. They are also more susceptible to accidental antihistamine overdose. Do not give Dimetapp to a child under 12 unless directed by your doctor.

Seniors

Older individuals should not take Dimetapp, which are extended-release tablets, until they have first tried a short-acting product containing the decongestant phenylpropanolamine and experienced no ill effects.

Seniors may be more sensitive to the side effects of antihistamines and decongestants. They may experience nervousness, irritability, restlessness, dizziness, sedation, blurred vision, constipation, urinary retention, confusion, hallucinations, seizures, and low blood pressure. Most mild reactions may be handled by switching to another product.

Seniors taking Dimetapp should be especially cautious about the amount of caffeine they ingest (see "Drug Interactions").

Drixoral Non-Drowsy (dricks-OR-al)

*see **Pseudoephedrine,** page 1002*

Brand Names

PediaCare Cough-Cold (PEE-dee-ah-care)
Triaminic Night Time (TRYE-ah-MIN-ik)

Generic Ingredients

Chlorpheniramine maleate
Dextromethorphan
Pseudoephedrine

Type of Drug

Antihistamine, decongestant, and antitussive (cough suppressant).

Used for

Relief of runny nose, sneezing, nasal congestion, itchy eyes, dry throat, and cough associated with cold and allergy in children.

General Information

Some OTC drugs use a combination of medications to relieve the many symptoms that can accompany colds and allergies. PediaCare Cough-Cold and Triaminic Nite Time contain an antihistamine, a decongestant, and an antitussive.

The antihistamine in these products is chlorpheniramine maleate. Antihistamines block the release of histamine in the body, relieving the sneezing and itching that often occur with colds and allergies. They may also help relieve a runny nose by reducing the secretions caused by histamine release.

Since histamine is only one of several substances released by the body during an allergic reaction, antihistamines can only reduce about 40% to 60% of allergic symptoms.

The decongestant in these products is pseudoephedrine, an oral decongestant. Decongestants work by narrowing or constricting the blood vessels. This reduces the puffiness and swelling of nasal and bronchial mucous membranes, thus relieving congestion. Unlike topical decongestants (decongestant nasal sprays) that act on local blood vessels, oral decongestants may constrict blood vessels throughout the body.

The ingredient in these products that reduces coughing is dextromethorphan, a common ingredient in OTC cough preparations. Dextromethorphan suppresses the cough reflex by acting directly on the cough center in the brain. Unlike some antitussives, dextromethorphan does not depress breathing and has a low potential for addiction.

These products will not cure or prevent your child's allergies or colds. The best you can hope for is symptomatic relief. Colds will usually go away in 1 to 2 weeks whether they are treated or not.

Cautions and Warnings

Do not give a child PediaCare Cough-Cold or Triaminic Nite Time for more than 7 days continuously unless under the supervision of a doctor. If symptoms do not improve or if fever is present, call your doctor.

If your child's cough lasts longer than 7 days or keeps coming back, contact your doctor. A persistent cough can be a sign of a more serious condition.

Do not exceed the recommended daily dosage of these products.

If your child experiences fever, rash, or persistent headache while taking these products, call your doctor.

These products should be used with caution if your child has a condition that causes breathing problems, such as emphysema, chronic bronchitis, or asthma. Its antihistamine ingredient, chlorpheniramine, acts to dry the mucous membranes. This in turn can inhibit the ability of the lungs to move or get rid of the excess secretions that these conditions produce.

These products should be used with caution in a child with glaucoma, hyperthyroidism, heart disease, high blood pressure, or diabetes, because it can worsen these conditions. If your child has one of these illnesses, give these products only upon the advice of a physician.

The antihistamine ingredient in these products acts as a depressant on the central nervous system (CNS), and can cause sleepiness or grogginess and interfere with your child's ability to concentrate.

Because productive coughing (coughing that brings up mucus) actually helps relieve the underlying condition, some doctors do not believe that suppressing a productive cough makes good sense. However, severe cough can interfere with sleep, and loss of sleep can contribute to the severity and duration of illness. For that reason, the most appropriate use of cough suppressants may be to relieve dry cough, especially at night.

These products should not be used for a chronic cough, such as that associated with asthma, chronic bronchitis, or emphesema, or for coughs associated with excessive mucus, unless directed by your doctor.

Possible Side Effects

- ▼ Most common: restlessness, nervousness, sleeplessness or drowsiness, dizziness, excitability, poor muscle coordination, headache, and upset stomach.
- ▼ Less common: dry eyes, nose, and mouth; blurred vision; difficulty urinating; irritability (at high doses); increased blood pressure; increased or irregular heart rate; and heart palpitations.
- ▼ Rare: nausea, breathing difficulty, anxiety, tremor, hallucinations, seizures, and cardiovascular collapse.

Drug Interactions

• The antihistamine ingredient in PediaCare Cough-Cold and Triaminic Nite Time can enhance the effect of other drugs that depress the CNS, such as barbiturates, tranquilizers, sleeping medications, and alcohol (present in many OTC preparations). Check with your doctor before giving these products to a child who is taking other depressant drugs.

• Antihistamines can also affect the results of skin and blood tests. Notify your health care professional before scheduling these tests if your child is taking these products.

• These products should not be used at the same time as a monoamine oxidase inhibitor (MAOI) or within 2 weeks of stopping treatment with an MAOI. MAOIs are used to treat depression, other psychiatric or emotional conditions, and Parkinson's disease. If you are not sure whether your child is or has been taking an MAOI, check with your doctor or pharmacist before giving your child these products.

• The effects of pseudoephedrine, the decongestant ingredient in these products, may combine with those of caffeine, a CNS stimulant found in many prescription and OTC drugs. This combination can cause disorientation, delirium, and other side effects.

• Taking these products along with another decongestant can increase the risk of adverse effects and toxicity. If your child is taking another decongestant, do not give these products without first asking your doctor.

Food Interactions

Decongestants interact adversely with caffeine (see "Drug Interactions"), which is found in many popular beverages, including coffee, tea, and cola, and in chocolate.

Usual Dose

To relieve the symptoms of allergy, it is best to take PediaCare Cough-Cold or Triaminic Nite Time on a schedule rather than as needed because histamine is released nearly continuously.

PediaCare Cough-Cold
Each tablet and each 5 ml (1 tsp.) of liquid contains 1 mg of chlorpheniramine, 15 mg of pseudoephedrine, and 5 mg of dextromethorphan.

Child (age 11–12): 3 tablets or 3 tsp. every 4–6 hours. Do not exceed 4 doses in a 24-hour period.

Child (age 9–10): 2 1/2 tablets or 2 1/2 tsp. every 4–6 hours. Do not exceed 4 doses in a 24-hour period.

Child (age 6–8): 2 tablets or 2 tsp. every 4–6 hours. Do not exceed 4 doses in a 24-hour period.

Child (under age 6): as directed by your doctor.

Triaminic Nite Time
Each 5 ml (1 tsp.) contains 1 mg of chlorpheniramine, 15 mg of pseudoephedrine, and 7.5 mg of dextromethorphan.

Adult and Child (age 12 and over): 4 tsp. every 6 hours. Do not exceed 4 doses in a 24-hour period.

Child (age 6–11): 2 tsp. every 6 hours. Do not exceed 4 doses in a 24-hour period.

Child (under age 6): as directed by your doctor.

You may minimize the disruptiveness of the sedative effects of these products by having your child take a full dose at bedtime or by using the smallest recommended doses during the day. You can establish the lowest dose necessary for effective relief by starting with the lowest dose when you first administer the drug, and gradually increasing the dosage as needed over several days.

If you forget a dose of these products, give it as soon as you remember. If it is almost time for the next dose, skip the one you forgot and continue with your regular schedule. Do not give your child a double dose.

Overdosage

Signs of overdose include fixed, dilated pupils; blurred vision; rapid rolling of the eyeballs; flushed face; dry mouth; nausea; vomiting; fever; excitability; dizziness; drowsiness; hallucinations; difficulty breathing; shallow breathing; delay in urinating; uncoordinated muscular movements; and seizures, stupor, toxic psychosis, and coma.

Even if the victim is not displaying any of the symptoms listed above, do the following in case of accidental overdose: If the victim is unconscious or having convulsions, call for an ambulance immediately. If you take the victim to an emergency room, be sure to bring the bottle or container with you. If the victim is conscious, call your local poison control center or a health care professional. The poison control center may suggest inducing vomiting with ipecac syrup (available without a prescription at any pharmacy). DO NOT induce vomiting unless specifically instructed to do so.

Special Populations

Pregnancy/Breast-feeding

Antihistamines are not recommended for use during pregnancy unless directed by your doctor. Antihistamines, decongestants, and acetaminophen are known to pass into the breast milk of nursing mothers and may cause side effects in infants. Check with your doctor before taking PediaCare Cough-Cold or Triaminic Nite Time if you are or might be pregnant, or if you are breast-feeding.

Infant/Children

Children may be more susceptible to the side effects of these products. They are also more susceptible to accidental antihistamine overdose. Do not give PediaCare Cough-Cold or Triaminic Nite Time to children under age 6 without consulting your doctor.

Seniors

Older persons may be more sensitive to the side effects of antihistamines and decongestants. They may experience nervousness, irritability, blurred vision, constipation, urinary retention, confusion, restlessness, dizziness, sedation, hallucinations, seizures, and low blood pressure. Most mild reactions may be handled by either lowering the dose or by switching to another product.

Seniors taking these products should be especially cautious about the amount of caffeine they ingest (see "Drug Interactions").

Pertussin CS Children's Strength Cough Relief (per-TUSS-in)

*see **Dextromethorphan,** page 784*

Pertussin DM Extra Strength Cough Relief (per-TUSS-in)

*see **Dextromethorphan,** page 784*

Robitussin (ROE-bih-TUSS-in)

*see **Guaifenesin,** page 833*

Brand Name

Robitussin CF (ROE-bih-TUSS-in)

Generic Ingredients

Dextromethorphan
Guaifenesin
Phenylpropanolamine

Type of Drug

Decongestant, antitussive (cough suppressant), and expectorant.

Used for

Temporary relief of cough and nasal congestion associated with colds, and loosening and thinning of bronchial secretions.

General Information

Some OTC products use a combination of drugs to relieve the symptoms associated with colds. Robitussin CF contains a decongestant, a cough suppressant, and an expectorant.

The decongestant ingredient in Robitussin CF is phenylpropanolamine, an oral decongestant. Decongestants relieve nasal congestion by narrowing or constricting blood vessels in the nose. This action reduces the blood supplied to the nose and decreases the swelling of nasal mucous membranes. Unlike topical decongestants (decongestant nasal sprays) that act on local blood vessels, oral decongestants may constrict blood vessels throughout the body.

The cough suppressant in Robitussin CF is dextromethorphan, a common antitussive in OTC cough preparations. Dextromethorphan suppresses the cough reflex by acting directly on the cough center in the brain. Unlike other cough suppressants, dextromethorphan does not depress breathing and has a low potential for addiction.

The expectorant ingredient in Robitussin CF is guaifenesin. Expectorants make mucus more watery and less sticky so that it is easier to bring up with coughing. Easier removal of secretions may indirectly reduce the impulse to cough. Guaifenesin is a common ingredient in OTC cough preparations; however, there is some controversy over its efficacy.

Some doctors have questioned the wisdom of combining an antitussive and an expectorant, since the action of the antitussive may make it harder for you to cough up the secretions loosened by the expectorant.

Robitussin CF will not cure or prevent your cold. The best you can hope for is symptomatic relief. Colds will usually go away in 1 to 2 weeks whether they are treated or not.

Cautions and Warnings

Do not use Robitussin CF for more than 7 consecutive days.

If a cough lasts longer than 7 days, or keeps coming back, consult your doctor. A persistent cough may be the sign of a more serious condition.

Do not exceed the recommended daily dosage of Robitussin CF.

If you experience fever, rash, or persistent headache while taking Robitussin CF, stop taking it immediately and call your doctor.

Robitussin CF should be used with caution by people with hyperthyroidism, heart disease, high blood pressure, diabetes, an enlarged prostate, asthma, or liver disease. If you have any of these conditions, ask your doctor before using Robitussin CF.

Because productive coughing (coughing that brings up mucus) actually helps relieve the underlying condition, some doctors do not believe that suppressing a productive cough makes good sense. However, a severe cough can interfere with sleep, and loss of sleep can contribute to the severity and duration of an illness. In the balance, the most appropriate use of cough suppressants may be to relieve a dry, nonproductive cough.

Unless directed by your doctor, do not use Robitussin CF if you have a chronic cough, such as that associated with smoking, asthma, chronic bronchitis, or emphysema, or for coughs associated with excessive mucus.

Dextromethorphan, the antitussive ingredient in Robitussin CF, is not recommended for people confined to bed rest or under sedation.

Possible Side Effects

- ▼ Most common: restlessness, nervousness, excitability, sleeplessness, dizziness, weakness, drowsiness, and headache.
- ▼ Less common: increased blood pressure, increased or irregular heart rate, heart palpitations, and loss of appetite.
- ▼ Rare: nausea, vomiting, severe headache, feelings of tightness in the chest, greatly elevated blood pressure, and heart contractions.

Drug Interactions

• Robitussin CF should not be used at the same time as a monoamine oxidase inhibitor (MAOI) or within 2 weeks of stopping treatment with an MAOI. MAOIs are used to treat depression, other psychiatric or emotional conditions, and Parkinson's disease. If you are not sure whether you are or have been taking an MAOI, check with your doctor or pharmacist before you use Robitussin CF.

• The effects of phenylpropanolamine, the decongestant in Robitussin CF, may combine with those of caffeine, a CNS stimulant found in many prescription and OTC drugs. This combination can cause disorientation, delirium, and other side effects.

• Taking Robitussin CF along with another decongestant can increase the risk of adverse effects and toxicity. If you are taking another decongestant, do not use Robitussin CF without first asking your doctor.

Food Interactions

The decongestant in Robitussin CF interacts adversely with caffeine (see "Drug Interactions"), which is found in many popular beverages, including coffee, tea, and cola, and in chocolate.

Usual Dose

Each 5 ml (1 tsp.) contains 12.5 mg of phenylpropanolamine, 10 mg of dextromethorphan, and 100 mg of guaifenesin.

Adult and Child (age 12 and over): 2 tsp. every 4 hours. Do not exceed 12 tsp. in a 24-hour period.

Child (age 6–11): 1 tsp. every 4 hours. Do not exceed 6 tsp. in a 24-hour period.

Child (age 2–5): 1/2 tsp. every 4 hours. Do not exceed 3 tsp. in a 24-hour period.

Child (under age 2): Consult your doctor.

Overdosage

Symptoms of overdose include nausea, vomiting, urinary retention, shallow breathing, blurred vision, rapid rolling of the eyeballs, loss of muscle coordination, confusion, drowsiness, dizziness, hallucinations, and coma.

Even if the victim is not displaying any of the symptoms listed above, do the following in case of accidental overdose: If the victim is unconscious or having convulsions, call for an ambulance immediately. If you take the victim to an emergency room, be sure to bring the bottle or container with you. If the victim is conscious, call your local poison

control center or a health care professional. The poison control center may suggest inducing vomiting with ipecac syrup (available without a prescription at any pharmacy). DO NOT induce vomiting unless specifically instructed to do so.

Special Populations

Pregnancy/Breast-feeding

It is not generally recommended that pregnant women take any drugs, particularly during the first 3 months after conception. Decongestants have been shown to pass into the breast milk of nursing mothers and may cause side effects in nursing infants. Check with your doctor before taking Robitussin CF if you are or might be pregnant, or if you are breast-feeding.

Infants/Children

Do not give Robitussin CF to a child under age 2 unless directed by your doctor.

Seniors

Older persons may be more sensitive to the side effects of Robitussin CF. They may experience nervousness, irritability, restlessness, dizziness, sedation, hallucinations, seizures, and low blood pressure. Most mild reactions may be handled by either lowering your dose or trying another product.

Seniors taking these products should be especially cautious about the amount of caffeine they ingest (see "Drug Interactions").

Brand Name

Robitussin Cold & Cough Liqui-Gels

(ROE-bih-TUSS-in)

Generic Ingredients

Dextromethorphan
Guaifenesin
Pseudoephedrine

Type of Drug

Decongestant, antitussive (cough suppressant), and expectorant.

Used for

Temporary relief of cough and nasal congestion associated with colds and allergies, and loosening and thinning of bronchial secretions.

General Information

Some OTC products use a combination of drugs to relieve the symptoms associated with coughs, colds, and allergies. Robitussin Cold & Cough Liqui-Gels contains a decongestant, a cough suppressant, and an expectorant.

The decongestant ingredient in Robitussin Cold & Cough is pseudoephedrine, an oral decongestant. Decongestants relieve nasal congestion by narrowing or constricting blood vessels in the nose. This action reduces the blood supplied to the nose and decreases the swelling of nasal mucous membranes. Unlike topical decongestants (decongestant nasal sprays) that act on local blood vessels, oral decongestants may constrict blood vessels throughout the body.

The cough suppressant in Robitussin Cold & Cough is dextromethorphan, a common antitussive in OTC cough preparations. Dextromethorphan suppresses the cough reflex by acting directly on the cough center in the brain. Unlike other cough supressants, dextromethorphan does not depress breathing and has a low potential for addiction.

The expectorant ingredient in Robitussin Cold & Cough is guaifenesin. Expectorants make mucus more watery and less sticky so that it is easier to bring up with coughing. Easier removal of secretions may indirectly reduce the impulse to cough. Guaifenesin is a common ingredient in OTC cough preparations; however, there is some controversy over how effective it is.

Some doctors have questioned the wisdom of combining an antitussive and an expectorant, since the action of the antitussive may make it harder for you to cough up the secretions loosened by the expectorant.

Robitussin Cold & Cough will not cure or prevent colds or allergies. The best you can hope for is symptomatic relief. Colds will usually go away in 1 to 2 weeks whether they are treated or not.

Cautions and Warnings

Do not use Robitussin Cold & Cough for more than 7

consecutive days. If a cough lasts longer than 7 days, or keeps coming back, consult your doctor. A persistent cough may be the sign of a more serious condition.

Do not exceed the recommended daily dosage of Robitussin Cold & Cough.

If you experience fever, rash, or persistent headache while taking Robitussin Cold & Cough, stop taking it immediately and call your doctor.

Robitussin Cold & Cough should be used with caution by people with hyperthyroidism, heart disease, high blood pressure, diabetes, an enlarged prostate, asthma, or liver disease. If you have any of these conditions, ask your doctor before using Robitussin Cold & Cough.

Because productive coughing (coughing that brings up mucus) actually helps relieve the underlying condition, some doctors do not believe that suppressing a productive cough makes good sense. However, a severe cough can interfere with sleep, and loss of sleep can contribute to the severity and duration of an illness. In the balance, the most appropriate use of cough suppressants may be to relieve a dry, nonproductive cough.

Unless directed by your doctor, do not use Robitussin Cold & Cough for a chronic cough, such as that associated with smoking, asthma, chronic bronchitis, or emphysema, or for coughs associated with excessive mucus.

Dextromethorphan, the antitussive ingredient in Robitussin Cold & Cough is not recommended for people confined to bed rest or under sedation.

Possible Side Effects

- ▼ Most common: restlessness, nervousness, excitability, sleeplessness, dizziness, weakness, drowsiness, and headache.
- ▼ Less common: increased blood pressure, increased or irregular heart rate, and heart palpitations.
- ▼ Rare: nausea, vomiting, difficulty breathing, difficulty or pain when urinating, anxiety, tremor, hallucinations, seizures, and cardiovascular collapse.

Drug Interactions

• Robitussin Cold & Cough should not be used at the same time as a monoamine oxidase inhibitor (MAOI) or within 2 weeks of stopping treatment with an MAOI. MAOIs are used to treat depression, other psychiatric or emotional conditions, and Parkinson's disease. If you are not sure whether you are or have been taking an MAOI, check with your doctor or pharmacist before you use Robitussin Cold & Cough.

• The effects of pseudoephedrine, the decongestant in Robitussin Cold & Cough Liqui-Gels, may combine with those of caffeine, a CNS stimulant found in many prescription and OTC drugs. This combination can cause disorientation, delirium, and other side effects.

• Taking Robitussin Cold & Cough along with another decongestant can increase the risk of adverse effects and toxicity. If you are taking another decongestant, do not use Robitussin Cold & Cough without first asking your doctor.

Food Interactions

The decongestant in Robitussin Cold & Cough interacts adversely with caffeine (see "Drug Interactions"), which is found in many popular beverages, including coffee, tea, and cola, and in chocolate.

Usual Dose

Each softgel contains 30 mg of pseudoephedrine, 10 mg of dextromethorphan, and 200 mg of guaifenesin.

Adult and Child (age 12 and over): 2 softgels every 4 hours. Do not exceed 8 softgels in a 24-hour period.

Child (age 6–11): 1 softgel every 4 hours. Do not exceed 4 softgels in a 24-hour period.

Child (under age 6): Consult your doctor.

Overdosage

Symptoms of overdose include nausea, vomiting, urinary retention, shallow breathing, blurred vision, rapid rolling of the eyeballs, loss of muscle coordination, confusion, drowsiness, dizziness, hallucinations, and coma.

Even if the victim is not displaying any of the symptoms listed above, do the following in case of accidental overdose: If the victim is unconscious or having convulsions, call for an ambulance immediately. If you take the victim to an

emergency room, be sure to bring the bottle or container with you. If the victim is conscious, call your local poison control center or a health care professional. The poison control center may suggest inducing vomiting with ipecac syrup (available without a prescription at any pharmacy). DO NOT induce vomiting unless specifically instructed to do so.

Special Populations

Pregnancy/Breast-feeding

It is not generally recommended that pregnant women take any drugs, particularly during the first 3 months after conception. Decongestants have been shown to pass into the breast milk of nursing mothers and may cause side effects in nursing infants. Check with your doctor before taking Robitussin Cold & Cough if you are or might be pregnant, or if you are breast-feeding.

Infants/Children

Do not give Robitussin Cold & Cough to a child under age 6 unless directed by your doctor.

Seniors

Seniors may be more sensitive to the side effects of Robitussin Cold & Cough. They may experience nervousness, irritability, restlessness, dizziness, sedation, hallucinations, seizures, and low blood pressure. Most mild reactions may be handled by either lowering your dose or trying another product.

Seniors taking these products should be especially cautious about the amount of caffeine they ingest (see "Drug Interactions").

Brand Names

Robitussin DM (ROE-bih-TUSS-in)
Vicks 44E (VIKS)

Generic Ingredients

Dextromethorphan
Guaifenesin

Type of Drug

Antitussive (cough suppressant) and expectorant.

Used for

Temporary relief of cough associated with colds; loosening of mucus and thinning of bronchial secretions.

General Information

Robitussin DM and Vicks 44E contain 2 types of drugs used to treat cough: an antitussive to suppress the cough reflex, and an expectorant to help thin and remove secretions from the lungs.

The antitussive ingredient in these products is dextromethorphan. It suppresses the cough reflex by acting directly on the cough center in the brain. Unlike some antitussives, dextromethorphan does not depress breathing and has a low potential for addiction.

The expectorant ingredient in these products is guaifenesin. Expectorants make mucus more watery and less sticky, so that it is easier to bring up with coughing. Easier removal of secretions may indirectly reduce the impulse to cough. Guaifenesin is a common ingredient in OTC cough preparations; however, there is some controversy over how effective it is.

The combination of a cough suppressant and an expectorant may actually be counterproductive. The action of the antitussive may make it harder for you to cough up the secretions loosened by the expectorant.

Cautions and Warnings

Do not take Robitussin DM or Vicks 44E for more than 7 consecutive days.

If your cough lasts longer than 7 days or keeps coming back, contact your doctor. A persistent cough can be a sign of a more serious condition.

Do not exceed the recommended daily dosage of Robitussin DM or Vicks 44E.

If you experience fever, rash, or persistent headache while taking these products, call your doctor.

These products should be used with caution if you have asthma or liver disease.

Because productive coughing (coughing that brings up mucus) actually helps relieve the underlying condition, some physicians do not believe that suppressing a productive cough makes good sense. However, a severe cough can interfere with sleep, and loss of sleep can contribute to the severity and duration of an illness. For that reason, the most appropriate use of cough suppressants may be to relieve dry cough, especially at night.

These products should not be used for persistent or chronic cough, such as that associated with smoking, asthma, chronic bronchitis, or emphysema, or for coughs associated with excessive mucus, except on the advice of a physician.

Dextromethorphan is not recommended for people confined to bed rest or under sedation.

Possible Side Effects

▼ Rare: headache, nausea, vomiting, slight drowsiness, and dizziness.

Drug Interactions

• These products should not be used at the same time as a monoamine oxidase inhibitor (MAOI) or within 2 weeks of stopping treatment with an MAOI. MAOIs are used to treat depression, other psychiatric or emotional conditions, and Parkinson's disease. If you are not sure whether you are or have been taking an MAOI, check with your doctor or pharmacist before you use Robitussin DM or Vicks 44E.

Food Interactions

None known.

Usual Dose

Robitussin DM
Each 5 ml (1 tsp.) contains 10 mg of dextromethorphan and 100 mg of guaifenesin.

Adult and Child (age 12 and over): 2 tsp. every 4 hours. Do not exceed 6 doses (12 tsp.) in a 24-hour period.

Child (age 6–11): 1 tsp. every 4 hours. Do not exceed 6 doses (6 tsp.) in a 24-hour period.

Child (age 2–5): 1/2 tsp. every 4 hours. Do not exceed 6 doses (3 tsp.) in a 24-hour period.

Child (under age 2): Consult your doctor.

Vicks 44E
Each 5 ml (1 tsp.) contains 6.67 mg of dextromethorphan and 66.7 mg of guaifenesin.

Adult and Child (age 12 and over): 3 tsp. every 4 hours. Do not exceed 6 doses in a 24-hour period.

Child (age 6–11): 1 1/2 tsp. every 4 hours. Do not exceed 6 doses in a 24-hour period.

Child (under age 6): Consult your doctor.

Overdosage

Signs of overdose include nausea, vomiting, drowsiness, dizziness, blurred vision, involuntary eye movements, uncoordinated muscular movements, shallow breathing, urinary retention, stupor, toxic psychosis, and coma.

Even if the victim is not displaying any of the symptoms listed above, do the following in case of accidental overdose: If the victim is unconscious or having convulsions, call for an ambulance immediately. If you take the victim to an emergency room, be sure to bring the bottle or container with you. If the victim is conscious, call your local poison control center or a health care professional. The poison control center may suggest inducing vomiting with ipecac syrup (available without a prescription at any pharmacy). DO NOT induce vomiting unless specifically instructed to do so.

Special Populations

Pregnancy/Breast-feeding

It is not generally recommended that pregnant women take any drugs, particularly during the first 3 months after conception. Check with your doctor before taking Robitussin DM or Vicks 44E if you are or might be pregnant, or if you are breast-feeding.

Infants/Children

The most appropriate use for cough suppressants in young children may be before bedtime to prevent the cough from disturbing their sleep.

Unless directed by your doctor, do not give Robitussin DM to a child under age 2, or Vicks 44E to a child under age 6.

Seniors

Seniors should exercise the same caution as younger adults when taking these products.

Brand Name

Robitussin PE (ROE-bih-TUSS-in) Robitussin Severe Congestion Liqui-Gels

Generic Ingredients

Guaifenesin
Pseudoephedrine

Type of Drug

Decongestant and expectorant.

Used for

Temporary relief of nasal congestion associated with colds and allergies, loosening and thinning of bronchial secretions, and management of cough.

General Information

Some OTC products use a combination of drugs to relieve the symptoms associated with colds and allergies. Robitussin PE and Robitussin Severe Congestion Liqui-Gels contain a decongestant and an expectorant.

The decongestant ingredient in Robitussin PE and Robitussin Liqui-Gels is pseudoephedrine, an oral decongestant. Decongestants relieve nasal congestion by narrowing or constricting blood vessels in the nose. This action reduces the blood supplied to the nose and decreases the swelling of nasal mucous membranes. Unlike topical decongestants (decongestant nasal sprays) that act on local blood vessels, oral decongestants may constrict blood vessels throughout the body.

The expectorant ingredient in these products is guaifenesin. Expectorants make mucus more watery and less sticky so that it is easier to bring up with coughing. Easier removal of secretions may indirectly reduce the impulse to cough. Guaifenesin is a common ingredient in OTC cough preparations; however, there is some controversy over its efficacy.

Robitussin PE and Robitussin Liqui-Gels will not cure or prevent cold or allergies. The best you can hope for is symptomatic relief. Colds will usually go away in 1 to 2 weeks whether they are treated or not.

Cautions and Warnings

Do not use Robitussin PE or Robitussin Liqui-Gels for more than 7 consecutive days.

If a cough lasts longer than 7 days, or keeps coming back, consult your doctor. A persistent cough may be the sign of a more serious condition.

Do not exceed the recommended daily dosage of these products.

If you experience fever, rash, or persistent headache while taking these products, stop taking them immediately and call your doctor.

Robitussin PE and Robitussin Liqui-Gels should be used with caution by people with hyperthyroidism, heart disease, high blood pressure, diabetes, and an enlarged prostate; if you have any of these conditions, ask your doctor before using them.

Because productive coughing (coughing that brings up mucus) actually helps relieve the underlying condition, some doctors do not believe that suppressing a productive cough makes good sense. However, a severe cough can interfere with sleep, and loss of sleep can contribute to the severity and duration of an illness. In the balance, the most appropriate use of cough suppressants may be to relieve a dry, nonproductive cough, especially at night.

Unless directed by your doctor, do not use Robitussin PE or Robitussin Liqui-Gels for a chronic cough, such as that associated with smoking, asthma, chronic bronchitis, or emphysema, or for coughs associated with excessive mucus.

Possible Side Effects

- ▼ Most common: restlessness, nervousness, excitability, sleeplessness, dizziness, weakness, drowsiness, and headache.
- ▼ Less common: increased blood pressure, increased or irregular heart rate, and heart palpitations.
- ▼ Rare: nausea, vomiting, difficulty breathing, difficulty or pain when urinating, anxiety, tremor, hallucinations, seizures, and cardiovascular collapse.

Drug Interactions

• Robitussin PE or Robitussin Liqui-Gels should not be used at the same time as a monoamine oxidase inhibitor (MAOI) or within 2 weeks of stopping treatment with an MAOI. MAOIs are used to treat depression, other psychiatric or emotional conditions, and Parkinson's disease. If you are not sure whether you are or have been taking an MAOI, check with your doctor or pharmacist before you use Robitussin PE or Robitussin Liqui-Gels.

• Taking these products along with another decongestant can increase the risk of adverse effects and toxicity. If you are taking another decongestant, do not use Robitussin PE or Robitussin Liqui-Gels without first asking your doctor.

• The effects of pseudoephedrine, the decongestant in these products, may combine with those of caffeine, a central nervous system stimulant found in many prescription and OTC drugs. This combination can cause disorientation, delirium, and other side effects.

Food Interactions

The decongestant in these products interacts adversely with caffeine (see "Drug Interactions"), which is found in many popular beverages, including coffee, tea, and cola, and in chocolate.

Usual Dose

Robitussin PE

Each 5 ml (1 tsp.) contains 30 mg of pseudoephedrine and 100 mg of guaifenesin.

Adult and Child (age 12 and over): 2 tsp. every 4 hours. Do not exceed 8 tsp. in a 24-hour period.

Child (age 6–11): 1 tsp. every 4 hours. Do not exceed 4 tsp. in a 24-hour period.

Child (age 2–5): 1/2 tsp. Every 4 hours. Do not exceed 2 tsp. in a 24-hour period.

Child (under age 2): Consult your doctor.

Robitussin Severe Congestion Liqui-Gels

Each softgel contains 30 mg of pseudoephedrine and 200 mg of guaifenesin.

Adult and Child (age 12 and over): 2 softgels every 4 hours. Do not exceed 8 softgels in a 24-hour period.

Child (age 6–11): 1 softgel every 4 hours. Do not exceed 4 softgels in a 24-hour period.

Child (under age 6): Consult your doctor.

Overdosage

Do the following in case of accidental overdose: If the victim is unconscious or having convulsions, call for an ambulance immediately. If you take the victim to an emergency room, be sure to bring the bottle or container with you. If the victim is conscious, call your local poison control center or a health care professional. The poison control center may suggest inducing vomiting with ipecac syrup (available without a prescription at any pharmacy). DO NOT induce vomiting unless specifically instructed to do so.

Special Populations

Pregnancy/Breast-feeding

It is not generally recommended that pregnant women take any drugs, particularly during the first 3 months after conception. Decongestants have been shown to pass into the breast milk of nursing mothers and may cause side effects in nursing infants. Check with your doctor before taking Robitussin PE or Robitussin Liqui-Gels if you are or might be pregnant, or if you are breast-feeding.

Infants/Children

Do not give Robitussin PE to a child under age 2 unless directed by your doctor. Do not give Robitussin Liqui-Gels to a child under age 6 unless directed by your doctor.

Seniors

Older persons may be more sensitive to the side effects of these products. They may experience nervousness, irritability, restlessness, dizziness, sedation, hallucinations, seizures, and low blood pressure. Most mild reactions may be handled by either lowering your dose or trying another product.

Seniors taking these products should be especially cautious about the amount of caffeine they ingest (see "Drug Interactions").

Brand Names

Sudafed Cold & Cough (SOO-dah-fed)
Tylenol Cold Severe Congestion (TYE-leh-nol)
Vicks DayQuil (VIKS DAY-kwill)

Generic Ingredients

Acetaminophen
Dextromethorphan
Guaifenesin
Pseudoephedrine

Type of Drug

Decongestant, analgesic (pain reliever), antipyretic (fever reducer), antitussive (cough suppressant), and expectorant.

Used for

Temporary relief of cough, nasal congestion, minor sore throat pain, headache, fever, and body aches due to cold or flu.

General Information

Some OTC drugs use a combination of medications to relieve the many symptoms that can accompany coughs, colds, and allergies. Sudafed Cold & Cough, Tylenol Cold Severe Congestion and Vicks DayQuil LiquiCaps combine a decongestant, an analgesic/antipyretic, a cough suppressant, and an expectorant.

The decongestant in these products (and the ingredient from which Sudafed gets its name) is pseudoephedrine, an oral decongestant. Decongestants work by narrowing or constricting the blood vessels. This relieves the puffiness and swelling of nasal and bronchial mucous membranes. Unlike topical decongestants (decongestant nasal sprays) that act on local blood vessels, oral decongestants may constrict blood vessels throughout the body.

Acetaminophen, the analgesic and antipyretic ingredient, relieves pain and fever associated with the common cold, flu, and viral infections.

Dextromethorphan is a very common antitussive used in OTC cough preparations. Dextromethorphan suppresses the cough reflex by acting directly on the cough center in the brain. Unlike other cough suppressants, it does not depress breathing and has a low potential for addiction.

The expectorant ingredient in these products is guaifenesin. Expectorants are used to make mucus more watery and less sticky, so that it is easier to bring up with coughing. Easier removal of secretions may indirectly reduce the impulse to cough. Guaifenesin is a common ingredient in OTC cough preparations; however, there is some controversy over its efficacy.

The combination of an expectorant and an antitussive, such as that found in these products, may be counterproductive. The action of the antitussive may make it harder for you to cough up the secretions loosened by the expectorant.

These products will not cure or prevent colds. The best you can hope for is symptomatic relief. Colds will usually go away in 1 to 2 weeks whether they are treated or not.

Cautions and Warnings

Do not take Sudafed Cold & Cough, Tylenol Severe Congestion, or DayQuil for more than 7 consecutive days (5 days for children) or, in the presence of fever, for more than 3 days, unless directed by your doctor.

If your cough lasts longer than 7 days, is recurrent, or is accompanied by fever, rash, or persistent headache, call your doctor. A persistent cough may be a sign of a serious condition.

Do not exceed the recommended daily dosage of these products.

These products should be used with caution by people with hyperthyroidism, heart disease, high blood pressure, diabetes, an enlarged prostate, asthma, or liver disease. If you have any of these conditions, ask your doctor before using Sudafed Cold & Cough, Tylenol Severe Congestion, or DayQuil.

In doses of more than 4 grams per day, acetaminophen, one of the active ingredients in these products, is potentially toxic to the liver. Use these products with caution if you have kidney or liver disease or viral infections of the liver.

Studies have shown that the risk of liver damage with acetaminophen is associated with fasting and alcohol use; people with liver disease who are taking other drugs that are potentially damaging to the liver, who do not eat regularly, or who drink alcohol (even moderately) are especially at risk. If you take these products regularly, avoid drinking alcoholic beverages and/or fasting.

Because productive coughing (coughing that brings up mucus) actually helps relieve the underlying condition, some doctors do not believe that suppressing a productive cough makes good sense. However, a severe cough can interfere with sleep, and loss of sleep can contribute to the severity and duration of an illness. For that reason, the most appropriate use of cough suppressants may be to relieve a dry cough, especially at night.

These products should not be used for a persistent or chronic cough, such as that associated with smoking, asthma, chronic bronchitis, or emphysema, or for coughs associated with excessive mucus.

Dextromethorphan, the antitussive ingredient in these products, is not recommended for people confined to bed rest or under sedation.

Possible Side Effects

- ▼ Most common: restlessness, nervousness, sleeplessness or drowsiness, dizziness, lightheadedness, excitability, poor muscle coordination, headache, and upset stomach.
- ▼ Less common: dry eyes, nose, and mouth; blurred vision; difficulty urinating; irritability (at high doses); increased blood pressure; increased or irregular heart rate; and heart palpitations.
- ▼ Rare: extreme fatigue; rash, itching, or hives; sore throat or fever; unexplained bleeding or bruising; anemia; yellowing of the skin or eyes; blood in urine; painful or frequent urination; decreased output of urine volume; vomiting; nausea; anxiety; breathing difficulty; tremor; hallucinations; seizures; and cardiovascular collapse.

Drug Interactions

• These products should not be used at the same time as a monoamine oxidase inhibitor (MAOI) or within 2 weeks of stopping treatment with an MAOI. MAOIs are used to treat depression, other psychiatric or emotional conditions, and Parkinson's disease. If you are not sure whether you are or have been taking an MAOI, check with your doctor or pharmacist before you use Sudafed Cold & Cough, Tylenol Severe Congestion, or DayQuil.

• The effects of pseudoephedrine, the decongestant in these products, may combine with those of caffeine, a central nervous system stimulant found in many prescription and OTC drugs. This combination can cause disorientation, delirium, and other side effects.

• Taking these products along with another decongestant can increase the risk of adverse effects and toxicity; if you are taking another decongestant, do not take these products without first asking your doctor.

• The effects of these products may be reduced by long-term use or large doses of barbiturate drugs; carbamazepine, an anticonvulsant; phenytoin (and other similar drugs), used to control epilepsy; rifampin, an antitubercular drug; and sulfinpyrazone, an antigout medication. These drugs may also increase the chances of liver toxicity if taken with Sudafed Cold & Cough, Tylenol Severe Congestion, or DayQuil. Taking acetaminophen with the antitubercular drug isoniazid may also increase the risk of liver damage.

• If Sudafed Cold & Cough, Tylenol Severe Congestion, or DayQuil is taken with an anticoagulant such as warfarin, it may increase the blood-thinning effect of the anticoagulant agent. This does not occur with occasional use.

• Avoid alcohol while taking Sudafed Cold & Cough, Tylenol Severe Congestion, or DayQuil LiquiCaps. (Be aware that alcohol is found in many OTC preparations.) Alcohol may contribute to the risk of liver damage associated with these products (see "Cautions and Warnings").

Food Interactions

Decongestants interact adversely with caffeine (see "Drug Interactions"), which is found in many popular beverages, including coffee, tea, and cola, and in chocolate.

Usual Dose

Sudafed Cold & Cough or Vicks DayQuil LiquiCaps
Each softgel contains 30 mg of pseudoephedrine, 250 mg of acetaminophen, 10 mg of dextromethorphan, and 100 mg of guaifenesin.

Adult and Child (age 12 and over): 2 softgels every 4 hours, not to exceed 8 softgels in 24 hours.

Child (under age 12): not recommended unless directed by your doctor.

Tylenol Cold Severe Congestion
Each caplet contains 30 mg of pseudoephedrine, 325 mg of acetaminophen, 15 mg of dextromethorphan, and 200 mg of guaifenesin.

Adult and Child (age 12 and over): 2 caplets every 6–8 hours. Do not exceed 8 caplets in a 24-hour period.

Child (age 6–11): 1 caplet every 6–8 hours. Do not exceed 4 caplets in a 24-hour period.

Child (under age 6): not recommended unless directed by your doctor.

Vicks DayQuil Liquid
Each 5 ml (1 tsp.) contains 30 mg of pseudoephedrine, 325 mg of acetaminophen, 10 mg of dextromethorphan, and 100 mg of guaifenesin.

Adult and Child (age 12 and over): 2 tsp. every 4 hours. Do not exceed 8 tsp. in a 24-hour period.

Child (age 6–11): 1 tsp. every 4 hours. Do not exceed 4 tsp. in a 24-hour period.

Child (under age 6): Consult your doctor.

Overdosage

Symptoms of overdose include nausea, vomiting, abdominal pain, urinary retention, low blood pressure, shallow breathing, blurred vision, rapid rolling of the eyeballs, loss of muscle coordination, confusion, hallucinations, drowsiness, dizziness, coma, yellowing of the skin and eyes, and liver damage. Symptoms may develop within 30 minutes, or may not be seen for as long as 2 days after the overdose.

Even if the victim is not displaying any of the symptoms listed above, do the following in case of accidental overdose: If the victim is unconscious or having convulsions, call for an ambulance immediately. If you take the victim to an emergency room, be sure to bring the bottle or container with you. If the victim is conscious, call your local poison control center or a health care professional. The poison control center may suggest inducing vomiting with ipecac syrup (available without a prescription at any pharmacy). DO NOT induce vomiting unless specifically instructed to do so.

Special Populations

Pregnancy/Breast-feeding

Sudafed Cold & Cough, Tylenol Severe Congestion, and DayQuil LiquiCaps are not recommended for pregnant women. Decongestants and acetaminophen are known to pass into the breast milk of nursing mothers and may cause side effects in infants. Check with your doctor before taking these products if you are breast-feeding.

Infants/Children

Children may be more susceptible to the side effects of Sudafed Cold & Cough, Tylenol Severe Congestion, and DayQuil LiquiCaps. Unless directed by your doctor, do not give Sudafed Cold & Cough to a child under age 12, or Tylenol Cold Severe Congestion and DayQuil LiquiCaps to a child under age 6.

Seniors

Seniors may be more sensitive to the side effects of Sudafed Cold & Cough, Tylenol Severe Congestion, and DayQuil LiquiCaps. They may experience nervousness, irritability, restlessness, dizziness, sedation, hallucinations, seizures, and low blood pressure. Most mild reactions may be handled by either lowering your dose or by switching to another product.

Seniors taking these products should be especially cautious about the amount of caffeine they ingest (see "Drug Interactions").

Sudafed Severe Cold Formula

(SOO-dah-fed)

*see **Alka-Seltzer Plus Flu & Body Aches Liqui-Gels**, page 142*

Theraflu Flu, Cold & Cough Medicine, Original Formula and Maximum Strength Night Time

(THER-uh-flu)

*see **Alka-Seltzer Plus Cold & Cough Medicine Liqui-Gels,** page 117*

Brand Name

Triaminic Expectorant

(TRYE-uh-MIN-ik)

Generic Ingredients

Guaifenesin
Phenylpropanolamine

Type of Drug

Decongestant and expectorant.

Used for

Temporary relief of nasal congestion associated with colds, loosening and thinning of bronchial secretions, and management of cough.

General Information

Some OTC products use a combination of drugs to relieve the symptoms associated with colds. Triaminic Expectorant contains a decongestant and an expectorant.

The decongestant ingredient in Triaminic Expectorant is phenylpropanolamine, an oral decongestant. Decongestants relieve nasal congestion by narrowing or constricting blood vessels in the nose, which reduces the blood supplied to the nose and decreases the swelling of nasal mucous membranes. Unlike topical decongestants (decongestant nasal sprays) that act on local blood vessels, oral decongestants may constrict blood vessels throughout the body.

The expectorant ingredient in Triaminic Expectorant is guaifenesin. Expectorants make mucus more watery and less sticky so that it is easier to bring up with coughing. Easier removal of secretions may indirectly reduce the impulse to cough. Guaifenesin is a common ingredient in OTC cough preparations; however, there is some controversy over its efficacy.

Triaminic Expectorant will not cure or prevent colds. The best you can hope for is symptomatic relief. Colds will usually go away in 1 to 2 weeks whether they are treated or not.

Cautions and Warnings

Do not use Triaminic Expectorant for more than 7 consecutive days.

If a cough lasts longer than 7 days, or keeps coming back, consult your doctor. A persistent cough may be the sign of a more serious condition.

Do not exceed the recommended daily dosage of Triaminic Expectorant.

If you experience fever, rash, or persistent headache while taking Triaminic Expectorant, stop taking it immediately and call your doctor.

Triaminic Expectorant should be used with caution by people with hyperthyroidism, heart disease, high blood pressure, diabetes, and an enlarged prostate. If you have any of these conditions, ask your doctor before using Triaminic Expectorant.

Unless directed by your doctor, do not use Triaminic Expectorant for a chronic cough, such as that associated with smoking, asthma, chronic bronchitis, or emphysema, or for coughs associated with excessive mucus.

Possible Side Effects

- ▼ Most common: restlessness, nervousness, excitability, sleeplessness, dizziness, weakness, drowsiness, and headache.
- ▼ Less common: increased blood pressure, increased or irregular heart rate, and heart palpitations.
- ▼ Rare: nausea, vomiting, severe headache, feelings of tightness in the chest, greatly elevated blood pressure, and heart contractions.

Drug Interactions

• Triaminic Expectorant should not be used at the same time as a monoamine oxidase inhibitor (MAOI) or within 2 weeks of stopping treatment with an MAOI. MAOIs are used to treat depression, other psychiatric or emotional conditions, and Parkinson's disease. If you are not sure whether you are or have been taking an MAOI, check with your doctor or pharmacist before you use Triaminic Expectorant.

• Taking Triaminic Expectorant along with another decongestant can increase the risk of adverse effects and toxicity. If you are taking another decongestant, do not use Triaminic Expectorant without first asking your doctor.

• The effects of phenylpropanolamine, the decongestant in Triaminic Expectorant, may combine with those of caffeine, a central nervous system stimulant found in many prescription and OTC drugs. This combination can cause disorientation, delirium, and other side effects.

Food Interactions

The decongestant in Triaminic Expectorant interacts adversely with caffeine (see "Drug Interactions"), which is found in many popular beverages, including coffee, tea, and cola, and in chocolate.

Usual Dose

Each 5 ml (1 tsp.) contains 6.25 mg of phenylpropanolamine and 50 mg of guaifenesin.

Adult and Child (age 12 and over): 4 tsp. every 4 hours. Do not exceed 24 tsp. in a 24-hour period.

Child (age 6–11): 2 tsp. every 4 hours. Do not exceed 12 tsp. in a 24-hour period.

Child (age 2–5): 1 tsp. every 4 hours. Do not exceed 6 tsp. in a 24-hour period.

Child (under age 2): Consult your doctor.

Overdosage

Do the following in case of accidental overdose: If the victim is unconscious or having convulsions, call for an ambulance immediately. If you take the victim to an emergency room, be sure to bring the bottle or container with you. If the victim is conscious, call your local poison control center or a health care professional. The poison control center may suggest inducing vomiting with ipecac syrup (available without a prescription at any pharmacy). DO NOT induce vomiting unless specifically instructed to do so.

Special Populations

Pregnancy/Breast-feeding

It is not generally recommended that pregnant women take any drugs, particularly during the first 3 months after conception. Decongestants have been shown to pass into the breast milk of nursing mothers and may cause side effects in nursing infants. Check with your doctor before taking Triaminic Expectorant if you are or might be pregnant, or if you are breast-feeding.

Infants/Children

Do not give Triaminic Expectorant to a child under age 2 unless directed by your doctor.

Seniors

Older persons may be more sensitive to the side effects of Triaminic Expectorant. They may experience nervousness, irritability, restlessness, dizziness, sedation, hallucinations, seizures, and low blood pressure. Most mild reactions may be handled by either lowering your dose or trying another product.

Seniors taking these products should be especially cautious about the amount of caffeine they ingest (see "Drug Interactions").

Triaminic Nite Time (TRYE-uh-MIN-ik)

*see **PediaCare Cough-Cold,** page 180*

Brand Name

Triaminic Cold & Cough

(TRYE-uh-MIN-ik)

Generic Ingredients

Chlorpheniramine maleate
Dextromethorphan
Phenylpropanolamine

Type of drug

Antihistamine, decongestant, and antitussive (cough suppressant).

Used for

Temporary relief of runny nose, sneezing, nasal congestion, itchy and watery eyes, itching of the nose or throat, and cough associated with colds and allergies.

General Information

Some OTC products use a combination of drugs to relieve symptoms that can accompany colds and allergies. Triaminicol contains an antihistamine, a decongestant, and an antitussive.

The antihistamine ingredient in Triaminicol is chlorpheniramine maleate. Antihistamines block the release of histamine in the body, relieving the sneezing and itching that often occurs with colds and allergies. They can also aid in stopping a runny nose by reducing the secretions caused by histamine release.

Since histamine is only one of several substances released by the body during an allergic reaction, antihistamines can only reduce about 40% to 60% of allergic symptoms.

The decongestant ingredient in Triaminicol is phenylpropanolamine, an oral decongestant. Decongestants relieve nasal congestion by narrowing or constricting blood vessels in the nose, which reduces the blood supplied to the nose and decreases the swelling of nasal mucous membranes. Unlike topical decongestants (decongestant nasal sprays) that act on local blood vessels, oral decongestants may constrict blood vessels throughout the body.

The cough suppressant in Triaminicol is dextromethorphan, which suppresses the cough reflex by acting directly on the cough center in the brain. Unlike some antitussives, dextromethorphan does not have pain-relieving effects, does not depress breathing, and has a low potential for addiction.

Triaminicol will not cure or prevent colds or allergies. The best you can hope for is symptomatic relief. Colds will usually go away in 1 to 2 weeks whether they are treated or not.

Cautions and Warnings

If symptoms do not improve after taking Triaminicol for 7 days continuously, see your doctor.

If a cough lasts longer than 7 days, or keeps coming back, consult your doctor. A persistent cough may be the sign of a more serious condition.

Do not exceed the recommended daily dosage of Triaminicol.

If you experience fever, rash, or persistent headache while taking Triaminicol, stop taking it immediately and call your doctor.

Triaminicol should be used with caution if you have a condition that causes breathing problems, such as emphysema, chronic bronchitis, or asthma. Consult your doctor before using Triaminicol if you have any of these conditions.

Triaminicol should be used with caution by people with glaucoma, hyperthyroidism, heart disease, high blood pressure, diabetes, an enlarged prostate, or liver disease. If you have any of these conditions, ask your doctor before using Triaminicol.

The antihistamine ingredient in Triaminicol acts as a depressant on the central nervous system (CNS), and can cause sleepiness or grogginess and interfere with the ability to concentrate. Your ability to perform activities that require your full alertness and coordination, such as driving a motor vehicle or operating machinery, may be affected. Refrain from drinking alcohol while you are taking Triaminicol, because alcohol aggravates these effects.

Because productive coughing (coughing that brings up mucus) actually helps relieve the underlying condition, some doctors do not believe that suppressing a productive cough makes good sense. However, a severe cough can interfere with sleep, and loss of sleep can contribute to the severity and duration of an illness. In the balance, the most appropriate use of cough suppressants may be to relieve a dry, nonproductive cough, especially at night.

Unless directed by your doctor, do not take Triaminicol if you have a chronic cough, such as that associated with smoking, asthma, chronic bronchitis, or emphysema, or for coughs associated with excessive mucus.

Dextromethorphan, the antitussive ingredient in Triaminicol, is not recommended for people confined to bed rest or under sedation.

Possible Side Effects

- ▼ Most common: restlessness, nervousness, sleeplessness or drowsiness, sedation, excitability, dizziness, poor coordination, and upset stomach.
- ▼ Less common: dry eyes, nose, and mouth; blurred vision; difficulty urinating; irritability (at high doses); increased blood pressure; increased or irregular heart rate; heart palpitations, and loss of appetite.
- ▼ Rare: nausea, severe headache, feelings of tightness in the chest, greatly elevated blood pressure, and heart contractions.

Drug Interactions

• The antihistamine ingredient in Triaminicol can enhance the effect of other drugs that depress the CNS, such as barbiturates, tranquilizers, sleeping medications, and alcohol (present in many OTC preparations). If you are taking other depressant drugs, check with your doctor before taking Triaminicol. Avoid drinking alcohol if you are taking Triaminicol.

• Antihistamines can affect the results of skin and blood tests. Notify your health care professional before scheduling these tests if you are taking Triaminicol.

• Triaminicol should not be used at the same time as a monoamine oxidase inhibitor (MAOI) or within 2 weeks of stopping treatment with an MAOI. MAOIs are used to treat depression, other psychiatric or emotional conditions, and Parkinson's disease. If you are not sure whether you are or have been taking an MAOI, check with your doctor or pharmacist before using Triaminicol.

• The effects of the decongestant in Triaminicol may combine with those of caffeine, a CNS stimulant found in many prescription and OTC drugs. This combination can cause disorientation, delirium, and other side effects.

• Taking Triaminicol along with another decongestant can increase the risk of adverse effects and toxicity. If you are taking another decongestant, do not use Triaminicol without first asking your doctor.

Food Interactions

The decongestant in Triaminicol interacts adversely with caffeine (see "Drug Interactions"), which is found in many popular beverages, including coffee, tea, and cola, and in chocolate.

Usual Dose

To relieve the symptoms of allergies, it is best to take Triaminicol on a schedule rather than as needed because histamine is released almost continuously.

Each 5 ml (1 tsp.) contains 1 mg chlorpheniramine, 6.25 mg of phenylpropanolamine, and 5 mg of dextromethorphan.

Adult and Child (age 12 and over): 4 tsp. every 4–6 hours. Do not exceed 6 doses in a 24-hour period.

Child (age 6–11): 2 tsp. every 4–6 hours. Do not exceed 6 doses in a 24-hour period.

Child (under age 6): not recommended unless directed by your doctor.

You may minimize the inconvenience of the sedative effects of Triaminicol by taking a full dose at bedtime and by using the smallest recommended dose during the day. You can establish the lowest dose necessary for effective relief by starting with the lowest dose when you begin taking the drug, and gradually increasing the dosage over several days as needed.

If you forget to take a dose of Triaminicol, do so as soon as you remember. If it is almost time for your next dose, skip the one you forgot and continue with your regular schedule. Do not take a double dose.

Overdosage

Symptoms of overdose include nausea, vomiting, urinary retention, shallow breathing, flushed face, dry mouth, blurred vision, dilated pupils, rapid rolling of the eyeballs, loss of muscle coordination, excitability, confusion, drowsiness, dizziness, hallucinations, seizures, and coma.

Even if the victim is not displaying any of the symptoms listed above, do the following in case of accidental overdose: If the victim is unconscious or having convulsions, call for an ambulance immediately. If you take the victim to an

emergency room, be sure to bring the bottle or container with you. If the victim is conscious, call your local poison control center or a health care professional. The poison control center may suggest inducing vomiting with ipecac syrup (available without a prescription at any pharmacy). DO NOT induce vomiting unless specifically instructed to do so.

Special Populations

Pregnancy/Breast-feeding

Antihistamines are not recommended for use during pregnancy unless directed by your doctor. Antihistamines and decongestants have been shown to pass into the breast milk of nursing mothers and may cause side effects in infants. Check with your doctor before taking Triaminicol if you are or might be pregnant, or if you are breast-feeding.

Infants/Children

Children may be more susceptible to the side effects of Triaminicol. They are also more susceptible to accidental antihistamine overdose. Do not give Triaminicol to a child under age 6 unless directed by your doctor.

Seniors

Older persons may be more sensitive to the side effects of Triaminicol. They may experience nervousness, irritability, and restlessness. Dizziness, sedation, and low blood pressure may also occur. Older men may experience difficulty in urinating. Most mild reactions may be handled by either lowering your dose or trying another antihistamine/decongestant combination.

Seniors taking Triaminicol should be especially cautious about the amount of caffeine they ingest (see "Drug Interactions").

Tylenol Cold Multi-Symptom Hot Medication (TYE-leh-nol)

*see **Alka-Seltzer Plus Cold & Cough Medicine Liqui-Gels,** page 117*

Tylenol Cold Non Drowsy Medication (TYE-leh-nol)

see *Alka-Seltzer Plus Flu & Body Aches Liqui-Gels*, *page 142*

Tylenol Cold Severe Congestion (TYE-leh-nol)

see *Sudafed Cold & Cough*, *page 201*

Tylenol Flu Maximum Strength Gelcaps (TYE-leh-nol)

see *Alka-Seltzer Plus Flu & Body Aches Liqui-Gels*, *page 142*

Vicks DayQuil (VIKS)

see *Sudafed Cold & Cough*, *page 201*

Brand Name

Vicks 44D (VIKS)

Generic Ingredients

Dextromethorphan
Pseudoephedrine

Type of Drug

Decongestant and antitussive (cough suppressant).

Used for

Temporary relief of cough and nasal congestion associated with colds.

General Information

Some OTC products use a combination of drugs to relieve symptoms that can accompany colds. Vicks 44D contains a decongestant and an antitussive.

The decongestant ingredient in Vicks 44D is pseudoephedrine, an oral decongestant. Decongestants relieve nasal congestion by narrowing or constricting blood vessels in the nose, which reduces the blood supplied to the nose and decreases the swelling of nasal mucous membranes. Unlike topical decongestants (decongestant nasal sprays) that act on local blood vessels, oral decongestants may constrict blood vessels throughout the body.

The cough suppressant in Vicks 44D is dextromethorphan, which suppresses the cough reflex by acting directly on the cough center in the brain. Unlike some antitussives, it does not depress breathing, and has a low potential for addiction.

Vicks 44D will not cure or prevent colds or flu. The best you can hope for is symptomatic relief. Colds will usually go away in 1 to 2 weeks whether they are treated or not.

Cautions and Warnings

Do not use Vicks 44D for more than 7 consecutive days.

If your cough lasts longer than 7 days, or keeps coming back, consult your doctor. A persistent cough may be the sign of a more serious condition.

Do not exceed the recommended daily dosage of Vicks 44D.

If you experience fever, rash, or persistent headache while taking Vicks 44D, stop taking it immediately and call your doctor.

Vicks 44D should be used with caution by people with hyperthyroidism, heart disease, high blood pressure, diabetes, an enlarged prostate, asthma, or liver disease. If you have any of these conditions, ask your doctor before using Vicks 44D.

Because productive coughing (coughing that brings up mucus) actually helps relieve the underlying condition, some doctors do not believe that suppressing a productive cough makes good sense. However, a severe cough can interfere with sleep, and loss of sleep can contribute to the severity and duration of an illness. In the balance, the most appropriate use of cough suppressants may be to relieve a dry, nonproductive cough, especially at night.

Unless directed by your doctor, do not use Vicks 44D if you have chronic cough, such as that associated with smoking, asthma, chronic bronchitis, or emphysema, or for coughs associated with excessive mucus.

Dextromethorphan, the antitussive ingredient in Vicks 44D, is not recommended for people confined to bed rest or under sedation.

Possible Side Effects

▼ Most common: restlessness, nervousness, excitability, sleeplessness, dizziness, weakness, drowsiness, and headache.

▼ Less common: increased blood pressure, increased or irregular heart rate, and heart palpitations.

▼ Rare: nausea, difficulty breathing, difficulty or pain when urinating, anxiety, tremor, hallucinations, seizures, and cardiovascular collapse.

Drug Interactions

• Vicks 44D should not be used at the same time as a monoamine oxidase inhibitor (MAOI) or within 2 weeks of stopping treatment with an MAOI. MAOIs are used to treat depression, other psychiatric or emotional conditions, and Parkinson's disease. If you are not sure whether you are or have been taking an MAOI, check with your doctor or pharmacist before you use Vicks 44D.

• The effects of the decongestant in Vicks 44D may combine with those of caffeine, a CNS stimulant found in many prescription and OTC drugs. This combination can cause disorientation, delirium, and other side effects.

• Taking Vicks 44D along with another decongestant can increase the risk of adverse effects and toxicity. If you are taking another decongestant, do not use Vicks 44D without first asking your doctor.

Food Interactions

The decongestant in Vicks 44D interacts adversely with caffeine (see "Drug Interactions"), which is found in many popular beverages, including coffee, tea, and cola, and in chocolate.

Usual Dose

Each 15 ml (3 tsp.) contains 60 mg of pseudoephedrine and 30 mg of dextromethorphan.

Adult and Child (age 12 and over): 3 tsp. every 6 hours. Do not exceed 4 doses in a 24-hour period.

Child (age 6–12): 1 1/2 tsp. every 6 hours. Do not exceed 4 doses in a 24-hour period.

Child (under age 6): Consult your doctor.

Overdosage

Symptoms of overdose include nausea, vomiting, urinary retention, shallow breathing, blurred vision, rapid rolling of the eyeballs, loss of muscle coordination, confusion, drowsiness, dizziness, hallucinations, and coma.

Even if the victim is not displaying any of the symptoms listed above, do the following in case of accidental overdose: If the victim is unconscious or having convulsions, call for an ambulance immediately. If you take the victim to an emergency room, be sure to bring the bottle or container with you. If the victim is conscious, call your local poison control center or a health care professional. The poison control center may suggest inducing vomiting with ipecac syrup (available without a prescription at any pharmacy). DO NOT induce vomiting unless specifically instructed to do so.

Special Populations

Pregnancy/Breast-feeding

It is not generally recommended that pregnant women take any drugs, particularly during the first 3 months of after conception. Decongestants have been shown to pass into the breast milk of nursing mothers and may cause side effects in infants. Check with your doctor before taking Vicks 44D if you are or might be pregnant, or if you are breast-feeding.

Infants/Children

Do not give Vicks 44D to a child under age 6 without your doctor's supervision.

Seniors

Older persons may be more sensitive to the side effects of Vicks 44D. They may experience nervousness, irritability, restlessness, dizziness, sedation, hallucinations, seizures, and low blood pressure. Most mild reactions may be handled by either lowering your dose or trying another product.

Seniors taking these products should be especially cautious about the amount of caffeine they ingest (see "Drug Interactions").

Vicks 44E (VIKS)

*see **Robitussin DM,** page 193*

Vicks NyQuil (VIKS)

*see **Alka-Seltzer Plus Night-Time Cold Medicine Liqui-Gels,** page 155*

Brand Name

Vicks Vapor Inhaler (VIKS)

Generic Ingredient

l-Desoxyephedrine

Type of Drug

Topical decongestant.

Used for

Temporary relief of nasal congestion due to colds and allergies.

General Information

Vicks Vapor Inhaler contains *l*-desoxyephedrine, which acts as a topical decongestant by narrowing or constricting blood vessels in the nose. This reduces the blood supplied to the nose and decreases the swelling of nasal mucous membranes.

Vicks Inhaler will not cure or prevent nasal congestion. The best you can hope for is symptomatic relief.

Cautions and Warnings

Do not use Vicks Inhaler for more than 3 consecutive days.

Do not exceed the recommended daily dosage of Vicks Inhaler.

Do not use Vicks Inhaler if you have hyperthyroidism, heart disease, high blood pressure, diabetes, or an enlarged prostate.

Frequent or prolonged use of Vicks Inhaler may cause nasal congestion to recur or worsen. You may experience rebound congestion; that is, you may still have a stuffy nose even though you have been using Vicks Inhaler for several days. The lining of your nose may swell and turn red, giving the appearance of allergic rhinitis. If this happens, stop using Vicks Inhaler and call your doctor. The signs of rebound congestion will usually go away within 7 days of not using the drug.

To prevent the spread of infection, a single Vicks Inhaler should not be used by more than one person.

Possible Side Effects

Vicks Inhaler may cause temporary stinging, burning, itching, or an increase in nasal discharge.

Drug Interactions

None known.

Food Interactions

None known.

Usual Dose

Each inhaler contains 50 mg of *l*-desoxyephedrine.

Adult and Child (age 12 and over): 2 inhalations in each nostril every 2 hours.

Child (6–11): 1 inhalation in each nostril every 2 hours, with adult supervision.

Child (under age 6): Consult your doctor.

Overdosage

Do the following in case of accidental ingestion or overdose If the victim is unconscious or having convulsions, call fo an ambulance immediately. If you take the victim to a emergency room, be sure to bring the bottle or containe with you. If the victim is conscious, call your local poiso control center or a health care professional. The poison con trol center may suggest inducing vomiting with ipecac syru (available without a prescription at any pharmacy). DO NO induce vomiting unless specifically instructed to do so.

Special Populations

Pregnancy/Breast-feeding

It is not generally recommended that pregnant women tak any drugs, particularly during the first 3 months after con ception. Check with your doctor before using Vicks Inhaler i you are or might be pregnant, or if you are breast-feeding.

Infants/Children

Do not use Vicks Inhaler for a child under age 6 unles directed by your doctor. Children over age 6 should onl use Vicks Inhaler with adult supervision.

Seniors

Seniors should exercise the same caution as younge adults when using Vicks Inhaler.

Chapter 3: Diet and Stomach Medicines

Weight

In the U.S., 1 out of every 4 persons is overweight. This is due to a number of factors: Supermarket shelves are loaded with plenty of high-calorie, high-fat foods, and most of us do not get enough exercise to burn off the excessive calories we consume during meals and frequent snacks. On the other hand, some people inherit a genetic problem or have a hormonal imbalance that disrupts body metabolism (the process of digesting food and using its energy).

Many overweight people are obese, which doctors define as being 20% above the ideal weight for a given age and height. For example, a person who, according to standard charts, should weigh 140 pounds but who tips the scales at 170 would be considered obese. Another way to measure obesity is the body mass index (see box). Excess body weight is a serious threat to health. It increases the risk of many conditions, including high blood pressure, stroke, coronary artery disease, adult-onset diabetes, and cancer.

At any given time, as many as 70% of American women and 50% of men are taking steps either to lose or to maintain their weight. In their desire to look and feel their best, some people will try anything. For decades, dieting—eating special foods or food combinations—has been one of the nation's great obsessions. Other strategies include everything from surgery to liposuction to hypnotism. The most effective technique is a change in lifestyle by reducing the intake of calories and participating in vigorous exercise, but that requires a combination of self-restraint, self-discipline, and physical effort that many people cannot manage.

Body Mass Index

The best way to determine obesity is by calculating your body mass index, (BMI). Because this number takes your size into account, nutritionists feel the BMI is a more accurate measurement than merely adding up pounds.

To determine your BMI, grab a calculator. Figure out your height in inches and multiply that number by itself (square it). Then divide your weight in pounds by that number and multiply the result by 705.

Example: Say you are 5′10″ tall and weigh 150 pounds. Your height in inches is 70; the square of 70 (70 x 70) is 4900. Divide 150 by 4900; the result is 0.0306122. Multiply that by 705 and you get a BMI of approximately 21.6.

Different experts interpret the results in various ways. However, as a rule of thumb, a BMI index above 26 for women or 28 for men indicates obesity.

Formula for calculating BMI:
(Weight in pounds ÷ height in inches squared) x 705 = BMI

We eat because we feel hungry. It makes sense, then, that reducing feelings of hunger, or appetite, would help to lower calorie intake and thus promote weight loss. Scientists conducting research to understand how the brain controls appetite have found that certain drugs act by turning off hunger signals. Most of these drugs, known as anorexiants, anorectics, or appetite suppressants, are available only with a prescription for people who are severely overweight. It is not yet certain whether such medicines will prove safe and effective in the long run, or whether they should be used by people who are just a few pounds over their ideal weight. What is known is that almost all people who lose weight with these drugs have regained it (and, often, more) 6 to 12 months after stopping the treatment.

Management of Weight

Not surprisingly, the concept that we might be able to swallow a pill and watch the pounds melt away has enormous appeal. Until recently, drugstores sold OTC products containing any one of more than 100 ingredients touted as weight-loss agents. The list includes everything from alfalfa to pineapple enzymes to vitamin A. In 1992, however, the FDA declared that none of these was safe and effective as a method for achieving weight control. Benzocaine, which is basically an anesthetic, is still found in some OTC products, but based on available data, the FDA also declared this ingredient ineffective. Most manufacturers have removed benzocaine from their weight loss products until further studies can be done to show whether it does any good.

For many years, dextroamphetamine was commonly available for use in controlling appetite. In most cases, however, this drug produces only mild weight loss, and the loss is sustained for only a few weeks. Any benefits are offset by the fact that dextroamphetamine can be highly addictive. Although amphetamines are officially approved for weight loss, they are no longer widely used for this purpose. Some states have even passed laws making them unavailable by prescription.

The only OTC drug currently approved for weight management is phenylpropanolamine hydrochloride (PPA). Although PPA is related to dextroamphetamine, it appears to act differently in the body. Instead of turning off the hunger signals directly, PPA may instead affect the body's overall metabolism. Scientists believe that the body has a kind of internal weight thermostat, which works by maintaining a certain weight level. This level, known as the setpoint, is different for each individual. The setpoint concept helps explain why so many dieters regain weight after a period of initial weight loss: The body's thermostat will increase or decrease appetite in order to maintain its steady, pre-established weight. Theoretically, use of PPA may lower that setpoint, just as we lower the thermostat in our homes to make them cooler. Another way PPA may work is by increasing body heat, which would help to burn off excess calories.

The maximum dose of PPA is 75 mg per day. Timed-release products deliver this dose over the course of the day; products with smaller doses (25 to 37.5 mg) can be taken 2 or 3 times a day. Studies show that use of PPA for up to 14 weeks can promote weight loss, but whether the drug is safe beyond that time is not fully known. Side effects include nervousness, insomnia, anxiety, headache, nausea, and increased blood pressure. The risk of adverse reactions increases if PPA is consumed at higher doses.

Given the fact that so many people are concerned about their weight, interest in weight loss products and programs is naturally very high. Controlling appetite and thus lowering calorie intake is an important part of a weight control program. Use of drugs may be helpful for a few weeks, but at best these products are just one part of an overall strategy. Behavioral changes, self-help programs, and increased exercise are other useful strategies.

OTC Product for Appetite Suppression
Phenylpropanolamine hydrochloride (PPA)

Constipation

Constipation means the infrequent and/or difficult passage of hard, dry stools. Often constipation occurs because the fecal material moves too slowly through the large intestines, allowing more time for water to be removed.

Sometimes people who feel constipated will say that they are irregular. They become concerned if they don't have daily bowel movements. But everybody has different patterns. Some people have bowel movements 3 times a day, while others have them 3 times a week. Frequency is not as important as whether the movements occur regularly and without discomfort or difficulty.

In most cases, constipation is a temporary problem resulting from a lack of sufficient liquid and fiber in the diet. Fiber, a component of fruits, vegetables, and whole grains, contributes bulk to the fecal material. Bulk stimulates the muscles of the intestine and helps them move the material along. Inadequate fluid intake may contribute to the problem by robbing the material of necessary lubrication and making the stools dry and hard. Lack of exercise can also affect the ability to have a comfortable bowel movement. Sometimes constipation results when people continually resist going to the toilet even though they feel the urge to do so. This is an occupational hazard for teachers and those in other occupations who are not always free to take breaks when the need arises.

In older people, constipation can arise due to weakness in pelvic and abdominal muscles, which makes it difficult to generate sufficient pressure during a bowel movement. Constipation can also result from other medical conditions, such as hemorrhoids, irritable bowel syndrome, hypothyroidism, intestinal cancer, and diverticular disease. Some of these illnesses can make bowel movements painful. Naturally, people who experience pain at such times will be afraid to have movements, which in turn contributes to constipation. Use of certain medications can also affect bowel function. Examples of drugs that list constipation as a side effect include analgesics (pain relievers), especially those containing narcotics; antidepressants; diuretics; and antihypertensives (blood pressure medications).

Seek medical attention if any of the following applies to you

- Persistent constipation arising after years of regular bowel habits
- Pain when having a bowel movement
- Loss of appetite
- Unexplained weight loss
- Chronic and worsening abdominal distention (bloating)
- Inadequate relief after appropriate use of laxatives
- Blood in the stool

Treatment for Constipation

Laxatives are products intended to provide temporary relief of constipation. Used appropriately, they can help restore regular bowel function (see box).

Laxatives are among the most frequently abused OTC medications. Sometimes people take them in doses that are too high or for too long a period. Some people use laxatives to make food pass more quickly from the body as a method of increasing weight loss. Over time, there is a strong chance that people will become dependent on laxatives because they believe that they cannot have a bowel movement without them. Ironically, chronic overuse of laxatives can severely disrupt the ability of the bowels to function normally and thus can actually make the constipation worse, in addition to posing a risk of other severe problems (see box).

Proper Use of Laxatives

- The best way to promote good bowel habits is to eat a healthy diet containing fiber; exercise; drink plenty of fluids; and try to use the toilet the same time each day and whenever the urge to have a bowel movement arises.
- Use laxatives only for temporary relief of occasional constipation. Once regular bowel movements have returned, discontinue use of laxatives.
- If a skin rash develops, discontinue laxative use and contact a physician.
- Do not use saline or stimulant laxatives on a daily basis.
- If you use a stimulant laxative, use the minimum dose needed to produce an effect.
- Do not give mineral oil laxatives to children under age 6 or to seniors.
- Do not use mineral oil in conjunction with emollient laxatives.
- Pregnant women should avoid mineral oil products.
- Do not use laxatives if you have abdominal pain, sores or irritation in the anal region, nausea, vomiting, bloating, or cramping; instead, contact your physician.
- Be aware that certain stimulant laxatives can cause stools or urine to turn pinkish or red.

Risks of Laxative Abuse

Severe diarrhea
Electrolyte imbalance (insufficient calcium, potassium, etc.)
Osteomalacia (bone wasting)
Steatorrhea (passage of fat in stools)
Colon dysfunction
Liver disease
Lung disease (lipid pneumonia in chronic mineral oil users)

There are different kinds of laxatives whose various ingredients produce different combinations of effects. They come in a number of forms: liquid, tablets, suppositories—even chewing gum and chocolate-flavored tablets. If you use a laxative, be sure to talk with your pharmacist to learn which one is right for your particular needs. Results from laxative use are usually seen within 12 to 24 hours, but some people may need to take laxatives for up to 3 days before they experience the expected benefits.

Types of Laxatives

Bulk-forming laxatives are usually the first choice for constipation relief. As the name suggests, these products contribute bulk, which is needed for normal passage of stools. Some laxatives contain natural bulking agents derived from agar, psyllium seeds, kelp, or other plants, while others contain synthetic ingredients, such as forms of cellulose or calcium polycarbophil. Bulk-forming laxatives work at least partly by increasing the amount of water absorbed in and retained by the stool. They are usually appropriate for use by seniors, by pregnant women and women who have recently undergone labor, and by those with conditions such as colostomies, irritable bowel syndrome, or diverticular disease. Since these products work best when taken with a full glass of water or juice, they may not be appropriate for individuals who must restrict fluid intake, such as those with kidney dysfunction. Generally, though, bulk-forming laxatives are quite safe and effective when used as directed.

Emollient laxatives are also known as stool softeners. The active ingredient in these products, docusate, increases the wetness of the feces to permit a smoother passage. These laxatives are best used to prevent constipation in people who need to avoid straining, such as those who have a hernia or who have undergone surgery for hemorrhoids. They are generally not effective in treating existing constipation. Emollient laxatives usually produce results within 1 to 2 days, but some people may need to use them for as long as 5 days. They are safe and may be used for up to 1 week; if longer use is needed, a physician should be consulted.

Lubricant laxatives achieve the same effect as emollients, but in a different way. They contain mineral or plant oils that coat the stool, preventing the water from being absorbed by the intestine. They are better at relieving an existing constipation problem than emollients, which are used primarily for preventing constipation. People who might consider a lubricant laxative include those who need to avoid straining, such as individuals who have recently undergone abdominal surgery. Emollient and lubricant laxatives should not be used at the same time because of the risk of adverse effects. Seniors, children under age 6, and patients who have a depressed gag reflex (e.g., stroke victims) may inadvertantly inhale small amounts of mineral oil; this can cause a lung inflammation known as lipid pneumonia.

Stimulant laxatives contain ingredients that activate the muscles and nerves in the intestines to increase passage of material. Some of these products may also trigger the release of water or other chemicals into the intestine to promote bowel movements. There are several types of stimulant laxatives available. One type contains such ingredients as cascara sagrada, casanthranol, and senna compounds. Generally these work within 12 hours; the liquid forms of these products are probably more effective than solid forms. Another group contains bisacodyl or phenolphthalein. These are typically used before gastrointestinal surgery and in patients with colostomies. A third type of stimulant laxative is castor oil, which is typically used only in severe cases requiring a complete and rapid evacuation of the entire bowel; it should not be used for less severe cases of constipation. Stimulant laxatives are effective, but they often work quickly and powerfully. Side effects include poorly functioning colon, fluid loss, discoloration (redness) of urine or stool, and worsening of hemorrhoids.

Glycerin is the main ingredient in laxative suppositories and some enemas. Use of a glycerin suppository usually stimulates a bowel movement within 30 minutes.

Saline laxatives are used when it is necessary to bring on an immediate bowel movement. Such products might be necessary in emergencies such as food or drug poisoning. They are also used in hospitals prior to certain medical procedures (e.g., colonoscopy). Saline laxatives are not used for normal cases of constipation.

OTC Products for Constipation

- Bulk-forming laxatives
  - Calcium polycarbophil
  - Methylcellulose
  - Oat bran
  - Psyllium seed husks + buckthorn bark
  - Psyllium, psyllium hydrophilic mucilloid or fiber
- Emollients and lubricants
  - Docusate calcium
  - Docusate potassium
  - Docusate sodium
  - Mineral oil
- Stimulants
  - Bisacodyl
  - Casanthranol
  - Cascara sagrada aromatic fluidextract
  - Cascara sagrada extract
  - Castor oil
  - Phenolphthalein, yellow phenolphthalein
  - Senna, senna concentrate
  - Sennosides
- Saline laxatives
  - Magnesium citrate
  - Magnesium oxide or hydroxide
  - Magnesium sulfate
  - Sodium phosphate
- Other
  - Glycerin suppositories
  - Lactulose

Diarrhea

Diarrhea is an increase in the frequency, fluidity, or quantity of stool passed in bowel movements. Normally, most of the water and fluid is absorbed during the stool's journey through the large intestine or colon, giving the stool the consistency of clay. If the material passes through too rapidly, however, or if excess fluid is secreted into the intestine as the result of irritation or inflammation, the water remains and causes the material to be expelled in a more liquid state. Usually diarrhea causes a sudden and uncontrollable urge to go to the bathroom. Frequent bowel movements usually lead to irritation and soreness in the anal region.

Diarrhea is not a disease in itself; instead, it is a symptom of some other underlying problem. Many cases of acute diarrhea are food-borne; that is, they are caused by consuming food or water contaminated by bacteria, viruses, or parasites. Often people who travel to other countries develop diarrhea because they ingest bacteria that are normally harmless but that interfere with the bacteria already living inside their digestive tract. In some cases, diarrhea can arise due to anxiety or stress.

Onset of acute infectious or toxin-induced diarrhea occurs within 2 to 48 hours, depending on the underlying cause. For example, staphylococcal infections—commonly arising from eating contaminated salads, dairy products, custard, sausage, ham, or poultry—can emerge within a few hours and are usually associated with nausea and vomiting in addition to diarrhea. Salmonella poisoning, which results from eating raw or undercooked foods such as ground beef or contaminated eggs, can take a day or two to show up. Diarrhea is also a symptom of shigellosis and amebic dysentery. People who are sensitive to certain foods such as spices or seeds or who are unable to digest foods such as the lactose (milk sugar) found in dairy products may develop diarrhea if they consume these items. Finally, diarrhea can also be a side effect of certain medications, including laxatives, stomach products (especially antacids) containing magnesium, and common broad-spectrum antibiotics such as ampicillin or tetracycline.

If diarrhea persists for 4 weeks or more, it is considered chronic. This condition may arise from a more serious disease, either in the gastrointestinal (GI) tract or elsewhere in the body. Diarrhea is a symptom of Crohn's disease, ulcerative colitis, AIDS, intestinal cancer, overactive thyroid, and irritable bowel syndrome. Laxative abuse can also lead to chronic diarrhea, as can stress. People with chronic diarrhea should be evaluated by a physician.

In most cases, acute diarrhea is merely unpleasant and inconvenient. The condition usually gets better within 1 to 3 days, even without treatment. However, persistent diarrhea causes the body to lose significant amounts of fluid, posing a risk of severe dehydration. In infants and children, severe diarrhea (8 to 10 bowel movements within 24 hours) can be fatal.

Seek medical attention if any of the following applies to you

- Diarrhea persisting for more than 2 days
- Diarrhea that gets worse
- Blood in the stool
- Fever
- Vomiting
- Dehydration
- Abdominal tenderness or cramping
- Loss of 5% or more of body weight

Pregnant women, children under age 3, people with other medical conditions, and those with a history of chronic illness such as heart disease or diabetes who experience diarrhea should see a doctor.

Treatment for Diarrhea

The immediate goal of treatment for diarrhea is to replenish lost fluids and restore lost electrolytes (salts such as calcium, sodium, and potassium). This is known as oral rehydration. One effective home remedy is to mix a teaspoon of table salt and 4 teaspoons of sugar in a quart of water, and drink 1 pint of the mixture every hour until the problem resolves. Do not eat solid food during this time.

Commercial products are also available to provide rehydration. These products, such as Pedialyte, contain potassium and other chemicals not found in table salt. Some come ready mixed; others must be mixed with water.

There are a number of other drugs that may be helpful in treating diarrhea or providing relief of its symptoms. Antiperistaltic agents work by slowing down the peristalsis (muscle movement) that propels stools through the intestines. Slowing the passage of the material permits more of the water and electrolytes to be reabsorbed into the body. Until recently, antiperistaltic agents containing opiates were available as OTC products. At this time, however, the only antiperistaltic drug available without a prescription is loperamide, found in such products as Imodium A-D. After the initial dose, further doses of the drug can be taken following each bowel movement. This medication helps relieve cramping and reduces the frequency of stools, but it should be taken for no more than 48 hours.

Adsorbents, another type of ingredient in antidiarrheal medications, work by causing other substances to stick to their surface and removing them from the digestive tract. The adsorbents currently available—attapulgite, kaolin, and pectin—are often used to treat mild acute diarrhea. Recently, however, concern has grown that these ingredients may remove too many of the good substances, such as nutrients and digestive enzymes, along with the bad ones, such as bacterial toxins. There is also a chance that these ingredients can interfere with other oral medications. As a result, the safety and efficacy of adsorbents are under review by the FDA. It is likely, for example, that pectin will no longer be approved as a treatment for diarrhea.

Bismuth subsalicylate—more commonly known by its brand name, Pepto-Bismol—relieves diarrhea by reducing the secretion of fluid into the intestine and by reducing the activity of bacteria.

Polycarbophil is a synthetic compound that absorbs excess water and thus reduces the amount of diarrhetic stool. This substance is available as a chewable tablet.

People who experience diarrhea because they cannot digest lactose may benefit from taking medications containing the digestive enzyme lactase.

In some cases, it may be possible to prevent traveler's diarrhea by using prescription antibiotics. Most experts do not recommend this strategy, however, because it is expensive and because overuse of antibiotic drugs can make them ineffective over time. Two tablets of Pepto-Bismol taken 4 times a day are also effective in preventing traveler's diarrhea. If traveler's diarrhea occurs, antibiotics are used to eradicate the cause of the problem, while fluid and electrolyte replacement, loperamide, and bismuth work to treat the symptoms.

OTC Products for Diarrhea

Antiperistaltic agent
- Loperamide

Adsorbents
- Attapulgite
- Kaolin and pectin

Other
- Bismuth subsalicylate
- Polycarbophil
- Digestive enzymes

Peptic Ulcer Disease

Peptic ulcer disease is the term for a group of chronic conditions that involve recurring, persistent ulcers—open sores arising on the surface of the mucous membranes that line the upper GI tract. The GI tract includes the esophagus (the tube from the mouth to the stomach), the stomach, and the duodenum (upper part of the small intestine). Ulcers in the stomach are called gastric ulcers; duodenal ulcers develop in the duodenum. Only in rare instances do ulcers form on the esophagus, although inflammation of the lower esophagus caused by acid reflux (acid-containing stomach contents return to the esophagus) is a common condition.

Normally, the membranes in the GI tract secrete mucus that serves as a protective barrier against the powerful acids and enzymes the body produces during digestion. If something occurs to weaken that barrier, these substances can eat away at the underlying tissue and produce an ulcer.

It used to be thought that excess stomach acid or spicy foods caused ulcers. In fact, however, the vast majority of peptic ulcers result from either one of two main factors: infection with a bacterium called *Helicobacter pylori* (which can be treated with antibiotics), or the long-term use of aspirin or other nonsteroidal anti-inflammatory drugs (NSAIDs) such as ibuprofen. The presence of the bacteria and the irritating effects of the drugs have been found to reduce the amount or the protective quality of the mucus. In rare cases, ulcers result from a tumor's secretion of a hormone that stimulates excess acid production.

Gastric ulcers, especially those caused by bacteria, usually (but not always) produce a dull, aching pain in the stomach or upper abdomen soon after eating. The pain may resemble a severe hunger pang. Duodenal ulcers may cause a gnawing pain a few hours after a meal. Strangely, the pain of duodenal ulcers usually gets better if the person eats again or has a glass of milk. The pain can feel as though it arises in the lower chest or the mid-back. In many cases, the pain continues for a few weeks and then disappears, only to return later. Pain is less often a symptom of ulcers caused by drugs. Gastric ulcers may cause nausea, vomiting, diarrhea, a sense of fullness, presence of blood in the stool, bloating, and in some cases, significant loss of body weight. Such symptoms are less common with duodenal ulcers.

In about 1 of 5 cases, the ulcer may cause bleeding. People with bleeding ulcers may not notice any pain, but they may have bowel movements that appear black and tar-like. Sometimes these individuals vomit a bloody material that resembles coffee grounds. Pain that is sharp, severe, and sudden in onset often indicates that the ulcer has eaten completely through the lining of the stomach or the duodenum. Such cases are called perforated ulcers.

The risk of peptic ulcer disease is higher in people who smoke, who drink alcohol, or who have a family history of the disorder.

Seek medical attention if any of the following applies to you

- Gnawing pain after eating
- Pain that is relieved by eating
- Black, tar-like stools
- Vomiting (especially vomiting of a material that looks like coffee grounds)
- Sharp, sudden, or severe pain

Treatment for Ulcers

In most cases, if you have peptic ulcer disease, you should not treat yourself with OTC products exclusively. Instead, you should be under the care of a physician. Research shows that use of prescription antibiotics to eliminate the bacterium that causes ulcers is an effective way to treat ulcers and to prevent their recurrence.

The same prescription medications used in the treatment of peptic ulcers are also available in OTC formulations. These drugs, classified as histamine$_2$-receptor antagonists (H_2RAs), include cimetidine (Tagamet HB), ranitidine (Zantac 75), and famotidine (Pepcid AC). However, in the low OTC doses available, these products are not effective for treatment of peptic ulcers. They are indicated only for the treatment of heartburn and acid indigestion, discussed in the next section. If you want to use one of these products for ulcer treatment, you need to get a prescription from your doctor for one of the higher-dose formulations, or use enough of the OTC drug to be equivalent to the prescription dose. This should be done under the direction of your physician.

OTC antacids appear to promote healing of peptic ulcers. Healing requires 4 to 6 weeks (longer for gastric ulcers). However, to be of much use, antacids must be taken very frequently (up to 7 times a day), which may not be very convenient or pleasant. Most clinicians believe the main role of antacids is to provide additional pain relief during the first week or 2 of prescription treatment for ulcers. Even if you do not experience symptoms, you should continue taking antacid treatment for the full length of time your doctor recommends. By the same token, you may continue to experience pain while taking antacids, even though the ulcer is healing well. Ulcers caused by drugs generally take longer to heal than those caused by bacteria. After the initial ulcers heal, antacids taken 2 to 4 times a day may reduce the risk that the ulcers will recur. Bismuth subsalicylate was formerly considered to be an antacid but it may now be used in the management of peptic ulcer disease and as one of the components of an anti-*H. pylori* regimen.

OTC Products for Ulcers

Antacids
Bismuth subsalicylate

Indigestion

Every week, at least 1 out of every 4 people experiences an episode of indigestion. There are several types of indigestion.

Gastroesophageal reflux disease (GERD) (also called acid reflux) is a condition in which the acidic contents of the stomach flow back into the esophageal tube. This is a normal, everyday occurrence in most people, not serious enough to cause symptoms of discomfort. In some cases, though, there is a chronic problem with the muscular valve that separates the esophagus from the stomach (see box). Conditions such as pregnancy, obesity, or hiatal hernia can also contribute to GERD. Sometimes the problem arises because of delayed gastric emptying—when digested food is moved out of the stomach into the small intestine abnormally slowly—or because of excess acid secretion.

During a reflux episode, the presence of acid can damage the delicate tissue of the esophagus, larynx, and respiratory system, leading to inflammation, ulcers, or abnormal growths. The pain caused by reflux, commonly known as heartburn, is a burning sensation in the lower chest, which can spread to other areas of the chest, back, or throat. Reflux usually occurs shortly after a meal, especially if you lie down or bend over. Many people also experience the problem during sleep; often the pain causes them to awaken. The severity of symptoms depends on how long the acid remains in contact with the tissue.

Occasionally the acidic material can flow upward into the mouth, causing a burning, bitter taste (sometimes called sour stomach). Left untreated, GERD can severely damage tissue, leading to esophageal ulcers, strictures (narrowings), respiratory inflammation, chronic cough, hoarseness, and even cancer.

Factors Contributing to Gastroesophageal Reflux Disease

- Weak esophageal valve, caused by
  - Smoking
  - Beverages and foods
    - Alcohol
    - Caffeine
    - Chocolate
    - Fatty foods
    - Mints
    - Citrus foods
  - Medications
    - NSAIDs
    - Tricyclic antidepressants
    - Certain blood pressure medications
    - Estrogen
    - Morphine and other narcotics
- Delayed gastric emptying, caused by
  - Motility disorder (slow passage of stool through intestine)
  - Medications
- Increased acid secretion, caused by
  - Smoking
  - Beverages and foods
    - Alcohol
    - Coffee
  - Medical conditions (e.g., duodenal ulcers)
- Increased pressure in the stomach, caused by
  - Lying down
  - Obesity
  - Tight-fitting clothing
  - Overeating

Gastritis refers to an inflammation of the stomach lining. Acute gastritis, which typically results from use of alcohol or NSAIDs, is a severe, short-term flare-up involving loss of tissue from the mucous membranes and the development of ulcers. Many people with acute gastritis will not experience pain or other symptoms. If symptoms do occur, the most common complication is bleeding in the upper GI tract. Sometimes the bleeding is severe, leading to black, tarlike stools and anemia. Gastritis can also be a more chronic condition involving inflammation but not ulcers. Chronic gastritis arises from the same bacterium that causes peptic ulcers, and in fact the 2 conditions often exist at the same time. If symptoms occur, they include pain, heartburn, and loss of appetite.

Dyspepsia is a general term for bad digestion; it can refer to a range of stomach ailments that do not result from the presence of peptic ulcers. Scientists are not sure what causes dyspepsia; the usual suspects—excess stomach acid, stress, smoking, caffeine use, and the presence of bacteria—have not proved to be at fault. Symptoms usually arise around mealtimes and include pain, nausea, belching, heartburn, indigestion, and bloating. The condition usually lasts for years but does not appear to increase the risk of ulcers or other more serious diseases.

Intestinal gas is a byproduct of digestion. Excess gas can cause belching, abdominal pain and discomfort, bloating, and flatulence.

Seek medical attention if any of the following applies to you

- Difficulty or pain when swallowing
- Chest pain that worsens with physical activity
- Heartburn that does not get better with antacids or nonprescription H_2RAs
- Vomiting of blood
- Black, tarlike stools

Treatment for Indigestion

People with mild to moderate GERD usually experience relief through the use of antacids, taken as needed. These products help by weakening the strength of stomach acid contents, thus dampening the fire of heartburn. They also appear to work by strengthening the esophageal valve to prevent the backward flow of acid. Antacids containing an ingredient called alginic acid form a protective nonacidic layer on top of the stomach contents. If reflux occurs, the material that enters the esophagus is less acidic, and is therefore less likely to cause pain and irritation. Relief from antacids usually occurs within minutes and lasts for up to 3 hours. Because of this relatively short duration of action, there is a chance that reflux will occur during the night. Antacids do nothing to heal esophageal tissue that has already been damaged. This occurs naturally over time once the underlying reflux is controlled, unless there is already scarring, which is irreversible.

The drugs classified as H_2RAs are prescribed for peptic ulcer disease. In lower doses, they are only available as OTC treatments for heartburn, acid indigestion, and sour stomach. All of the OTC H_2RAs are helpful in treating and preventing reflux. Relief may not occur until an hour or 2 after taking the drug. For that reason, many people may prefer to stick with the faster-acting (and cheaper) antacids. However, cimetidine and its cousins provide relief for 6 to 10 hours, which is an advantage for nighttime treatment. Like antacids, H_2RAs do not heal damaged tissue. If the problem persists, see a doctor.

Bismuth subsalicylate was formerly considered to be an antacid, but at this time its main use is in the treatment of diarrhea and for occasional relief of upset stomach.

Acute gastritis usually improves once consumption of alcohol or NSAIDs stops. Antacids or H_2RAs may provide relief of symptoms. If bleeding is present, you must consult your physician. Since bacterial infection is usually the cause of chronic gastritis, you should see a physician for an antibiotic prescription.

People with dyspepsia may find relief from taking antacids or H_2RAs, but there is little scientific proof that these medications do much good for this condition.

Excess intestinal gas can be treated with products known as antiflatulents. The main ingredient in most antiflatulents for upper intestinal gas is simethicone, a form of silicon.

This agent reduces the surface tension of gas bubbles, making them easier to pop so the gas can be adsorbed by the simethicone. For lower intestinal gas, products containing the adsorbent activated charcoal may help. Many OTC antacids also contain simethicone. A newer form of antiflatulent, alpha-galactosidase, is an enzyme that breaks down sugars before they are digested and turned into gas by intestinal bacteria. People who consume a high-fiber diet (including whole grains, lentils, broccoli, peas, and cabbage) might benefit from taking alpha-galactosidase along with their meal, although its safety and efficacy are not fully established. However, this product is a way to prevent gas from developing; treatment of an existing problem calls for the use of simethicone.

OTC Products for Indigestion

- Antacid products
  - Alginic acid
  - Aluminum salts
  - Calcium carbonate
  - Magaldrate
  - Magnesium salts
  - Sodium bicarbonate
- Antigas products
  - Simethicone
  - Alpha-galactosidase
- H_2RAs
  - Cimetidine
  - Famotidine
  - Nizatidine
  - Ranitidine
- Other
  - Bismuth subsalicylate

Antidiarrheal Products

BRAND NAME	ADSORBENT			OTHER ACTIVE INGREDIENTS			
	attapulgite	pectin	polycarbophil	bismuth subsalicylate	enzyme (lactase)	kaolin	loperamide HCl
Dairy Ease (caplet)					x		
Dairy Ease (drops)					x		
Dairy Ease (tablet)					x		
Diar Aid							2mg
Diarrhea and Cramp Relief	600g/15ml						
Diasorb (liquid)	750mg/5ml						
Diasorb (tablet)	750mg						
Donnagel (suspension)	600mg/5ml						
Donnagel (tablet)	600mg						
Equalactin			500mg				
Imodium A-D (caplet)							2mg
Imodium A-D (liquid)							1mg/5ml
Kaodene A-D							2mg
Kaodene NN (Non-Narcotic)		195mg/30ml		30mg/30ml		3.89g/30ml	
Kaolin Pectin [S]		130.2mg/30ml				5.7g/30ml	
Kaopectate	750mg/15ml						
Kaopectate, Children's	750mg						
Kao-Spen		260mg/30ml				5.2g/30ml	
K-C		260mg/30ml		260mg/30ml		5.2g/30ml	
Lactaid (caplet)					x		
Lactaid (drops) [S]					x		
Lactaid Extra Strength					x		
Lactrase					x		

BRAND NAME	ADSORBENT			OTHER ACTIVE INGREDIENTS			
	attapulgite	pectin	polycarbophil	bismuth subsalicylate	enzyme (lactase)	kaolin	loperamide HCl
Maalox Anti-Diarrheal							2mg
Parepectolin	600mg/15ml						
Pepto Diarrhea Control							2mg
Pepto-Bismol (caplet)				262.5mg			
Pepto-Bismol (tablet)				262.5mg			
Pepto-Bismol Cherry				262.39mg			
Pepto-Bismol Maximum Strength				1050mg/30ml			
Pepto-Bismol Original Strength				525mg/30ml			
Percy Medicine				959mg/10ml			
Rheaban	750mg						

Antacid and Antireflux Products

BRAND NAME	ANTACID				
	aluminum hydroxide	calcium carbonate	magaldrate	magnesium salts (carbonate, hydroxide, oxide, etc.)	sodium bicarbonate
Acid-X		250mg			
Alamag	225mg/5ml			200mg/5ml	
Alka-Mints		850mg			
Alka-Seltzer (caplet)		380mg			
Alka-Seltzer (gelcap)		500mg			
Alka-Seltzer Extra Strength					1985mg
Alka-Seltzer Gold					958mg
Alka-Seltzer, Lemon-Lime					1700mg

Alka-Seltzer Original				1916mg
Alkets		500mg		
Alkets Extra Strength		750mg		
Almora			500mg mag. gluconate dihydrate; 2.8mg mag. stearate	
ALternaGEL	600mg			
Alu-Cap	400mg			
Alu-Tab	500mg			
Amitone		350mg		
Amphojel (suspension)	320mg/5ml			
Amphojel (tablet)	300mg; 600mg			
Antacid Extra Strength		750mg		
Antacid Liquid (gelcap)		311mg	232mg	
Antacid Liquid (liquid)	400mg/5ml		400mg/5ml	
Arm & Hammer Pure Baking Soda [S]				100%
Basaljel (capsule)	500mg			
Basaljel (suspension)	400mg			
Basaljel (tablet)	500mg			
Bell/ans				520mg
Bromo-Seltzer				2.78mg
Chooz		500mg		
Citrocarbonate				2.34g
Dialume	500mg			
Dicarbosil		500mg		
Equilet		500mg		
Gaviscon	80mg		20mg	70mg
Gaviscon ESRF [S]	50.8mg/ml		47.5mg/ml	
Gaviscon Extra Strength	160mg		105mg/ml	x

BRAND NAME	ANTACID				
	aluminum hydroxide	calcium carbonate	magaldrate	magnesium salts (carbonate, hydroxide, oxide, etc.)	sodium bicarbonate
Gaviscon Liquid	31.5mg/5ml			119.5mg/ml	
Gaviscon-2	160mg			40mg	140mg
Genalac		420mg			
Losopan			540mg/5ml		
Maalox (caplet)		311mg		232mg	
Maalox (suspension)	225mg/5ml			200mg/5ml	
Maalox Heartburn relief	140mg/5ml			175mg/5ml	
Maalox Therapeutic Concentrate	600mg/5ml			300mg/5ml	
Magnalox	225mg/5ml			200mg/5ml	
Mag-Ox 400				400mg	
Marblen (suspension)		520mg/5ml		400mg/5ml	
Marblen (tablet)		520mg		400mg	
Milk of Magnesia (Pharmaceutical Association)				390mg/5ml	
Milk of Magnesia (Roxane Labs)				400mg/5ml	
Milk of Magnesia Concentrate (Pharmaceutical Association)				1165mg/5ml	
Milk of Magnesia Concentrate (Roxane Labs)				1200mg/5ml	
Mylanta		550mg		125mg	
Mylanta Double Strength		700mg		300mg	
Mylanta Regular Strength		350mg		150mg	
Mylanta Soothing		600mg			
Nephrox	320mg/5ml				
Phillips' Milk of Magnesia (suspension)				400mg/5ml	
Phillips' Milk of Magnesia (tablet)				311mg	
Phillips' Milk of Magnesia Concentrate				800mg/5ml	

Riopan		108mg/ml	
Rolaids (fruit flavors)	550mg		
Rolaids (mint flavors)	412mg		80mg
Titralac	420mg		
Titralac Extra Strength	750mg		
Tums	500mg		
Tums E-X Extra Strength	750mg		
Tums Ultra	1000mg		
Tylenol Headache Plus Extra Strength	250mg		
Uro-Mag			140mg

Histamine 2 Receptor Antagonists

BRAND NAME	ACTIVE INGREDIENT
Axid AR	nizatidine 75mg
Pepcid AC	famotidine 10mg
Tagamet HB	cimetidine 100mg
Zantac 75	ranitidine HCl 84mg

Antiflatulent Products

BRAND NAME	ACTIVE INGREDIENT	
	simethicone	alpha galactosidase
Alka-Seltzer Anti-Gas	125mg	
Antacid Liquid	40mg/5ml	

BRAND NAME	ACTIVE INGREDIENT	
	simethicone	alpha galactosidase
Beano		X
Di-Gel (liquid)	20mg/ml	
Di-Gel (tablet)	20mg	
Gas-X	80mg	
Gas-X Extra Strength [S]	125mg	
Gelusil	25mg	
Genasyme (drops)	40mg/0.6ml	
Genasyme (tablet)	80mg	
Kudrox	40mg/5ml	
Little Tummy Infant Gas Relief [S]	20mg/0.3ml	
Losopan Plus	20mg/5ml	
Maalox Antacid Plus Anti-Gas	25mg	
Maalox Antacid Plus Anti-Gas Extra Strength	30mg	
Maalox Anti-Gas	80mg	
Maalox Anti-Gas Extra Strength	150mg	
Maalox Extra Strength Antacid/Anti-Gas [S]	200mg/5ml	
Mylanta	20mg/5ml	
Mylanta Double Strength	40mg/5ml	
Mylanta Gas Relief (gelcap)	62.5mg	
Mylanta Gas Relief (tablet)	80mg	
Mylanta Gas Relief Maximum Strength	125mg	
Mylicon, Infant's	40mg/0.6ml	
Phazyme Gas Relief (drops)	40mg/0.6ml	
Phazyme Gas Relief (tablet)	95mg	
Phazyme Gas Relief Maximum Strength	125mg	
Riopan Plus (suspension)	40mg/5ml	

Riopan Plus (tablet)	20mg
Riopan Plus Double Strength (suspension)	40mg/5ml
Riopan Plus Double Strength (tablet)	20mg
Simaal Gel	20mg/5ml
Simaal 2 Gel	40mg/5ml
Tempo Drops	20mg
Titralac Plus (liquid)	20mg/5ml
Titralac Plus (tablet)	21mg
Tums Anti-Gas/Antacid	20mg

Appetite Suppressants

BRAND NAME	phenylpropanolamine HCl
Acutrim 16 Hour Steady Control	75mg
Acutrim Late Day Strength	75mg
Acutrim Maximum Strength	75mg
Amfed T.D.	75mg
Control	75mg
Dexatrim Caffeine Free Extended Duration C	75mg
Dexatrim Caffeine Free Maximum Strength C	75mg
Dexatrim Caffeine Free Plus Vitamins C	75mg
Dexatrim Caffeine Free with Vitamin C C	75mg
Dieutrim	75mg
Mini Slims	75mg
Permathene Maximum Strength Chromium Picolinate	75mg
Permathene with Calcium	25mg

BRAND NAME	phenylpropanolamine HCl
Permathene-12	75mg
Permathene-12 Maximum Strength with Vitamin C	75mg
Permathene-16	75mg
Protrim	37.5mg
Protrim S.R.	75mg
Super Odrinex	25mg
Thinz Back-To-Nature	75mg
Thinz Span	75mg

Laxative Products/Bulk Agents

BRAND NAME	BULK AGENT							
	calcium poly-carbophil	methyl-cellulose	oat bran, psyllium seed husks	psyllium	psyllium hydrophilic fiber	psyllium hydrophilic mucilloid	psyllium mucilloid	psyllium seed husks, buckthorn bark
Citrucel		2g/tbsp						
Citrucel Sugar Free [S]		2g/tbsp						
Fiber	625mg							
Fiberall	1250mg							
Fiberall Fruit & Nut						3.4g		
Fiberall, Natural						3.4g		
Fiberall, Oatmeal Raisin						3.4g		
Fiberall, Orange						3.4g		
FiberCon [S]	625mg							
Garfields Tea •								x
GenFiber						3.4g/7g		

Hydrocil Instant			95%			
Innerclean Herbal						x
Konsyl [S]					100%	
Konsyl Fiber	625mg					
Konsyl-D				50%		
Konsyl-Orange				28%		
Metamucil Fiber Apple Crisp/Cinnamon Spice				3.4g/2 wafers		
Metamucil Original Texture				3.4g/tsp		
Metamucil Original Texture, Effervescent Sugar Free [S]				3.4g/packet		
Metamucil Smooth Texture				3.4g/tsp		
Metamucil Smooth Texture Sugar-Free [S]				3.4g/packet		
Modane Bulk				50%		
Natural Bulk (regular, orange)				3.4g/tsp		
Natural Fiber (citrus, orange)				3.5g/tsp		
Perdiem			3.25g/tsp			
Perdiem Fiber			4g/tsp			
Serutan				2.5mg/tsp		
Swiss Kriss [S]		x				
V-Lax				50%		

Emollient/Lubricant

BRAND NAME	docusate calcium	docusate potassium	docusate sodium	mineral oil
Agoral				x
Colace (capsule)			50mg; 100mg	
Colace (liquid)			50mg/ml	
Colace (syrup)			20mg/5ml	

BRAND NAME	docusate calcium	docusate potassium	docusate sodium	mineral oil
Correctol Extra Gentle			100mg	
DC 240	240mg			
Dialose			100mg	
Dialose Plus		100mg		
Dioctolose		100mg		
Doxidan	60mg			
Ducolax			x	
Ex-Lax Extra Gentle			75mg	
Femilax			100mg	
Fleet Mineral Oil Enema				100%
Fleet Mineral Oil Oral Lubricant [A]				100%
Genasoft			100mg	
Genasoft Plus			100mg	
Gentlax S			50mg	
Haleys M-O [A]			25%	
Kasof		240mg		
Kondremul				55%
Liqui-Doss [A]				x
Milkinol				x
Mineral oil				x
Modane Plus			100mg	
Modane Soft			100mg	
Peri-Colace (capsule)			100mg	
Peri-Colace (syrup)			20mg/5ml	
Peri-Dos			100mg	
Phillips'			83mg	
Pro-Cal-Sof	240mg			

Pro-Sof		100mg; 250mg
Pro-Sof Plus		100mg
Regulace		100mg
Regulax SS		100mg; 200mg
Senokot-S		50mg
Sof-lax		100mg
Sof-lax Overnight		100mg
Surfak 240mg	240mg	
Therevac Plus [A]		283mg
Therevac-SB [A]		283mg
Unilax [S]		230mg
Woman's Gentle Laxative		100mg

Stimulant

BRAND NAME	bisacodyl	casan-thranol	cascara sagrada	castor oil	phenolph-thalein	senna	yellow phenolphthalein
Agoral					65.67mg/5ml		
Alophen					60mg		
Bisco-Lax	10mg						
Bisco-Lax Enteric Coated	5mg						
Caroid			50mg		32.4mg		
Correctol	5mg						
Correctol Herbal Tea						30mg/teabag	
Deficol Enteric Coated	5mg						
Dialose Plus							65mg
Docu-K Plus		30mg					

BRAND NAME	bisacodyl	casan-thranol	cascara sagrada	castor oil	phenolph-thalein	senna	yellow phenolphthalein
Doxidan							65mg
Dr. Caldwell Senna						166.5mg/5ml	
Ducolax	5mg						
Emulsoil				95%			
Espotabs							97.2mg
Evac-Q-Kwik (suppository)	10mg						
Evac-Q-Kwik (tablet)					130mg		
Evac-U-Gen (tablet)							97.2mg
Ex-Lax Chocolate							90mg
Ex-Lax Extra Gentle							65mg
Ex-Lax Gentle Nature Natural						20mg	
Ex-Lax Maximum Relief Formula							135mg
Ex-Lax Regular Strength							90mg
Feen-A-Mint	5mg						
Femilax					65mg		
Fleet Bisacodyl Enema	10mg						
Fleet Laxative (suppository)	10mg						
Fleet Laxative (tablet)	5mg						
Fleet Magnesium Citrate Prep Kit 4	20mg/4 tablets; 10mg/suppository						
Fleet Magnesium Citrate Prep Kit 5	20mg/4 tablets						
Fleet Magnesium Citrate Prep Kit 6	20mg/4 tablets; 10mg/enema						
Fleet Prep Kit 1	20mg/4 tablets; 10mg/suppository						
Fleet Prep Kit 2	20mg/4 tablets						

Fleet Prep Kit 3	20mg/4 tablets; 10mg/enema						
Fletcher's Castoria						166.5mg/5ml	
Fletcher's, Children's							0.3%
Garfields Tea						610mg/0.5tsp	
Genasoft Plus		30mg					
Gentle Laxative	5mg						
Gentlax S						187mg	
Innerclean Herbal						x	
Kellogg's Tasteless Castor Oil							100%
Kondremul				x			
Lax-Pills					90mg		
Medilax					120mg		
Milk of Magnesia Cascara (Pharmaceutical Assoc.)			5ml				
Milk of Magnesia Cascara (Roxane)			5ml				
Milk of Magnesia Cascara Concentrate			5ml				
Modane					130mg		
Modane Plus					60mg		
Nature's Remedy			150mg (+aloe 100mg)				
Neoloid				36.4%			
Perdiem						0.74g/tsp	
Peri-Colace (capsule)		30mg					
Peri-Colace (syrup)		10mg/5ml					
Peri-Dos		30mg					
Phillips'					90mg		
Pro-Sof Plus		30mg					
Prulet					60mg		
Purge [S]				95%			

BRAND NAME	bisacodyl	casan- thranol	cascara sagrada	castor oil	phenolph- thalein	senna	yellow phenolphthalein
Regulace		30mg					
Reliable Gentle Laxative	5mg						
Senna-Gen						217mg	
Senokot (granules)						15mg/tsp	
Senokot (suppository)						652mg	
Senokot (syrup)						8.8mg/5ml	
Senokot (tablet)						8.6mg	
Senokot Children's [A]						8.8mg/5ml	
Senokot-S						8.6mg	
SenokotXTRA						17mg	
Senolax						187mg	
Sof-lax Overnight		30mg					
Swiss Kriss [S]						52.5%	
Unilax [S]							130mg
Woman's Gentle Laxative							65mg

Other Laxatives

BRAND NAME	glycerin	magnesium citrate	magnesium hydroxide	magnesium oxide	magnesium sulfate	sodium phosphate
Agoral	x					
Doxidan	x					
Ducolax	x					

Epsom salt					40mEq/mg	
Evac-Q-Kwik (liquid)		25mEq/30ml				
Fiberall Fruit & Nut	x					
Fiberall, Oatmeal Raisin	x					
Fleet Babylax [A]	x					
Fleet Glycerin Adult Size	x					
Fleet Glycerin Child Size	x					
Fleet Glycerin Rectal Applicators [A]	7.5ml					
Fleet Magnesium Citrate Prep Kit 4		18.7g				
Fleet Magnesium Citrate Prep Kit 5		18.7g				
Fleet Magnesium Citrate Prep Kit 6		18.7g				
Fleet Prep Kit 1						45ml
Fleet Prep Kit 2						45ml
Fleet Prep Kit 3						45ml
Fleet Ready-to-Use Enema						x
Fleet Ready-to-Use Enema for Children						x
Fletcher's Castoria	x					
Fletcher's, Children's	x					
Glycerin	x					
Haleys M-O [A]			6%			
Kasof	x					
Kondremul	x					
Mag-Ox 400				400mg		
Metamucil Smooth Texture Sugar-Free [S]					x	
Milk of Magnesia (Pharmaceutical Association)			400mg/5ml			
Milk of Magnesia (Roxane) [A]			390mg/5ml			
Milk of Magnesia (Schein)			405mg/5ml			
Milk of Magnesia Cascara (Pharmaceutical Assoc.)			400mg/5ml			

BRAND NAME	glycerin	magnesium citrate	magnesium hydroxide	magnesium oxide	magnesium sulfate	sodium phosphate
Milk of Magnesia Cascara (Roxane)			390mg/5ml			
Milk of Magnesia Cascara Concentrate			800mg/5ml			
Milk of Magnesia Concentrate [A] (Roxane)			1165mg/5ml			
Milk of Magnesia Concentrate (Pharmaceutical Assoc.)			1200mg/5ml			
Modane Soft	x					
Phillips' Milk of Magnesia (suspension) [A]			400mg/5ml			
Phillips' Milk of Magnesia (tablet)			311mg			
Phillips' Milk of Magnesia Concentrate [A]			800mg/5ml			
Phospho-soda Buffered Saline						3.3g/5ml
Sani-Supp	x					
Surfak 240mg	x					
Therevac Plus [A]	x					
Therevac-SB [A]	x					
Uro-Mag				140mg		

Alka-Seltzer Original Effervescent Antacid Pain Reliever (AL-kuh-SELTZ-er)

see page 43

Alka-Seltzer Extra Strength Antacid Pain Reliever (AL-kuh-SELTZ-er)

see page 43

Brand Name

Axid AR (AX-id)

Generic Ingredient

Nizatidine (nye-ZA-tuh-deen)

Type of Drug

Acid reducer.

Used for

Relief of occasional heartburn, acid indigestion, and sour stomach.

General Information

There are currently 4 histamine H_2-receptor antagonists (H_2RAs) available for prescription use in the United States: cimetidine, ranitidine, famotidine, and nizatidine. Tagamet was the first to be introduced, in 1977. Prescription-strength H_2RAs are used to treat peptic ulcer disease (PUD) and gastroesophageal reflux disease (GERD).

As of May 1996, all 4 H_2RAs have been approved for OTC use (under the brand names Tagamet HB, Zantac 75, Pepcid AC, Mylanta AR, and Axid AR) in substantially lower doses than those indicated in the management of PUD and GERD. The OTC-strength H_2RAs are not indicated for the treatment of ulcer disease, are unlikely to provide sufficient relief for people with moderate-to-severe GERD, and will not provide relief for people with complications from GERD. They are taken for the same reasons that antacids are: to provide relief for individuals with heartburn, acid indigestion, or sour stomach. It has been reported that 25% of U.S. adults have at least 1 episode of abdominal discomfort in an average 2-week period, which partly accounts for the annual sales of antacids exceeding $1 billion. It is estimated that the OTC H_2RAs will soon be used as often as antacids for self-medication of these conditions.

H_2RAs work by reducing the production of stomach acid. The degree and duration of acid suppression depend upon the dose and length of time the drug stays in the bloodstream. H_2RAs usually begin to provide relief within 1 hour of ingestion. The duration of acid suppression reported for Axid AR (75 mg) is 6 to 8 hours.

In treating acid indigestion, sour stomach, and heartburn, antacids provide more rapid relief than H_2RAs and, if used at the recommended doses for 2 weeks, cost about 4 times less. But for people who find taking multiple doses of antacids undesirable, H_2RAs, with their longer duration of action, may be preferable.

Cautions and Warnings

Do not take the maximum daily dosage of Axid AR for more than 2 weeks continuously except under the advice and supervision of a doctor. Contact your doctor if your symptoms persist after 2 weeks of self-medication with Axid AR.

Do not exceed the recommended daily dosage of Axid AR.

If you have trouble swallowing or persistent abdominal pain, see your doctor promptly. You may have a serious condition that may need a different treatment.

Because nizatidine, the ingredient in Axid and Axid AR, is eliminated through the kidneys and metabolized in the liver, prescription-strength Axid is used with caution and in reduced dosage in individuals with kidney and/or liver dysfunction. OTC Axid AR is used in a lower dose, so a further reduction is probably unnecessary. Talk to your doctor or pharmacist before self-medicating with Axid AR if you have impaired liver or kidney function.

Axid AR—unlike its prescription-strength counterpart, Axid—is not approved for treatment of peptic ulcer disease. Do not take more than the recommended dosage of Axid AR to self-medicate an ulcer. If you have or believe you have an ulcer, consult a physician.

Possible Side Effects

▼ Rare: headache, dizziness, drowsiness, insomnia, abnormal dreams, somnolence, anxiety, nervousness, constipation, diarrhea, nausea, vomiting, abdominal pain/discomfort, dry mouth, tooth disorder, rash, sinusitis, increased cough, back or chest pain, fever, infection, impotence, small reductions in blood pressure and heart rate, hematologic effects, and, rarely, serious central nervous system reactions, including confusion, agitation, and hallucinations.

Drug Interactions

- Prescription-strength Axid has been noted to reduce the bioavailability of enoxacin, cefpodoxime, proxetil, itraconazole, and ketoconazole. While these interactions have not been studied in Axid AR, there is always the possibility that they may occur. Consult your doctor or pharmacist before self-medicating with Axid AR if you are taking one of these drugs.
- Antacids may slightly reduce the bioavailability of Axid AR. Separate the dose of Axid AR from doses of antacid by at least 1 hour.

Food Interactions

None known.

Usual Dose

Each tablet contains 75 mg of nizatidine.

Adult and Child (age 12 and over): 1 tablet with water. Do not exceed the maximum daily dosage of 2 tablets. For prevention of heartburn or indigestion, take 1 tablet 1 hour before eating.

Child (under age 12): not recommended unless directed by a doctor.

Overdosage

Do the following in case of accidental overdose: If the victim is unconscious or having convulsions, call for an ambulance immediately. If you take the victim to an emergency room, be sure to bring the bottle or container with you. If the victim is conscious, call your local poison control center or a health care professional. The poison control center may suggest inducing vomiting with ipecac syrup (available without a prescription at any pharmacy). DO NOT induce vomiting unless specifically instructed to do so.

Special Populations

Pregnancy/Breast-feeding

It is not generally recommended that pregnant women take any drugs, particularly during the first 3 months after conception. Check with your doctor before self-medicating with Axid AR if you are or might be pregnant.

Nizatidine passes into breast milk. If you must take Axid AR, bottle-feed your baby with formula.

Infants/Children

Axid AR should not be given to children younger than age 12 unless directed by a doctor.

Seniors

Seniors may safely self-medicate with Axid AR. The OTC dose is low enough that a dosage reduction is not necessary to compensate for age-related reductions in elimination and breakdown.

Seniors with impaired kidney function should talk to their doctor or pharmacist before self-medicating with Axid AR.

Brand Name

Basaljel (BAY-zuhl-gell)

Generic Ingredient

Aluminum carbonate (a-LOU-min-um kar-BON-ate)

Type of Drug

Antacid.

Used for

Relief of heartburn, sour stomach, and acid indigestion; and to control or manage hyperphosphatemia (too much phosphorus in the blood).

General Information

All antacids work in the same way, by neutralizing gastric acid. However, they differ in potency: Aluminum antacids such as aluminum carbonate are among the least potent of these products, after calcium carbonate, sodium bicarbonate, and magnesium antacids. The higher the potency of an antacid, the less of it you will need to take to achieve the desired effect.

Antacids also vary according to adverse effects and drug interactions, as well as onset and duration of action. Aluminum antacids dissolve more slowly in stomach acid than do sodium bicarbonate and magnesium hydroxide, and thus may take longer to begin working. It can take up to 30 minutes for the acid-neutralizing effect of an aluminum antacid to begin working.

How long an antacid product works depends on how long it remains in the stomach. Possibly because they delay gastric emptying, aluminum antacids have a longer duration of action than sodium bicarbonate or magnesium antacids. In general, an antacid taken on an empty stomach leaves the stomach rapidly and works for only 20 to 40 minutes. However, when taken after a meal, it leaves the stomach more slowly. When taken 1 hour after a meal, an antacid can work for up to 3 hours.

Aluminum carbonate is one of 4 types of aluminum antacid; the others are aluminum hydroxide, aluminum phosphate, and aluminum aminoacetate. Aluminum hydroxide is the most potent of the group.

Basaljel is available in suspension (liquid), capsule, and tablet form. While the suspension is more potent than the tablet or capsule, some people do not like the taste of the liquid and also prefer the convenience of the pill form when taking multiple doses throughout the day.

Cautions and Warnings

Do not take the maximum daily dosage of Basaljel for more than 2 weeks continuously except under a doctor's supervision. Antacids may relieve symptoms of a serious condition such as peptic ulcer disease. If you take Basaljel for a prolonged period, you run the risk of unknowingly masking the symptoms of a serious gastrointestinal (GI) disease and delaying its diagnosis.

Do not exceed the recommended daily dosage of Basaljel.

Call your doctor if you do not get relief from Basaljel, or if your stool is black or tarry, which may indicate bleeding in the intestines or stomach. These may be signs of a serious GI disorder that cannot and should not be treated with an OTC product without your doctor's supervision .

Because some of the aluminum in aluminum carbonate is absorbed into the bloodstream and then eliminated from the body through the kidneys, people with impaired kidney function should not take this product for prolonged periods. In those individuals, long-term use of Basaljel may lead to accumulation of aluminum in bones, lungs, and brain tissue.

Excessive amounts of an aluminum antacid taken for a prolonged period can lead to low blood phosphate levels, which are characterized by loss of appetite, malaise, and muscle weakness.

Possible Side Effects

▼ Most common: constipation.

Drug Interactions

• Aluminum carbonate decreases the absorption of the following drugs, reducing their effects: allopurinol, an antigout medication; nitrofurantoin, an antibiotic; tetracycline antibiotics; quinolone antibiotics, such as ciprofloxacin; cimetidine and ranitidine, used to treat peptic ulcers, heartburn, and acid indigestion; indomethacin, a nonsteroidal anti-inflammatory drug (NSAID); digoxin, used to treat congestive heart failure; iron; ticlopidine, an anticoagulant (blood thinning) drug; and thyroid hormones. It may also decrease the bioavailability of the beta blocker atenolol, used to treat high blood pressure. If you are taking Basaljel at the same time as any of these drugs, separate your dose of each drug by at least 2 hours; with quinolone antibiotics, 4 to 6 hours is preferable.

• Aluminum carbonate increases the absorption of the benzodiazepine diazepam, increasing its sedative effect. If you are taking diazepam, consult your doctor before taking Basaljel.

• Aluminum carbonate increases the body's elimination of aspirin and other salicylates, reducing their effect. Conversely, it increases the absorption of enteric-coated or buffered aspirin.

Food Interactions

Basaljel is best taken after meals (see "General Information").

Usual Dose

Adult and Child (age 6 and over): 2 capsules or tablets, or 2 tsps. of the suspension in water or fruit juice, as often as every 2 hours (up to 12 times a day). Do not exceed the recommended daily dosage specified on the package. If you are taking the chewable tablet, be sure to chew it completely and drink a full glass of water afterward to ensure maximum benefit. Shake the suspension well prior to use.

Child (under age 6): Consult your doctor.

Overdosage

Do the following in case of accidental overdose: If the victim is unconscious or having convulsions, call for an ambulance immediately. If you take the victim to an emergency room, be sure to bring the bottle or container with you. If the victim is conscious, call your local poison control center or a health care professional. The poison control center may suggest inducing vomiting with ipecac syrup (available without a prescription at any pharmacy). DO NOT induce vomiting unless specifically instructed to do so.

Special Information

Patients with a history of diarrhea may choose Basaljel over other antacids because it is more likely to cause constipation.

Because magnesium antacids may cause diarrhea, they are often taken concurrently with aluminum carbonate to regulate bowel function.

Storage Instructions

The suspension form of Basaljel may be stored at room temperature, but to improve its taste, refrigerate it. Do not freeze Basaljel in suspension form.

Special Populations

Pregnancy/Breast-feeding

It is not generally recommended that pregnant women take any drugs, particularly during the first 3 months after conception. However, antacids can be safely taken in small doses for short periods of time during pregnancy and while breast-feeding. Check with your doctor before using Basaljel if you are or might be pregnant, or if you are breast-feeding.

Infants/Children
The safety of antacid use in infants and children has not been established. Children under age 6 should not be given Basaljel unless directed by a doctor.

Seniors
Seniors may safely take antacids. However, be advised that many older patients are at high risk for complications from ulcers, yet often do not show classic ulcer symptoms. You may want to discuss with your pharmacist the possible causes of your gastric discomfort before self-medicating with an antacid. Be aware of possible interactions with other medications you may be taking.

Because constipation is a common complaint in seniors, Basaljel may not be the preferred antacid for this age group.

Brand Name

Beano (BEE-noe)

Generic Ingredient

Alpha-galactosidase (AL-fah gah-LACK-toe-SID-aze)

Type of Drug

Antiflatulent.

Used for

Relief of intestinal gas caused by high-fiber foods.

General Information

The enzyme alpha-galactosidase is made from *Aspergillus niger* mold. When added to high-fiber foods such as oats, wheat, beans, broccoli, and cabbage, alpha-galactosidase breaks down their complex sugars into the simple sugars glucose, galactose, and fructose and the disaccharide sucrose. The transformation makes these foods easier to digest and helps to reduce or eliminate gas and bloating; it does not affect the fiber content of the foods. Several recent studies have documented the effectiveness of alpha-galactosidase in reducing intestinal gas production. Alpha-galactosidase is intended to be used as a preventative measure against gas; it will not relieve gas symptoms that you are already experiencing or gas symptoms that are associated with causes other than high-fiber foods. In those situations you should choose another antiflatulent product. Beano is available in tablet and drop form. The amount of alpha-galactosidase in 1 tablet is equal to that in 5 drops.

Cautions and Warnings

This enzyme has been used in food processing for many years and is considered to be safe by the FDA. However, the amount of alpha-galactosidase contained in Beano is probably much greater than that in processed foods.

If you have diabetes, you should be aware that alpha-galactosidase will make the simple sugars in high-fiber foods available to be metabolized by your body.

People with galactosemia (accumulation of galactose in the blood due to an inability to break it down to glucose) should not use Beano.

Possible Side Effects

None known.

Drug Interactions

• If you are taking a monoamine oxidase inhibitor (MAOI) (used to treat depression, other psychiatric or emotional conditions, and Parkinson's disease) you should use Beano with caution. If you are not sure whether you are taking an MAOI, check with your doctor before you use Beano.

Usual Dose

Each 5 drop dosage or tablet contains 150 Ga/u (galactosidase units) of alpha-galactosidase.

Adult and Child (age 5 and over): Add 5–8 drops to the first bite of problem food immediately before eating, or swallow or chew 2–3 tablets per meal (defined as 2–3 servings of problem foods) immediately before eating. The tablets may also be crumbled onto the food. Children who tend to eat less than 2–3 servings of problem foods per meal should take 1–2 tablets per serving of problem food.

In some cases more or less enzyme will be needed depending on how much food you eat, the type of food, and how much gas you normally produce. Several studies have suggested that alpha-galactosidase's effect is dose-dependent, and that the higher recommended dose (8 drops) is more effective than lower doses.

Because temperatures higher than 130°F may inactivate alpha-galactosidase, it should be added only after your food has cooled. Do not add Beano while the food is cooking.

Overdosage

Do the following in case of accidental overdose: If the victim is unconscious or having convulsions, call for an ambulance immediately. If you take the victim to an emergency room, be sure to bring the bottle or container with you. If the victim is conscious, call your local poison control center or a health care professional. The poison control center may suggest inducing vomiting with ipecac syrup (available without a prescription at any pharmacy). DO NOT induce vomiting unless specifically instructed to do so.

Special Populations

Allergies

Because alpha-galactosidase is derived from a mold, people who are sensitive to molds may also react to this enzyme.

Pregnancy/Breast-feeding

If you are pregnant or nursing, check with your doctor or other health care professional before using Beano.

Infants/Children

Beano has not been proven to be safe or effective in infants and children under age 5. Children under 5 should not be given Beano unless directed by a doctor.

Seniors

Seniors should exercise the same caution as younger adults when using Beano.

Brand Name

Dulcolax (DULL-koh-lax)

Generic Ingredient

Bisacodyl

Type of Drug

Laxative.

Used for

Relief of occasional constipation (irregularity).

General Information

The average, healthy individual defecates anywhere from 3 times a day to 3 times a week. Constipation is determined not necessarily by the frequency of bowel movements, but by the consistency of the stool, how difficult it is to eliminate, and symptoms such as dull headache, low back pain, and abdominal distention (swelling). Evaluate your condition carefully and discuss your symptoms and their possible causes with your pharmacist before self-medicating with a laxative. Laxatives are not always necessary, and when used improperly can either prevent the desired effect or result in laxative dependency. If you are indeed constipated, your condition may be best managed through proper diet, adequate fluid intake, and exercise. If you must use a laxative, choose the mildest effective product.

Laxatives may be classified by their mechanism of action: bulk-forming, emollient (stool softeners), lubricant, saline, hyperosmotic, and stimulant. The active ingredient in Dulcolax is bisacodyl, a stimulant laxative. According to different studies, stimulant laxatives work by either increasing the propulsive activity of the intestine or stimulating the secretion of water and electrolytes in the intestine, thus leading to evacuation of the colon.

Dulcolax should produce a bowel movement in 8 to 12 hours if taken at bedtime or within 6 hours if taken before breakfast.

Cautions and Warnings

Do not use Dulcolax for more than 7 days unless directed by your doctor. Long-term use of laxatives has been linked with laxative dependence, chronic constipation, and loss of normal bowel function. Using laxatives too frequently can result in persistent diarrhea, hypokalemia (abnormally low potassium in the blood), loss of essential nutrients, and dehydration.

Do not exceed the recommended daily dosage of Dulcolax. Of all the types of laxatives, stimulant laxatives such as bisacodyl, the active ingredient in Dulcolax, are particularly habit-forming, and are the most likely to cause diarrhea, gastrointestinal (GI) irritation, and fluid and electrolyte depletion with long-term use.

Do not take Dulcolax if you have abdominal pain, nausea, vomiting, or kidney disease, unless directed by your doctor.

If you notice a marked change in bowel habits lasting for more than 2 weeks, do not take Dulcolax until you have spoken to your doctor. Also contact your doctor if there is blood in your stool, so that colon cancer or other significant disease can be ruled out before you begin self-medication with Dulcolax.

If you have had a disease or surgery affecting the GI tract, using Dulcolax may affect your condition adversely.

If you have rectal bleeding after using Dulcolax, or if you do not have a bowel movement after 7 days of using Dulcolax, you may have a serious condition. Stop using Dulcolax and call your doctor.

Dulcolax may affect the absorption of other drugs that pass through the GI tract (see "Drug Interactions").

Dulcolax is coated to prevent stomach irritation. Do not chew the tablets; doing so increases the risk that the medication will irritate your stomach and cause vomiting. People who cannot swallow pills without chewing or crushing them should not take Dulcolax unless directed by a doctor.

Possible Side Effects

- ▼ Most common: abdominal discomfort, faintness, nausea, cramps, pinching and spasmodic pain in the bowels, colic, and increased mucus secretion.
- ▼ Less common (chronic use of Dulcolax only): metabolic acidosis or alkalosis (imbalances of acid and base in body fluids); hypocalcemia (too little calcium in the blood); tetany (characterized by foot spasms, muscular twitching, and cramps); electrolyte and fluid deficiencies (characterized by vomiting and muscle weakness); impaired intestinal absorption of nutrients; cathartic colon (weak or dilated colon).

Drug Interactions

• All laxatives potentially affect the absorption rate of any oral drug taken at the same time. If you are currently taking any oral medication, including OTC products, talk to your doctor or pharmacist before using Dulcolax.

• To avoid stomach irritation and possible vomiting, do not take Dulcolax within 1 hour of taking an antacid.

• Dulcolax should not be taken with drugs that increase gastric pH, such as cimetidine and ranitidine (used to treat peptic ulcers, heartburn, and acid indigestion), and omeprazole, a proton pump inhibitor (used to treat ulcers).

Food Interactions

To avoid stomach irritation and possible vomiting, do not take Dulcolax within 1 hour of drinking milk.

Usual Dose

Each tablet contains 5 mg of bisacodyl.

Adult and Child (age 12 and over): 2–3 tablets taken in a single dose once daily. Do not chew or crush tablets.

Child (age 6–11): 1 tablet once daily.

Child (under age 6): Consult your doctor.

Dulcolax Tablets are not recommended for individuals (especially children) who may have trouble swallowing the tablets whole.

Overdosage

Symptoms of overdosage include persistent diarrhea and dehydration.

Even if the victim is not displaying any of these symptoms, do the following in case of accidental overdose: If the victim is unconscious or having convulsions, call for an ambulance immediately. If you take the victim to an emergency room, be sure to bring the bottle or container with you. If the victim is conscious, call your local poison control center or a health care professional. The poison control center may suggest inducing vomiting with ipecac syrup (available without a prescription at any pharmacy). DO NOT induce vomiting unless specifically instructed to do so.

Special Populations

Pregnancy/Breast-feeding

Products containing stimulant laxatives such as Dulcolax should be avoided during pregnancy. Only bulk-forming or emollient laxatives are recommended for pregnant women. Consider talking to your doctor about diet and mild exercise as alternative ways to manage constipation.

Bisacodyl passes into breast milk in very small amounts, but this drug has not been reported to cause problems in nursing infants.

Check with your doctor before using Dulcolax if you are breast-feeding.

Infants/Children

Observe your child carefully for patterns of bowel movements and the pain or difficulty with which the bowel movements are made before deciding whether the child is actually constipated. As is true of adults, "normal" bowel habits vary in children. If your child is indeed constipated, increasing fluid intake and adding fiber to his or her diet offer effective ways to manage the condition. In general, the use of laxatives should be avoided in children.

Do not give Dulcolax to children under age 6 unless directed by a doctor.

Seniors

Older individuals commonly experience constipation, and consequently are at risk of becoming laxative-dependent. Avoid chronically turning to laxatives to ease constipation, and instead look to diet, exercise, and increased fluid intake as therapeutic measures.

Products containing stimulant laxatives such as Dulcolax may not be the best choice for this group because they alter fluid and electrolyte balance, placing some seniors at risk for side effects. Bulk-forming laxatives are usually preferred for seniors.

Ex-Lax Chocolate (EX-laks)
Ex-Lax Regular Strength

*see **Phenolphthalein,** page 967*

FiberCon [$] (FYE-bur-kon)

*see **Calcium Polycarbophil,** page 729*

Gaviscon Extra Strength Tablets
(GAV-iss-con)

Generic Ingredients

Alginic acid
Aluminum hydroxide
Magnesium trisilicate
Sodium bicarbonate

Type of Drug

Antacid.

Used for

Relief of heartburn, sour stomach, and acid indigestion.

General Information

All antacids work in the same way, by neutralizing gastric acid. Gaviscon consists of 3 antacid ingredients: aluminum hydroxide, magnesium trisilicate, and sodium bicarbonate.

Alginic acid works by reacting with sodium bicarbonate and saliva to produce a foam-like layer that floats on the surface of the stomach acid. In the event of reflux of the stomach contents into the esophagus, it is the foam rather than the gastric acids that comes into contact with the delicate tissues in the throat. This minimizes possible irritation and discomfort and helps maintain the normal digestive process.

The efficiency of these combination medications has not been well studied; in fact, the FDA considers alginic acid to be of questionable value.

Cautions and Warnings

Do not take the maximum daily dosage of Gaviscon for more than 2 weeks continuously except under a doctor's supervision. Antacids may relieve symptoms of a serious condition such as peptic ulcer disease. If you take an antacid for a prolonged period, you run the risk of unknowingly masking the symptoms of a serious gastrointestinal (GI) disease and delaying diagnosis.

Do not exceed the recommended dosage of Gaviscon.

Call your doctor if you do not get relief from Gaviscon, or if your stool is black or tarry or looks life coffee grounds, which indicates bleeding in the intestines or stomach. These may be signs of a serious GI disorder that cannot and should not be treated unsupervised with Gavison.

Because some of the magnesium and aluminum in Gaviscon is absorbed into the bloodstream and then eliminated through the kidneys, people with impaired kidney function should not take Gaviscon. Excretion of magnesium and aluminum is decreased during chronic use by these people, and the magnesium and aluminum may accumulate in bones, lungs, and nerve tissue.

Unlike other antacids, sodium bicarbonate, one of the active ingredients in Gaviscon, is completely absorbed into the blood stream. When taken in large doses or by people with impaired kidney function, it can cause systemic metabolic alkalosis (a condition in which the blood becomes low in acidity, affecting the kidney, blood, and slat balance).

Large doses of sodium bicarbonate, when combined with milk or calcium, can cause milk-alkali syndrome, which occurs when there is a high intake of calcium combined with anything producing alkalosis (imbalance of acid and base in body fluids). Symptoms include headache, nausea, irritability, vertigo (dizziness), and vomiting. Left unchecked, the syndrome can cause irreversible kidney damage.

Prolonged use of Gaviscon may result in the development of silicate kidney stones.

Excessive amounts of Gaviscon taken for a prolonged period can lead to low blood phosphate levels, which are characterized by loss of appetite, malaise, and muscle weakness.

Do not use Gavison if you are on a sodium-restricted diet, or if you have hypertension (abnormally high blood pressure), edema (fluid retention), congestive heart failure, kidney failure, or cirrhosis.

Do not take Gaviscon if you are overfull from eating or drinking.

Possible Side Effects

▼ Most common: constipation, diarrhea, abdominal swelling, flatulence (gas), fluid retention, and weight gain.

Drug Interactions

• Gaviscon decreases the absorption of the following drugs, reducing their effect: allopurinol, an antigout medication; nitrofurantoin, an entibiotic tetracycline antibiotic; quinolone antibiotics, such as ciprofloxacin; cimetidine and ranitidine, used to treat peptic ulcers, heartburn, and acid indigestion; indomethacin, a nonsteroidal anti-inflammatory drug (NSAID); isoniazid, used to treat tuberculosis; digoxin, used to treat congestive heart failure; iron; and ketoconazole, an antifungal agent. It may also decrease the bioavailability of the beta blocker atenolol, used to treat high blood pressure. If you are taking Gaviscon at the same time as any of these drugs, separate your dose of each drug by at least 2 hours; with quinolone antibiotics, 4 to 6 hours is preferable.

• Gaviscon decreases the elimination of amphetamine, used to treat narcolepsy and obesity; and quinidine, an antiarrhytmic, leading to possible retention of these drugs and intoxication. Do not use Gaviscon at the same time as either of these products.

• Concurrent use of Gaviscon with sodium polystyrene sulfonate, a potassium remover, may be dangerous. Separate your dose of each drug by at least 2 hours.

• Gaviscon increases the absorption of the anticonvulsant valproic acid, creating the potential for valproic acid toxicity, and of the benzodiazepine, diazepam, increasing its sedative effect. If you are taking valproic acid or diazepam, consult your doctor before taking Gaviscon.

• Gaviscon increases the body's elimination of aspirin and other salicylates, reducing their effect. Conversely, it increases the absorption of enteric-coated aspirin.

Food Interactions

Gaviscon is best taken after meals (see "General Information").

Usual Dose

Each tablet contains 200 mg of alginic acid, 80 mg of aluminum hydroxide, 47.5 mg of magnesium carbonate, and 70 mg of sodium bicarbonate.

Adult and Child (age 12 or over): Chew 2(4 tablets 4 times a day, not to exceed 16 tablets in 24 hours. Follow immediately with 4–5 oz. of liquid. Do not swallow whole.

Child (under age 12): Consult a doctor.

Overdosage

Do the following in case of accidental overdose: If the victim is unconscious or having convulsions, call for an ambulance immediately. If you take the victim to an emergency room, be sure to bring the bottle or container with you. If the victim is conscious, call your local poison control center or a health care professional. The poison control center may suggest inducing vomiting with ipecac syrup (available without a prescription at any pharmacy). DO NOT induce vomiting unless specifically instructed to do so.

Special Populations

Pregnancy/Breast-feeding

It is not recommended that pregnant women take any drugs, especially during the first 3 months after conception. However, antacids can be safely taken in small doses for short periods of time during pregnancy and while breast-feeding. Pregnant women who increase their milk or calcium intake should be especially aware of the risk of milk-alkali syndrome (see "Cautions and Warnings") before using Gaviscon.

Check with your doctor before self-medicating with Gaviscon if you are or might be pregnant, or if you are breast-feeding.

Infants/Children

The safety of antacid use in infants and children has not been established. Children under age 12 should not be given Gaviscon unless directed by a doctor.

Seniors

Seniors may safely take antacids. However, be advised that many older patients are at high risk for complications from ulcers, yet often do not show classic ulcer symptoms. Discuss the possible causes of your gastric discomfort with your pharmacist before self-medicating with an antacid and possibly delaying diagnosis of an ulcer. Be aware of possible interactions with other medications you may be taking.

Imodium A-D (IM-o-dee-um)

*see **Loperamide Hydrochloride,** page 871*

Kaopectate (Kay-oh-PEK-tate)

*see **Attapulgite,** page 679*

Brand Name

Maalox Antacid (MAY-lox)

Generic Ingredients

Aluminum hydroxide
Magnesium hydroxide

Type of Drug

Antacid.

Used for

Relief of heartburn, sour stomach, acid indigestion, and upset stomach associated with these symptoms.

General Information

All antacids work in the same way, by neutralizing gastric acid. Maalox antacid contains 2 ingredients: magnesium hydroxide and aluminum hydroxide.

How long an antacid product works depends on how long it remains in the stomach. In general, an antacid taken on an empty stomach leaves the stomach rapidly, and works for only 20 to 40 minutes. However, when taken after a meal, it leaves the stomach more slowly. When taken 1 hour after a meal, an antacid can work for up to 3 hours.

Cautions and Warnings

Do not take the maximum daily dosage of Maalox Antacid for more than 2 weeks continuously except under a doctor's supervision. Maalox Antacid may relieve symptoms of a serious condition such as peptic ulcer disease. If you take Maalox Antacid for a prolonged period, you run the risk of unknowingly masking the symptoms of a serious gastrointestinal (GI) disease and delaying diagnosis.

Do not exceed the recommended daily dosage of Maalox Antacid.

Call your doctor if you do not get relief from Maalox Antacid, or if your stool is black or tarry or looks like coffee grounds, which indicates bleeding in the intestines or stomach. These may be signs of a serious GI disorder that cannot and should not be treated unsupervised with Maalox Antacid.

Because some of the magnesium and aluminum in Maalox Antacid is absorbed into the bloodstream and then eliminated through the kidneys, people with impaired kidney function should not use Maalox Antacid. Excretion of magnesium and aluminum is decreased during chronic use by these people, and the magnesium and aluminum may accumulate in bones, lungs, and nerve tissue.

Excessive amounts of Maalox Antacid taken for a prolonged period can lead to low blood phosphate levels, which are characterized by loss of appetite, malaise, and muscle weakness.

Possible Side Effects

▼ Most common: constipation and diarrhea.

▼ Less common: abdominal cramping, increased urination, nausea, vomiting, and dehydration.

Drug Interactions

• Maalox Antacid decreases the absorption of the following drugs, reducing their effect: allopurinol, an antigout medication; nitrofurantoin, an antibiotic; tetracycline antibiotics; quinolone antibiotics, such as ciprofloxacin; cimetidine and ranitidine, used to treat peptic ulcers, heartburn, and acid indigestion; indomethacin, a nonsteroidal anti-inflammatory drug (NSAID); digoxin, used to treat congestive heart failure; iron; and ketoconazole, an antifungal agent. It may also decrease the bioavailability of the beta blocker atenolol, used to treat high blood pressure. If you are taking aluminum hydroxide at the same time as any of these drugs, separate your dose of each drug by at least 2 hours; with quinolone antibiotics, 4 to 6 hours is preferable.

• Maalox Antacid increases the absorption of the anticonvulsant valproic acid, creating the potential for valproic acid toxicity, and of the benzodiazepine, diazepam, increasing its sedative effect. If you are taking valproic acid or diazepam, consult your doctor before taking Maalox Antacid.

• Maalox Antacid increases the body's elimination of aspirin and other salicylates, reducing their effect. Conversely, it increases the absorption of enteric-coated aspirin.

• Maalox Antacid decreases the elimination of the antiarrhythmic quindine, raising the serum concentration of quinidine to possibly dangerous levels. If you are taking quinidine, consult your doctor before taking Maalox Antacid.

• Concurrent use of Maalox Antacid with sodium polystyrene sulfonate, a potassium remover, may be dangerous. Separate your dose of each drug by at least 2 hours.

Food Interactions

Maalox Antacid is best taken after meals (see "General Information").

Usual Dose

Each teaspoonful (5 ml) contains 200 mg of magnesium hydroxide and 225 mg of aluminum hydroxide.

Adult and Child (age 12 and over): 2–4 tsp. 4 times a day.
Child (under 12): consult your doctor.

Take Maalox Antacid as symptoms occur, but do not exceed 16 tsp. per day.

Overdosage

Do the following in case of accidental overdose: If the victim is unconscious or having convulsions, call for an ambulance immediately. If you take the victim to an emergency room, be sure to bring the bottle or container with you. If the victim is conscious, call your local poison control center or a health care professional. The poison control center may suggest inducing vomiting with ipecac syrup (available without a prescription at any pharmacy). DO NOT induce vomiting unless specifically instructed to do so.

Storage Instructions

Maalox Antacid may be stored at room temperature, but to improve its taste, refrigerate it. Do not freeze it.

Special Populations

Pregnancy/Breast-feeding

Antacids can be safely taken in small doses for short periods of time during pregnancy and while breast-feeding. However, it is not generally recommended that pregnant women take any drugs, particularly during the first 3 months after conception. Check with your doctor before self-medicating with Maalox Antacid if you are, or might be, pregnant, or if you are breast-feeding.

Infants/Children

The safety of antacid use in infants and children has not been established. Children under age 12 should not be given Maalox Antacid unless directed by a doctor.

Seniors

Seniors may safely take Maalox Antacid. However, you should be advised that many older patients are at high risk for complications from ulcers, yet often do not show classic ulcer symptoms. Discuss the possible causes of your gastric discomfort with your pharmacist before self-medicating with Maalox Antacid and possibly delaying diagnosis of an ulcer. You should also be aware of possible interactions with other medications you may be taking.

Brand Names

Maalox Antacid/Antigas Tablets
Mylanta Liquid (my-LAN-tuh)
Mylanta Maximum Strength Liquid

Generic Ingredients

Aluminum hydroxide gel
Magnesium hydroxide
Simethicone

Type of Drug

Antiflatulent, antacid.

Used for

Relief from the pain and pressure symptoms of excess stomach acid and gas in the digestive tract.

General Information

Stomach gas is frequently caused by excessive swallowing of air or by eating foods that irritate the stomach lining. The retention of gas may also be a problem during recovery from surgery or from such medical conditions as peptic ulcer, spastic or irritable colon, and diverticulosis. Excess gas is often accompanied by complaints of bloating, distention, fullness, pressure, pain, cramps, and excess anal flatus (gas).

Products such as Maalox Antacid/Antigas, Mylanta, and Mylanta Maximum Strength contain simethicone, a chemical that works by preventing pockets of gas from forming in the gastrointestinal (GI) tract and relieving gas trapped in both the stomach and the intestines. The freed gas is then eliminated through belching or passing flatus.

Simethicone is regarded by the FDA and clinicians as a safe and effective antiflatulent, but there is no conclusive evidence that it relieves the symptoms of immediate postprandial upper abdominal distress, a condition that occurs within 30 minutes after a meal and is characterized by GI bloating, distention, fullness or pressure with abdominal discomfort; nor of intestinal distress, which is abdominal discomfort not accompanied by constipation or diarrhea. While both of these conditions are commonly thought to be caused by excess gas, this has not been proven in either case.

Aluminum hydroxide is a neutralizing salt compound that acts in the GI tract to change excess stomach acid into an aluminum salt (that causes less discomfort) and water. It does not effect the amount of gastric acid secreted. Instead, it can act only on acid already present in the stomach. Aluminum hydroxide dissolves more slowly than some other antacids, taking from 10 to 30 minutes to begin acting. However, this chemical also delays the emptying of stomach contents by relaxing the stomach's smooth musculature, and is therefore available to provide relief for a longer period of time than other antacids.

Magnesium hydroxide is another neutralizing compound that acts in much the same manner as aluminum hydroxide. It is a faster-acting antacid but is also eliminated from the stomach more quickly.

Due to the differences in the time it takes to obtain and maintain relief from aluminum and magnesium neutralizing compounds, they are quite often combined in OTC drugs of this nature.

Liquid preparations generally dissolve more easily in gastric acid than do tablets or powders, and may provide relief of your symptoms more quickly.

Cautions and Warnings

If your condition persists for a period of more than 2 weeks without significant improvement, consult your doctor. Gastric pain and acid imbalances can be signs of a more serious underlying condition.

Do not exceed the recommended dosage of Maalox, Mylanta, or Mylanta Maximum Strength.

Accumulation of aluminum and magnesium can occur in people with impaired kidney function resulting in significant and severe adverse reactions. If you have impaired renal function or are on dialysis, consult your doctor before taking these products.

The aluminum hydroxide in these products forms insoluble phosphate salts which are excreted in the feces. Even in people with normal renal function, this process can affect the body's natural ability to gather phosphates, which can cause calcium to be depleted from bones. In those taking large doses, a condition called osteomalacia, (gradual softening and bending of the bones) may occur.

Magnesium is a potent central nervous system depressant, and in large doses can cause depressed reflexes, muscle paralysis, nausea, vomiting, hypotension (abnormally low blood pressure), respiratory depression, coma, and death in persons with serious renal impairment.

Possible Side Effects

▼ Less common: diarrhea, constipation, and vomiting.

Drug Interactions

• The antacids in Maalox, Mylanta, and Mylanta Maximum Strength have been reported to interfere with the action of some 30 prescription drugs, usually by preventing the absorption or the timely elimination of the other medications. Consult your doctor before taking Maalox, Mylanta, or Mylanta Maximum Strength if you are taking other drugs for the maintenance of your health. Methods of compensating for this interaction include adjusting the dosage of the antacid and monitoring the times at which it is taken in relation to your other medications.

• Do not take these products if you are presently taking a prescription antibiotic drug containing any form of tetracycline.

Food Interactions

The duration of the antacid effect in your stomach depends largely upon the amount of food that is in your stomach at the time Maalox, Mylanta, or Mylanta Maximum Strength is administered. If taken on an empty stomach, antacids are rapidly eliminated within 20 to 40 minutes. However, if taken on a full stomach, they will neutralize gastric acid for up to 3 hours.

Usual Dose

Mylanta

Each 5 ml (1 tsp.) of Mylanta contains 200 mg of magnesium hydroxide, 200 mg of aluminum hydroxide, and 20 mg of simethicone.

Each 5 ml (1 tsp.) of Mylanta Maximum Strength contains 400 mg of magnesium hydroxide, 400 mg of aluminum hydroxide, and 40 mg of simethicone.

Adult and Child (age 12 and over): 2–4 tsps. at bedtime and 20 minutes to 1 hour after meals; not to exceed 24 teaspoons of Mylanta or 12 teaspoons of Mylanta Maximum Strength in 24 hours.

Child (under age 12): Consult a doctor.

Maalox

Each tablet contains 200 mg of magnesium hydroxide, 200 mg of aluminum hydroxide, and 25 mg of simethicone.

Adult and Child (age 12 and over): 1–3 tablets, 4 times a day.

Child (under age 12): Consult a doctor.

Overdosage

Symptoms of an overdose may include loss of appetite, general discomfort, muscle weakness, intestinal obstruction, hemorrhoids, fecal impaction, depressed reflexes, muscle paralysis, nausea, vomiting, hypotension, respiratory depression, coma, and death.

Even if the victim is not displaying any of the symptoms listed above, do the following in case of accidental overdose: If the victim is unconscious or having convulsions, call for an ambulance immediately. If you take the victim to an emergency room, be sure to bring the bottle or container with you. If the victim is conscious, call your local poison control center or a health care professional. The poison control center may suggest inducing vomiting with ipecac syrup (available without a prescription at any pharmacy). DO NOT induce vomiting unless specifically instructed to do so.

Special Populations

Pregnancy/Breast-feeding

Heartburn is a common occurrence during late pregnancy. The magnesium and aluminum hydroxide antacids contained in Maalox, Mylanta, and Mylanta Maximum Strength have been reported to cause congenital defects in fetal development. Consult your doctor for a more appropriate treatment for heartburn or other related symptoms.

The antacids in this OTC drug do not enter the breast milk in significant amounts, and there have been no reports of complications for infants of nursing mothers. However, there is no data regarding simethicone and breast-milk content. Check with your doctor before taking these products if you are breast-feeding.

Infants/Children

There is limited information on the safety of simethicone use in children and infants, although in general, Maalox, Mylanta, and Mylanta Maximum Strength are apparently nontoxic.

Consult your doctor before giving these products to a child under the age of 12.

Seniors

Older individuals are more prone to GI disorders, such as ulcers, yet often they do not show classic ulcer symptoms. Consult your doctor before taking Maalox, Mylanta, or Mylanta Maximum Strength to avoid masking important symptoms of a more serious and possibly life-threatening condition.

Brand Name

Mylanta AR (mye-LAN-tuh)
Pepcid AC (PEP-sid)

Generic Ingredient

Famotidine (fa-MOW-tuh-deen)

Type of Drug

Acid reducer.

Used for

Relief of occasional heartburn, acid indigestion, and sour stomach; prevention of heartburn or indigestion.

General Information

There are currently 4 histamine H_2-receptor antagonists (H_2RAs) available for prescription use in the United States: cimetidine, ranitidine, famotidine, and nizatidine. Tagamet was the first to be introduced, in 1977. Prescription-strength H_2RAs are used to treat peptic ulcer disease (PUD) and gastroesophageal reflux disease (GERD).

As of May 1996, all 4 H_2RAs have been approved for OTC use (under the brand names Tagamet HB, Zantac 75, Pepcid AC, Mylanta AR, and Axid AR) in substantially lower doses than those indicated in the management of PUD and GERD. The OTC-strength H_2RAs are not indicated for the treatment of ulcer disease, are unlikely to provide sufficient relief for people with moderate-to-severe GERD, and will not provide relief for people with complications from GERD. They are taken for the same reasons that antacids are: to provide relief for individuals with heartburn, acid indigestion, or sour stomach. It has been reported that 25% of U.S. adults have at least 1 episode of abdominal discomfort in an average 2-week period, which partly accounts for the annual sales of antacids exceeding $1 billion. It is estimated that the OTC H_2RAs will soon be used as often as antacids for self-medication.

H_2RAs work by reducing the production of stomach acid. The degree and duration of acid suppression depend upon the dose and length of time the drug stays in the bloodstream. H_2RAs usually begin to provide relief within 1 hour of ingestion.

The duration of acid suppression reported for Pepcid AC (10 mg) or Mylanta AR (10mg) is 8 to 10 hours.

In treating acid indigestion, sour stomach, and heartburn, antacids provide more rapid relief than H_2RAs and, if used at the recommended doses for 2 weeks, cost about 4 times less. But for people who find taking multiple doses of antacids undesirable, H_2RAs, with their longer duration of action, may be preferable.

Cautions and Warnings

Do not take the maximum daily dosage of Pepcid AC for more than 2 weeks continuously except under the advice and supervision of a doctor. Contact your doctor if your symptoms persist after 2 weeks of self-medication with Pepcid AC.

Do not exceed the recommended daily dosage of Pepcid AC.

If you have trouble swallowing or persistent abdominal pain, see your doctor promptly. You may have a serious condition that may need a different treatment.

Because famotidine, the ingredient in Pepcid AC and Mylanta AR, is eliminated through the kidneys and metabolized in the liver, prescription-strength famotidine is used with caution and in reduced dosage in individuals with kidney and/or liver dysfunction. OTC famotidine is used in a lower dose, so a further reduction is probably unnecessary. Still, you may want to talk to your doctor or pharmacist before self-medicating with Pepcid AC or Mylanta AR if you have impaired kidney or liver function.

Pepcid AC and Mylanta AR are not approved for the treatment of peptic ulcer disease. Do not take more than the recommended dosage of Pepcid AC or Mylanta AR to self-medicate an ulcer. If you have or believe you have an ulcer, consult a physician.

Possible Side Effects

- ▼ Less common: drowsiness, weakness, fatigue, insomnia, depression, confusion, anxiety, agitation, decreased libido, constipation, vomiting, abdominal pain/discomfort, flatulence, belching, dry mouth, heartburn, rash, fever, hypertension, flushing, ringing in the ears, small reductions in blood pressure and heart rate, hematologic effects.
- ▼ Rare: serious central nervous system reactions, including confusion, agitation, and hallucinations.

Drug Interactions

• Pepcid AC and Mylanta AR may reduce the bioavailability of enoxacin, cefpodoxime, proxetil, itraconazole, and ketoconazole. If you are taking one of these drugs, consult your doctor or pharmacist before self-medicating with Pepcid AC or Mylanta AR.

• Antacids may slightly reduce the bioavailability of Pepcid AC and Mylanta AR. Separate the dose of Pepcid AC or Mylanta AR from doses of antacid by at least 1 hour.

Food Interactions

None known.

Usual Dose

Each Pepcid AC and Mylanta AR tablet contains 10 mg of famotidine.

Adult and Child (age 12 and over): 1 tablet with water. Do not exceed the maximum daily dosage of 2 tablets. For prevention of heartburn or indigestion, take 1 tablet 1 hour before eating.

Child (under age 12): not recommended.

Overdosage

Do the following in case of accidental overdose: If the victim is unconscious or having convulsions, call for an ambulance immediately. If you take the victim to an emergency room, be sure to bring the bottle or container with you. If the victim is conscious, call your local poison control center or a health care professional. The poison control center may suggest inducing vomiting with ipecac syrup (available without a prescription at any pharmacy). DO NOT induce vomiting unless specifically instructed to do so.

Special Populations

Pregnancy/Breast-feeding

It is not generally recommended that pregnant women take any drugs, particularly during the first 3 months after conception. Check with your doctor before self-medicating with Pepcid AC or Mylanta AR, if you are or might be pregnant, or if you are breast-feeding.

Infants/Children

Pepcid AC and Mylanta AR should not be given to children younger than age 12 unless directed by a doctor.

Seniors

Seniors may safely self-medicate with Pepcid AC or Mylanta AR. The OTC dose is low enough that a dosage reduction is not necessary to compensate for age-related reductions in elimination and breakdown.

Brand Names

Mylanta Double Strength Tablets (My-LAN-tuh)
Rolaids (ROE-lades)

Generic Ingredients

Calcium carbonate
Magnesium hydroxide

Type of Drug

Antacid.

Used for

Relief of heartburn, sour stomach, acid indigestion, upset stomach, and flatulence (gas) associated with these symptoms. Calcium carbonate has also been recommended as a source of extra calcium to prevent osteoporosis.

General Information

All antacids work in the same way, by neutralizing gastric acid. However, they differ in potency. Rolaids and Mylanta Double Strength Tablets contain a combination of 2 antacid ingredients: calcium carbonate and magnesium hydroxide. Calcium carbonate is the most potent of the antacids, however it dissolves slowly in stomach acid. In these products, it is combined with magnesium hydroxide, a much faster acting antacid, to provide rapid relief.

How long an antacid product works depends on how long it remains in the stomach. In general, an antacid taken on an empty stomach leaves the stomach rapidly, and works for only 20 to 40 minutes. However, when taken after a meal, it leaves the stomach more slowly. When taken 1 hour after a meal, an antacid can work for up to 3 hours.

Cautions and Warnings

Do not take the maximum daily dosage of Rolaids or Mylanta Tablets for more than 2 weeks continuously except under a doctor's supervision. Antacids may relieve symptoms of a serious condition such as peptic ulcer disease. If you take an antacid for a prolonged period, you run the risk of unknowingly masking the symptoms of a serious gastrointestinal (GI) disease and delaying diagnosis.

Do not exceed the recommended daily dosage of Rolaids or Mylanta.

Call your doctor if you do not get relief from these product or if your stool is black or tarry or looks like coffee grounds, which indicates bleeding in the intestines or stomach. These may be signs of a serious GI disorder that cannot and should not be treated with an OTC product without your doctor's supervision.

Due to its calcium carbonate content, these products can have a rebound effect; that is, more gastric acid is secreted after the drug has been emptied by the stomach. This limits long-term use.

Large doses of these products may lead to hypercalcemia (an excess of calcium in the blood), which can cause nausea, vomiting, loss of appetite, weakness, headache, dizziness, bone weakness, and change in mental state.

Calcium carbonate, one of the active ingredients in these products, has also caused milk-alkali syndrome, which occurs when there is a high intake of calcium combined with anything producing alkalosis (imbalance of acid and base in body fluids). Symptoms include headache, nausea, irritability, dizziness, and vomiting. Left unchecked, the syndrome can cause irreversible kidney damage. Hypercalcemic and milk-alkali syndrome are more likely to occur in people with impaired kidney function.

Because some of the magnesium in these products is absorbed into the bloodstream and eliminated through the kidneys, people with impaired kidney function should not use them. Such people are at high risk for magnesium toxicity, which can lead to muscle paralysis, severe hypotension (abnormally low blood pressure), respiratory depression, and other life-threatening complications.

Possible Side Effects

▼ Most common: constipation, diarrhea, belching, and flatulence.

Drug Interactions

• Because antacids interact with a number of orally administered drugs, it is best to separate doses of other medications by 1 to 2 hours (or check with your pharmacist about possible interactions).

• Rolaids and Mylanta Tablets decrease the absorption of the following drugs, reducing their effect: tetracycline antibiotics; quinolone antibiotics such as ciprofloxacin; isoniazid (INH), an antibiotic used to treat tuberculosis; phenytoin, an anticonvulsant; dexamethasone, a corticosteroid; indomethacin, a nonsteroidal anti-inflammatory drug (NSAID); digoxin, used to treat congestive heart failure; and iron. It may also decrease the bioavailability of the beta blocker atenolol, used to treat high blood pressure. If you are taking Rolaids or Mylanta Tablets at the same time as any of these drugs, separate your dose of each drug by at least 2 hours; with quinolone antibiotics, 4 to 6 hours is preferable.

• Rolaids and Mylanta Tablets increase the absorption of the anticonvulsant valproic acid, creating the potential for valproic acid toxicity. If you are taking valproic acid, consult your doctor before taking these products.

• These products increase the body's elimination of aspirin and other salicylates, reducing their effect.

• Rolaids and Mylanta Tablets decrease the elimination of the antiarrhythmic quinidine, raising the serum concentration of quinidine to potentially dangerous levels. If you are taking quinidine, consult your doctor before taking these products.

• Taking Rolaids or Mylanta Tablets at the same time as sodium polystyrene sulfonate, a potassium remover, may be dangerous. Separate your dose of each drug by at least 2 hours.

Food Interactions

Rolaids or Mylanta Tablets are best taken after meals (see "General Information").

Usual Dose

Each Mylanta Double Strength Tablet contains 700 mg of calcium carbonate and 300 mg of magnesium hydroxide. Each

Rolaids tablet contains 412 mg of calcium carbonate and 80 mg of magnesium hydroxide.

Adult and Child (age 12 and over): 1–2 tablets chewed as symptoms appear. The dose can be repeated hourly but should not exceed 14 tablets per day.

Child (under age 12): Consult a doctor.

Overdosage

Do the following in case of accidental overdose: If the victim is unconscious or having convulsions, call for an ambulance immediately. If you take the victim to an emergency room, be sure to bring the bottle or container with you. If the victim is conscious, call your local poison control center or a health care professional. The poison control center may suggest inducing vomiting with ipecac syrup (available without a prescription at any pharmacy). DO NOT induce vomiting unless specifically instructed to do so.

Special Information

Patients with a history of constipation or hemorrhoids may choose Rolaids or Mylanta Tablets over other antacids because it can cause diarrhea. Diarrhea associated with magnesium hydroxide, one of the active ingredients in these products, unlike diarrhea brought on by other causes, does not necessarily cause stomach cramps or nocturnal bowel movements.

Special Populations

Pregnancy/Breast-feeding

It is not generally recommended that pregnant women take any drugs, particularly during the first 3 months after conception. However, antacids can be safely taken in small doses for short periods of time during pregnancy and while breast-feeding. Since pregnant women often increase their milk or calcium intake, they should be especially aware of the risk of milk-alkali syndrome (see "Cautions and Warnings") before taking Rolaids or Mylanta Tablets.

Check with your doctor before taking these products if you are or might be pregnant, or if you are breast-feeding.

Infants/Children

The safety of antacid use in infants and children has not been established. Children under age 12 should not be given Rolaids or Mylanta Tablets unless directed by a doctor.

Seniors
Seniors may safely take antacids. However, be advised that many older patients are at a high risk for complications from ulcers, yet often do not show classic ulcer symptoms. Discuss with your pharmacist the possible causes of your gastric discomfort before self-medicating with an antacid and possibly delaying diagnosis of an ulcer. Be aware of possible interactions with other medications you may be taking.

Seniors may be more likely than younger adults to have diarrhea caused by Rolaids or Mylanta Tablets.

Mylanta Liquid (My-LAN-tuh)
Mylanta Double Strength Liquid

*see **Maalox Antacid/Antigas Tablets,** page 281*

Pepcid AC (PEP-sid)

*see **Mylanta AR,** page 285*

Pepto-Bismol (PEP-toe-BIZ-moll)

*see **Bismuth Subsalicylate,** page 703*

Brand Name
Phillips' Gelcaps (FILL-ips)

Generic Ingredients

Docusate sodium
Phenolphthalein

Type of Drug

Laxative, emollient fecal softener.

Used for

Relief of occasional constipation (irregularity).

General Information

The average, healthy individual defecates anywhere from 3 times a day to 3 times a week. Constipation is determined not necessarily by the frequency of bowel movements, but by the consistency of the stool, how difficult it is to eliminate, and symptoms such as dull headache, low back pain, and abdominal distention (swelling). Evaluate your condition carefully and discuss your symptoms and their possible causes with your pharmacist before taking a laxative. Laxatives are not always necessary, and when used improperly can either prevent the desired effect or result in laxative dependency. If you are indeed constipated, it may be best managed through proper diet, adequate fluid intake (6 to 8 glasses of water daily), and exercise. If you must use a laxative, choose the mildest effective product.

Laxatives may be classified by their mechanism of action: bulk-forming, emollient (stool softeners), lubricant, saline, hyperosmotic, and stimulant. Phillips' Gelcaps consist of 2 laxatives, phenolphthalein, a stimulant laxative, and docusate, an emollient laxative. According to different studies, stimulant laxatives work by either increasing the propulsive activity of the intestine or stimulating the secretion of water and electrolytes in the intestine, thus leading to evacuation of the colon. Phenolphthalein also increases the activity of the small intestine.

Docusate works by drawing water into fecal material, thus softening it and easing defecation. Docusate has no stimulant properties.

Cautions and Warnings

Do not use Phillips' Gelcaps for more than 7 days, unless directed by your doctor. Long-term use of laxatives has been linked with laxative dependence, chronic constipation, loss of normal bowel function, and, in severe cases, nerve, muscle, and tissue damage to the intestines. Using laxatives too frequently can result in persistent diarrhea, hypokalemia (abnormally low potassium in the blood), loss of essential nutrients, and dehydration.

Do not exceed the maximum daily dosage of Phillips'.

Of all the types of laxatives, stimulant laxatives such as phenolphthalein, one of the active ingredients in Phillips', are particularly habit-forming, and are the most likely to cause adverse effects such as diarrhea, gastrointestinal (GI) irritation, and fluid and electrolyte depletion with long-term use.

Phillips' may continue its laxative effect for several days after it has been taken.

Overuse of Phillips' can impair the absorption of vitamin D and calcium. This can cause osteomalacia (softening of the bones), which is characterized by pain, tenderness, muscular weakness, loss of appetite, and weight loss.

Do not take Phillips' if you have abdominal pain, nausea, vomiting, or kidney disease, unless directed by your doctor.

If you notice a marked change in bowel habits lasting for more than 2 weeks, do not take Phillips' until you have spoken to your doctor. Also, contact your doctor if there is blood in your stool, so that colon cancer or other significant disease can be ruled out before you begin self-medication with Phillips'.

If you have had a disease or surgery affecting the GI tract, using Phillips' may affect your condition adversely.

If you have rectal bleeding after using Phillips', or if you do not have a bowel movement after 7 days of using Phillips', you may have a serious condition such as intestinal blockage. Stop using Phillips' and call your doctor.

Phenolphthalein can cause 3 types of allergic reactions in susceptible people. One is a pink or purple skin rash. The other, associated with large doses, causes diarrhea, colic, cardiac and respiratory distress, or circulatory collapse. If you experience any of these reactions, stop using Phillips' and call your doctor or pharmacist.

Phillips' may affect the absorption of other drugs that pass though the GI tract (see "Drug Interactions").

Possible Side Effects

▼ Most common: abdominal discomfort, faintness, nausea, cramps, pinching and spasmodic pain in the bowels, colic, and increased mucus secretion.

Possible Side Effects ***(continued)***

- ▼ Less common: metabolic acidosis or alkalosis (imbalances of acid and base in body fluids associated with chronic use of phenolphthalein), hypocalcemia (too little calcium in the blood), tetany (characterized by foot spasms, muscular twitching and cramps), electrolyte and fluid deficiencies (characterized by vomiting and muscle weakness), impaired intestinal absorption of nutrients, and cathartic colon (weak or dilated colon).
- ▼ Rare: rash.

Drug Interactions

• Laxatives may affect the absorption of many orally administered drugs. Consult your doctor or pharmacist before taking Phillps' Gelcaps if you are currently taking any other medication, including OTC products.

• Phillips' should not be taken at the same time as oral mineral oil.

• Taking docusate, an active ingredient in Phillips', with aspirin has reportedly caused greater intestinal damage of the mucous membranes than taking aspirin alone.

Food Interactions

None known.

Usual Dose

Each gelcap contains 90 mg of phenolphthalein and 83 mg of docusate sodium.

Adult and Child (age 12 and over): 1–2 gelcaps daily with 8 oz. of liquid.

Child (under age 12): not recommended unless directed by a doctor.

Overdosage

Symptoms of overdosage include persistent diarrhea and dehydration.

Even if the victim is not displaying any of these symptoms, do the following in case of accidental overdose: If the victim is unconscious or having convulsions, call for an ambulance immediately. If you take the victim to an emergency room, be sure to bring the bottle or container with you. If the victim is conscious, call your local poison control center or a health care professional. The poison control center may suggest inducing vomiting with ipecac syrup (available without a prescription at any pharmacy). DO NOT induce vomiting unless specifically instructed to do so.

Special Information

Phenolphthalein, one of the active ingredients in Phillips' Gelcaps, may cause your urine or feces to appear pink or red. This is not a cause for alarm.

Special Populations

Allergies

Phenolphthalein has been known to cause 2 types of allergic reactions in susceptible people (see "Cautions and Warnings"). Do not take Phillips' Gelcaps if you have ever had an unusual or allergic reaction to a phenolphthalien product.

Pregnancy/Breast-feeding

Products containing stimulant laxatives such as Phillips' Gelcaps should be avoided during pregnancy. Only bulk-forming or emollient laxatives are recommended for pregnant women. Consider talking to your doctor about diet and mild exercise in the management of constipation.

It is not known whether the active ingredients in Phillips' pass into breast milk. Check with your doctor before using Phillips' if you are breast-feeding.

Infants/Children

Observe your child carefully for patterns of bowel movements and the pain or difficulty with which the bowel movements are made before deciding whether the child is actually constipated. As with adults, "normal" bowel habits vary in children. If your child is indeed constipated, increasing fluid intake and adding fiber to his or her diet may help to manage the condition. In general, the use of laxatives should be avoided in children.

Do not give Phillips' to children under 12 years of age unless directed by a doctor.

Seniors

Seniors commonly experience constipation, and consequently may become laxative-dependent. Be cautious of chronically turning to laxatives to ease constipation, and instead look to diet, exercise, and increased fluid intake as therapeutic measures.

Phillips' may not be the best choice for this group because it may alter fluid and electrolyte balance, placing some seniors at risk for side effects. Bulk-forming laxatives are usually preferred for seniors.

Phillips' Milk of Magnesia [A]

(FILL-ips)

*see **Magnesium Hydroxide,** page 888*

Rolaids (ROE-lades)

*see **Mylanta Double Strength Tablets,** page 289*

Rolaids Calcium Rich/Sodium Free

(ROE-lades)

*see **Calcium Carbonate,** page 724*

Brand Name

Tagamet HB (TAG-uh-met)

Generic Ingredient

Cimetidine

Type of Drug

Acid reducer.

Used for

Relief of occasional heartburn, acid indigestion, and sour stomach; prevention of heartburn or indigestion.

General Information

There are currently 4 histamine H_2-receptor antagonists (H_2RAs) available for prescription use in the United States: cimetidine, ranitidine, famotidine, and nizatidine. Tagamet was the first to be introduced, in 1977. Prescription-strength H_2RAs are used to treat peptic ulcer disease (PUD) and gastroesophageal reflux disease (GERD).

As of May 1996, all 4 H_2RAs have been approved for OTC use (under the brand names Tagamet HB, Zantac 75, Pepcid AC, Mylanta AR, and Axid AR) in substantially lower doses than those indicated in the management of PUD and GERD. The OTC strength H_2RAs are not indicated for the treatment of ulcer disease, are unlikely to provide sufficient relief for people with moderate-to-severe GERD, and will not provide relief for people with complications from GERD. They are taken for the same reasons that antacids are: to provide relief for individuals with heartburn, acid indigestion, or sour stomach. It has been reported that 25% of U.S. adults have at least 1 episode of abdominal discomfort in an average 2-week period, which partly accounts for the annual sales of antacids exceeding $1 billion. It is estimated that the OTC H_2RAs will soon be used as often as antacids for self-medication.

H_2RAs work by reducing the production of stomach acid. The degree and duration of acid suppression depend upon the dose and the length of time the drug stays in the bloodstream. H_2RAs usually begin to provide relief within 1 hour of administration. The duration of acid suppression reported for Tagamet HB (200 mg) is 6 hours.

In treating acid indigestion, sour stomach, and heartburn, antacids provide more rapid relief than H_2RAs and, if used at the recommended doses for 2 weeks, cost about 4 times less. But for people who find taking multiple doses of antacids undesirable, H_2RAs, with their longer duration of action, may be preferable.

Cautions and Warnings

Do not take the maximum daily dosage of Tagamet HB for more than 2 weeks continuously except under the advice and supervision of a doctor. Contact your doctor if your symptoms persist after 2 weeks of self-medication with Tagamet HB.

Do not exceed the recommended daily dosage of Tagamet HB.

If you have trouble swallowing or persistent abdominal pain, see your doctor promptly. You may have a serious condition that may need a different treatment.

Consult your doctor before taking Tagamet HB if you are taking the oral asthma medicine theophylline, the blood thinner warfarin, or the seizure medication phenytoin (see "Drug Interactions").

Because cimetidine, the ingredient in Tagamet and Tagamet HB, is eliminated through the kidneys and metabolized in the liver, prescription-strength Tagamet is used with caution and in reduced dosage in individuals with kidney and/or liver dysfunction. OTC Tagamet HB is already much lower in dose, so a further reduction is probably unnecessary. Consult your doctor or pharmacist before self-medicating with Tagamet HB if you have impaired liver or kidney function.

Tagamet HB—unlike its prescription-strength counterpart, Tagamet—is not approved for treatment of PUD (see "General Information"). It is simply a less potent version of Tagamet. If you have or believe you have an ulcer, consult a physician. Do not take more than the recommended dosage of Tagamet HB to self-medicate an ulcer.

Possible Side Effects

- ▼ Most common: headache, diarrhea, and nausea.
- ▼ Rare: drowsiness, constipation, vomiting, abdominal pain/discomfort, small reductions in blood pressure and heart rate, hematologic effects, and, rarely, serious central nervous system reactions, including confusion, dizziness, agitation, and hallucinations.

  Tagamet HB is the only one of the H_2RAs to have a mild antiandrogenic effect, which may cause impotence or gynecomastia (excessive development of male breasts). However, this effect, which is reversible upon discontinuation of the drug, occurs primarily in men receiving higher prescription doses of the drug per day, and is highly unlikely to occur at the approved OTC dose.

Drug Interactions

• Tagamet HB has the greatest potential to interact with other drugs compared to Axid AR, Pepcid AC, Mylanta AR, or Zantac 75. If you are taking any prescription medication, check with your physician or pharmacist to make sure you can take Tagamet HB.

• Consult your doctor before taking Tagamet HB if you are currently taking the oral asthma medicine theophylline, the blood thinner warfarin, or the seizure medication phenytoin. Because Tagamet HB binds to certain enzymes, it impairs the metabolism of these drugs. Your drug doses may have to be adjusted, or you may need to switch to another H_2RA.

• Interactions have been reported between prescription-strength Tagamet and tricyclic antidepressants, benzodiazepines, beta blockers, calcium channel blockers, lidocaine, and quinidine. Prescription-strength Tagamet has also been noted to increase the absorption of the antihypertensive nifedipine; reduce the bioavailability of enoxacin, a fluoroquinolone anti-infective; cefpodoxime, a cephalosporin antibiotic; and the antifungals, itraconazole and ketoconazole; and impair the elimination of procainamide, an antiarrhythmic. While these interactions have not been studied in Tagamet HB, there is always the possibility that they may occur.

• Antacids may slightly reduce the bioavailability of Tagamet HB. Separate the dose of Tagamet HB from doses of antacid by at least 1 hour.

Food Interactions

None known.

Usual Dose

Each tablet contains 100 mg of cimetidine.

Adult and Child (age 12 and over): 2 tablets, as needed, up to twice daily. Do not exceed the maximum daily dosage of 4 tablets. For prevention of heartburn or indigestion, take 2 tablets 1 hour before eating.

Child (under age 12): not recommended unless directed by a doctor.

Overdosage

Do the following in case of accidental overdose: If the victim is unconscious or having convulsions, call for an ambulance immediately. If you take the victim to an emergency room, be sure to bring the bottle or container with you. If the victim is conscious, call your local poison control center or a health care professional. The poison control center may suggest inducing vomiting with ipecac syrup (available without a prescription at any pharmacy). DO NOT induce vomiting unless specifically instructed to do so.

Special Populations

Pregnancy/Breast-feeding

It is not generally recommended that pregnant women take any drugs, particularly during the first 3 months after conception. Check with your doctor if you are or might be pregnant.

Cimetidine passes into breast milk. If you must take Tagamet HB, bottle-feed your baby with formula.

Infants/Children

Tagamet HB should not be given to children younger than 12 years of age unless directed by a doctor.

Seniors

Seniors may safely self-medicate with Tagamet HB. The OTC dose is low enough that a dosage reduction is not necessary to compensate for age-related reductions in elimination and metabolism. However, seniors should make certain that they are not taking any medications that interact with Tagamet HB (see "Drug Interactions").

Tums

see ***Calcium Carbonate,*** *page 724*

Tums E-X Sugar Free

see ***Calcium Carbonate,*** *page 724*

Brand Name

Tylenol Headache Plus Extra Strength (TYE-leh-nol)

Generic Ingredients

Acetaminophen
Calcium Carbonate

Type of Drug

Analgesic (pain reliever) and antacid.

Used for

Relief of heartburn, sour stomach, acid indigestion, upset stomach, flatulence (gas), and pain associated with these symptoms.

General Information

Tylenol Headache Plus contains acetaminophen, an analgesic, and calcium carbonate, an antacid, to relieve the pain and stomach upset from indigestion.

Acetaminophen is used to relieve pain associated with the common cold, flu, viral infections, or other disorders (neuritis, neuralgia, bursitis, arthritis, rheumatism, simple headache, menstrual cramps, tooth and periodontic pain, sprains, and minor muscular aches). All antacids work in the same way, by neutralizing gastric acid. This may take up to 30 minutes with Tylenol Headache Plus.

How long an antacid product works depends on how long it remains in the stomach. In general, an antacid taken on an empty stomach leaves the stomach rapidly and works for only 20 to 40 minutes. However, when taken after a meal, it leaves the stomach more slowly. When taken 1 hour after a meal, an antacid can work for up to 3 hours.

Cautions and Warnings

Do not take Tylenol Headache Plus for more than 10 consecutive days or, in the presence of fever, for more than 3 days, unless directed by your doctor. Antacids may relieve symptoms of a serious condition such as peptic ulcer disease. If you take Tylenol Headache Plus for a prolonged period, you run the risk of unknowingly masking the symptoms of a serious gastrointestinal (GI) disease and delaying diagnosis.

Call your doctor if you do not get relief from calcium carbonate, or if your stool is black or tarry or looks like coffee grounds, which indicates bleeding in the intestines or stomach. These may be signs of a serious GI disorder that cannot and should not be treated with Tylenol Headache Plus without your doctor's supervision.

Do not exceed the recommended daily dosage of Tylenol Headache Plus.

In doses of more than 4 grams per day, the acetaminophen ingredient in Tylenol Headache Plus is potentially toxic to the liver. Use Tylenol Headache Plus with caution if you have kidney or liver disease or viral infections of the liver. Studies have shown that the risk of liver damage with acetaminophen is associated with fasting and alcohol use. People with pre-existing liver disease who are taking other drugs that are potentially damaging to the liver, who do not eat regularly, or who drink alcohol (even moderately) are especially at risk. If you take Tylenol Headache Plus regularly, avoid drinking alcoholic beverages and/or fasting.

The effectiveness of Tylenol Headache Plus may be decreased if you smoke, and you may need a higher dose to achieve the desired effect.

Calcium carbonate, the antacid ingredient in Tylenol Headache Plus, can have a rebound effect; that is, more gastric acid is secreted after the drug has been emptied by the stomach. This limits long-term use.

Large doses of calcium carbonate may lead to hypercalcemia (an excess of calcium in the blood), which can cause nausea, vomiting, loss of appetite, weakness, headache, dizziness, and change in mental state.

Calcium carbonate has also caused milk-alkali syndrome, which occurs when there is a high intake of calcium combined with anything producing alkalosis (imbalance of acid and base in body fluids). Symptoms include headache, nausea, irritability, dizziness, and vomiting. Left unchecked, the syndrome can cause irreversible kidney damage.

Hypercalcemic and milk alkali syndrome are more likely to occur in people with impaired kidney function.

Possible Side Effects

- ▼ Most common: lightheadedness, constipation and diarrhea.
- ▼ Less common: trembling and pain in lower back or side, belching, and flatulence.
- ▼ Rare: extreme fatigue, rash, itching, or hives; sore throat or fever; unexplained bleeding or bruising; anemia; yellowing of the skin or eyes; blood in urine; painful or frequent urination; and decreased output of urine volume.

Drug Interactions

• The effects of Tylenol Headache Plus may be reduced by long-term use or large doses of barbiturate drugs; the anticonvulsants carbamazepine and phenytoin (and other similar drugs); rifampin, used to treat tuberculosis (TB) and sulfinpyrazone, used to treat gout. These drugs may also increase the chances of liver toxicity if taken with acetaminophen.

• Taking chronic, large doses of Tylenol Headache Plus with isoniazid (used to treat TB) may increase the risk of liver damage.

• If Tylenol Headache Plus is taken with an anticoagulant such as warfarin, it may increase the blood-thinning effect of the anticoagulant agent. This does not occur with occasional use.

• Alcohol increases the liver toxicity caused by large doses of acetaminophen, one of the active ingredients in Tylenol Headache Plus (see "Cautions and Warnings"). If you take Tylenol Headache Plus regularly, avoid alcohol.

• It has been reported that patients with acquired immunodeficiency syndrome (AIDS) and AIDS-related complex taking zidovudine (AZT) with acetaminophen have an increased incidence of bone marrow suppression. However, studies performed to try to determine if a harmful interaction exists have not shown that short-term use of acetaminophen (less than 7 days) increases the risk of bone marrow suppression or causes a decrease in white blood cells in AIDS patients taking AZT.

• Because antacids interact with a number of orally administered drugs, it is best to separate doses of other medications by 1 to 2 hours (or check with your pharmacist about possible interactions).

• Tylenol Headache Plus decreases the absorption of the following drugs, reducing their effect: tetracycline antibiotics, quinolone antibiotics, such as ciprofloxacin; and iron. It may also decrease the bioavailability of the beta blocker atenolol, used to treat high blood pressure.

• If you are taking Tylenol Headache Plus at the same time as any of these drugs, separate your dose of each drug by at least 2 hours; with quinolone antibiotics, 4 to 6 hours is preferable.

• Tylenol Headache Plus increases the body's elimination of aspirin and other salicylates, reducing their effect.

• Tylenol Headache Plus decreases the elimination of the antiarrhythmic quinidine, raising the serum concentration of quinidine to potentially dangerous levels. If you are taking quinidine, consult your doctor before taking Tylenol Headache Plus.

• Concurrent use of Tylenol Headache Plus with sodium polystyrene sulfonate, a potassium remover, may be dangerous. Separate your dose of each drug by at least 2 hours.

Food Interactions

None known.

Usual Dose

Each caplet contains 500 mg of acetaminophen and 250 mg of calcium carbonate.

Adult and Child (age 12 and over): 2 caplets every 6 hours. Do not take more than 8 caplets in 24 hours.

Child (under age 12): not recommended.

Overdosage

The first signs of overdose, which can include nausea, vomiting, drowsiness, confusion, and abdominal pain, usually occur within 2 to 3 hours but may not be seen for as long as 2 days after the overdose is taken. Other effects of overdose include low blood pressure, yellowing of the skin and eyes, and liver damage.

Even if the victim is not displaying any of the symptoms listed above, do the following in case of accidental overdose: If the victim is unconscious or having convulsions, call for an ambulance immediately. If you take the victim to an emergency room, be sure to bring the bottle or container with you. If the victim is conscious, call your local poison control center or a health care professional. The poison control center may suggest inducing vomiting with ipecac syrup (available without a prescription at any pharmacy). DO NOT induce vomiting unless specifically instructed to do so.

Special Populations

Pregnancy/Breast-feeding

It is not generally recommended that pregnant women take any drugs, particularly during the first 3 months after conception. Although taking normal dosages of acetaminophen is considered relatively safe for the expectant mother and her baby, taking continual high doses may cause birth defects or interfere with the baby's development.

Acetaminophen is considered acceptable for use during breast-feeding by the American Academy of Pediatrics. Although acetaminophen does pass into breast milk when taken by nursing mothers, the only side effect reported in infants is a rash that goes away when the mother stops taking the drug.

Antacids may also be safely taken in small doses for short periods of time during pregnancy and while breast-feeding. Since pregnant women often increase their milk or calcium intake, they should be especially aware of the risk of milk-alkali syndrome (see "Cautions and Warnings") before choosing Tylenol Headache Plus.

Check with your doctor before taking Tylenol Headache Plus if you are or might be pregnant, or if you are breast-feeding.

Infants/Children

Tylenol Headache Plus is not recommended for children under the age of 12.

Seniors

Because acetaminophen may clear the body more slowly in older adults, the side effects of Tylenol Headache Plus may be more noticeable.

Seniors taking Tylenol Headache Plus should be advised that many older patients are at high risk for complications from ulcers, yet often do not show classic ulcer symptoms.

Discuss the possible causes of your gastric discomfort with your pharmacist before using an antacid and possibly delaying diagnosis of an ulcer. Be aware of possible interactions with other medications you may be taking.

Seniors may be more likely than younger adults to have diarrhea caused by Tylenol Headache Plus.

Brand Name

Zantac 75 (ZAN-tack)

Generic Ingredient

Ranitidine hydrochloride (ra-NIT-tuh-deen HYE-droe-KLOR-ide)

Type of Drug

Acid reducer.

Used for

Relief of occasional heartburn, acid indigestion, and sour stomach.

General Information

There are currently 4 histamine H_2-receptor antagonists (H_2RA) available for prescription use in the United States: cimetidine, ranitidine, famotidine, and nizatidine. Tagamet was the first to be introduced, in 1977. Prescription-strength H_2RAs are used to treat peptic ulcer disease (PUD) and gastroesophageal reflux disease (GERD).

As of May 1996, all 4 H_2RAs have been approved for OTC use (under the brand names Tagamet HB, Zantac 75, Pepcid AC, Mylanta AR, and Axid AR) in substantially lower doses than those indicated in the management of PUD and GERD. The OTC-strength H_2RAs are not indicated for the treatment of ulcer disease, are unlikely to provide sufficient relief for people with moderate-to-severe GERD, and will not provide relief for people with complications from GERD. They are taken for the same reasons that antacids are: to provide relief for individuals with heartburn, acid indigestion, or sour stomach. It has been reported that 25% of U.S. adults have at least 1 episode of abdominal discomfort in an average 2-week period, which partly accounts for the annual sales of antacids exceeding $1 billion. It is estimated that the OTC H_2RAs will soon be used as often as antacids for self-medication.

H_2RAs work by reducing the production of stomach acid. The degree and duration of acid suppression depend upon the dose and length of time the drug stays in the bloodstream. H_2RAs usually begin to provide relief within 1 hour of administration. The duration of acid suppression reported for Zantac 75 (75 mg) is 6 to 8 hours.

In treating acid indigestion, sour stomach, and heartburn, antacids provide more rapid relief than H_2RAs and, if used at the recommended doses for 2 weeks, cost about 4 times less. But for people who find taking multiple doses of antacids undesirable, H_2RAs, with their longer duration of action, may be preferable.

Cautions and Warnings

Do not take the maximum daily dosage of Zantac 75 for more than 2 weeks continuously except under the advice and supervision of a doctor. Contact your doctor if your symptoms persist after 2 weeks of self-medication with Zantac 75.

Do not exceed the recommended daily dosage of Zantac 75.

If you have trouble swallowing or persistent abdominal pain, see your doctor promptly. You may have a serious condition that may need a different treatment. Because ranitidine, the ingredient in Zantac and Zantac 75, is eliminated through the kidneys and metabolized in the liver, prescription-strength Zantac is used with caution and in reduced dosage in individuals with kidney and/or liver dysfunction. OTC Zantac 75 is already much lower in dose, so a further reduction is probably unnecessary. Still, you may want to talk to your doctor or pharmacist before self-medicating with Zantac 75 if you have impaired liver or kidney function.

Zantac 75—unlike its prescription-strength counterpart, Zantac—is not approved for treatment of peptic ulcer disease. Do not take more than the recommended dosage of

Zantac 75 to self-medicate an ulcer. If you have or believe you have an ulcer, consult a physician.

Possible Side Effects

▼ Rare: headache, dizziness, drowsiness, insomnia, vertigo, constipation, diarrhea, nausea, vomiting, abdominal pain/discomfort, rash, small reductions in blood pressure and heart rate, hematologic effects, and, rarely, serious central nervous system reactions, including confusion, agitation, and hallucinations.

Drug Interactions

• Zantac 75 may impair the metabolism of the oral asthma medicine theophylline, the blood-thinner warfarin, and the seizure medication phenytoin. Check with your doctor or pharmacist before taking Zantac 75 if you are taking one of these drugs.

• Zantac 75 may increase the absorption of the antihypertensive nifedipine. It may reduce the bioavailability of enoxacin, a fluoroquinolone anti-infective, cefpodoxime, a cephalosporin antibiotic, and the antifungals, itraconazole, and ketoconazole. It may impair the elimination of procainamid, an antiarrhythmic. If you are taking one of these drugs consult your doctor or pharmacist before self-medicating with Zantac 75.

• Antacids may slightly reduce the bioavailability of Zantac 75. Separate the dose of Zantac 75 from doses of antacid by at least 1 hour.

Food Interactions

None known.

Usual Dose

Each tablet contains 75 mg of ranitidine.

Adult and Child (age 12 and over): 1 tablet with water. Do not exceed the maximum daily dosage of 2 tablets.

Child (under age 12): not recommended unless directed by a doctor.

Overdosage

Do the following in case of accidental overdose: If the victim is unconscious or having convulsions, call for an ambulance immediately. If you take the victim to an emergency room, be sure to bring the bottle or container with you. If the victim is conscious, call your local poison control center or a health care professional. The poison control center may suggest inducing vomiting with ipecac syrup (available without a prescription at any pharmacy). DO NOT induce vomiting unless specifically instructed to do so.

Special Information

Cigarette smoking appears to decrease the efficacy of prescription-strength Zantac.

Special Populations

Pregnancy/Breast-feeding

It is not generally recommended that pregnant women take any drugs, particularly during the first 3 months after conception. Check with your doctor before self-medicating with Zantac 75 if you are or might be, pregnant.

Ramitidine passes into breast milk. If you must take Zantac 75 bottle-feed your baby with formula.

Infants/Children

Zantac 75 should not be given to children younger than 12 years of age unless directed by a doctor.

Seniors

Seniors may safely self-medicate with Zantac 75. The OTC dose is low enough that a dosage reduction is not necessary to compensate for age-related reductions in elimination and breakdown.

Chapter 4: Skin Care

The skin, the largest organ of the body, is a complex structure responsible for many functions. It protects internal organs from the environment; regulates body temperature; permits passage of air, moisture, and light; secretes oils and perspiration; and allows us to sense heat, cold, and movement. Melanin (pigment) in the skin blocks out harmful radiation.

Skin contains a number of layers. The outermost group of layers is called the epidermis. The surface of the skin consists of dead cells, which contain a material called keratin and which are constantly being sloughed off. Hair, fingernails, and toenails are basically made of keratin. Below the epidermis is the dermis, a thicker layer that contains connective tissue, nerves, small blood vessels, sweat glands, oil glands, and hair follicles. The innermost layer, the hypodermis or subcutaneous tissue, contains connective and fatty tissues and is important for controlling temperature, storing energy, and providing cushioning.

Because it is the body's first line of defense, the skin is vulnerable to a wide range of problems: cuts, scrapes, infections, diseases, allergies, rashes, bites, and stings. This chapter describes the various OTC products available to relieve, as Hamlet put it, "the thousand natural shocks that flesh is heir to."

Acne

Inside the dermis are thousands of glands that produce an oily, waxy substance called sebum. Normally, the sebaceous glands secrete this material through the hair follicles (small tube-like glands or sacs from which hair grows) or through pores (tiny holes) in the skin. Sebum coats the surface of skin and hair and helps to prevent loss of moisture. If the pores or follicles become blocked, however, the material can build up and cause small swellings on the skin surface. These swellings are the characteristic features of acne (see box).

Acne Blemishes

Type	Description
Whitehead	Small, white, noninflammatory skin elevation
Blackhead	Small, black, noninflammatory skin elevation
Pimple	Prominent, inflamed swelling of the skin
Pustule	Inflamed swelling filled with pus

Acne usually develops as a result of the increased level and activity of sex hormones during puberty. These hormones stimulate the sebaceous glands to grow and produce increased amounts of sebum. At the same time, the wall of the hair follicle starts shedding larger numbers of cells. These cells can stick together, forming a plug that blocks the pore and prevents the sebum from reaching the skin surface. This produces a white swelling known as a whitehead. Sometimes the plug rises through the pore and emerges on the surface; such swellings are called blackheads. (Contrary to popular belief, the black color is not dirt; it is melanin, the chemical that gives skin its color.) If a whitehead grows large enough, it can stretch the cell wall that lines the hair follicle or pore. Bacteria trapped inside the pore produce fatty acids that irritate the cells. At that point the swelling becomes inflamed, red, and sore—that is, it develops into an acne pimple. To fight the infection, the body's immune system sends white cells to the area. As the cells accumulate, they create a yellowish pus-filled sac called a pustule. In serious cases, the pimples can develop into fluid-filled pockets called cysts. After the cysts heal, they can leave permanent pits or scars.

Acne is the most common skin disorder among adolescents. It affects as many as 8 out of 10 people at some time between the ages of 12 and 25. For most men, the chances are good that the condition will eventually clear up on its own. In women, however, there is a risk that acne will persist until after menopause. The blemishes appear in areas with the highest concentration of sebaceous glands: the face, center of the chest, upper back, shoulders, and neck.

Acne is not a life-threatening condition, but it occurs at a time of life when young people are going through enormous physical and emotional changes. The eruption of pimples on the face can threaten self-esteem, sap confidence, and cause social problems.

The main type of acne discussed here is acne vulgaris, common acne, although other forms are described (see box).

Types of Acne

Name	Cause
Acne vulgaris	Blocked sebaceous glands
Tropical acne	Exposure to a hot, humid climate
Chemical acne	Exposure to chemicals
Acne cosmetica	Use of makeup
Acne mechanica	Irritation and friction from rough or tight-fitting clothing, athletic equipment, headgear straps, etc.
Pomade acne	Use of hair dressings containing petrolatum
Drug-induced acne	Use of medications including oral contraceptives, thyroid drugs, antipsychotics, steroids, etc.
"French-fryer's" acne	Exposure to oil particles circulating in the air

Seek medical attention if any of the following applies to you

- Inflammatory acne
- Ten or more blemishes on either side of the face

Treatment for Acne

There is no cure for acne, and experts disagree about whether acne can be prevented. Evidence does not suggest, for example, that avoiding foods such as chocolate will reduce the risk of acne. People with inflammatory acne should seek treatment from a physician, because there is a risk of permanent scarring. There are many steps you can take to control acne (see box).

Controlling Acne

- Use water-based (rather than oil-based) cosmetics.
- Use a water-based shampoo formulated for oily hair.
- Wash the face 2 or 3 times a day with a mild facial soap (perhaps a mildly abrasive soap) and soft washcloth; pat dry (do not rub dry).
- Avoid environmental factors such as dirt, dust, oil, or chemicals that seem to exacerbate the problem.
- Never squeeze, pinch, or pick at acne blemishes—especially pimples—doing so can cause acne to spread or become infected and may result in permanent scarring.

Mild or moderate acne—defined as no more than 10 whiteheads or blackheads on either side of the face—can probably be treated using OTC products. The main ingredients in these products are benzoyl peroxide, salicylic acid, sulfur, and resorcinol. These chemicals all work in essentially the same way, by sloughing off (removing dead cells) from the skin.

Benzoyl peroxide is an effective antiacne chemical that acts by mildly irritating the skin. This increases the skin's ability to shed cells inside the hair follicles and then slough the cells off from the surface, thus opening the blocked pores. Benzoyl peroxide also kills bacteria, which reduces the risk that a blemish will become irritated and develop into a pimple. It is available in concentrations ranging from 2.5% to 20% and is found in various forms, including lotions, gels, creams, and soaps. Products that contain an alcohol-gel base may offer increased drying action, but these are generally available only by prescription. Soaps and cleansers that contain benzoyl peroxide may not be of value because they do not remain on the surface of the skin long enough to work effectively. Recent research has raised the concern that benzoyl peroxide may promote the growth of cancerous tumors that result from exposure to ultraviolet (UV) radiation. For this reason, the FDA is re-examining whether the ingredient is still safe to use.

Salicylic acid removes keratin-containing cells from the surface of the skin. Some studies have found that pads containing salicylic acid are better than those with benzoyl peroxide at clearing acne blemishes and preventing their return. Generally, salicylic acid products should not be used over large areas for long periods of time.

Sulfur helps clear up whiteheads and blackheads in the short run. There is some concern, however, that over time sulfur can actually cause these blemishes to develop. Sulfur products have an unpleasant odor that some people find unacceptable.

Resorcinol (in concentrations of 2%) or resorcinol monoacetate (3%) is effective only when combined with sulfur (concentrations of 3% to 8%). Resorcinol is the sole antiacne ingredient in some products, but at concentrations that are not thought to be very effective.

As is true of all skin medications, the active drug in acne products needs to be able to break free of the rest of the ingredients in the product (called the vehicle) if it is to penetrate the cells and do its job. For that reason, the vehicle can make a big difference in the effectiveness of the drug. Vehicles in antiacne products include cleansing bars, liquids, suspensions, lotions, creams, and gels. Gels generally work best, especially for those with darker skin, but lotions and creams may be better for those with dry or sensitive skin or for use during dry, cold weather; creams are also recommended for those with lighter skin. As noted previously, cleansing products do not leave enough of the active ingredient behind to be of much use.

OTC Products for Acne

Benzoyl peroxide
Salicylic acid
Sulfur
Resorcinol (+ sulfur)

Burns and Sunburn

Burns are among the most common household accidents, accounting for 2% of all injuries in the U.S. each year. The major types of burns are thermal (resulting from exposure to heat or open flame, steam or other hot gases, or boiling water), chemical, and electrical. The most common causes of burns indoors include misuse of fire sources (such as playing with matches); inadvertently touching a hot surface such as the oven rack or a heated dish or iron; faulty or misused heating or electrical equipment; and carelessness when smoking. About two-thirds of burns occur on the hands and arms and the rest on the face and legs.

Experts classify the severity of burns according to the depth to which the damage penetrates the skin (see box).

Severity of Burns

Degree	Characteristics
1st	Affects epidermis Causes redness and local pain No blisters or scars Heals within 3 to 10 days
2nd	Affects epidermis and upper portion of dermis Causes redness and local pain Blisters Little or no permanent damage Usually heals fully in 3 to 4 weeks without scarring
3rd	Affects entire epidermis and dermis Extensive and usually permanent damage Skin has leathery or white mottled appearance Damage is too great for blisters to form Sometimes less painful than 1st or 2nd degree burns due to nerve damage Risk of infection Requires months to heal Scarring likely; skin grafts may be needed
4th	Affects all layers of skin, underlying tissue, and muscle Charred, dry skin Serious risk of infection Requires many months to heal Skin grafts necessary for survival

Sunburn results from exposure to UV radiation, not from heat; it is possible to get a sunburn on a chilly ski slope in the dead of winter. Sunburn is the most common burn occurring outside the home. When exposed to UV rays, the skin gets thicker and releases higher amounts of melanin to block the rays from penetrating too deeply. (This increased pigment is why you get a tan.) Within as little as an hour after overexposure to sunlight, the skin turns red and begins to peel. Some people may experience pain and low-grade fever. In serious cases, sunburn causes more severe pain, swelling, skin tenderness, and possibly blistering. If the burn affects most of the body's surface area, the person may experience fever, chills, weakness, and shock. Response to sun exposure varies among different types of people. Because blonds and redheads generally have less skin pigment, they are more prone to burn, but even very dark skin can develop sunburn after prolonged exposure. For several weeks following a sunburn, people are much more likely to burn again when exposed to sunlight even for short periods. Many common medications can also cause people to experience toxic or allergic reactions to sunlight exposure (see box).

Seeing the Light

If you are taking any drugs, it's a good idea to ask your pharmacist whether they carry a potential increased risk of adverse reactions following sun exposure. Among the drugs associated with toxic reactions are:

- antibiotics, particularly fluoroquinolones, sulfa drugs, or tetracyclines
- anticancer drugs
- antidepressants
- antihistamines
- antihypertensives (blood pressure) medications
- diuretics
- estrogen preparations

Seek medical attention if any of the following applies to you

- Blisters
- Infection
- Burn caused by contact between a chemical and the eyes
- High fever
- Mental confusion
- Weakness
- Convulsions

Anyone experiencing any electrical burn (other than a very minor one) should see a physician, since the damage to the body may not be apparent.

Treatment for Burns and Sunburn

Minor (first-degree) burns that do not cover an extensive area and that do not involve the eyes, ears, face, feet, or rectal area can be effectively treated with OTC products. So can some very small second-degree burns (those involving 1% or less of the body area). Usually such burns heal well and do not cause long-term problems. More serious burns should be treated by a physician, since there is a significant risk of scarring or infection in damaged skin.

The goal of OTC treatment for burns is to provide relief of symptoms and promote healing. Ingredients used for burn treatment include protectants, analgesics (pain relievers), local anesthetics, antimicrobials, and other products (see box).

As their name suggests, protectants are substances intended to guard the burned area to prevent further injury or irritation and to reduce pain. By coating the skin, they also prevent dryness and restore moisture to the epidermis. These ingredients protect skin and relieve burn symptoms, but they do not directly heal the burn. Available protectant agents deemed safe and effective include allantoin, cocoa butter, petrolatum, and shark liver oil.

Analgesics are effective in reducing the pain resulting from burns. Nonsteroidal anti-flammatory drugs (NSAIDs) such as aspirin, naproxen, and ibuprofen reduce swelling and redness; acetaminophen relieves pain, but not inflammatory symptoms. In cases of sunburn, NSAIDs typically reduce inflammation for only about 24 hours. Some people experience more prolonged relief of sunburn pain using a combination of a topical corticosteroid and oral ibuprofen or another NSAID. (For more information on NSAIDs, see chapter 1.)

Local anesthetics relieve pain by numbing the nerve endings that send pain signals to the brain. The most common ingredients for this purpose are benzocaine (available in concentrations ranging from 5% to 20%) and lidocaine (0.5% to 4%). Other options include dibucaine (0.25% to 1%), butamben picrate (1%), and pramoxine (0.5% to 1%). Higher concentrations are used if the skin is intact; lower concentrations are indicated if the skin is broken. Unfortunately, pain relief from local anesthetics usually lasts only about 15 to 45 minutes. As a rule, these products should be applied no more than 3 to 4 times a day; thus they do not provide round-the-clock relief. Using higher doses or using local anesthetics for longer than a few days poses an increased risk of adverse effects.

Antimicrobials are drugs that fight infection. Usually infection is not a major risk in first-degree burns, especially if the skin is not broken. However, many OTC burn medications contain antimicrobial ingredients. These probably will not do much good, but they won't do much harm either—although an allergic reaction may develop with prolonged or repeated use. (For more information, see the section on wounds later in this chapter.)

Other products used in the treatment of minor burns include topical hydrocortisone ointment or cream (1%), which can reduce inflammation but should not be used if the skin is broken. Higher-potency corticosteroids should not be used for treatment of skin wounds, because they can delay the healing process. Vitamin C supplements (up to 2 grams a day) may improve wound healing, since vitamin C is an essential ingredient in the connective tissue found throughout the body. People with poor diets may also benefit from taking vitamins A and B, copper, and zinc during their recovery from a burn.

Burn treatments are available in various formulations. Aerosols and pump sprays allow you to apply medication without touching the affected areas. However, these products do not provide the surface protection available in an ointment, lotion, or cream. Ointments should not be used if the skin is broken, because they can trap moisture and promote bacterial growth inside the wound; in this instance, creams are preferred. Lotions are easy to apply, but they can sometimes cause dryness in the affected area.

OTC Products for Burns and Sunburn

- Protectants
  - Allantoin
  - Cocoa butter
  - Petrolatum
  - Shark liver oil
- Analgesics (specifically, NSAIDs)
- Anesthetics
  - Benzocaine
  - Benzyl alcohol
  - Butamben picrate
  - Dibucaine
  - Lidocaine
  - Pramoxine
- Antimicrobials
  - Benzalkonium chloride
  - Benzethonium chloride
  - Cetylpyridinium chloride
  - Chloroxylenol
  - 8-Hydroxyquinoline
  - Oxyquinolone
  - Phenol

Corns, Calluses, Bunions, and Warts

Since the time humans began wearing shoes, we've been plagued by problems affecting our feet. Among the most prevalent—and annoying—of these problems are corns, calluses, and bunions. Each of these conditions is the result of pressure or friction on the skin. The increased friction stimulates cells from lower layers of skin to migrate to the upper layers at a higher rate than normal, causing excess growth on the epidermis.

A corn is a small, thickened bump arising on the skin on the upper surface of the toes. Corns have a characteristic appearance: round, yellowish-gray in color, and with a distinct center. The top of the corn points inward and presses on the nerves in the skin below. That pressure is what makes the corn so painful. Corns come in 2 varieties: hard and soft. Hard corns usually erupt on the top of the toes or the outside of the little toe and have a shiny, almost polished appearance. Soft corns emerge in the moist tissue between toes, usually between the fourth and fifth toes. They are whiter, wetter, and less rigid, resembling a blister. Most corns arise because of a defect in the underlying bone, such as a bone spur or a bony tumor, coupled with pressure from ill-fitting shoes. Narrow or high-heeled shoes severely crowd the toes, especially the little toes, which is where most corns develop. Corns are also more likely to occur in people whose feet have high arches, since they experience greater pressure on their toes while walking.

Skin calluses are areas of thickened skin that develop in places exposed to constant pressure or rubbing. (The word *callus* is also used to describe a growth of new bone along the site of a fracture; doctors distinguish these conditions by using the terms *skin callus* and *bony callus*.) Skin calluses often develop on the soles of the feet, especially if the shoes are too loose. Other causes of calluses include walking barefoot, or having abnormally shaped legs or feet or unevenly distributed body weight. People who work a lot with their hands may get calluses on their palms. Guitarists and violinists actively try to develop calluses on their fingertips to make it easier to press on the instrument's strings. Corns are basically calluses that develop on the toes, but whereas hard corns contain a distinctive center, calluses have an even appearance.

A bunion is a fluid-filled, inflamed, often painful swelling arising on the outside of the big toe, just above the joint at the base (when these occur on the little toe, they are called bunionettes). As is true of corns and calluses, bunions result from pressure and friction, especially in people whose big toes are abnormally shaped.

The primary symptom of these conditions is pain, which can range from dull and aching to sharp and stabbing. Most calluses do not cause pain unless pressure is applied directly. Likewise, bunions do not always cause symptoms, but they can become painful, swollen, and tender.

Warts are a different, usually less serious problem. These growths, which can arise just about anywhere on the skin or mucous membranes, are the result of infections caused by human papilloma viruses. There are several kinds of warts (see box). Although the virus is contagious, the growths are harmless; most of them typically cause no symptoms.

Plantar warts are an exception. These growths, which erupt on the soles of the feet, are common in children and adolescents but can also occur in adults. Calluses and plantar warts look similar and can appear in the same regions, but plantar warts feel tender when pressure is applied. Another difference is that plantar warts contain tiny black dots, which are clotted blood from blood vessels that have stopped functioning due to the growth of the tissue. Also, warts growing on weight-bearing parts of the foot do not usually emerge above the surface of the skin the way calluses do. Several plantar warts may develop at the same place; their edges may grow together to look like one large wart. Over time, plantar warts can cause discomfort and may limit movement.

Most warts are not permanent. About 1 out of every 3 warts will vanish by itself within 6 months, and most of the rest disappear within 5 years.

Warts and All

- Common warts affect the hands, fingers, and sometimes the face.
- Plantar warts affect soles of the feet.
- The following must not be treated with OTC medication:
  - Periungual and subungual warts (develop on fingernail and toenail beds).
  - Juvenile (flat) warts (occur on the face, neck, hands, wrists, and knees of children).
  - Venereal warts (develop on the genitalia and anus).

Seek medical attention if any of the following applies to you

- Foot complications from diabetes or rheumatoid arthritis
- Circulatory problems
- Infection or inflammation at the site
- Bleeding or oozing from the site
- Body deformity or uneven weight distribution
- Extensive warts (especially plantar) at one site
- Warts on anus or genitalia
- Warts under toenails or fingernails
- Warts on the face, neck, hands, wrists, or knees of a child
- Warts that persist despite 4 to 12 weeks of self-treatment

Treatment for Corns, Calluses, Bunions, and Warts

Since corns, calluses, and bunions arise from pressure and friction, the sensible approach is to eliminate the source of the problem by wearing well-fitting shoes. People with leg or foot deformities might benefit from special corrective footwear.

The only approved product deemed safe and effective for the treatment of corns and skin calluses is salicylic acid. This substance works by promoting the shedding of excess cells from the epidermis. It also increases the water content of the cells, helping the skin return to its normal softness.

For corns and calluses, salicylic acid is available in 2 vehicles: collodion and plaster. Collodion is a liquid that dries to a strong film, somewhat like rubber cement. This helps prevent moisture from evaporating and increases the ability of the medication to penetrate the skin. The substance is applied once or twice per day as needed for up to 14 days. The film should be peeled away periodically to help speed up removal of the cells.

The plaster vehicle is a pastelike material that is mixed with water and placed on a pad, which is then applied to the affected area and held in place with adhesive tape. The product also comes in ready-cut disks, which are easier to handle than the cut-it-yourself variety. The plaster form contains a higher concentration of salicylic acid than colloidal vehicles and allows prolonged contact of the drug to the tissue. Pads are applied for 48 hours and then removed; up to 5 such treatments can be used in a 2-week period.

There are no OTC medications approved for the treatment of bunions; instead, relief is achieved by reducing friction and pressure. This can be accomplished by wearing properly fitting shoes, discarding high heels, and covering the affected area with padding for part of the day. A product such as Bunion Guard is a soft, self-adhesive pad containing a cushioning gel; the pad can be applied and removed daily over a 3-month period.

Salicylic acid is the only OTC treatment for warts. This drug does not cure warts, but it can promote their removal and relieve pain. The FDA has approved salicylic acid only for treatment of common warts and plantar warts. Other types of warts (and multiple plantar warts) must be treated by a physician. Salicylic acid for wart treatment is available in plaster and collodion vehicles. Treatment is applied for 48 hours and then removed for another 48 hours; the process is repeated for up to 12 weeks. Another formulation contains a vehicle called karaya gum and glycol plaster. This product is designed to be applied at bedtime and left in place for 8 hours. The treatment is repeated each day for up to 12 weeks.

OTC Products for Corns, Calluses, Bunions, and Warts

Salicylic acid
Protective pads

Dermatitis, Eczema, and Dry Skin

The terms *dermatitis* and *eczema* are used (often interchangeably) to refer to a group of skin conditions that involve inflammation, redness, and itching. Dermatitis can result from a number of causes: exposure to an allergen (a substance that provokes an allergic response), irritation, infections, or perhaps even emotional stress. In many cases, however, the exact cause of these common skin problems is unknown. There are several types of dermatitis (see box.)

Types of Dermatitis

Atopic dermatitis

The word *atopic* basically means "allergic" and indicates that the problem arises from a genetic trait, not from a contagious or infectious agent. Atopic dermatitis is the most common skin condition affecting children; most cases begin as early as age 2 months. Typically, affected areas include the face and the skin folds inside the knees and elbows. The main symptom is intense itching and scratching, accompanied by inflammation and, in some cases, scaly skin. Attacks of atopic dermatitis can be triggered by a number of factors, including irritants (e.g., smoke, fumes, and paints), rapid and severe changes of temperature and humidity, dry skin, emotional stress, and skin infections. Allergens that may trigger episodes include pollen and certain plant or animal proteins in foods.

Contact dermatitis

As the name indicates, this skin condition arises from direct contact with an allergen or an irritating substance. Irritants may include everything from soaps, detergents, and cosmetics to nickel (found in many items of jewelry), chemicals in rubber gloves, certain medications, skin creams, smoke particles, and pet dander. Perhaps the most common cause is exposure to poison ivy, oak, or sumac (see the section on these conditions later in this chapter). Different irritants produce somewhat different types of rashes, but, as is true of all forms of dermatitis, the main symptoms are itching, redness, and swelling.

Hand dermatitis

This form of dermatitis—sometimes called dishpan hands or housewives' eczema—is limited to the hands and occurs most often in people who wash their hands frequently or who work with moist products or chemicals, such as hairdressers, bartenders, and food handlers. Often the problem begins when moisture remains trapped under the person's ring. Untreated, it can spread to other fingers, the palm, and the other hand.

Symptoms of dermatitis include itching, redness, and swelling. In some cases the swelling involves the appearance of small fluid-filled blisters called vesicles. If the surface skin of the vesicles breaks due to irritation or scratching, they can leak fluid or ooze. As the material dries, it creates a crust or scales. If the condition persists for a long time, the affected area can develop a dry, scaly appearance and can become cracked and sore. Severe scratching can cause the skin to become thick and full of ridges; scratching can also lead to infections. Sometimes the skin in the affected area becomes darker or loses its color.

Xerosis (dry skin) is a condition that results when the skin, especially on the hands, forearms, and lower legs, is unable to retain sufficient moisture. As in dermatitis, the dryness causes itching, pain, and inflammation, and can make the area more susceptible to bacterial infection. The problem does not arise from exposure to an irritant, however; instead it may result from excessive bathing and use of soap, low humidity and high wind, or damage to the outer layer of skin. Dry skin is often a complication of aging.

Seek medical attention if any of the following applies to you

- The skin problem does not improve after 1 to 2 weeks of appropriate self-treatment.
- Symptoms are severe.
- The problem affects a large area of the body.

Children under age 2 who have skin rashes should be treated by a physician.

Treatment for Dermatitis, Eczema, and Dry Skin

Dermatitis causes the skin to become dry; thus a sound approach to self-treatment is to restore moisture to the area. However, frequent bathing and use of soap can increase dryness and make the problem worse. Some experts suggest bathing less frequently (every other day, for example) and using sponge baths with lukewarm water. In the winter, when dry skin is at its worse, wash only the genital area, the underarms, and the feet: Skip the rest except perhaps once or twice weekly.

On the other hand, it is often necessary to promote dryness in areas where the dermatitis produces oozing sores. One method is to apply a soft cloth soaked in tap water to the area for 20 minutes, 4 to 6 times a day, then gently pat the area dry. If the area is not infected, you may want to apply topical hydrocortisone afterward to reduce inflammation. This corticosteroid is the only steroid product approved for treatment of dermatitis. Hydrocortisone has anti-inflammatory and antipruritic (anti-itch) properties and decreases inflammation, thus reducing redness, heat, pain, swelling, and itch. To be effective, a concentration of at least 1% should be used. Hydrocortisone ointment products are best for rehydrating the skin, but people with atopic dermatitis may do better using a cream, which is less likely to cause sweating in the affected area. Hydrocortisone topical products should never be used for self-medication longer than 7 days. If the condition worsens or persists, a physician should be consulted. Products that contain an astringent (drying agent) such as aluminum acetate also relieve dermatitis symptoms by reducing blood flow to the affected area, thus easing swelling and inflammation.

For contact dermatitis, the best approach is to figure out what substance is causing the problem and then avoid it whenever possible. Usually the problem clears up soon after contact with the irritant has stopped. If treatment is needed, skin moisturizing strategies plus use of a topical hydrocortisone can be tried.

Other products available for keeping skin moist include colloidal oatmeal or bath oil. Oil-based emollients (moisturizers) can be applied while the skin is still damp. Emollients work by preventing the escape of water already present inside skin cells. Another type of ingredient in OTC skin care products is a humectant, which actually increases the amount of water entering the cells by absorbing it from the atmosphere or from nearby skin tissue. More severe cases may require use of products containing skin-softening ingredients such as urea or lactic acid.

Itching may be relieved through the use of local anesthetics, topical antihistamines, or hydrocortisone. Do not use a topical antihistamine or anesthetic for more than a week without checking with your doctor. Some experts suggest taking an oral antihistamine as a way of relieving the itching associated with dermatitis, but this strategy is controversial. Sometimes, however, the itching is so severe that it can keep you awake at night. An oral antihistamine that causes drowsiness may help you sleep more soundly, even if it doesn't have any direct effect on improving the itch.

OTC Products for Dermatitis, Eczema, and Dry Skin

Dermatitis
- Hydrocortisone (0.5% to 1%)
- Astringents

Dry skin
- Emollients (e.g., lanolin)
- Humectants (e.g., glycerin, propylene glycol)
- Keratin-softening agents (e.g., urea, lactic acid)
- Petrolatum creams

Skin Infections

Skin infections can result when a pathogen (a microscopic disease-causing agent) invades the tissue and begins to reproduce. The cause of most common skin infections is most often bacterial or fungal; organisms such as viruses or parasites can also cause infection. Often, though, symptoms result because of the toxic products the pathogens release. When the body's immune system recognizes the presence of an invader, it sets off a complex chain of events in an effort to fight and destroy it. In many cases, the symptoms of an infectious disease (such as fever or inflammation) are actually signs that the body is at work eliminating the source of illness.

Bacterial infections: Bacteria are single-celled organisms that are found everywhere, including the surface of the body and in the lining of the intestines. Of the thousands of kinds of bacteria, most are harmless. But if certain germs, such as staphylococcus or streptococcus, penetrate the defensive layer of skin—through a cut or wound, for example—they can multiply quickly and produce an infection.

Fungal infections: A fungus is a single-celled organism that cannot manufacture its own food. A parasite, it must invade and live off other creatures to survive. Fungi like to grow in dark, moist regions, which is why they are so good at taking up residence at certain sites in the human body. Types of fungal infections are shown in the box. The infections known as *tinea versicolor, tinea capitis,* and *tinea corporis* are often called ringworm, but this name is misleading, since the cause is not a worm but a fungus. Yeast is also a form of fungus; yeast infections are a common problem for men, women, and children.

Common Fungal Infections

Name	Common Name(s)	Site(s)	Pathogen(s)
Candidiasis	Yeast infection, thrush	Genitals, armpits, under the breasts, mouth, and corners of the mouth	*Candida*
Tinea capitis	Ringworm of the scalp	Head	*Microsporum, Trichophyton*
Tinea corporis	Ringworm of the body	Various sites	*Microsporum, Trichophyton*
Tinea cruris	Jock itch	Groin, upper and inner thigh	*Epidermophyton, Trichophyton*
Tinea pedis	Athlete's foot	Between the toes; soles of the feet	Various
Tinea versicolor	Ringworm	Trunk, neck	*Pityrosporon*

Athlete's foot is the most common fungal skin infection in humans, affecting about 10% of the population (most of them male) at any one time. This condition causes itching that can range from mild to severe, as well as inflammation, cracking, oozing, stinging, odor, and loss of skin. The exact symptoms and location of the infection vary depending on the species of fungus involved. Athlete's foot is easily transmitted to other people who share bathrooms, swimming pool decks, or other places where an infected person has walked. The infection is more likely to take hold if the fungus can enter skin through a blister or other wound.

Jock itch is a similar problem, with a different location. This infection—also more common among men—arises in the folds of the genital area and spreads across the inside of the thighs and to the genitals. It causes redness, itching, and irritation.

Tinea corporis causes round, itchy patches with distinct borders in different locations of the body. Tinea capitis—more common among children—produces one or more round itchy areas on the scalp, sometimes causing loss of hair. Tinea versicolor gets its name because it produces patches of differently colored flaking skin on the trunk and the neck.

Candidiasis (yeast infection) is a common problem, especially among women, but can develop in anyone. The yeast invades the mucous membranes, such as those of the vagina or, less frequently, the mouth. Symptoms of vaginal yeast infection include a thick, white discharge from the vagina, itching, and, occasionally, burning discomfort while urinating. In men, especially those who are not circumcised, it can cause inflammation under the foreskin and on the head of the penis. It can also contribute to diaper rash in infants. (For more information on vaginal yeast infection, see chapter 10.)

Viral infections: Viruses are among the strangest entities on the planet—not quite plants, not quite animals, not quite even living. They are tiny chunks of protein with a maddeningly powerful ability to invade cells and hijack the nucleus to make new copies of themselves. Without a cell for their home, viruses can do nothing. Once they take over, however, they can cause all sorts of problems.

Warts are among the most common viral skin infections and are caused by the various kinds of human papilloma viruses. (For more information, see the section on corns, calluses, and warts in this chapter.)

Another common viral skin infection is caused by the herpes virus. Herpes simplex type 1 causes small groups of painful, burning vesicles (blisters)—also known as cold sores or fever blisters—to appear on the mucous membranes of the mouth, lips, or nose. Over the course of a week or 10 days, the blisters can grow, become inflamed, and develop pus. They often ooze or burst, forming a crust, and then disappear. Herpes simplex type 2 causes infections that most often arise on the genitals. Usually people with herpes feel itching or tingling at the site a few days before the lesions form.

Another form of herpes virus, varicella-zoster, causes chicken pox. Usually a disease of childhood, chicken pox produces small red spots on the skin and mucous membranes. The spots can develop into vesicles and pustules that become crusted over. Other symptoms include itching, fever, and general weakness. The same virus can be reactivated later in life to cause shingles, an extremely painful condition in which redness and vesicles erupt along the distribution of a nerve. The disease can cause itching, tenderness, and nerve pain that may persist for weeks.

Molluscum contagiosum, a viral infection of the skin and mucous membranes, produces scattered tumors (growths) that resemble pink or white pimples with a small central dimple, usually on the abdomen, inner thigh, or anal region. The disease can take up to 3 years to run its course.

Treatment of Skin Infections

The choice of treatment needs to target the specific cause of the infection. Generally, if bacteria are the culprits, antibiotics are called for; antifungals work against fungal infections (see box). Antibiotics that have a broad spectrum of activity are effective against a wide variety of bacteria. A chemical disinfectant or an agent such as chlorine or iodine can kill both bacteria and fungi. Antibiotics are discussed in more detail in the section on wounds later in this chapter.

Antifungal medications are effective both in relieving the symptoms of infection and in eliminating the fungus at the root of the problem. Certain of these products work better against some species than others. For example, tolnaftate is an effective treatment for tinea pedis, tinea cruis, and tinea corporis but it does not work against tinea versicolor or candidiasis. When selecting a product, talk to your doctor and pharmacist to make sure you choose the one that is most likely to work for your condition.

Antifungals come in various formulations, including ointments, liquid solutions, creams, powders, and aerosol sprays. As a rule, creams and liquids work best because they can more easily penetrate the cracks and crevices where fungi like to grow. Powders and aerosols do not usually get rubbed in sufficiently to do the best jobs, but since powders absorb moisture, they are good to use during the day on the feet or under the breasts. If you use an antifungal medication, first wash and dry the area thoroughly, then massage the medication in completely. To reduce the risk of spreading the infection, make sure to cover not just the affected area but nearby skin as well. In treating athlete's foot, for example, apply the antifungal to all the toes, the skin around the toenail, and the entire soles of both feet.

There are no nonprescription medications that directly treat viral infections. However, other products can sometimes provide effective relief of symptoms caused by viruses. As discussed elsewhere in this chapter, salicylic acid can promote healing of warts, although it does nothing to eradicate the virus that causes warts. People with chicken pox may take baths containing oatmeal or starch to promote drying of the vesicles. Calamine lotion and oral antihistamines may alleviate itching, and analgesics (such as acetaminophen) can be taken to reduce fever. In cases of shingles, it often helps to cover the affected area with a protective bandage. NSAIDs may reduce pain, but some people may need prescription pain relievers. Topical capsaicin may work to reduce pain along the nerve. Oral antihistamines can help control itching, while topical antibiotics and antifungals may treat or prevent infection. Use of sunscreens containing paraaminobenzoic acid (PABA) can prevent outbreaks of fever blisters triggered by sun exposure. If the blisters erupt, ice can reduce the swelling, while petrolatum can prevent cracking and bleeding. Using drying agents such as alcohol or topical corticosteroids is not a good idea; such products may actually encourage the virus to spread.

OTC Products for Skin Infections

Antibiotics
- Bacitracin
- Mupirocin
- Neomycin
- Polymyxin B sulfate
- Tetracycline combinations
- Chlortetracycline
- Oxytetracycline combinations

Antifungals
- Clioquinol
- Clotrimazole
- Haloprogin
- Miconazole
- Povidone-iodine
- Tolnaftate
- Undecylenates

Antivirals
- (None)

Insect Bites and Stings

Insects are 6-legged creatures; their 8-legged cousins, such as ticks and spiders, are technically classified as arachnids. For the sake of simplicity, we refer to all of these beings as insects.

These critters are small, but they can pack a wallop. Insects bite in order to suck blood and obtain a meal. The most notorious biting insects are mosquitoes. When they land, they cut through the skin with their jaws, insert a long strawlike organ, and begin to drink. The saliva from the insect's mouth contains a substance that keeps blood from clotting. This material and other components in the saliva trigger an allergic reaction, producing the redness, itching, and blisters or nodules that make mosquito bites so annoying.

Mosquitoes are not the only biting insects. Fleas are tiny wingless beasts that hop onto their hosts. Their bites also cause redness and itching. Bedbugs, which get their name because they strike at night, have barbed mouths. Their bites can be so severe they can cause bleeding at the site.

Lice are voracious 8-legged parasites that cling to hair and that bite their hosts several times a day. The 3 main kinds that infest humans are head lice, body lice, and pubic lice (crabs). Head lice, a common problem among children in schools and day care centers, are transmitted by direct contact or by sharing combs, towels, and clothing (see chapter 5). Nits (baby lice) literally glue themselves to the hair, so they can be very difficult to remove. Body lice live in the seams and folds of clothing, while pubic lice like to nestle into the pubic area, armpits, or other moist hairy areas.

Mites are tiny 8-legged animals that do not bite but instead burrow into the upper layer of skin, laying eggs and depositing feces, which produces inflammation and intense itching. The itching can irritate the skin and lead to bacterial infections. Infection from a mite called *Sarcoptes scabiei* is known as scabies.

Ticks, another form of parasite, have teeth that curve backward, which can make them very difficult to dislodge. Once in place, the tick sucks blood and swells up like a balloon. When full, it lets go and drops off to digest its meal.

The pain, itching, scratching, and irritation caused by hungry insects are usually minor annoyances. Of greater concern is the fact that many insects harbor bacteria or parasites that can spread other much more serious diseases when they enter the bloodstream of another animal. Mosquitoes, for example, carry malaria. Fleas can spread the bubonic plague, and the deer tick carries the bacterium that causes Lyme disease, which produces a rash and flulike symptoms, including fever, headache, fatigue, and muscle and joint pain.

Stinging insects include bees, wasps, and certain kinds of ants. These animals sting only as an act of self-defense. The venom they inject during a sting can be very powerful.

Honeybees have stingers with barbed edges. When they poke the stinger into the skin, poison flows from a gland inside their bodies. When the bee flies away, the barb stays attached to the skin, and the poison sac is ripped out of the bee's body. The bee dies, but the sac continues to pump venom into the victim for another 2 or 3 minutes. Wasps have smooth stingers that do not remain in the wound; they can sting their victims many times. Fire ants, which in recent years have invaded the southwestern U.S., bite their victims so they can hold on while stinging repeatedly. Their stings cause intense burning, itching, blistering, and tissue damage.

Some people are more sensitive to insect bites and stings than others. Almost everyone develops redness, itching, and raised patches or wheals (bumps). Usually these symptoms arise immediately and fade away in a few hours, but sometimes they can take a few days to develop and can last for weeks. Scratching the area can make the problem worse by spreading the inflammatory material or by promoting secondary infections. Where the bite occurs on the body can also make a difference. For example, bites on the legs and ankles tend to be more severe, and stings on the head or neck are more dangerous than those on the arms or legs. Stings that inject poison directly into a blood vessel can cause systemic (whole-body) reactions. After being stung, some individuals develop fever or general body aches and pains. People who are severely allergic to the poison can die from a single bee sting. This is known as anaphylactic shock. More people die each year due to bites or stings from insects than from all other poisonous animals.

Seek medical attention if any of the following applies to you

- Shortness of breath
- Abdominal cramps
- Dizziness
- Profuse sweating
- Nausea

People who know they are hypersensitive to insect bites should ask a physician about undergoing desensitization therapy to reduce the risk of serious allergic reactions. For emergency treatment, they should also carry an epinephrine auto-injector (e.g., Epipen), available by prescription only.

Treatment for Insect Bites and Stings

Products available to treat insect bites contain various ingredients designed to ease pain, reduce itching, and relieve inflammation. Medications that relieve symptoms fall into 3 groups.

Counterirritants are substances that cause the skin to produce other sensations, such as warmth or cooling, which help mask the pain of the injury and reduce itching or irritation. Examples include camphor, menthol, and methyl salicylate.

Local anesthetics numb pain by blocking nerve signals. The most commonly available local anesthetics are benzocaine, dibucaine, and phenol. These products should be applied no more than 4 times a day and for no more than 5 consecutive days.

Antipruritics are chemicals that reduce the itching that results from inflammation. Topical antihistamines such as diphenhydramine are absorbed through the skin. Hydrocortisone, a topical corticosteroid, prevents or decreases swelling, redness, and tenderness, which in turn reduces itching. This product should be applied up to 4 times a day. However, hydrocortisone should not be used for treatment of scabies because it can make the problem worse.

Like burn medications, some treatments also contain skin protectants. Examples include aluminum acetate, glycerin, and zinc oxide. These substances help dry skin and absorb fluid from irritated areas.

Antibacterials prevent or treat infection that may arise when people scratch the affected area and expose the wound to bacteria.

Some people use a paste made of dissolved aspirin applied directly to the insect sting. This method may reduce the formation of wheals, which in turn relieves itching and irritation. There are other steps you can take to reduce the effect of an insect bite (see box).

Lice can be treated with a pediculicide (antilice medicattion) such as 1% permethrin cream rinse. This medication kills not just the adult creature, but also the eggs it lays. In most cases, a single application does the trick; some people may require a second dose a week later. Another option is to use a combination product containing pyrethrins and piperonyl butoxide; these are available as gels, liquids, and shampoos.

Are Insect Bites Bugging You?

To get maximum relief from insect bites, try the following strategies:

- Do not wear rough or irritating clothing, especially clothes made of wool.
- Avoid strong soaps with perfumes or dyes and harsh detergents.
- Apply bandages or other protection to the affected area after bathing.
- Soak the area in cool water for 10 to 20 minutes.
- Resist the temptation to scratch.

OTC Products for Insect Bites and Stings

Counterirritants
- Camphor
- Menthol
- Methyl salicylate

Local anesthetics
- Benzocaine
- Dibucaine
- Phenol

Antipruritics
- Antihistamines (e.g., diphenhydramine)
- Hydrocortisone

Protectants
- Aluminum acetate
- Glycerin
- Hamamelis water (witch hazel)
- Zinc oxide

Antibacterials
- Benzalkonium chloride
- Benzethonium chloride

Pediculicides
- Permethrin
- Pyrethrins + piperonyl butoxide
- Gamma benzene hexachloride

Poison Ivy, Oak, and Sumac

Anyone who spent time as a Girl Scout or Boy Scout remembers the old expression: "Leaves of 3, let it be." That simple slogan reminds hikers and campers to stay away from poison ivy, a shrub or vine with 3-leafed branches, and its cousins, poison oak and poison sumac. The leaves of these plants contain a toxic resin. If damaged or torn leaves come into contact with human skin, the resin can produce a severe allergic reaction.

Poison ivy is one of the most common forms of contact dermatitis, causing up to 50 million cases a year in the U.S. alone. The resin of this plant is persistent. It can stick to another surface, such a shoe or an animal's fur. If you touch that surface—even weeks or months later—you can still develop the rash. As many campers and firefighters have discovered to their dismay, inhaling smoke from burning poison ivy can cause severe irritation of the lungs and nasal passage.

Symptoms can develop wherever the resin touches the skin, but the hands, ankles, legs, face, and neck are the most common sites. It is possible to spread the rash from place to place; one person can even pass it on to another if the resin has not been washed off. The first symptoms are usually redness, itching, and burning, followed by raised lesions and the appearance of fluid-filled vesicles (these are not contagious). The affected area becomes hot and swollen; oozing develops, followed by drying and crusting. Breaks in the skin increase the risk of secondary bacterial infection. Without treatment, poison ivy dermatitis can persist for up to 2 or 3 weeks, depending on how intense the initial exposure was.

The Boy Scout motto "Be prepared" is good advice for dealing with poison ivy, oak, or sumac. People who work or play outdoors should be prepared to recognize—and avoid—poisonous plants. Wearing protective clothing and gloves is a good idea; after an outing, clothes should be laundered in hot water, and you should immediately shower and carefully wash all over to remove any resin. Herbicides can be used to kill poison ivy, oak, or sumac in the garden; if the plant is removed by hand, it should be buried, not burned. Although many OTC products are available that claim to prevent poison ivy, oak, or sumac infection, most of these have not proved to be of much value.

Seek medical attention if any of the following applies to you

- Severe, widespread lesions
- Swelling
- Lesions near the eye

Treatment for Poison Ivy, Oak, or Sumac

Treatment of mild poison ivy is much the same as for other forms of contact dermatitis or minor skin conditions (see box). Use of astringents such as calamine lotion or zinc oxide can relieve pain and itching and reduce the development of vesicles. Soaking the area in an aluminum acetate solution can be soothing. Local anesthetics, topical antihistamines, and topical hydrocortisone also reduce pain and itching. Cream or lotion formulations are better for this purpose than ointments, which can prevent drying of vesicles (see box).

More severe cases may require other steps. Moisturizing creams (with a neutral pH) may help prevent crusting, scaling, and thickening of the affected area. Wet dressings can be applied to lesions on the face; cold compresses with dilute boric acid solution can be applied to lesions on the eyelids. Lukewarm baths with oatmeal can be soothing.

Severe cases may require treatment with prescription medications, including corticosteroids or other anti-inflammatory drugs. Oral antihistamines may help reduce itching.

For more information on products used in treating poison ivy, see the sections on dermatitis and insect bites earlier in this chapter.

OTC Products for Poison Ivy, Oak, and Sumac

Astringents
- Calamine lotion
- Zinc oxide
- Aluminum acetate solution

Local anesthetics
- Benzocaine
- Pramoxine

Antipruritics
- Topical antihistamines
- Topical hydrocortisone
- Counterirritants

Other products
- Moisturizing cream
- Oatmeal baths

Psoriasis

Psoriasis is a disease that causes the body to produce new skin cells at a much faster rate then usual while shedding old cells at a normal rate. This results in inflamed, red patches covered with dry, flaking, silvery scales. If the scales are removed, they usually develop a characteristic small spot of bleeding. Itching is not always a symptom of the disease. About 2 of every 100 people develop psoriasis, usually between the ages of 10 and 30.

Most patches of psoriasis erupt on the scalp, ears, lower back, and genital region, or over bony areas such as the knees and elbows. Scales can also develop over areas where the skin has been damaged, such as at vaccination sites or over surgical scars. In mild cases, the affected regions are small and localized, but sometimes the condition can affect large areas of the body.

Psoriasis is usually episodic; that is, attacks can develop fairly quickly and then fade away for a period of time. Sometimes, though, the scales develop and remain for months or years. Some attacks are more severe than others. People with psoriasis often develop a type of arthritis that causes painful swelling and stiffness. In moderate to severe cases, psoriasis can be disfiguring, leading to discomfort and social embarrassment.

Scientists do not know what causes psoriasis. It is not contagious, but it can be hereditary; about 3 of every 10 people with psoriasis have a family history of the disease. Attacks of psoriasis can be triggered by a number of factors, including infections or other illnesses, emotional stress, cold weather, or injury to the skin. Use of certain medications, including beta blockers and lithium, can trigger episodes.

Seek medical attention if any of the following applies to you

- Moderate to severe psoriasis
- Scales affecting a large portion of the body
- Episodes of psoriasis that do not improve after 1 to 2 weeks of self-treatment

Treatment for Psoriasis

There is no known cure for psoriasis, but there are several effective approaches that provide symptomatic relief. If skin is dry and itchy, emollients and soothing baths can help. After a bath, when the skin is soft, scales can be removed by gently rubbing the area with a soft cloth. Keratolytics (drugs that help remove surface layers of skin) may also be used if thick scales are present. The most common forms of keratolytic products are salicylic acid and sulfur. The scaly area should be soaked in warm water for 10 to 20 minutes, then the drugs should be applied and the area covered with a dressing to promote absorption. Keratolytics help loosen cells, and sulfur stimulates increased sloughing of the cells. (For more information, see the section on corns, calluses, bunions, and warts earlier in this chapter; also see chapter 8.)

Coal tar, another ingredient used as a nonprescription ingredient for treatment of psoriasis, is available in creams, ointments, pastes, lotions, bath oils, shampoos, soaps, and gels. The reason for all these different formulations is that coal tar has some unpleasant properties, including its color, odor, and tendency to leave stains. The many product formulations are attempts to get around these problems. The gel form is easy to apply, and, because it is not greasy, almost colorless, and nonstaining, it is usually cosmetically acceptable. It tends to be drying, however, so you may want to use an emollient at the same time. Some people develop dermatitis as a reaction to using coal tar. Use of topical hydrocortisone can reduce this risk.

Some people with psoriasis find relief from exposure to UV radiation, either from the sun or in measured doses in tanning salons, especially in combination with the use of coal tar. UV radiation poses some risks, including an increased risk of skin cancer. Talk to your doctor before undergoing UV treatment for psoriasis.

OTC Products for Psoriasis

Emollients
Lubricating bath products
Keratolytics
Coal tar
Topical hydrocortisone

Wounds

The skin is the shield that protects the body from the outside world. Because the skin comes into contact with so many objects during the course of the day, it is naturally vulnerable to nicks, cuts, burns, scrapes, or other minor wounds. Fortunately, our skin is usually remarkably quick to heal on its own. Clots form to stop the flow of blood; scabs develop to protect the area; and in a short while the skin grows back together, ready to fend off another assault.

Wounds that heal quickly (within a few days or weeks) are known as acute wounds. Types of acute wounds include abrasions (scrapes), punctures, or lacerations (cuts). Acute wounds require different treatment approaches than chronic wounds, which persist for longer periods or recur frequently. Pressure or rubbing can cause chronic wounds such as bed sores or bunions (see the section on corns, calluses, bunions, and warts earlier in this chapter). Some chronic wounds are the result of seepage from weak blood vessels just below the skin.

Even tiny wounds can represent a serious breach in the body's defense against infection. It doesn't take a very large opening to allow microscopic creatures such as bacteria or viruses to penetrate and take up residence. For this reason, it is important to use common sense in helping the wound heal as quickly and as completely as possible.

Seek medical attention if any of the following applies to you

- The wound is slow to heal or gets worse.
- Self-treatment doesn't work.
- Infection develops.
- Fever or malaise or both occur.
- The infection occurs secondary to another skin condition (such as dermatitis).
- You haven't had a tetanus shot in the last 10 years (5 years for deep, dirty wounds).
- The area surrounding the wound becomes red and hot, and the size of the red area rapidly increases.
- The wounds are deep or extensive or require sutures (closing).

Treatment for Wounds

For most of this century, people believed that the best way to promote wound healing was to keep the site exposed to the air. Today, experts think a better strategy is to keep the wound covered and moist while using appropriate medications that clean the site, prevent infection (triple-antibiotic ointment is an excellent choice), and treat the symptoms.

Antiseptics are chemicals that stop infection from spreading. Some antiseptics kill microorganisms, but many simply slow down their growth. The main purpose of an antiseptic is to clean the undamaged surface skin around the edge of a wound so that any germs lurking nearby won't reach the exposed area. However, antiseptics should be used sparingly because they can also interfere with the cells that manage the body's own healing process. The 2 main types of antiseptics available over the counter are hand cleansers and first aid products for treatment of minor scrapes, cuts, and burns. There are dozens of antiseptic products available in many formulations, but most of these contain some combination of the same few ingredients (see box).

Antiseptics

Alcohol (ethanol)
Isopropyl alcohol
Iodine topical solution
Iodine tincture
Povidone-iodine
Hydrogen peroxide
Phenol
Hexylresorcinol
Ammonium compounds

Antibiotics are drugs that can arrest or kill microorganisms. Some antibiotics work only against specific germs, but others can destroy many kinds of bacteria and fungi. The OTC antibiotics available are intended as first aid for use on the skin only. Oral antibiotics for internal diseases such as bronchitis require a prescription.

Once the wound is clean and the infection is in check, the wound should be covered with a bandage as soon as possible. As mentioned, the modern strategy for covering a wound is to use a dressing that protects the site against friction from irritants while retaining moisture and reducing—but not eliminating—contact with the air. This method promotes healing and reduces the risk of scarring. There are many types of dressings available, ranging from sprays and gels to medicated pads.

OTC Products for Wounds

- Antiseptics
- Antibiotics
  - Bacitracin
  - Mupirocin
  - Neomycin
  - Polymyxin B sulfate
  - Tetracycline
  - Chlortetracycline
  - Oxytetracycline combinations
- Dressings
  - Sprays
  - Gels
  - Adhesive bandages
  - Transparent films
  - Occlusive wafers
  - Calcium alginates
  - Polyurethane foams
  - Moistened gauze

Acne Products

BRAND NAME	ANTIACNE INGREDIENTS				
	benzoyl peroxide	sulfur	resorcinol	salicylic acid	other
Acne-5	5%				
Acne-10	10%				
Acno		3%		2%	
Acnomel		8%	2%		
Acnotex		8%	2%		
AMBI 10 Acne Medication	10%				
AMBI 10 Acne Pads				2%	
Aveeno Medicated Cleanser				2%	
Benoxyl 5	5%				
Benoxyl 10	10%				
Betadine Skin Cleanser					povidone-iodine 7.5%
Clean & Clear Invisible Blemish Treatment				2%	
Clean & Clear Invisible Blemish Treatment, Sensitive Skin				0.5%	
Clean & Clear Oil Controlling Astringent				2%	
Clean & Clear Oil Controlling Astringent, Sensitive Skin				0.5%	
Clean & Clear Persa-Gel Extra Strength	5%				
Clean & Clear Persa-Gel Maximum Strength	10%				
Clear By Design	2.5%				
Clearasil Clearstick Maximum Strength				2%	
Clearasil Clearstick Regular Strength				1.25%	
Clearasil Clearstick Sensitive Skin				2%	
Clearasil Double Textured Maximum Strength				2%	
Clearasil Double Textured Regular Strength				2%	
Clearasil Maximum Strength	10%				
Clearasil Medicated Deep Cleanser				0.5%	

Drytex			2%	
ExACT Adult Medication	2.5%			
ExACT Pore Treatment			2%	
ExACT Vanishing	5%			
Fostex 10% BPO	10%			
Fostex 10% BPO Wash	10%			
Fostex Medicated			2%	
Fostex Medicated Cleansing			2%	
Fostril		2%		
Ionax Astringent			x	
Liquimat		4%		
Loroxide	5.5%			
Neutrogena Acne	5%			
Neutrogena Clear Pore Treatment			2%	
Neutrogena Oil-Free Wash			2%	
Noxzema 2 in 1 Maximum Strength			2%	
Noxzema 2 in 1 Regular Strength			0.5%	
Noxzema Oily Astringent			2%	
On-the-Spot	2.5%			
Oxy Deep Cleansing, Maximum Strength			2%	
Oxy Deep Cleansing, Regular Strength			0.5%	
Oxy Deep Cleansing, Sensitive Skin			0.5%	
Oxy Medicated Cleanser			0.5%	
Oxy Medicated Face Wash	10%			
Oxy Medicated Soap				triclosan 1.0%
Oxy Moisturizing Face Wash				triclosan 0.6%
Oxy Night Watch Maximum Strength			2%	
Oxy Sensitive Skin, Vanishing	2.5%			

BRAND NAME	ANTIACNE INGREDIENTS				
	benzoyl peroxide	sulfur	resorcinol	salicylic acid	other
Oxy-10 Maximum Strength	10%				
Pan Oxyl 5	5%				
Pan Oxyl 10	10%				
Pernox		2%		1.5%	
Propa pH Acne Medication				2%	
Propa pH Astringent Cleanser				0.5%	
Propa pH Astringent Cleanser Maximum Strength				2%	
Propa pH Foaming Face Wash				2%	
Propa pH Peel-Off				2%	
Propa pH Perfectly Clear Cleansing, Oily Skin				0.6%	
Propa pH Perfectly Clear Cleansing, Sensitive Skin				0.5%	
Rezamid Acne Lotion		5%	2%		
SalAc Cleanser				2%	
SAStid Soap		10%			
Seales Lotion-Modified		6.4%			
Sebasorb				2%	
Stri-Dex Clear				2%	
Stri-Dex Maximum Strength				2%	
Stri-Dex Regular Strength				0.5%	
Stri-Dex Sensitive Skin				0.5%	
Stri-Dex Super Scrub				2%	
Sulforcin		5%	2%		
Sulmasque		6.4%			
Sulpho-Lac		5%			
Sulpho-Lac Soap		5%			
Sulray Acne Treatment		3%			

Sulray Facial Cleanser		3%	
Sulray Soap		5%	
Therac		10%	2.35%
Thylox Acne Treatment Soap		3%	
Vanoxide	5%		

Burn and Sunburn Products

BRAND NAME	ANESTHETIC						ANTIMICROBIAL								OTHER
	benzocaine	benzyl alcohol	butamben picrate	dibucaine	lidocaine	pramoxine	8-hydroxyquinoline	benzalkonium chloride	benzethonium chloride	cetylpyridinium chloride	chloroxylenol	oxyquinoline	phenol	resorcinol	
A & D Ointment															vitamin A & D
ActiBath Soak Oatmeal Treatment															oatmeal
Aerocaine	13.6%								0.5%						
Aerotherm	13.6%								0.5%						
Americaine First Aid	20%								0.1%						
Anti-Itch						1%			x						
Aveeno Bath Treatment Moisturizing Formula															oatmeal
Aveeno Bath Treatment Soothing Formula															oatmeal
Bactine First Aid					2.5%			0.13%							
Banana Boat Sooth-A-Caine					x										

BRAND NAME	ANESTHETIC						ANTIMICROBIAL								OTHER
	benzo-caine	benzyl alcohol	butam-ben picrate	dibu-caine	lido-caine	pram-oxine	8-hydroxy-quinoline	benzal-konium chloride	benze-thonium chloride	cetylpyri-dinium chloride	chlor-oxylenol	oxy-quin-oline	phenol	resor-cinol	
Bicozene External Analgesic Creme	6%													1.67%	
Boil Ease	5%												x		
Burnamycin					0.5%										
Burn-O-Jel					0.5%										menthol
Burntame	20%						x								
Cala-gel Clearly Calamine									15%						
Delazinc															zinc oxide 25%
Dermacoat	x										x				
Dermoplast	20%														menthol 0.5%
Dibucaine				1%											
DML Lotion		x													
Family Medic					2.5%			0.13%							
Family Medic Afterburn					2.5%										
First Aid Cream										x					
First Aid Medicated Powder															zinc oxide
Foille Medicated First Aid (aerosol)	5%	x									0.6%	x			
Foille Medicated First Aid (ointment)	5%	x									0.1%	x			
Foille Plus	5%								0.15%						

Foille Plus Medicated First Aid	5%						0.4%	
Gold Bond Medicated Anti-Itch			x					
Itch-X		10%		1%				
Lagol	5%							
Lanacane	20%					0.1%		
Medicated First Aid Burn	5%						0.4%	
Medi-Quik First Aid			2%		0.13%			
Neosporin Plus Maximum Strength (cream)			40mg/g					
Neosporin Plus Maximum Strength (ointment)			40mg/g					
No More Burn			2.3%			0.13%		
No More Ouchies			2.3%			0.13%		
Outgro Pain Relieving	20%							
Pramegel		x		1%				
Prax				1%				
Solarcaine Aloe Extra Burn Relief			0.5%					
Solarcaine Medicated First Aid Spray	20%							
Unguentine								1%
Unguentine Plus			2%					0.5%
Vaseline Medicated Anti-Bacterial Petroleum Jelly							0.53%	x

Corns, Calluses, Warts

BRAND NAME	SALICYLIC ACID	OTHER INGREDIENTS		
		alcohol	ether	other analgesic
Clear Away One Step Wart Remover	40%			
Clear Away Plantar Wart Remover	40%			
Compound W Wart Remover	17%	67.5%		camphor
Corn Fix	12%	21.2%	63.5%	camphor
Dr. Scholl's Advanced Pain Relief Callus Removers	40%	33%	65.5%	
Dr. Scholl's Advanced Pain Relief Corn Removers	40%			
Dr. Scholl's Callus Removers (disc)	40%			
Dr. Scholl's Corn Removers (disc)	40%			
Dr. Scholl's Corn/Callus Remover (liquid)	12.6%	18%	55%	
Dr. Scholl's Moisturizing Corn Remover Kit	40%			
Dr. Scholl's One Step Callus Remover (disk)	40%			
Dr. Scholl's One Step Corn Removers (strip)	40%			
Dr. Scholl's Wart Remover Kit	17%	17%	52%	
DuoFilm Liquid Wart Remover	17%	15.8%	42.6%	
DuoFilm Patch System Wart Removers	40%			
DuoPlant Plantar Wart Remover	17%	57.6%	16.42%	
Freezone Corn and Callus Remover	13.6%	20.5%	64.8%	
Fung-O	17%			acetone, camphor, menthol
Gordofilm	16.7%			
Mosco Corn & Callus Remover	17%	23%		
Mosco-Cain		alcohol 40-60%		benzocaine 20%
Occlusal HP	17%	x	x	
OFF-Ezy Corn and Callus Remover Kit	17%			
OFF-Ezy Wart Remover	17%			

Sal-Acid Wart Remover	40%		
Salactic Film	17%		
Sal-Plant	17%		
Trans-Ver-Sal 12mm "Adult Patch"	15%		
Trans-Ver-Sal 20mm "PlantarPatch"	15%		
Trans-Ver-Sal 6mm "PediaPatch"	15%		
Wart Fix	12%	33%	65.5%
Wart-Off	17%	X	X

Dermatitis Products

BRAND NAME	STEROID	ASTRINGENT						
	hydro-cortisone	alcohol	aluminum sulfate	calcium acetate	cetearyl alcohol	cetyl alcohol	hydrocortisone alcohol	stearyl alcohol
Aquanil HC	1%					X		X
Bactine Hydrocortisone 1%	1%	X	X		X		X	
Caldecort	1%							
Cortaid FastStick	1%	55%						
Cortaid Maximum Strength (cream)	1%					X		
Cortaid Maximum Strength (ointment)	1%							
Cortaid Maximum Strength (spray)	1%	55%						
Cortaid Sensitive Skin Formula	0.5%							
Corticaine	0.5%							
Cortizone-10 (cream)	1%		X	X				

BRAND NAME	STEROID	ASTRINGENT						
	hydro-cortisone	alcohol	aluminum sulfate	calcium acetate	cetearyl alcohol	cetyl alcohol	hydrocortisone alcohol	stearyl alcohol
Cortizone-10 (ointment)	1%							
Cortizone-10 Scalp Itch	1%							
Cortizone-5 (cream)	0.5%		x	x				
Cortizone-5 (ointment)	0.5%							
Dermarest DriCort	1%							
DermiCort	0.5%							
Dermtex	1%							
Dermtex HC	1%							
Hytone	1%					x		
Kericort 10	1%					x		x
Lanacort	0.5%							
Lanacort 10	1%							
Neutrogena T/Scalp Anti-Pruritic	1%							
No More Itchies	1%	45%						
Preparation H Hydrocortisone 1% Anti-Itch	1%							
Procort	1%							
Scalp Relief Medicine	1%							
Scalpicin Anti-Itch	1%							
Scalpmycin	1%	x						

First Aid Skin Care

BRAND NAME	ANTIBIOTIC INGREDIENTS				
	bacitracin	bacitracin zinc	neomycin sulfate	polymyxin B sulfate	Lidocaine HCL
Baciguent	500 IU/g				
Betadine First Aid Antibiotics + Moisturizer		500 IU/g		10000 IU/g	
Campho-phenique Triple Antibiotic		500 IU/g	5mg/g	10000 IU/g	40mg/g
Clomycin	500 IU/g		3.5mg/g	5000 IU/g	40mg/g
Lanabiotic	500 IU/g		5mg/g	10000 IU/g	
Medi-Quik Triple Antibiotic	500 IU/g		3.5mg/g	5000 IU/g	
Myciquent			3.5mg/g		
Mycitracin		500 IU/g	5mg	10000 IU/g	40mg/g
Mycitracin Plus		500 IU/g	3.5mg/g	10000 IU/g	
Neosporin		400 IU/g	3.5mg/g	5000 IU/g	
Neosporin Plus Maximum Strength (cream)			3.5mg/g	10000 IU/g	40mg/g
Neosporin Plus Maximum Strength (ointment)		500 IU/g	3.5mg/g	10000 IU/g	40mg/g
Polysporin		500 IU/g		10000 IU/g	
Tribiotic Plus	600 IU/g		3.85mg/g	5500 IU/g	40mg/g

Antiseptic Ingredients

KEY:
8-hy = 8-hydroxyquinoline
bza = benzalkonium chloride
bze = benzethonium chloride
bis = bismuth formic iodide
cam = camphor
cet = cetylpyridinium chloride
chl = chlorhexidine gluconate
hex = hexylresorcinol
hyd = hydrogen peroxide
iod = iodine
mer = merbromin
pep = oil of peppermint
phen = phenol
pov = povidone-iodone
sda = SD alcohol
sdi = sodium diacetate
shy = sodium hypochlorite
sio = sodium iodide
thi = thimerosal

The products in italics also contain an analgesic ingredient listed below.

BRAND NAME	ANTISEPTIC INGREDIENTS																	
	8-hy	bza	bze	bis	cam	cet	chl	hex	hyd	iod	mer	pep	phe	pov	sda	sdi	shy	sio	thi
Aerocaine			0.5%																
B.F.I.				16%															
Bactine		0.13%																	
Benzalkonium Chloride		17%		16%															
Buro-Sol Antiseptic			4.4%													0.23%			
Campho-phenique Pain Relieving Antiseptic					10.8%								4.7%						
Castellani Paint, Modified													1.5%		x				
Dakins 1/2 Strength																	0.25%		
Dakins Full Strength																	0.5%		
Dr. Tichenor's Antiseptic												x			70%				
Efodine											1%								
First Aid Cream						x													
Hibiclens							4%												
Hibiclens Sponge Brush							4%												
Hibiclens Towelette							0.5%												
Iodine Topical										2%								2.5%	

Mercurochrome			2%		
Mersol					0.1%
New Skin Liquid Bandage	1%				
Oxyzal Wet Dressing		0.05%			
Unguentine				1%	
Unguentine Plus				0.5%	

Other (Analgesic) Ingredients

BRAND NAME	OTHER (ANALGESIC)
Aerocaine	benzocaine 13.6%
Bactine	lidocaine HCl 2.5%
Unguentine	eucalyptus oil
Unguentine Plus	lidocaine HCl 2%

Antifungal Products

BRAND NAME	ANTIFUNGAL INGREDIENT									
	8-hydroxy-quinoline	calcium undecy-lenate	chlor-oxylenol	clotri-mazole	miconazole nitrate	povidone-iodine	tolnaftate	undecy-lenate	undecy-lenic acid	zinc undecy-lenate
Aerodine						x				
Aftate							1%			
Aftate Jock Itch							1%			
Aftate Spray Liquid							1%			

BRAND NAME	ANTIFUNGAL INGREDIENT									
	8-hydroxy-quinoline	calcium undecy-lenate	chlor-oxylenol	clotri-mazole	miconazole nitrate	povidone-iodine	tolnaftate	undecy-lenate	undecy-lenic acid	zinc undecy-lenate
Betadine						10%				
Betadine First Aid						5%				
Blis-To-Sol (liquid)							1%			
Blis-To-Sol (powder)										12%
Breezee Mist					2%					
Care-Creme Cream			0.8%							
Cruex Antifungal (aerosol)								19%		
Cruex Antifungal (cream)								20%		
Cruex Antifungal Squeeze Powder		10%								
Desenex AF (aerosol)					2%					
Desenex AF (cream)				1%						
Desenex AF Spray Liquid					2%					
Desenex Antifungal (aerosol)								25%		
Desenex Antifungal (cream, ointment)								25%		
Desenex Antifungal (powder)								25%		
Desenex Antifungal Spray Liquid							1%			
FungiCure (gel)							1%			
FungiCure (liquid)									10%	
Fungoid Tincture					2%					
Genaspor							1%			
Isodine Antiseptic						10%				
Lagol	0.0377%									
Lotrimin AF (aerosol)					2%					
Lotrimin AF (cream)				1%						

Lotrimin AF (powder)			2%					
Lotrimin AF (solution)		1%						
Lotrimin AF Jock Itch (aerosol)			2%					
Lotrimin AF Jock Itch (lotion)		1%						
Lotrimin AF Spray Liquid			2%					
Micatin (aerosol)			2%					
Micatin (cream, powder)			2%					
Micatin Liquid			2%					
Minidyne				10%				
NP-27 Cream					1%			
NP-27 Solution					1%			
NP-27 Spray Powder					1%			
Polydine				10%				
Tetterine			2%					
Tinactin (cream)					1%			
Tinactin (powder)					1%			
Tinactin (solution)					1%			
Tinactin Jock Itch					1%			
Tinactin Spray Liquid					1%			
Tinactin, Deodorant or Regular					1%			
Ting Antifungal					1%			
Ting Antifungal Spray Liquid					1%			
Undelenic (ointment)							x	x
Undelenic (tincture)							x	
Vaseline Medicated Anti-Bacterial Petroleum Jelly	0.53%							
Zeasorb-AF			2%					

Athlete's Foot Products

BRAND NAME	ANTIFUNGAL INGREDIENTS					
	benzioc acid	calcium undecylenate	chlorthymol	miconazole nitrate	resorcinol	tolnaftate
Absorbine Jr. Antifungal Foot (aerosol)				2%		
Absorbine Jr. Antifungal Foot (cream, powder)						1%
Absorbine Jr. Antifungal Foot Spray Liquid						1%
Athlete's Foot Antifungal				2%		
Desenex Foot & Sneaker Deodorant Plus		10%				
Dr. Scholl's Athlete's Foot (aerosol)						1%
Dr. Scholl's Athlete's Foot (powder)						1%
Dr. Scholl's Athlete's Foot Spray Liquid						1%
Johnson's Odor-Eaters						1%
Odor-Eaters Antifungal						1%
Rid-Itch	1%		1%		1%	

Insect Bites and Stings

BRAND NAME	ANESTHETICS, ANTIPRURITICS, and COUNTERIRRITANTS											
	alum-inum	am-monia	benzo-caine	benzyl alcohol	cam-phor	dibu-caine	diphenhy-dramine	lido-caine	menthol	methylsali-cylate	oatmeal	pramox-ine	resor-cinol
ActiBath Soak Oatmeal Treatment											20%		
Aerocaine			13.6%										
After-Bite		3.6%											
Americaine First Aid			20%										
Americaine Topical Anesthetic			20%										
Anti-Itch												1%	

Aveeno Anti-Itch				0.3%						x	1%	
Bactine Antiseptic/Anesthetic First Aid							2.5%					
Bicozene External Analgesic Creme		6%										1.67%
Blue Star				x								
Burnamycin							5%					
Buro-Sol Antiseptic	46.8%											
Caladryl											1%	
Caladryl Clear											1%	
Cala-gel Clearly Calamine						1.8%		0.11%				
Chiggerex		2%										
Chigger-Tox		2.1%										
Dermamycin (cream)						1%		1%				
Dermamycin (spray)						2%						
Dermarest						2%						
Dermarest Plus						2%		1%				
Dermoplast		20%										
Dermtex								0.5%				
Dermtex HC								1%				
Di-Delamine Double Antihistamine								0.1%				
Domeboro	x											
Gold Bond Medicated								x	x			
Gold Bond Medicated Anti-Itch							x	x				
HC-DermaPax			1%			0.5%						
Itch-X			10%								1%	
Lanacort 10												
Nupercainal (cream)					0.5%							
Nupercainal (ointment					1%							

BRAND NAME	ANESTHETICS, ANTIPRURITICS, and COUNTERIRRITANTS												
	alum-inum	am-monia	benzo-caine	benzyl alcohol	cam-phor	dibu-caine	diphenhy-dramine	lido-caine	menthol	methylsali-cylate	oatmeal	pramox-ine	resor-cinol
Outgro Pain Relieving			20%										
Pedi-Boro Soak Paks	x												
Pramegel				x					0.5%			1%	
Rhuli (gel)				2%	0.3%				0.3%				
Rhuli (spray)			5%	x	0.7%								
Rhuli Bite-Aid			10%	10%									
Sarna					0.5%				0.5%				
Solarcaine Medicated First Aid			20%										
Sting-Eze			x		x								

Hydrocortisone

BRAND NAME	HYDROCORTISONE
Bactine Hydrocortisone 1%	1%
Cortaid FastStick	1%
Cortaid Maximum Strength	1%
Cortaid Sensitive Skin Formula	0.5%
Dermarest DriCort	1%
Dermtex	1%
Dermtex HC	1%
HC-Dermapax	0.5%
Kericort 10	1%
Lanacort 10	1%
Preparation H Hydrocortisone 1% Anti-Itch	1%

Poison Ivy, Oak, and Sumac Relief

BRAND NAME	ANALGESIC/ANTIPRURITIC									
	benzocaine	benzyl alcohol	camphor	hydrocortisone	lidocaine	menthol	oatmeal	phenol	pramoxine HCl	resorcinol
ActiBath Soak Oatmeal Treatment							x			
Anti-Itch									1%	
Aveeno Anti-Itch			0.3%				x		1%	
Aveeno Bath Treatment Moisturizing Formula							43%			
Aveeno Bath Treatment Soothing Formula							100%			
Aveeno Moisturizing		x					1%			
Benadryl Itch Stopping Extra Strength (gel)			x							
Benadryl Itch Stopping Regular Strength (gel)			x							
Blue Star			x							
Caladryl (cream)									1%	
Caladryl (lotion)									1%	
Caladryl Clear									1%	
Cala-gel Clearly Calamine						0.11%				
Calamycin									1%	
Dermamycin (spray)						1%				
Dermapax		1%								
Dermarest Plus						1%				
Dermoplast	20%					0.5%				

BRAND NAME	ANALGESIC/ANTIPRURITIC									
	benzo-caine	benzyl alcohol	camphor	hydro-cortisone	lidocaine	menthol	oatmeal	phenol	pramoxine HCl	resorcinol
Dermtex						1%				
Di-Delamine						0.1%				
Gold Bond Medicated						x				
Gold Bond Medicated Anti-Itch					x	x				
HC-DermaPax		1%								
Itch-X		10%							1%	
Lanacane	20%									
Lanacane Creme	6%									
Nutra Soothe Oatmeal Bath							100%			
Ostiderm			x					x		
Ostiderm Roll-On			x					x		
Pramegel		x				0.5%			1%	
Resinol Medicated										2%
Rhuli (gel)		2%	0.3%			0.3%				
Rhuli (spray)	5%	x	0.7%							
Sarna			0.5%			0.5%				

Antihistamine

BRAND NAME	ANTIHISTAMINE		
	diphenhydramine	methyl salicylate	tripelennamine
Benadryl Itch Stopping Extra Strength (cream)	2%		
Benadryl Itch Stopping Extra Strength (gel)	2%		
Benadryl Itch Stopping Extra Strength (spray)	2%		
Benadryl Itch Stopping Extra Strength (stick)	2%		
Benadryl Itch Stopping Regular Strength (cream)	1%		
Benadryl Itch Stopping Regular Strength (gel)	1%		
Benadryl Itch Stopping Regular Strength (spray)	1%		
Cala-gel Clearly Calamine	1.8%		
Cala-gen Clear	1%		
Dermamycin (cream)	1%		
Dermamycin (spray)	2%		
Dermapax	0.5%		
Dermarest	2%		
Dermarest Plus	2%		
Di-Delamine	1%		0.5%
Gold Bond Medicated		x	
Gold Bond Medicated Anti-Itch		x	
HC-DermaPax	0.5%		
Hydrosal	1%		

Astringents and Hydrocortisone

BRAND NAME	ASTRINGENTS					HYDROCORTISONE
	alcohol-based	aluminum acetate	calamine	witch hazel	zinc acetate (or zinc oxide)	
Aveeno Anti-Itch			3%			
Bactine Hydrocortisone 1%	x					1%
Benadryl Itch Stopping Extra Strength (cream)	x				0.1%	
Benadryl Itch Stopping Extra Strength (gel)	x				1%	
Benadryl Itch Stopping Extra Strength (spray)	73.5%				0.1%	
Benadryl Itch Stopping Extra Strength (stick)	73.5%				0.1%	
Benadryl Itch Stopping Regular Strength (cream)	x				0.1%	
Benadryl Itch Stopping Regular Strength (gel)	x				1%	
Benadryl Itch Stopping Regular Strength (spray)	73.6%				0.1%	
Buro-Sol Antiseptic		0.23%				
Caladryl (cream)	x		8%			
Caladryl (lotion)	x		8%			
Caladryl Clear	x				0.1%	
Cala-gel Clearly Calamine					0.21%	
Cala-gen Clear					2%	
Calamycin					0.1%	
CaldeCORT						1%
Cortaid FastStick	55%					1%
Cortaid Maximum Strength (cream)	55%					1%
Cortaid Maximum Strength (cream)	x					1%
Cortaid Sensitive Skin Formula						0.5%
Cortizone-10						1%

Cortizone-5					0.5%
Cortizone-5 for Kids					0.5%
Dermapax	35%				
Dermarest DriCort					1%
DermiCort					1%
Dermoplast	x				
Dermtex					1%
Dermtex HC					1%
Dickenson's Witch Hazel Formula	14%		x		
FoilleCort	x				0.5%
Gold Bond Medicated				x (oxide)	
Gold Bond Medicated Anti-Itch	x			x (oxide)	
HC-DermaPax				x	0.5%
Hydrosal				x	
Ivarest 8-Hour Medicated		14%			
Kericort 10	x				1%
Lanacort 10					1%
Lanacort 5					0.5%
No More Itchies	x				1%
Ostiderm				x (oxide)	
Pramegel	x				
Preparation H Hydrocortisone 1% Anti-Itch					1%
Resinol Medicated		6%		12% (oxide)	
Rhuli (gel)	31%				
Rhuli (spray)	70%	13.8%			

Brand Name

Benadryl Itch-Stopping Cream Extra Strength (BEN-uh-drill)

Generic Ingredients

Diphenhydramine hydrochloride
Zinc acetate

Type of Drug

Antihistamine and antipruritic.

Used for

Temporary relief of itching and pain associated with insect bites, minor skin irritations, and rash due to poison ivy, oak, or sumac.

General Information

Histamine is one of the substances released by the body tissues during an allergic reaction. This substance causes a variety of symptoms, including itching. Antihistamines block the effects of histamine, effectively relieving the symptoms of allergic reactions. Oral antihistamines work to relieve runny nose, itchy eyes, and other allergic reactions. Applied topically (to the skin), antihistamines relieve itching that arises in response to contact with an allergen. The antihistamine in Benadryl Itch-Stopping Cream Extra Strength is diphenhydramine hydrochloride.

The most common contact allergen is urushiol, a resin found in poison ivy, oak, and sumac. A number of metals such as cobalt, chromium, and nickel can also cause allergic reactions in some individuals. However, because antihistamines do not work against the other substances released by the body during an allergic reaction, they can reduce only about 40% to 60% of symptoms. Benadryl will not cure skin inflammation, which must run its natural course before the skin heals. Benadryl is able to inhibit the activity of histamine at the site of inflammation, acting as a local anesthetic and temporarily relieving the urge to scratch and possibly irritate the skin even further.

Zinc acetate is used in Benadryl for its astringent (drying) effects.

Cautions and Warnings

If your condition does not improve or worsens within 7 days, or if your symptoms last more than 7 days or clear up and return within a few days, stop using Benadryl and call your doctor.

Do not exceed the recommended daily dosage of Benadryl.

Do not use Benadryl on chicken pox, measles, blisters, or on extensive areas of skin except as directed by your doctor.

Avoid contact with the eyes.

Do not use any other oral or topical drugs containing diphenhydramine while using Benadryl.

Used topically for prolonged periods, Benadryl can irritate skin—the result of a secondary allergic reaction to diphenhydramine, the active ingredient in Benadryl. The original symptom may disappear but skin irritation will continue so long as the medication is being used. Once you develop such an allergic reaction to Benadryl, future oral administration of products containing diphenhydramine may cause skin irritation to recur. To avoid this problem (known as sensitization), do not use Benadryl for more than 7 consecutive days. If rash, burning, or irritation develops or worsens, stop using Benadryl (remove by washing with soap and water) and contact your doctor or pharmacist.

Side Effects

▼ Rare: rash, burning, and skin irritation.

Drug Interactions

• Benadryl should not be used at the same time as other oral or topical medications containing diphenhydramine.

Usual Dose

Benadryl contains diphenhydramine hydrochloride 2.0% and zinc acetate 0.1%.

Because histamine is released nearly continuously, it is best to apply Benadryl on a regular schedule rather than occasionally as needed.

Adult and Child (age 12 and over): Apply sparingly over the affected area no more than 3–4 times per day.

Child (under age 12): Consult your doctor.

If you forget to apply a dose of Benadryl, do so as soon as you remember. If it is almost time for your next dose, skip the one you forgot and continue with your regular schedule. Do not take a double dose.

Overdosage

Do the following in case of accidental ingestion: If the victim is unconscious or having convulsions, call for an ambulance immediately. If you take the victim to an emergency room, be sure to bring the bottle or container with you. If the victim is conscious, call your local poison control center or a health care professional. The poison control center may suggest inducing vomiting with ipecac syrup (available without a prescription at any pharmacy). DO NOT induce vomiting unless specifically instructed to do so.

Special Populations

Pregnancy/Breast-feeding
It is not generally recommended that pregnant women take any drugs, particularly during the first 3 months after conception. Check with your doctor if you are or might be pregnant, or if you are breast-feeding, before using Benadryl.

Infants/Children
Do not use Benadryl on children under age 12 without consulting your doctor.

Seniors
Seniors should exercise the same caution as younger adults when using Benadryl.

Clearasil (CLEER-uh-sill)

see ***Benzoyl Peroxide,*** *page 693*

Cortaid (COURT-aid)

see ***Hydrocortisone,*** *page 836*

Cortizone (CORE-ti-sone)

see ***Hydrocortisone,*** *page 836*

Dr. Scholl's (SHOLES)

*see **Salicylic Acid,** page 1029*

Brand Name

Ivy Block

Generic Ingredients

Bentoquatam

Type of Drug

Skin protectant

Used for

Helps protect against poison-ivy, poison-oak, or poison-sumac rash when applied before contact.

General Information

Bentoquatam, applied topically, has been proven to be effective in preventing or reducing the effects of contact with poison ivy, poison oak, or poison sumac, by stopping the absorption of the allergen into the skin.

Cautions and Warnings

Do not exceed the recommended daily dosage of Ivy Block.

Ivy Block must be applied at least 15 minutes prior to possible contact with poison ivy, poison oak, or poison sumac.

Avoid contact with eyes.

Do not use Ivy Block if you already have a rash from poison ivy, poison oak, or poison sumac.

Ivy Block contains alcohol and is flammable; it remains flammable on the skin until it dries. When applying Ivy Block, keep away from heat or open flame until it dries.

Possible Side effects

▼ Rare: temporary reddening of the skin in the area where Ivy Block is applied.

Drug Interactions

None known.

Usual Dose

Adult and Child (age 6 and over): every 4 hours or as needed to maintain protective coating. Rub lotion into skin; leave a smooth wet film. Coating will remain visible after it dries.

Child (under age 6): not recommended unless directed by a doctor.

Overdosage

Do the following in case of accidental ingestion: If the victim is unconscious or having convulsions, call for an ambulance immediately. If you take the victim to an emergency room, be sure to bring the bottle or container with you. If the victim is conscious, call your local poison control center or a health care professional. The poison control center may suggest inducing vomiting with ipecac syrup (available without a prescription at any pharmacy). DO NOT induce vomiting unless specifically instructed to do so.

Storage Instructions

Ivy Block contains alcohol and is flammable. Cap bottle tightly and store away from heat and open flame.

Special Populations

Pregnancy/Breast-feeding

It is not generally recommended that pregnant women take any drugs, particularly during the first 3 months after conception. Check with your doctor if you are or might be pregnant, before using Ivy Block.

It is not known whether Ivy Block passes into breast-milk. If you must use Ivy Block, bottle feed your baby with formula.

Children/Infants

The use of Ivy Block is not recommended for children under age 6, unless directed by a doctor.

Seniors

Seniors should exercise the same caution as younger adults when using Ivy Block.

Lotrimin AF Antifungal Cream

(LOE-tri-min)

see ***Clotrimazole,*** *page 769*

Oxy 10

see ***Benzoyl Peroxide,*** *page 693*

Preparation H Anti-Itch Cream

see ***Hydrocortisone,*** *page 836*

Chapter 5: Hair and Scalp Care

This chapter deals with 3 common problems that affect the hair and scalp. Two of these, dandruff and seborrhea, are forms of scaly dermatosis, conditions in which the body sheds skin cells in the form of flakes or scales. Dandruff is the more common and less serious, whereas seborrhea is somewhat more troubling. Another type of scaly dermatosis is psoriasis, which can also appear in many places on the body and which can be severely disfiguring. Psoriasis is discussed in detail in chapter 4. Hair loss and head lice are discussed in this chapter.

Dandruff

The outermost layer of our skin, the epidermis, is made up of dead cells that form a protective barrier, our first line of defense against the outside environment. When new cells form in the lower layers of skin, the older cells get pushed to the top. As they age, the cells become flatter; they lose water and become more compact. Eventually the cells die and are sloughed off (shed). Sloughing is important for maintaining healthy skin. If we didn't shed unneeded cells, our skin would continue to grow thicker. A complete cycle of turnover—cell birth, death, and shedding—takes about 4 to 6 weeks.

Generally, the scalp (the skin covering the top of the skull) goes through the turnover process at a somewhat faster rate than the skin on the rest of the body. Dandruff is a condition in which the dead skin is shed from the scalp at an even faster rate (about twice the normal pace) and appears as visible flakes or scales. It is not a disease, but an exaggerated form of the natural skin turnover process. Dandruff is usually a chronic condition, meaning that it persists for a long time or recurs frequently, and it seems to be less severe in the summer. About 1 out of every 5 people has visible dandruff. Usually the problem begins at puberty, peaks at early adulthood, and declines with age. However, it can occur among older adults and for some reason is more likely in people who have had strokes. Dandruff is a cosmetic concern, not a threat to health, but many people find the flakes that appear on the collar and shoulders to be annoying and embarrassing.

The only real symptom of dandruff is the shedding of large flakes. Much of the material in dead cells is a protein called keratin. These cells (called keratinized cells) form an outer layer of scalp skin that is relatively hard and tough. Normally, during shedding, this outer layer breaks up into tiny pieces. In people with dandruff, however, the outer layer is different. There are fewer normal dead cells and larger numbers of cells that do not contain keratin. The outer layer develops cracks, which cause the layer to break into larger pieces—the characteristic flakes of dandruff. Usually, dandruff affects most or all of the scalp. It does not form obvious patches, the way psoriasis or other skin conditions usually do. Nor does dandruff involve inflammation (itching and redness). If those symptoms are present, the problem may actually be seborrhea or psoriasis (see box).

Characteristics of the Scaly Dermatoses

	Dandruff	**Seborrhea**	**Psoriasis**
Location	Scalp	Head, trunk, back, skin folds	Scalp, elbows, knees, trunk, legs
Appearance of scales	Dry, white, small	Oily, yellow or gray, small	Dry, silvery, large
Extent	Evenly distributed	Distinct patchy areas	Symmetrical red patchy areas with distinct border
Inflammation	No	Possibly	Yes
Skin cell turnover rate	2x normal	5-6x normal	5-6x normal

The cause of the accelerated cell growth seen in dandruff is not known. Although many people assume that dandruff is the result of dry skin, the opposite is true. Mild dandruff is more common among people with oily skin. Some experts believe more serious cases of dandruff may be the result of increased growth of microorganisms, such as a type of yeast called *Pityrosporum ovale,* which is normally present on the scalp in small numbers. Perhaps the excess oil in the skin creates an environment in which the yeast can flourish. Men tend to be more likely to have dandruff than women. It may be that men's increased levels of the male hormone testosterone promote oil production in the skin.

If the dandruff is severe, and if other symptoms such as itching occur, the problem may involve one of the other scaly dermatoses, seborrhea (discussed below) or psoriasis.

Seek medical attention if any of the following applies to you

- Dandruff does not improve despite appropriate self-treatment.
- Greasy, waxy patches are apparent.
- The condition affects parts of the body other than the scalp.
- The scalp becomes irritated or severely itchy.

Treatment for Dandruff

There is no cure for dandruff. The problem will likely recur often throughout life. However, OTC products are usually effective. Dandruff is one of the 10 most common medical problems that people are likely to treat using OTC products (see box).

The most basic approach to controlling mild dandruff is simply to wash the hair using ordinary (nonmedicated) shampoo every day, or perhaps only every other day. While shampooing, be sure to rub the lather in gently but completely. Massage the scalp with your fingertips to loosen and remove flakes. Rinse carefully, and repeat the process. Avoid use of greasy mousses or styling gels, because these can make the problem worse.

If shampoo doesn't control the problem, you may want to step up to a medicated product that contains one or more of the approved ingredients. These ingredients are available in various forms, including shampoos, rinses, and special dandruff treatment products that are applied to the scalp and left in place for a while before being rinsed off. Any medicated product should be left on the scalp for at least a minute and then rinsed off thoroughly. Many products direct the user to repeat the application and rinse again. A sensible strategy in cases of mild dandruff is to use a regular shampoo one day and a medicated product the next. Once dandruff is under control, you might want to go back to using a regular shampoo. Should the dandruff return—a pretty sure bet—you can switch back to the medicated variety.

Shampoos that only wash away dandruff are considered cosmetic products, while those that claim to actually treat the condition are classified as drugs. Until the 1990s, there were dozens of ingredients available claiming to be of benefit in preventing or managing dandruff. However, the FDA reviewed the scientific claims for these products and found that most of them were not safe or effective. Consequently, the only ingredients now approved for treatment of dandruff are coal tar, pyrithione zinc, selenium sulfide, salicylic acid, and sulfur. The first 3 of these are classified as cytostatic agents, which means that they help slow down the rate of cell growth and skin turnover. The other 2 ingredients are keratolytic agents, which soften skin and help promote loosening and removal of the flakes. Coal tar shampoos are effective, but they have a tendency to discolor light (either natural or bleached) hair. They may also cause discoloration of clothing and jewelry.

OTC Products for Dandruff

Regular (nonmedicated) shampoos
Medicated hair care products containing
- Coal tar
- Pyrithione zinc
- Salicylic acid
- Selenium sulfide
- Sulfur

Seborrhea

Oil glands (also called sebaceous glands) are found throughout the body except the palms of the hands and the soles of the feet. These glands are especially common near all types of body hair, especially on the scalp and face and in the nose. They release a fatty, waxy substance called sebum, which lubricates skin and keeps it supple and flexible. Sebum also prevents skin from becoming waterlogged when immersed in water and protects against drying, cracking, and infection.

Some people produce excess amounts of sebum, resulting in increased oiliness on the face. If pores become blocked with sloughed skin cells, the sebum can accumulate and produce skin blemishes such as acne (see chapter 4). Excess sebum can create a greasy buildup on the scalp, a condition generally known as seborrhea. Sometimes oversecretion of sebum, coupled with rapid growth of skin cells, causes the eruption of waxy patches of scaly skin. The patches may be inflamed and mildly itchy; this more severe form of seborrhea is often referred to as seborrheic dermatitis. For simplicity, the term seborrhea will be used here to refer to both conditions.

Seborrhea affects about 12 million people in this country. It is more prevalent in men, especially those who are middle-aged or elderly, but it can also occur in newborns, causing a condition commonly called cradle cap. Seborrhea is a complication of such illnesses as Parkinson's disease, obesity, zinc deficiency, infection with human immunodeficiency virus (HIV) and cardiovascular conditions such as stroke or heart attack.

The condition causes clearly marked, dull, yellow-red lesions and oily yellow scales to erupt on the skin. Usually these patches appear on the scalp, but they can also appear in other areas with lots of sebaceous glands, such as the back and mid-chest. In severe cases, the scalp patches may extend into the middle third of the face and may affect the eyelids, eyebrows, and ears. Sometimes the problem extends to the navel and the skin folds under the arms, breasts, groin, or buttocks.

Most, but not all, experts believe that seborrhea is simply a more serious form of the same skin condition that causes dandruff. Others argue that it is a different disorder entirely. Dandruff tends to be a stable problem, remaining at about the same level of severity over time. Seborrhea, however, can fluctuate in intensity and tends to worsen during times of stress. Also, unlike dandruff, seborrhea may involve the eyebrows and eyelids, causing redness, swelling, and crusting.

Doctors are not quite sure what causes seborrhea, but some people appear to inherit a tendency to develop the problem. In addition to its association with emotional stress, seborrhea can worsen when other medical illnesses are present. Some cases may arise due to food allergies, vitamin deficiencies, or climatic factors such as low humidity. Seborrhea does not increase the risk of getting other skin diseases, nor does it progress to or cause skin cancer.

The most serious form of scaly dermatosis is psoriasis, discussed in chapter 4. One way to distinguish seborrhea from psoriasis is the location of the scaly patches. Seborrhea is usually confined to the scalp and the face and seldom appears on the arms and legs. Psoriasis usually affects the scalp, but it also appears on the elbows and knees and seldom arises on the face. The scales of seborrhea are oily and have a yellowish color, whereas the scales seen in psoriasis are dry and silvery. If you gently scrape away a flake of psoriasis, you would see a tiny spot of bleeding; this characteristic does not occur in seborrhea. A common fungal infection, tinea capitis (ringworm of the scalp), may also resemble seborrhea. It is important to know what is causing the symptoms, because antifungal treatment mistakenly applied to seborrhea can actually make the problem worse.

Treatment for Seborrhea

The same medicated products used for dandruff are often effective in mild cases of seborrhea (see section on dandruff, above). Frequent use of shampoos containing selenium sulfide, however, can sometimes stimulate excess oil production, which may make the problem worse.

If medicated products don't work, and if the seborrhea involves inflammation, treatment with lotions containing a topical corticosteroid, such as hydrocortisone, may provide relief. These OTC products are usually applied 2 or 3 times a day until the symptoms clear up. If the problem returns, the same medication can be used again to provide relief. For best results, the product should be applied after a shampoo, because damp skin absorbs the medication better. The hair is pulled to one side, and lotion is applied directly to the affected area of the scalp and massaged carefully into the skin.

The use of a topical corticosteroid lotion should continue for no longer than a week, because there is a risk that with longer use the seborrhea will flare up in a more serious form when the medication is stopped. If the lotion does not provide sufficient relief, a doctor can prescribe a more potent form of topical corticosteroid.

OTC Products for Seborrhea

Medicated hair care products
Topical corticosteroid (e.g., hydrocortisone)

Seek medical attention if any of the following applies to you

- Seborrhea affects parts of the body other than the scalp, especially the eyelashes, eyelids, or ear canals.
- The problem persists despite 7 days of treatment with a topical corticosteroid (see "Treatment for Seborrhea").

Hair Loss

About 1 man in 3 and 1 woman in 6 will suffer from hair loss at some point during their lifetimes. The problem is usually hereditary, passed on in the genes at the moment of conception. Despite popular belief, the tendency to become bald is actually inherited from the mother's side of the family, not the father's. (For other causes, see box.)

Causes of Hair Loss

- Heredity
- Scalp infection
- Nutritional deficiencies
- Hormonal changes (such as during pregnancy)
- Hypothyroidism or other endocrine disorders
- Mental illnesses causing hair-pulling behavior
- Misuse of harsh hair care products
- Side effects of medication, such as chemotherapy for cancer

Hairs grow inside pouchlike indentations in the skin called follicles. It takes about 2 to 5 years for a hair to grow. However, a mature hair only "lives" for about 100 days before it falls out. Normally, the human head sheds about 100 hairs each day, but only about 10 new hairs will grow to take their place.

The rate of growth and loss is determined by our genes. People with hereditary baldness have hair that "matures" and falls out more quickly than normal. These hairs are not replaced, or are replaced at a much slower rate than in people who do not have hereditary hair loss.

The pattern of hair loss is determined by sex. Male-pattern hereditary baldness arises at the top rear of the head (the area where a skullcap would be worn) and progresses forward along the top of the scalp. In women, hair loss typically begins at the top center of the scalp. Hereditary hair loss is not a health problem, but it is a cosmetic concern.

Treatment for Hair Loss

There are countless techniques promoted for restoring scalp hair, from weaves to implants to transplants. The only OTC hair restorative available is minoxidil. It is indicated only for treatment of adult hair loss due to hereditary factors. The brand-name version of minoxidil, Rogaine, is labeled for use by both men and women, but the generic versions are labeled only for treatment of male-pattern baldness.

Minoxidil, applied twice a day, apparently works by stimulating the hair-growth cells inside the follicles, perhaps by increasing the flow of blood to the cells of the scalp. It also seems to prolong the growth phase of the hair-growth cycle. The drug may increase the amount of time the hair stays in place or cause thicker hairs to grow. The best time to start using minoxidil is before the baldness has become too extensive—that is, when less than one-fourth of the scalp in men or one-third of the scalp in women has started to show hair loss. The longer the hair loss has existed, the less likely it is that the drug will work. Even when started early, minoxidil will not usually cause all of the hair to regrow. At best, it will slow down the rate of loss. Once use of the drug begins, it must be continued indefinitely to maintain the effects.

Increasing the dosage will not increase the results.

After about a year of use, only about 1 man in 4 and 1 woman in 5 will notice moderate effects from minoxidil. Some new hair may grow, but it will not be dense or thick enough to cover the bald patch completely. About 1 person in 3 will not experience any significant results from the product.

OTC Product for Treating Hair Loss
Topical minoxidil

Head Lice

Head lice are tiny, brown 8-legged creatures that infest and thrive on the human scalp. Different types of lice occupy other regions of the body, such as the pubic area, but head lice are the most common form of infestation. (For more information about lice, see chapter 4.) Approximately 10 million Americans, most of them school-age children, carry head lice. Infestation is not a sign of poor hygiene or poor housekeeping. No amount of bathing will dislodge these tenacious critters. Lice are widespread parasites that can show up in people regardless of their economic or social status.

Lice live among hairs on the head, especially along the hairline at the back of the neck, and feed on blood. Their bites and their droppings irritate the skin, causing persistent and annoying itching. Scratching can cause further irritation and can strip away the outer layer of skin, leaving the scalp more vulnerable to bacterial infections. The itching may not show up until 2 weeks after the lice invade, by which point they may have already laid their eggs.

Lice eggs, known as nits, look like tiny flakes of yellow, gray, or brownish dandruff. Unlike dandruff, however, nits are affixed to strands of hair with a powerfully sticky substance and are very difficult to dislodge. After the egg has hatched, the empty shell remains attached to the hair. If you see your child scratching persistently, check the scalp carefully. In such circumstances, it pays to be a nitpicker.

Because lice cannot jump or fly, the infestation is spread by direct contact: rubbing up against the person's head or shoulders; sharing hats, caps, combs, or hair fasteners; or in some cases, lying on a carpet or sitting in a chair where an infested person has been. As long as any of the lice or nits are alive, it is possible for another person to become infested. To help cut down on the risk of spreading infestations, take precautionary measures (see box).

Preventing Head Lice

- Change and wash clothing regularly.
- Wash clothes and bedding in hot water (over 130°F).
- Do not allow children to share clothes (especially headwear), brushes, combs, and so on.
- Inspect children's heads for signs of lice or nits once a week.
- If you see lice, notify school authorities so other parents can check their children.
- Soak combs, brushes, and hair clips for 10 minutes in hot soapy water or in a lice control solution.

Treatment for Head Lice

Because lice and their nits cling so strongly to the scalp, ordinary shampooing will not eliminate them. It is usually necessary to use a pediculicide (a product containing ingredients designed to kill the pests). Some of these products are available without a prescription.

The best choice is a cream rinse containing 1% permethrin, which acts to paralyze and kill both the lice and their eggs. The effects of the medication last even after it is rinsed off. Virtually all cases of head lice can be eradicated following a single application of permethrin rinse. If the lice remain, a second treatment applied a week later will usually be effective. Other products contain a combination of pyrethrins and piperonyl butoxide in a nonaerosol spray. Pyrethrins paralyze the lice; piperonyl butoxide does not kill directly but helps by enhancing the effectiveness of the pyrethrins.

Results are best if treatment is given after use of a regular shampoo that does not contain a cream rinse or conditioner. Make sure any traces of oil-based mousses or other hair products have been washed away. Dry the hair thoroughly. Then apply the product so that it saturates the hair and especially the scalp. Long hair requires using more of the medication. Shampoos should be left in place for at least 4 minutes, other formulations for at least 10 minutes. The medication is then removed with careful rinsing with warm water. Afterward, the hair should be combed using a specially designed fine-toothed comb to remove lice, nits, and shells. The lotion may cause temporary itching, burning, or stinging. The spray does not usually cause adverse reactions.

Rinsing the hair with a mixture of white vinegar and water can help loosen the nits. Part the hair into small sections and comb as close to the scalp as possible, wiping any nits from the comb as you go along. After combing, rinse the head again.

It may take as long as 2 days for the lice to die. If a second treatment is needed, wait a week. It may be best to switch to another product for the second dose.

Seek medical attention if

- Head lice infestation does not clear up despite 2 doses of appropriate treatment.

OTC Products for Head Lice

Pediculicides
- Permethrin
- Pyrethrins + piperonyl butoxide

Dandruff, Seborrhea, and Psoriasis Products

BRAND NAME	KERATOLYTIC AGENT		CYTOSTATIC AGENT		COAL TAR (FORM)
	salicylic acid	sulfur	pyrithione zinc	selenium sulfide	
Balnetar					2.5%
Brylcreem Anti-Dandruff			1%		
Cutar					1.5%
Denorex Dandruff for Dry Scalp					(extract) 2%
Denorex Medicated					(solution) 9%
Denorex Medicated Extra Strength					(solution) 12.5%
Denorex Medicated Mountain Fresh Scent					(solution) 9%
DHS Sal	3%				
DHS Tar					0.5%
DHS Tar Gel					0.5%
DHS Zinc			2%		
Doak Oil					(distillate) 2%
Doak Tar (lotion)					(distillate) 5%
Doak Tar (shampoo)					(distillate) 3%
Doctar					0.5%
Duplex-T					(solution) 10%
Estar					5%
Glover's Dandruff Control Medicine		2.5%			(pine tar oil)
Glover's Medicated					(solution) 5%
Glover's Medicated Dandruff Soap		2.08%			(pine tar)
Glover's Medicated for Dandruff	3%	5%			
Grandpa's Pine Tar Soap					(pine tar oil) 2.7%
Head & Shoulders Dandruff			1%		
Head & Shoulders Dandruff 2-in-1			1%		

Grandpa's Pine Tar Shampooing					(pine tar oil) 1%
Head & Shoulders Dry Scalp			1%		
Head & Shoulders Intensive Treatment				1%	
Ionil	2%				
Ionil Plus	2%				
Ionil T					(solution) 5%
Ionil T Plus					(crude coal tar)
Meted	3%	5%			
MG217 for Psoriasis (lotion)					(solution) 5%
MG217 for Psoriasis (ointment)					(solution) 10%
Neutrogena Healthy Scalp Anti-Dandruff	1.8%				
Neutrogena T/Derm					1.2%
Neutrogena T/Gel					0.5%
Neutrogena T/Gel Extra Strength Therapeutic					4%
Neutrogena T/Sal Maximum Strength Therapeutic	3%				
Oxipor VHC					(solution) 25%
P&S	2%				
Pentrax					4.3%
Pentrax Gold					2%
Polytar (cleansing bar)					0.5%
Polytar (shampoo)					0.5%
Poslam Psoriasis	2%	5%			
Psor-A-Set	2%				
Psoriasin					1.25%
Psoriasis Tar					(solution) 5%
Psorigel					(solution) 8.8%
Scalpicin Maximum Strength	3%				

BRAND NAME	KERATOLYTIC AGENT		CYTOSTATIC AGENT		COAL TAR (FORM)
	salicylic acid	sulfur	pyrithione zinc	selenium sulfide	
Sebucare	1.8%				
Sebulex Conditioning with Protein	2%	2%			
Sebulex Medicated	2%	2%			
Sebulon			2%		
Sebutone	1.5%	1.5%			0.5%
Sebutone Cream	1.5%	1.5%			0.5%
Selsun Blue				1%	
Selsun Gold for Women				1%	
SLT Lotion					(distillate) 2.5%
Sulfoam Medicated Antidandruff		2%			
Sulray		5%			
Sulray Dandruff		2%			
Taraphilic					(distillate) 1%
Tarsum					(solution) 10%
Tegrin (cleansing bar)					(extract) 2%
Tegrin (cream)					(solution) 5%
Tegrin (shampoo)					(solution) 7%
X-Seb			1%		
X-Seb Plus			1%		
X-Seb T Pearl					(solution) 10%
X-Seb T Plus					(solution) 10%
Zetar					(whole colloidal) 1%
Zincon			1%		
ZNP Bar			2%		

Hair Loss Products

BRAND NAME	MINOXIDIL
Rogaine for Men	2%
Rogaine for Women	2%

Lice Products

BRAND NAME	ACTIVE INGREDIENTS			
	permethrin	piperonyl butoxide	pyrethrins or pyrethrum extract	resmethrin
A-200 Lice Control for Dogs and Household	0.5%			
A-200 Lice Killing		4%	0.33%	
A-200 Lice Treatment Kit (shampoo)		4%	0.33%	
A-200 Lice Treatment Kit (spray)	0.5%			
Barc		2.2%	0.18%	
End-Lice		4%	0.33%	
InnoGel Plus		4%	0.33%	
Lice Treatment		3%	0.3%	
Lice Treatment Kit				0.5%
Licetrol		4%	0.33%	
Licetrol 600		3%	0.3%	
Licide (shampoo)		3%	0.3%	
Licide (spray)		1%	0.2%	
Licide Blue			0.2%	

BRAND NAME	ACTIVE INGREDIENTS			
	permethrin	piperonyl butoxide	pyrethrins or pyrethrum extract	resmethrin
Nix	1%			
Pronto Lice Killing (shampoo)		4%	0.33%	
Pronto Lice Killing (spray)			0.4%	
R&C Shampoo		3%	0.33%	
R&C Spray			0.4%	
RID Lice Control for Dogs and Household	0.5%			
RID Lice Elimination Kit (shampoo)		4%	0.33%	
RID Lice Elimination Kit (spray)	0.5%			
RID Lice Killing		4%	0.33%	
Tegrin-LT Lice Treatment		3%	0.33%	
Tisit (liquid)		2%	0.3%	
Tisit (shampoo)		3%	0.3%	
Tisit Blue		3%	0.3%	

Head & Shoulders Dandruff

*see **Pyrithione Zinc,** page 1020*

Head & Shoulders Dry Scalp

*see **Pyrithione Zinc,** page 1020*

Head & Shoulders 2 in 1

*see **Pyrithione Zinc,** page 1020*

Rogaine for Men (ROE-gain)

*see **Minoxidil,** page 931*

Rogaine for Women (ROE-gain)

*see **Minoxidil,** page 931*

Chapter 6: Sleep Aids and Stimulants

Insomnia

It is a widespread—but mistaken—belief that everyone needs to get 8 hours of sleep a night. In fact, the amount of sleep each person needs to stay healthy and alert varies widely. Some people do fine sleeping 6 hours at a stretch, while others require 9 or even 10 hours. On average, most adults need 7 to 8 hours of sleep a night; children and adolescents typically need more.

Quantity of sleep is not as important as quality. Ideally, sleep is restful, refreshing, and restorative. Sleep that is interrupted frequently or that is too shallow to reach the dream stage (REM, or rapid eye movement, stage) will not provide adequate rest.

When we can't get to sleep, we call it insomnia. There are several kinds of insomnia (see box). It is the third most common ailment, behind headaches and the common cold, and it affects about 1 out of 3 people at some time in their lives. For 1 person in 10, the problem is severe, with devastating effects on health and productivity.

Types of Insomnia

- *Difficulty falling asleep.* Normally people drop off to sleep within 5 or 10 minutes of going to bed. With this kind of insomnia, however, people toss and turn for 30 minutes or more. The harder they try to fall asleep, the more anxious they become, and the harder it is for them to get to sleep.
- *Frequent nighttime awakenings and difficulty returning to sleep.* People with this form of insomnia wake up many times during the night, due to a physical problem such as the need to urinate or because of an emotional concern such as anxiety.
- *Early morning waking.* This pattern, a common symptom of depression, causes people to wake up 2 to 4 hours earlier than normal and makes them unable to fall back to sleep.
- *Unrestful sleep.* With this pattern, people may get some sleep but it is shallow and fitful. The next day, they feel draggy, irritable, and unable to concentrate.

Insomnia falls into different patterns, depending on how long it persists:

- *Short-term* (or *transient*) insomnia lasts from 1 night to several weeks.
- *Intermittent* insomnia involves several incidents of short-term insomnia over the course of a year or 2.
- *Chronic* insomnia disrupts sleep on most nights for a month or more.

A number of factors can cause or contribute to insomnia. Sleep problems are more common in people over age 60. It is commonly—but wrongly—believed that seniors have a decreased need for sleep. What actually happens is that, as our bodies age, our ability to get a good night's sleep declines. Women are more likely to be affected than men, especially after menopause. Physical or emotional problems may contribute to insomnia.

Short-term and intermittent insomnia often result from temporary conditions such as:

- stress
- poor sleep environment (too much noise or light; too hot or cold)
- change in the sleep environment (such as hospitalization or moving to a new house)
- sleep schedule problems (e.g., travel, jet lag, or adjusting to a new work schedule)
- side effects of medication
- alcohol and caffeine abuse

If these temporary conditions persist, there is a risk that they will develop into a longer-term problem that is more difficult to treat.

Chronic insomnia tends to be the result of a combination of factors. Not surprisingly, physical illnesses that disrupt the body's ability to function can also cause problems with sleep. The long list of conditions that may lead to insomnia includes arthritis, chronic pain, kidney disease, heart failure, asthma, Parkinson's disease, and hyperthyroidism. Psychiatric illnesses can also cause insomnia, as can many prescription and OTC medications. People in withdrawal from addiction to drugs or alcohol frequently have sleep disorders.

Behavior plays a key role in the ability to get a good night's sleep. Poor sleep hygiene—irregular hours, participating in stimulating activities such as exercise just prior to bedtime, misuse of alcohol, cigarette smoking, excessive caffeine consumption in the evening—can interfere with sleep patterns. Daytime or evening naps can be restful and restorative, but excessive napping can lead to chronic insomnia.

Treatment for Insomnia

If you have ever taken an OTC medication for relief of cold allergy symptoms, you have probably noticed the warnings that some of these products may cause drowsiness. The ingredients that cause this unwanted side effect in allergy treatment antihistamines also produce the sleep-promoting benefit of sleep aids.

When a viral or bacterial infection strikes the body, or when the tissue is damaged, many of the cells release histamine, one of the chemicals that cause the irritation, itching, and inflammation associated with allergies, infections, or injuries. Histamine also causes blood vessels to dilate (widen), allowing fluid to leak out and producing redness and swelling. As their name suggests, antihistamines provide relief by blocking the activity of histamine. Through a mechanism not fully understood, certain antihistamines also cause sleepiness.

The only antihistamine that the FDA has declared safe and effective for OTC use as a sleep aid is diphenhydramine. Two available forms of this antihistamine are diphenhydramine hydrochloride and diphenhydramine citrate. Doses in sleep aids range from 25 to 50 milligrams. Another antihistamine, doxylamine, can also be found in a few sleep aids on the market, but evidence for its safety is not as well established.

Some sleep aids also contain acetaminophen or magnesium. The acetaminophen is intended to provide relief of pain that can contribute to insomnia. Use products with added acetaminophen only if you are experiencing pain while trying to fall asleep.

As a rule, sleep aids should be used only for short periods of time—no more than 7 to 10 consecutive nights—as a means of restoring a normal sleep pattern. If the problem persists for longer than 10 days, see a doctor to determine if there is an underlying medical problem or if a stronger prescription medication (such as a benzodiazepine) may be needed.

Another form of sleep disorder is sleep apnea, which causes sudden and repeated interruptions in breathing during sleep. In their struggle to regain breath, people with apnea may snore extremely loudly, snort, choke, cough, or gasp. This strenuous effort to get the lungs working again rouses them from deep sleep to light sleep for a few seconds, but does not necessarily cause them to awaken to full consciousness. The next day, people with apnea (unaware of their nighttime apnea and fragmented sleep) may be excessively sleepy, often falling asleep at inappropriate or potentially dangerous times (e.g., in meetings or while driving).

Sleep aids containing antihistamines should not be used for treatment of sleep apnea because they can actually worsen the problem. For the same reason, alcohol and tobacco should also be avoided; all of these drugs can reduce the ability of the brain to regulate nighttime breathing.

Seek medical attention if any of the following applies to you

- Daytime sleepiness
- Frequent daytime napping
- Difficulty concentrating
- Difficulty staying awake while driving
- Sleep apnea

OTC Treatment for Insomnia

Sedating antihistamines

Stimulants

People who feel sleepy during the day often feel the need to take a stimulant to help them stay awake and alert. Caffeine, the most common drug used for this purpose, is an ingredient in many beverages, including coffee, tea, cola, and hot chocolate. Chocolate candy also contains caffeine (see table).

Sources of Caffeine

Product	Serving size	Caffeine (mg)
Instant coffee	1 cup	66 mg
Coffee (percolated)	1 cup	110 mg
Coffee (drip brewed)	1 cup	146 mg
Decaf coffee	1 cup	5 mg
Tea (brewed 1 minute)	1 cup	25 mg
Tea (brewed 5 minutes)	1 cup	46 mg
Cocoa	1 cup	13 mg
Jolt Cola	12-ounce can	120 mg
Coca-Cola	12-ounce can	60 mg
Dr. Pepper	12-ounce can	60 mg
Tab	12-ounce can	49 mg
Pepsi Cola	12-ounce can	43 mg
Mountain Dew	12-ounce can	55 mg
Chocolate bar	approx. 2 ozs.	25 mg

OTC stimulant products contain caffeine in doses ranging from 100 mg to 250 mg. In varying doses, caffeine is also an ingredient in certain headache and cold remedies, menstrual pain relief products, and diet aids.

Of course, too much stimulation can disrupt sleep, leading to a vicious cycle of insomnia and daytime sleepiness. To avoid sleep problems, it's a good idea to avoid consuming caffeine in any form at least 6 hours before bedtime.

Despite its widespread availability, caffeine is not always a safe and benign substance. Some people appear to become tolerant to caffeine; that is, they must consume higher doses to achieve the same effect they used to achieve with lower doses. Caffeine also causes physical dependence, in which people experience cravings for the substance and believe they need it to function normally. The substance may affect mood by increasing anxiety or panic symptoms and by worsening symptoms of premenstrual syndrome (PMS). When they stop consuming caffeine, many people experience withdrawal, the main symptoms of which are headache and fatigue. It is possible to consume an overdose of caffeine. At high doses (250 to 500 mg), caffeine can cause shakiness, nervousness, headache, irritability, rapid heartbeat, and gastrointestinal problems. Some prescription medications can interact with caffeine, making its effects even stronger or longer-acting. Check with your physician or pharmacist if you have any questions about your medicine and caffeine.

Sleep Aid Products

BRAND NAME	ANTIHISTAMINE		ANALGESIC	
	diphenhydramine HCl *diphenhydramine citrate	doxylamine succinate	acetaminophen	aspirin
Anacin P.M. Aspirin Free	25mg		500mg	
Arthriten PM	25mg		250mg	
Arthritis Foundation Nighttime	25mg		500mg	
Backaid PM Pills	25mg			500mg
Bayer PM Extra Strength	25mg		500mg	
Bayer Select Aspirin-Free Night Time Pain Relief	25mg		500mg	
Compoz (gelcap)	25mg			
Compoz (tablet)	50mg			
Doan's P.M. Extra Strength	25mg			
Dormarex	50mg			
Dormarex 2	50mg			
Dormin	25mg			
Doxylamine Succinate	25mg			
Excedrin PM	38mg*		500mg	
Excedrin PM LiquiGels	25mg		500mg	
Legatrin PM	50mg		500mg	
Midol PM Night Time Formula	25mg		500mg	
Nervine Nighttime Sleep-Aid	25mg			
Night-Time Sleep-Aid		25mg		
NiteGel		6.25mg	250mg	
Nytol	25mg			
Nytol Maximum Strength		25mg		
Sleep Rite	25mg			

BRAND NAME	ANTIHISTAMINE		ANALGESIC	
	diphenhydramine HCl *diphenhydramine citrate	doxylamine succinate	acetaminophen	aspirin
Sleep-Eze 3	25mg			
Sleepinal	50mg			
Snooze Fast	50mg			
Sominex Maximum Strength	50mg			
Sominex Original	25mg			
Sominex Pain Relief Formula	25mg		500mg	
Tranquil	25mg			
Tranquil Plus	25mg		250mg	
Twilite	50mg			
Tylenol PM Extra Strength	25mg		500mg	
Unisom Nighttime Sleep Aid		25mg		
Unisom Pain Relief	50mg		650mg	
Unisom Sleepgels	50mg			

Stimulant Products

BRAND NAME	CAFFEINE
20/20	200mg
357 Magnum II	200mg
Caffedrine	200mg
Dexitac	250mg
King of Hearts	200mg
No Doz	100mg
No Doz Maximum Strength	200mg
Overtime	200mg
Pep-Back	100mg
Pep-Back Ultra	200mg
Quick-Pep	150mg
Vivarin	200mg

Brand Name

Bayer PM (BAY-er)

Generic Ingredients

Aspirin
Diphenhydramine

Type of Drug

Nonsteroidal anti-inflammatory drug (NSAID), analgesic (pain reliever) and antipyretic (fever reducer), and antihistamine.

Used for

Temporary relief of occasional headache and minor aches and pains, with accompanying sleeplessness.

General Information

Some OTC products use a combination of drugs to relieve symptoms. Bayer PM contains an analgesic/antipyretic and an antihistamine.

NSAID is the general term for a group of drugs that reduce inflammation and pain. Aspirin is also a member of the group of drugs called salicylates. Aspirin reduces inflammation, relieves pain, and reduces fever.

Aspirin's effects on pain and inflammation are thought to be related to its ability to prevent the manufacture of complex hormones called prostaglandins, which sensitize pain receptors and stimulate the inflammatory response. Of all the salicylates, aspirin has the greatest effect on prostaglandin production.

Aspirin reduces fever by acting on the heat-regulating center in the brain. This causes the blood vessels in the skin to dilate which allows heat to leave the body more rapidly.

Bayer PM also contains the antihistamine diphenhydramine. Antihistamines block the release of histamine in the body, and are generally used to relieve the sneezing and itching that can occur with colds and allergies. However, diphenhydramine has several other uses, including the short-term management of insomnia. Diphenhydramine has been shown to be effective both in reducing the amount of time it takes to fall asleep and in increasing the depth and quality of sleep.

Cautions and Warnings

Unless directed by your doctor, do not take Bayer PM for more than 10 days continuously, or in the presence of fever, for more than 3 days continuously.

Do not exceed the recommended daily dosage of Bayer PM.

If you have insomnia that lasts longer than 2 weeks, call your doctor. Insomnia may be a sign of a serious underlying physical, emotional, or psychological condition that needs medical attention.

If dizziness, hearing loss, ringing or buzzing in the ears, or continuous stomach pain occur while using Bayer PM or any other aspirin product, stop taking the drug immediately and call your doctor.

Children with the flu or chicken pox who are given aspirin or other salicylates may develop Reye's syndrome, a life-threatening condition characterized by vomiting, progressive damage to the central nervous system, liver injury, and abnormally low blood sugar. Up to 30% of children who develop Reye's syndrome die, and permanent brain damage is possible in those who survive. Because of the risk of Reye's syndrome, do not give Bayer PM to children under age 16.

Aspirin is associated with gastrointestinal (GI) irritation, erosion and bleeding. Unless directed by a doctor, people with GI bleeding or a history of peptic ulcers should not take Bayer PM. Be aware that the risk of aspirin-related ulcers is increased by alcohol.

People with liver or kidney damage should avoid aspirin.

To reduce the risk of bleeding, aspirin should be avoided prior to surgery. Ask your doctor how long before surgery you should avoid taking Bayer PM and any other aspirin product.

Bayer PM should be used with caution if you have a condition that causes breathing problems, such as emphysema, chronic bronchitis, or asthma. Patients with a history of asthma, nasal polyps, or rhinitis should not use aspirin without checking with a doctor. In addition, Bayer PM's antihistamine ingredient can dry the mucous membranes. This in turn can inhibit the ability of the lungs to move or get rid of the excess secretions that these conditions produce.

Because of its antihistamine ingredient, Bayer PM should be used with caution by people with glaucoma, hyperthyroidism, heart disease, high blood pressure, or an enlarged prostate. If you have any of these conditions, consult your doctor before using Bayer PM.

The antihistamine ingredient in Bayer PM acts as a depressant on the central nervous system (CNS), and can cause sleepiness or grogginess and interfere with the ability to concentrate. Your ability to perform activities that require your full alertness and coordination, such as driving a motor vehicle or operating machinery, may be affected. Drinking alcohol while you are taking Bayer PM can aggravate these effects.

Possible Side Effects

▼ Most common: nausea, upset stomach, heartburn, loss of appetite; small amounts of blood in the stool, restlessness, nervousness, sedation, excitability, dizziness, and poor coordination.

▼ Less common: dry eyes, nose, and mouth; blurred vision; difficulty urinating; irritability (at high doses); and increased or irregular heart rate.

▼ Rare: rashes, hives, liver damage, fever, thirst, and difficulty breathing.

Drug Interactions

• Bayer PM should not be taken by individuals currently taking methotrexate, used to treat cancer, severe psoriasis, severe rheumatoid arthritis, and to induce abortion; or valproic acid, an anticonvulsant. The aspirin in Bayer PM can increase the toxicity of these drugs.

• Aspirin should also not be taken with anticoagulant (blood-thinning) drugs, such as warfarin and dicumarol. It will exaggerate the effects of these drugs and increase the risk of abnormal bleeding.

• The possibility of a stomach ulcer is increased if aspirin is taken together with alcoholic beverages; an adrenal corticosteroid, such as hydrocortisone; or phenylbutazone, another NSAID. Taking Bayer PM with another NSAID has no benefit and carries a greatly increased risk of side effects.

• The aspirin in Bayer PM will counteract the effects of the antigout medications probenecid and sulfinpyrazone, and may counteract the effects of angiotensin-converting enzyme (ACE) inhibitors and beta blockers, which work to lower blood pressure. Aspirin may also counteract the effects of some diuretics in people with severe liver disease.

• Combining nitroglycerin tablets and aspirin may lead to an unexpected drop in blood pressure.

• People with AIDS and AIDS-related complex who take zidovudine (AZT) should avoid using Bayer PM because the aspirin in it may increase the risk of bleeding.

• Diphenhydramine, the antihistamine ingredient in Bayer PM, can enhance the effect of other drugs that depress the CNS, such as barbiturates, tranquilizers, sleeping medications, and alcohol (present in many OTC preparations). If you are taking other depressant drugs, check with your doctor before taking Bayer PM.

• Because of its antihistamine ingredient, Bayer PM should not be used at the same time as a monoamine oxidase inhibitor (MAOI) or within 2 weeks of stopping treatment with an MAOI. MAOIs are used to treat depression, other psychiatric or emotional conditions, and Parkinson's disease. If you are not sure whether you are or have been taking an MAOI, check with your doctor or pharmacist before you use Bayer PM.

• The antihistamine ingredient in Bayer PM can also affect the results of skin and blood tests. Notify your health care professional before scheduling these tests if you are taking Bayer PM.

Food Interactions

Taking Bayer PM along with food, milk, or water reduces the risk of upset stomach or GI bleeding.

Usual Dose

Each Bayer PM caplet contains 500 mg of aspirin and 25 mg of diphenhydramine.

Adult (age 16 and over): 2 caplets at bedtime, or as directed by your doctor.

Child (under age 16): not recommended because of the risk of Reye's syndrome (see "Cautions and Warnings").

Overdosage

Symptoms of overdose include ringing or buzzing in the ears, rapid and deep breathing, rapid heartbeat, sweating, fever, dry mouth, flushed face, thirst, headache, nausea, vomiting, and diarrhea, dilated pupils, loss of muscle coordination, excitability, confusion, drowsiness, dizziness, seizures, liver or kidney failure, and bleeding.

Severe overdose may cause dilated pupils, dry mouth, fever, excitability, confusion, hallucinations, loss of muscle coordination, coma, seizures, liver or kidney failure, and bleeding.

Even if the victim is not displaying any of the symptoms listed above, do the following in case of accidental overdose: If the victim is unconscious or having convulsions, call for an ambulance immediately. If you take the victim to an emergency room, be sure to bring the bottle or container with you. If the victim is conscious, call your local poison control center or a health care professional. The poison control center may suggest inducing vomiting with ipecac syrup (available without a prescription at any pharmacy). DO NOT induce vomiting unless specifically instructed to do so.

Special Populations

Pregnancy/Breast-feeding

Do not take Bayer PM if you are or might be pregnant.

Aspirin and antihistamines are known to pass into the breast milk of nursing mothers and may cause side effects in infants. Check with your doctor before taking Bayer PM if you are breast-feeding.

Infants/Children

Aspirin should not be used by children under 16 unless directed by your doctor, because of the risk of Reye's syndrome (see "Cautions and Warnings"). Children are also more susceptible to accidental antihistamine overdose. Do not give Bayer PM to a child under age 16 unless directed by your doctor.

Seniors

Older individuals may find aspirin irritating to the stomach, especially in large doses.

Older adults with liver disease or severe kidney impairment should not use aspirin.

Older adults may also be more sensitive to the side effects of the antihistamine ingredient in Bayer PM. They may experience nervousness, irritability, and restlessness. Dizziness, sedation, and low blood pressure may also occur. Older men may experience difficulty in urinating.

Persons over age 80 and those with acute physical disorders or dementia may be at risk of developing delerium from even small doses of the antihistamine diphenhydramine.

Brand Name

Excedrin PM (ex-SED-rin)
Tylenol PM (TYE-leh-nol)

Generic Ingredients

Acetaminophen
Diphenhydramine

Type of Drug

Analgesic (pain reliever) and antipyretic (fever reducer), and antihistamine.

Used for

Temporary relief of occasional headache and minor aches and pains, with accompanying sleeplessness.

General Information

Some OTC products use a combination of drugs to relieve symptoms. Excedrin PM and Tylenol PM contain an analgesic/antipyretic and an antihistamine.

The analgesic/antipyretic ingredient in Excedrin PM and Tylenol PM, acetaminophen, relieves pain and reduces fever.

Excedrin PM and Tylenol PM also contain the antihistamine diphenhydramine. Antihistamines block the release of histamine in the body, and are generally used to relieve the sneezing and itching that can occur with colds and allergies. However, diphenhydramine has several other uses, including the short-term management of insomnia. Diphenhydramine has been shown to be effective both in reducing the amount of time it takes to fall asleep and in increasing the depth and quality of sleep.

Cautions and Warnings

Unless directed by your doctor, do not take Excedrin PM or Tylenol PM for more than 10 days continuously, or in the presence of fever, for more than 3 days continuously.

Do not exceed the recommended daily dosage of Excedrin PM or Tylenol PM.

If you have insomnia that lasts longer than 2 weeks, call your doctor. Insomnia may be a sign of a serious underlying physical, emotional, or psychological condition that needs medical attention.

In doses of more than 4 grams per day, acetaminophen is potentially toxic to the liver. Use Excedrin PM and Tylenol PM with caution if you have kidney or liver disease or viral infections of the liver. Studies have shown that the risk of liver damage with acetaminophen is associated with fasting and alcohol use. People with liver disease who are taking other drugs that are potentially damaging to the liver, people who do not eat regularly, or who drink alcohol (even moderately) are especially at risk. If you take Excedrin PM or Tylenol PM regularly, avoid drinking alcohol and/or fasting.

Excedrin PM and Tylenol PM should be used with caution if you have a condition that causes breathing problems, such as emphysema, chronic bronchitis, or asthma. Their antihistamine ingredient, diphenhydramine, can dry the mucous membranes. This in turn can inhibit the ability of the lungs to move or get rid of the excess secretions that these conditions produce.

Because of their antihistamine ingredient, Excedrin PM and Tylenol PM should be used with caution by people with glaucoma, hyperthyroidism, heart disease, high blood pressure, or an enlarged prostate; if you have any of these conditions, consult your doctor before using them.

The antihistamine ingredient in these products acts as a depressant on the central nervous system (CNS), and can cause sleepiness or grogginess and interfere with the ability to concentrate. Your ability to perform activities that require your full alertness and coordination, such as driving a motor vehicle or operating machinery, may be affected. Drinking alcohol while you are taking Excedrin PM or Tylenol PM can aggravate these effects.

Possible Side Effects

- ▼ Most common: lightheadedness, restlessness, nervousness, sleeplessness, sedation, excitability, dizziness, poor coordination, and upset stomach.
- ▼ Less common: dry eyes, nose, and mouth; blurred vision; difficulty urinating; irritability (at high doses); and increased or irregular heart rate.

Possible Side Effects ***(continued)***

▼ Rare: extreme fatigue, rashes, hives, sore throat, fever, unexplained bleeding or bruising, anemia, yellowing of the skin or eyes, blood in the urine, painful or frequent urination, and decreased output of urine volume.

Drug Interactions

• Acetaminophen's effects may be reduced by long-term use or large doses of barbiturate drugs; the anticonvulsants carbamazepine and phenytoin (and other similar drugs); rifampin, used to treat tuberculosis (TB) and sulfinpyrazone, used to treat gout. These drugs may also increase the chances of liver toxicity if taken with acetaminophen. Chronically taking large doses of acetaminophen with isoniazid (used to treat TB) may increase the risk of liver damage.

• If Excedrin PM or Tylenol PM are taken with an anticoagulant such as warfarin, the acetaminophen in them may increase the blood-thinning effect of the anticoagulant agent. This does not occur with occasional use.

• People with acquired immunodeficiency syndrome (AIDS) and AIDS-related complex who are taking zidovudine (AZT) may experience increased suppression of bone marrow production if they also take products that contain acetaminophen, such as Excedrin PM and Tylenol PM. However, studies have not shown that short-term use (less than 7 days) of acetaminophen increases the risk of bone marrow suppression or causes a decrease in white blood cells in people taking AZT. Acetaminophen, when taken on a short-term basis or only as needed, is the recommended OTC pain-relieving drug for people with AIDS who are taking AZT, but you should contact your doctor for proper monitoring of AZT and acetaminophen interaction.

• The antihistamine ingredient in Excedrin PM and Tylenol PM can enhance the effect of other drugs that depress the CNS, such as barbiturates, tranquilizers, sleeping medications, and alcohol (present in many OTC preparations). If you are taking other depressant drugs, check with your doctor before taking Excedrin PM or Tylenol PM.

• Because of their antihistamine ingredient, neither Excedrin PM nor Tylenol PM should be used at the same time as a monoamine oxidase inhibitor (MAOI) or within 2 weeks of stopping treatment with an MAOI. MAOIs are used to treat depression, other psychiatric or emotional conditions, and Parkinson's disease. If you are not sure whether you are or have been taking an MAOI, check with your doctor or pharmacist before you use Excedrin PM or Tylenol PM.

• The antihistamine ingredient in Excedrin PM and Tylenol PM can affect the results of skin and blood tests. Notify your health care professional before scheduling these tests if you are taking Excedrin PM or Tylenol PM.

• Avoid alcohol while taking Excedrin PM or Tylenol PM. (Be aware that alcohol is found in many OTC preparations.) Alcohol interacts with acetaminophen and may contribute to liver damage; it also increases the sedative effects of antihistamines (see "Cautions and Warnings").

Food Interactions

None known.

Usual Dose

Each Excedrin PM tablet, caplet, and liquigel contains 500 mg of acetaminophen and 38 mg of diphenhydramine.

Each Tylenol PM caplet, geltab, and gelcap contains 500 mg of acetaminophen and 25 mg of diphenhydramine.

Adult and Child (age 12 and over): At bedtime: 2 Excedrin PM tablets, caplets, or liquigels; or 2 Tylenol PM caplets, geltabs, or gelcaps; or as directed by your doctor.

Child (under age 12): Consult your doctor.

Overdosage

Symptoms of overdose include nausea, vomiting, abdominal pain, low blood pressure, fever, flushed face, dry mouth, dilated pupils, loss of muscle coordination, confusion, excitability, hallucinations, drowsiness, coma, seizures, yellowing of the skin and eyes, and liver damage. Symptoms may develop within 30 minutes, but may not be seen for as long as 2 days after the overdose.

Even if the victim is not displaying any of the symptoms listed above, do the following in case of accidental overdose: If the victim is unconscious or having convulsions, call for an ambulance immediately. If you take the victim to an emergency room, be sure to bring the bottle or container with you. If the victim is conscious, call your local poison control center or a health care professional. The poison control center may suggest inducing vomiting with ipecac syrup (available without a prescription at any pharmacy). DO NOT induce vomiting unless specifically instructed to do so.

Special Populations

Pregnancy/Breast-feeding

Antihistamines, are not recommended for use during pregnancy unless directed by your doctor. Antihistamines and acetaminophen are known to pass into the breast milk of nursing mothers and may cause side effects in infants. Check with your doctor before taking Excedrin PM or Tylenol PM if you are or might be pregnant, or if you are breast-feeding.

Infants/Children

Children may be more susceptible to the side effects of Excedrin PM and Tylenol PM. They are also more susceptible to accidental antihistamine overdose. Do not give either Excedrin PM or Tylenol PM to a child under age 12 unless directed by your doctor.

Seniors

Because acetaminophen may clear the body more slowly in older adults, side effects of Excedrin PM or Tylenol PM may be more noticeable in seniors.

Older adults may also be more sensitive to the side effects of the antihistamine ingredient in Excedrin PM and Tylenol PM. They may experience nervousness, irritability, and restlessness. Dizziness, sedation, and low blood pressure may also occur. Older men may experience difficulty in urinating.

Persons over age 80 and those with acute physical disorders or dementia may be at risk of developing delerium from even small doses of the antihistamine diphenhydramine.

Nervine Nighttime Sleep-Aid

(NER-vine)

*see **Diphenhydramine,** page 796*

Tylenol PM (TYE-leh-nol)

*see **Excedrin PM,** page 409*

Vivarin (VYE-var-in)

*see **Caffeine,** page 715*

Chapter 7: Allergy and Sinus Pain Relief

An allergy is a condition in which the body becomes very sensitive to certain substances in the environment. These substances, called allergens, are harmless to most people. But in those susceptible to them, exposure to allergens causes the body's immune system to respond by trying to destroy or counteract the irritating substance. This immune response, however, is far out of proportion to the actual threat to the person's health. The exaggerated response produces the typical symptoms of allergies.

A common type of chronic allergy is rhinitis, also called allergic rhinitis or hay fever. Despite its name, hay fever is not caused by hay and does not involve fever. Hay fever produces a range of symptoms (see box).

Hay Fever Symptoms

- Sneezing
- Itchy, watery, red eyes
- Puffy eyes
- Runny nose
- Nasal congestion (leading to mild sore throat)
- Postnasal drip (continuous trickle of mucus from the back of the nose into the throat)
- Loss of taste
- Loss of smell
- Earache
- Sinus headache
- Itching in the mouth and throat
- Malaise
- Fatigue

Although colds and flu share some of the same symptoms as many allergies, those conditions result from infection by bacteria or viruses, while allergies are a response to allergens. (Colds are sometimes called acute infectious rhinitis; for more information, see chapter 2.)

Other allergies can involve local reactions on the surface of the skin or the bronchial tubes, causing asthma. People frequently develop allergies to certain foods, such as dairy products, wheat products (e.g., breads and cereals), and peanuts. Allergies to both prescription and OTC drugs can also occur. Allergies can contribute to a range of other health problems, including ear infections, related hearing loss, sinusitis, recurrent sore throat, cough, headache, fatigue, irritability, loss of sleep, and poor performance on the job or at school. In severe cases, such as allergy to venom from bee stings, the condition can be fatal.

The Allergy-Sinus Connection

Sinus headache occurs when an infection or blockage of the sinuses causes swelling of the sensitive sinus cavity walls. Pain is usually felt upon waking and may lessen after the sufferer has been upright for some time. Blowing one's nose or leaning over may increase the pain.

Sinusitis (sinus infection) is caused by an infection of the sinus cavity lining. Chronic allergic rhinitis often causes sinusitis because infections can start in the mucus present in the nose and easily travel to the sinuses. Chronis sinusitis is often the result of frequent sinus infections that have been left untreated. Scarring from previous infections can cause the sinus opening to narrow or close, making it difficult for the sinuses to drain properly.

Allergies are very common. In the U.S., as many as 1 person in 7 suffers from some form of allergy. Allergies are the fifth most common chronic condition, accounting for about 10% of all visits to a doctor's office. Although allergies can develop at any age, they usually first appear between ages 5 and 30. Boys are more likely to be allergic than girls, but among adults the rate is about the same.

It is not clear what causes allergies. In about 60% of cases, allergies appear to be inherited, passed on from parents to children. Other cases may be related to various factors such as use of tobacco, a history of viral infections, hormonal conditions, and environmental factors. Generally, though, scientists are not sure why some people have allergies and others do not.

Onset of Allergies

An allergy develops following a series of events. The first thing that must happen is exposure to an allergen such as pollen from ragweed. (You can't be allergic to something you've never encountered, although the exposure may be unknown to you; e.g., you can become sensitized to antibiotics used in cow and cattle feed when you drink milk or eat beef.) When the allergen is inhaled, it comes into contact with the mucous membranes of the nose or throat. Allergens consumed in food enter the bloodstream during the process of digestion.

The surface of the allergen molecule is studded with various proteins, like cloves on a ham. As they circulate in the body, those proteins come into contact with cells of the immune system. If this is the first time the allergen is present in the body, cells called lymphocytes create a blueprint of the invader so it will be recognized the next time it shows up.

Over the next few weeks, the immune system uses this blueprint to manufacture thousands of copies of antibodies. These are specialized proteins designed to recognize one and only one type of allergen. Antibodies are technically called immunoglobulins. There are several kinds of immunoglobulins; the one most often involved in allergic reactions is immunoglobulin E, or IgE. Everybody produces IgE to some extent, but for some reason, people with a genetic tendency to produce higher amounts are the ones who develop allergies. Substances that trigger allergic reactions on the skin, such as poison ivy, or environmental irritants, such as smoke or perfumes, cause the body to produce other types of immunoglobulins.

Like alert sentries, the antibodies circulate in the bloodstream, waiting for the invader or antigen to reappear. Once the antibodies are present in large numbers, the body has become sensitized to the allergen. Each person has thousands of different antibodies, all waiting for the call to action against its one specific allergen.

The next time the same allergen appears in the body, it eventually bumps into the antibody assigned to it. The antibody becomes activated, sending out chemical signals alerting the other antibody molecules in the vicinity that trouble is brewing. The stimulated antibodies then attach themselves to certain cells called mast cells. Mast cells are found throughout the body, especially in connective tissue such as skin, the lining of the nose and lungs, the gastrointestinal tract, and the reproductive system. Each mast cell contains hundreds of little pockets filled with more than 2 dozen chemicals, including histamine. When the antibodies attach to mast cells, they cause the cells to release histamine and other chemicals into the bloodstream. Histamine is responsible for allergy symptoms: It irritates nearby nerves, leading to itching; causes blood vessels to expand; and allows fluids to leak out of cells into the surrounding tissue, producing congested or runny nose, watery eyes, and swelling.

Causes of Allergies

Allergies can be seasonal, coming and going at different times of the year, or they can be perennial, occurring year-round. The major cause of seasonal allergies is pollen. Pollen grains are reproductive cells released by the male organs of plants. The pollen is carried by the wind until it happens to land on the female organs of another plant of the same species. This fertilizes the plant's seeds, allowing it to reproduce.

In the U.S., the pollen responsible for about 75% of cases of hay fever is ragweed. A ragweed plant can release up to a billion pollen particles in a single season. Other plants, including grasses, trees, and flowers, also release pollen. The pollen from flowers is not usually a cause of allergies because such particles are usually too heavy to be carried by the breeze. Allergies arising in spring are usually due to tree pollen; those in early summer tend to be caused by grass, while allergies in fall are usually due to weeds.

There are other sources of allergens. The most prevalent cause of perennial allergies worldwide is the dust mite. These microscopic 8-legged creatures are found in every temperate climate. To survive and reproduce, dust mites require an environment where the temperature stays above

65°F and the relative humidity is at least 50%—coincidentally, the same conditions found in most people's homes year-round. If you were to sweep the floor and collect a pile of dust weighing about the same as a paper clip, you would find at least 100 to 500 dust mites among the particles. The presence of dust mites is not a sign of poor housekeeping; it is virtually impossible to prevent these creatures from taking up residence.

Dust mites live between the fibers in bedding, mattresses, clothing, carpeting, and upholstered furniture. They thrive by eating the particles of dead skin that we humans shed constantly. Actually, the mites themselves are not what cause allergies. It's their feces, little balls of sticky stuff that cling to the fibers of bedclothes, rugs, and other fabrics. If allergic people inhale these particles, they develop a reaction to the proteins the material contains. Dust can be stirred up by walking across the carpet, by changing the bedclothes, and especially, by vacuuming carpets or drapes. The particles can circulate in the air as long as a half hour after being disturbed. The dust mite season peaks in the summer, but the allergy symptoms can be triggered throughout the year. Feces from cockroaches is another common allergen found in urban environments.

Other allergens that cause hay fever include mold, which is commonly found in bathrooms, damp basements, around window moldings, and in air conditioners and their vents. It is also a component in decaying vegetation, such as rotting logs, mulch, and compost piles.

Pet dander is a major cause of allergy. Dander is made of tiny flakes from an animal's skin, hair, or feathers. These tiny flakes float in the air and make up a significant portion of dust found in the homes where they live. The actual substance that triggers allergic reactions to cats is protein in their saliva. Cats lick their fur; the saliva remains on the hairs after they are shed. In some cases, animal urine or droppings can also trigger allergic reactions. Pets most likely to cause allergies are cats, dogs, rodents, and birds. Ideally, for the sake of their health, people who are allergic should not keep pets, especially ones with hair, fur, or feathers. Safe pets—animals that do not cause allergies—include fish, turtles, lizards, hermit crabs, and snakes. (see box).

Managing Pet Allergies

If you are allergic to your pet but cannot bear to give it up, there are some steps you can take to minimize your risk of developing allergy symptoms.

- Do not allow the animal in the bedroom or other rooms where you spend a lot of time.
- Once the animal has been removed from the bedroom, replace linens, bedding, and carpeting.
- Keep the animal outside whenever possible.
- Keep the pet well groomed to reduce shedding; ask someone who is not allergic to be responsible for grooming.
- Do not clean the litter box or cage yourself.
- Talk to your doctor about getting allergy shots to prevent symptoms from developing.
- Get fresh air whenever possible.
- Install an air filtration system.
- Use allergy medications when needed to control symptoms.

Seek medical attention if any of the following applies to you

- Difficulty breathing
- Symptoms that do not improve despite appropriate self-treatment
- Fever, significant sore throat, vomiting, or diarrhea

Treatment for Allergies

The best way to reduce the risk of allergies is to avoid the substances that trigger symptoms: pollen, dust, mold, and animal dander (see box).

If allergens cannot be avoided, or if symptoms arise despite avoidance, OTC medications can provide significant relief. The mainstays of treatment for allergy symptoms are antihistamines and decongestants.

As their name indicates, antihistamines counteract the effects of histamine, the main chemical released by cells in response to an allergen. Seasonal allergies are easier to treat than perennial ones, because the cause of the allergy will eventually disappear, and with it, the misery.

For best results, antihistamines should be taken prior to the start of allergy season or immediately after exposure to the allergen, so that the drug can block the effects of histamine and thus prevent symptoms from developing. These drugs do not cure the allergy, nor do they prevent release of histamine from cells. Even at their best, antihistamines reduce symptoms by only about 50%, because they do not counteract any of the other symptom-causing chemicals that the mast cells release. But they do help relieve the main symptoms, especially itching, sneezing, and nasal irritation. They are less effective at drying up mucus production, and they do not relieve nasal congestion.

A newly approved OTC medication for allergies—cromolyn sodium (Nasalcrom)—works differently than antihistamines. With regular use, it suppresses inflammatory cell activity and stabilizes mast cells in the nose.

There are literally hundreds of products available for treatment of allergies, colds, and the flu. Each product contains one of several dozen types of antihistamines. The choice of OTC medication depends on the exact combination of active ingredients you need for your particular symptoms, the formulation you prefer, and the length of time you anticipate needing the medication. Antihistamines can be administered in liquid eyedrop solutions, or they can be taken orally as tablets or liquids. Certain products start to work immediately and are short-acting (4 to 6 hours). Timed-release formulations may deliver the medication for up to 12 hours, providing longer-lasting relief.

The most common side effect of antihistamines, especially the older ones, is daytime sedation or drowsiness. (It is this ability of antihistamines to induce sleep that led to their use as sleeping aids; for more information, see chapter 6.) Products labeled for nighttime use contain more sedating forms of antihistamine, such as diphenhydramine, doxylamine, and phenyltoloxamine. The least sedating antihistamines (but still a problem for many people) are chlorpheniramine, brompheniramine, and pheniramine. Other potential side effects include dryness of the nose, mouth, and eyes, blurred vision, rapid heartbeat, impaired mental performance, and difficulty urinating in men with enlarged prostates.

Avoiding Allergies

To reduce the risk of exposure to pollen, mold, and other allergens, consider taking the following steps:

- Avoid going outside, especially on windy days and in the morning, when pollen counts tend to be at their highest.
- Install and use air conditioners in the home; use the air conditioner in the car when necessary. (Note: this will help you avoid pollen allergies only; it may make mold allergies worse).
- Use dehumidifiers to keep humidity low and reduce the dust mite population.
- Install an air cleaner with a high-efficiency or electrostatic filter.
- Shower or bathe to remove pollen after being outdoors.
- Do not keep houseplants (a potential source of mold).
- Clean shower curtains, bathroom walls, toilet, sink, and tub regularly using a mixture of water and chlorine bleach.
- Repair areas around the home where dry rot has occurred.
- Waterproof your basement.
- Improve ventilation in kitchens and bathrooms.
- Decorate using mold-proof paint instead of wallpaper.
- Avoid use of carpets or rugs, especially in bathrooms or other damp rooms.
- Discard old and unwanted shoes, clothes, and bedding.
- Use window shades instead of fabric drapes or venetian blinds.
- Wear a mask when doing household cleaning chores or gardening, or ask (or hire) other people to handle these chores for you.
- Use a damp mop on floors and wipe furniture and shelves with a damp cloth to keep down dust.
- Use a vacuum cleaner with specially designed filters for trapping dust and dust mites.
- Vacuum furniture and drapes as well as floors.

Avoiding Allergies (*continued*)

- Use cleaners such as benzyl benzoate or tannic acid spray when washing carpets and upholstery.
- Wash bedding in hot water (more than 130°F) every 7 to 10 days.
- Do not hang clothes outdoors to dry.
- Do not use mattress pads.
- Use plastic slipcovers on mattresses, chairs, and sofas.
- Reduce the number of places where dust can collect, such as shelves and knickknack displays.

More recently discovered products (the second-generation antihistamines) are more selective in their actions—that is, they affect fewer systems in the body—and are thus less likely to cause drowsiness and other adverse reactions. At this writing, however, second-generation antihistamines such as cetirizine (Zyrtec) are still available in the U.S. only with a prescription.

For some people, antihistamines seem to become less effective if they are used for prolonged periods. This loss of efficacy may be the result of factors other than resistance to the medication, such as exposure to higher amounts of allergen or development of similar symptoms from a second medical disease. However, if you find that an OTC medication is not providing you with the same level of relief you are accustomed to, you might consider switching to another type of antihistamine.

The other main active ingredient available in many allergy products is a decongestant. These drugs work by shrinking swollen blood vessels to reduce tissue swelling and sinus pressure.

Side effects seldom result from the use of topical decongestants (those that are inhaled or applied directly to the nostrils), although they can sometimes cause minor irritation. However, these products, especially the short-acting variety, should not be used for longer than 3 to 5 days because they can actually make congestion worse. For that reason, systemic (whole-body) decongestants, taken orally, are better for use in chronic allergies. As a rule, these drugs tend to be short acting (4 to 6 hours). However, a relatively new product, Efidac/24, is designed to release the decongestant over a 24-hour period, thus providing relief throughout the day and night. Potential side effects of systemic decongestants include increased blood pressure, rapid or irregular heart rate, headache, and urine retention in older men with enlarged prostates.

Some OTC allergy products contain guaifenesin, a drug classified as an expectorant. Expectorants help break up mucus and make it easier to expel through coughing. Cough, however, is seldom a major symptom of allergic rhinitis, and it is not clear whether this medication actually does much good. By the same token, if you suffer from allergies, it is probably not necessary to take a medication that contains an antitussive (cough suppressant). Many products also contain various pain relievers, such as acetaminophen or ibuprofen.

If you do not experience adequate relief from OTC allergy products, talk to your physician. You may be a candidate for treatment with prescription medications. Options include inhaled corticosteroids, which reduce inflammation, mucus secretion, and swelling. If you have perennial allergies, ask about immunotherapy (allergy shots). This treatment, which helps up to 85% of people who take it, is the only available therapy that provides long-lasting protection against allergies.

OTC Products for Allergies

- Allergy preventative
  - Cromolyn sodium
- Systemic antihistamines
  - Brompheniramine
  - Chlorcyclizine
  - Chlorpheniramine
  - Clemastine
  - Dexbrompheniramine
  - Dexchlorpheniramine
  - Diphenhydramine
  - Doxylamine
  - Phenindamine
  - Pheniramine
  - Pyrilamine
  - Thonzylamine
  - Triprolidine
- Topical decongestants
  - Drops, sprays
    - Short acting (4 to 6 hours)
      - Ephedrine
      - Epinephrine
      - Naphazoline
      - Phenylephrine
      - Tetrahydrozaline
    - Intermediate acting (6 to 10 hours)
      - Xylometazoline
    - Long acting (10 or more hours)
      - Oxymetazoline
  - Inhalers
    - Deoxyephedrine
    - Prophylhexedrine
- Systemic decongestants
  - Ephedrine
  - Phenylephrine
  - Phenylpropanolamine
  - Pseudoephedrine
- Ophthalmic (eye) decongestants
  - Epinephrine
  - Naphazoline
  - Oxymetazoline
  - Phenylephrine
  - Tetrahydrozaline
- Analgesics

Antihistamines

Check the chart in chapter 2 for antihistamine combination products.

BRAND NAME	ANTIHISTAMINES					
	brompheniramine maleate	chlorpheniramine maleate	clemastine fumarate	diphenhydramine HCl	phenira-mine	pyrilamine maleate
A.R.M.		5mg				
AllerMax (caplet)				50mg		
Aller-med				25mg		
Antihist-1			1.34mg			
Benadryl Allergy (capsule)				25mg		
Benadryl Allergy (chewable tablet)				12.5mg		
Benadryl Allergy (liquid) [A]				12.5mg/5ml		
Benadryl Allergy (tablet)				25mg		
Benadryl Allergy Dye-Free [A]				6.25mg/5ml		
Benadryl Allergy Dye-Free Liqui-gels				25mg		
Chlor-Trimeton Allergy [A]		2mg/5ml				
Chlor-Trimeton 8-Hour Allergy		8mg				
Chlor-Trimeton 4-Hour Allergy		4mg				
Chlor-Trimeton 12-Hour Allergy		12mg				
Codimal (capsule) [A]		2mg				
Codimal (tablet)		2mg				
Codimal DM [A]						8.3mg/5ml
Codimal PH [A]						8.3mg/5ml
Diabetic Tussin Allergy Relief [A]		2mg				
Dimetane Allergy Extentabs	12mg					
Dimetapp Allergy	4mg					

Dimetapp Allergy Liqui-Gels	4mg				
Diphenadryl				12.5mg/5ml	
Efidac 24 Chlorpheniramine		16mg			
Genahist (capsule)				25mg	
Genahist (elixir)				12.5mg/5ml	
Hydramine Cough				12.5mg/5ml	
Nolahist					25mg
Tavist-1 Antihistamine			1.34mg		

Brand Name

Actifed Cold & Allergy (AK-tif-ed)

Generic Ingredients

Pseudoephedrine
Triprolidine hydrochloride

Type of Drug

Antihistamine and decongestant.

Used for

Relief of runny nose, sneezing, nasal congestion, itchy and watery eyes, and itching of the nose or throat associated with colds and allergies.

General Information

Some OTC products use a combination of drugs to relieve the many symptoms that can accompany colds and allergies. Actifed Cold & Allergy contains an antihistamine and a decongestant.

The antihistamine in Actifed Cold & Allergy is tripolidine hydrochloride. Antihistamines block the release of histamine, a chemical substance released by the body during an allergic reaction, thus relieving the sneezing and itching that often occur with colds and allergies. They can also aid in stopping a runny nose by reducing the secretions caused by histamine release.

Because histamine is only one of several substances released during an allergic reaction, antihistamines can reduce only about 40% to 60% of allergic symptoms.

The decongestant in Actifed Cold & Allergy is pseudoephedrine, an oral decongestant. Decongestants work by narrowing or constricting the blood vessels. This relieves the swelling of mucous membranes of the nose and sinuses. Unlike topical decongestants (decongestant nasal sprays), which act on local blood vessels, oral decongestants may constrict blood vessels throughout the body.

Actifed Cold & Allergy will not cure or prevent allergies or colds. The best you can hope for is symptomatic relief. Colds will usually go away in 1 to 2 weeks whether they are treated or not.

Cautions and Warnings

Do not take Actifed Cold & Allergy for more than 7 days continuously. If symptoms do not improve, or if fever is present, see a doctor.

Do not exceed the recommended daily dosage of Actifed Cold & Allergy.

Actifed Cold & Allergy should be used with caution if you have a condition that causes breathing problems, such as emphysema, chronic bronchitis, or asthma. Its antihistamine ingredient, triprolidine, acts to dry the mucous membranes. This in turn can inhibit the ability of the lungs to move or get rid of the excess secretions that these diseases produce.

Actifed Cold & Allergy should be used with caution by people with glaucoma, hyperthyroidism, heart disease, high blood pressure, diabetes, or an enlarged prostate, because it can worsen these conditions. If you have any of these conditions, take Actifed Cold & Allergy only on the advice of a physician.

The antihistamine ingredient in Actifed Cold & Allergy acts as a depressant on the central nervous system (CNS), and can cause sleepiness or grogginess and interfere with the ability to concentrate. Use caution when driving a motor vehicle or operating machinery. Refrain from drinking alcohol while taking Actifed Cold & Allergy, because alcohol makes the drowsiness worse. Be aware that many drugs available by prescription or OTC contain alcohol.

Possible Side Effects

- ▼ Most common: restlessness, nervousness, sleeplessness or drowsiness, dizziness, excitability, poor muscle coordination, headache, and upset stomach.
- ▼ Less common: blurred vision; difficulty urinating; irritability (at high doses); increased blood pressure; increased or irregular heart rate; dry eyes, nose, and mouth; and heart palpitations.
- ▼ Rare: anxiety, tremors, hallucinations, seizures, and cardiovascular collapse.

Drug Interactions

• The antihistamine ingredient in Actifed Cold & Allergy can enhance the effect of other CNS depressants, such as barbiturates, tranquilizers, sleeping medications, and alcohol (present in many OTC preparations). If you drink alcohol, or if you are taking any drugs that contain alcohol or any other depressant drugs, check with your doctor before taking Actifed Cold & Allergy.

• Antihistimines can also affect the results of skin and blood tests. Notify your health care professional before scheduling these tests if you are taking Actifed Cold & Allergy.

• Actifed Cold & Allergy should not be used at the same time as a monoamine oxidase inhibitor (MAOI) or within 2 weeks of stopping treatment with an MAOI. MAOIs are used to treat depression, other psychiatric or emotional conditions, and Parkinson's disease. If you are not sure whether you are or have been taking an MAOI, check with your doctor or pharmacist before you use Actifed Cold & Allergy.

• Taking Actifed Cold & Allergy along with another decongestant can increase the risk of adverse effects and toxicity. If you are taking another decongestant, do not take Actifed Cold & Allergy without first asking your doctor.

• The effects of the decongestant in Actifed Cold & Allergy may combine with those of caffeine, a CNS stimulant found in many prescription and OTC drugs. This combination can cause disorientation, delirium, and other side effects.

Food Interactions

Decongestants interact adversely with caffeine (see "Drug Interactions"), which is found in many popular beverages, including coffee, tea, and cola, and in chocolate.

Usual Dose

To relieve the symptoms of allergy, it is best to take Actifed Cold & Allergy on a schedule rather than as needed, because histamine is released almost continuously.

Each tablet contains 60 mg of pseudoephedrine and 2.5 mg of triprolidine hydrochloride.

Adult and Child (age 12 and over): 1 tablet every 4–6 hours. Do not exceed 4 doses in 24 hours.

Child (age 6–11): 1/2 tablet every 4–6 hours. Do not exceed 4 doses in 24 hours.

Child (under age 6): Consult your doctor.

You may minimize the inconvenience of the sedative effects of Actifed Cold & Allergy by taking a full dose at bedtime and using the smallest recommended doses during the day. You can establish the lowest dose necessary for effective relief by starting with the lowest dose when you begin taking the drug, and gradually increasing the dosage over several days, as needed.

If you forget to take a dose of Actifed Cold & Allergy, do so as soon as you remember. If it is almost time for your next dose, skip the one you forgot and continue with your regular schedule. Do not take a double dose.

Overdosage

Symptoms of overdose in children include dilated pupils, flushed face, dry mouth, fever, excitability, hallucinations, loss of muscle coordination, and seizures.

In adults, severe overdose can cause drowsiness or coma, which may be followed by excitability or seizures. Eventually fluid can build up in the brain; the kidneys may fail, and the heart and lungs may stop working, resulting in death. Symptoms may develop within 30 minutes to 2 hours following an overdose, and death may occur within 18 hours.

Even if the victim is not displaying any of the symptoms listed above, do the following in case of accidental overdose: If the victim is unconscious or having convulsions, call for an ambulance immediately. If you take the victim to an emergency room, be sure to bring the bottle or container with you. If the victim is conscious, call your local poison control center or a health care professional. The poison control center may suggest inducing vomiting with ipecac syrup (available without a prescription at any pharmacy). DO NOT induce vomiting unless specifically instructed to do so.

Special Populations

Pregnancy/Breast-feeding

Antihistamines are not recommended for use during pregnancy unless directed by your doctor. Antihistamines and decongestants are known to pass into the breast milk of nursing mothers and may cause side effects in infants.

Check with your doctor before taking Actifed Cold & Allergy if you are or might be pregnant, or if you are breast-feeding.

Infants/Children
Children may be more susceptible to the side effects of Actifed Cold & Allergy. They are also more susceptible to accidental antihistamine overdose. Do not give Actifed Cold & Allergy to a child under 6 unless directed by your doctor.

Seniors
Seniors may be more sensitive to the side effects of antihistamines and decongestants. They may experience nervousness, irritability, restlessness, dizziness, sedation, hallucinations, seizures, and low blood pressure. Most mild reactions may be handled by either lowering the dose or switching to another product.

Seniors taking Actifed Cold & Allergy should be especially cautious about the amount of caffeine they ingest (see "Drug Interactions").

Afrin 12-Hour Nasal Spray (AFF-rin)

*see **Oxymetazoline Hydrochloride,** page 947*

Benadryl Allergy (BEN-uh-drill)

*see **Diphenhydramine,** page 796*

Brand Name

Benadryl Allergy Decongestant Tablets (BEN-uh-drill)

Generic Ingredients

Diphenhydramine
Pseudoephedrine

Type of drug

Antihistamine and decongestant.

Used for

Temporary relief of runny nose, sneezing, nasal congestion, itchy and watery eyes, and itching of the nose and throat associated with colds and allergies.

General Information

Some OTC products use a combination of drugs to relieve symptoms that can accompany colds and allergies. Benadryl Allergy Decongestant contains an antihistamine and a decongestant.

The antihistamine ingredient in Benadryl Allergy Decongestant is diphenhydramine. Antihistamines block the release of histamine in the body, relieving the sneezing and itching that often occurs with colds and allergies. They can also aid in stopping a runny nose by reducing the secretions caused by histamine release.

Because histamine is only one of several substances released by the body during an allergic reaction, antihistamines can only reduce about 40% to 60% of allergic symptoms.

The decongestant ingredient in Benadryl Allergy Decongestant is pseudoephedrine, an oral decongestant. Decongestants relieve congestion by narrowing or constricting blood vessels. This relieves the swelling of the mucous membranes of the nose and sinuses. Unlike topical decongestants (decongestant nasal sprays) that act on local blood vessels, oral decongestants may constrict blood vessels throughout the body.

Benadryl Allergy Decongestant will not cure or prevent colds or allergies. The best you can hope for is symptomatic relief. Colds will usually go away in 1 to 2 weeks whether they are treated or not.

Cautions and Warnings

Do not take Benadryl Allergy Decongestant for more than 7 days continuously. If symptoms do not improve or if fever is present, see your doctor.

Do not exceed the recommended daily dosage of Benadryl Allergy Decongestant.

Benadryl Allergy Decongestant should be used with caution if you have a condition that causes breathing problems, such as emphysema, chronic bronchitis, or asthma. Its antihistamine ingredient dries the mucous membranes. This in turn can inhibit the ability of the lungs to move or get rid of the excess secretions that these conditions produce.

Benadryl Allergy Decongestant should be used with caution by people with glaucoma, hyperthyroidism, heart disease, high blood pressure, diabetes, or an enlarged prostate. If you have any of these conditions, ask your doctor before using Benadryl Allergy Sinus.

The antihistamine ingredient in Benadryl Allergy Decongestant acts as a depressant on the central nervous system (CNS), and can cause sleepiness or grogginess and interfere with the ability to concentrate. Your ability to perform activities that require your full alertness and coordination, such as driving a motor vehicle or operating machinery, may be affected. Refrain from drinking alcohol while you are taking Benadryl Allergy Decongestant, because alcohol aggravates these effects.

Possible Side Effects

- ▼ Most common: restlessness, nervousness, sleeplessness or drowsiness, sedation, excitability, dizziness, poor coordination, headache, and upset stomach.
- ▼ Less common: dry eyes, nose, and mouth; blurred vision; difficulty urinating; irritability (at high doses); increased blood pressure; increased or irregular heart rate; and heart palpitations.
- ▼ Rare: anxiety, tremor, hallucinations, seizures, breathing difficulty, and cardiovascular collapse.

Drug Interactions

- The antihistamine ingredient in Benadryl Allergy Decongestant can enhance the effect of other drugs that depress the CNS, such as barbiturates, tranquilizers, sleeping medications, and alcohol (present in many OTC preparations). If you are taking other depressant drugs, check with your doctor before taking these products. Avoid drinking alcohol if you are taking Benadryl Allergy Decongestant.
- The antihistamine ingredient in Benadryl Allergy Decongestant can affect the results of skin and blood tests.

Notify your health care professional before scheduling these tests if you are taking Benadryl Allergy Decongestant.

• Benadryl Allergy Decongestant should not be used at the same time as a monoamine oxidase inhibitor (MAOI) or within 2 weeks of stopping treatment with an MAOI. MAOIs are used to treat depression, other psychiatric or emotional conditions, and Parkinson's disease. If you are not sure whether you are or have been taking an MAOI, check with your doctor or pharmacist before you use Benadryl Allergy Decongestant.

• Taking Benadryl Allergy Decongestant along with another decongestant can increase the risk of adverse effects and toxicity; if you are taking another decongestant, do not use Benadryl Allergy Decongestant without first asking your doctor.

• The effects of pseudoephedrine, the decongestant in Benadryl Allergy Decongestant may combine with those of caffeine, a CNS stimulant found in many prescription and OTC drugs. This combination can cause disorientation, delirium, and other side effects.

Food Interactions

Decongestants interact adversely with caffeine (see "Drug Interactions"), which is found in many popular beverages, including coffee, tea, and cola, and in chocolate.

Usual Dose

If you are taking Benadryl Allergy Decongestant for allergies, it is best to take it on a schedule rather than as needed because histamine is released almost continuously.

Each tablet contains 25 mg diphenhydramine and 30 mg of pseudoephedrine.

Adult and Child (age 12 and over): 1 tablet every 4–6 hours. Do not take more than 4 tablets in a 24-hour period.

Child (under age 12): Consult your doctor.

You may minimize the inconvenience of the sedative effects of Benadryl Allergy Decongestant by taking a full dose at bedtime and by using the smallest recommended dose during the day. You can establish the lowest dose necessary for effective relief by starting with the lowest dose when you begin taking the drug, and gradually increasing the dosage over several days as needed.

If you forget to take a dose of Benadryl Allergy Decongestant, do so as soon as you remember. If it is almost time for your next dose, skip the one you forgot and continue with your regular schedule. Do not take a double dose.

Overdosage

Symptoms of overdose in children include dilated pupils, flushed face, dry mouth, fever, excitability, hallucinations, loss of muscle coordination, and seizures.

In adults, severe overdose can cause drowsiness or coma, which may be followed by excitability or seizures. Eventually fluid can build up in the brain; the kidneys may fail, and the heart and lungs stop working, resulting in death. Symptoms may develop within 30 minutes to 2 hours following an overdose, and death may occur within 18 hours.

Even if the victim is not displaying any of the symptoms listed above, do the following in case of accidental overdose: If the victim is unconscious or having convulsions, call for an ambulance immediately. If you take the victim to an emergency room, be sure to bring the bottle or container with you. If the victim is conscious, call your local poison control center or a health care professional. The poison control center may suggest inducing vomiting with ipecac syrup (available without a prescription at any pharmacy). DO NOT induce vomiting unless specifically instructed to do so.

Special Populations

Pregnancy/Breast-feeding

Antihistamines are not recommended for use during pregnancy unless directed by your doctor. Antihistamines and decongestants are known to pass into the breast milk of nursing mothers and may cause side effects in infants. Check with your doctor before taking Benadryl Allergy Sinus if you are or might be pregnant, or if you are breast-feeding.

Infants/Children

Children may be more susceptible to the side effects of Benadryl Allergy Decongestant. They are also more susceptible to accidental antihistamine overdose. Do not give Benadryl Allergy Decongestant to a child under age 12 unless directed by your doctor.

Seniors

Older persons may be more sensitive to the side effects of Benadryl Allergy Decongestant. They may experience nervousness, irritability, and restlessness. Dizziness, sedation, and low blood pressure may also occur. Older men may experience difficulty in urinating. Most mild reactions may be handled by either lowering your dose or trying another antihistamine/decongestant combination. However, persons over age 80 and those with acute physical disorders or dementia may be at risk of developing delirium from even small doses of diphenhydramine.

Seniors taking Benadryl Allergy Decongestant should be especially cautious about the amount of caffeine they ingest (see "Drug Interactions").

Brand Name

Benadryl Allergy Sinus Headache

(BEN-uh-drill)

Generic Ingredients

Acetaminophen
Diphenhydramine
Pseudoephedrine

Type of drug

Antihistamine, decongestant, and analgesic (pain reliever).

Used for

Temporary relief of runny nose, sneezing, nasal and sinus congestion, itchy and watery eyes, itching of the nose and throat, headache, and minor pains associated with colds and allergies.

General Information

Some OTC products use a combination of drugs to relieve symptoms that can accompany colds and allergies. Benadryl Allergy Sinus Headache contains an antihistamine, a decongestant, and an analgesic to relieve pain.

The antihistamine ingredient in Benadryl Allergy Sinus Headache is diphenhydramine. Antihistamines block the release of histamine in the body, relieving the sneezing and itching that often occurs with colds and allergies. They can also aid in stopping a runny nose by reducing the secretions caused by histamine release.

Because histamine is only one of several substances released by the body during an allergic reaction, antihistamines can only reduce about 40% to 60% of allergic symptoms.

The decongestant ingredient in Benadryl Allergy Sinus Headache is pseudoephedrine, an oral decongestant. Decongestants relieve congestion by narrowing or constricting blood vessels. This relieves the swelling of the mucous membranes of the nose and sinuses. Unlike topical decongestants (decongestant nasal sprays) that act on local blood vessels, oral decongestants may constrict blood vessels throughout the body.

Acetaminophen, the analgesic ingredient in Benadryl Allergy Sinus Headache, relieves pain and headache.

Benadryl Allergy Sinus Headache will not cure or prevent colds or allergies. The best you can hope for is symptomatic relief. Colds will usually go away in 1 to 2 weeks whether they are treated or not.

Cautions and Warnings

Do not take Benadryl Allergy Sinus Headache for more than 10 days continuously, or 3 days continuously in the presence of fever. If symptoms do not improve, see your doctor.

Do not exceed the recommended daily dosage of Benadryl Allergy Sinus Headache.

Benadryl Allergy Sinus Headache should be used with caution if you have a condition that causes breathing problems, such as emphysema, chronic bronchitis, or asthma. Its antihistamine ingredient dries the mucous membranes. This in turn can inhibit the ability of the lungs to move or get rid of the excess secretions that these conditions produce.

Benadryl Allergy Sinus Headache should be used with caution by people with glaucoma, hyperthyroidism, heart disease, high blood pressure, diabetes, or an enlarged prostate. If you have any of these conditions, consult your doctor before using Benadryl Allergy Sinus Headache.

The antihistamine ingredient in Benadryl Allergy Sinus Headache acts as a depressant on the central nervous system (CNS), and can cause sleepiness or grogginess and interfere with the ability to concentrate. Your ability to perform activities that require your full alertness and coordination, such as driving a motor vehicle or operating machinery, may be affected. Refrain from drinking alcohol while you are taking Benadryl Allergy Sinus Headache, because alcohol aggravates these effects.

In doses of more than 4 grams per day, the acetaminophen ingredient in Benadryl Allergy Sinus Headache is potentially toxic to the liver. Use Benadryl Allergy Sinus Headache with caution if you have kidney or liver disease or viral infections of the liver. Studies have shown that the risk of liver damage with acetaminophen is associated with fasting and alcohol use. People with liver disease who are taking other drugs that are potentially damaging to the liver, people who do not eat regularly, or who drink alcohol (even moderately) are especially at risk. If you take Benadryl Allergy Sinus Headache regularly, avoid drinking alcohol and/or fasting.

Possible Side Effects

- ▼ Most common: restlessness, nervousness, sleeplessness or drowsiness, sedation, excitability, dizziness, lightheadedness, poor coordination, headache, and upset stomach.
- ▼ Less common: dry eyes, nose, and mouth; blurred vision; difficulty urinating; irritability (at high doses); increased blood pressure; increased or irregular heart rate; and heart palpitations.
- ▼ Rare: extreme fatigue; rash, itching, or hives; sore throat or fever; unexplained bleeding or bruising; anemia; yellowing of the skin or eyes; blood in the urine; painful or frequent urination; decreased output of urine volume; anxiety, tremor, hallucinations, seizures, breathing difficulty, and cardiovascular collapse.

Drug Interactions

• The antihistamine ingredient in Benadryl Allergy Sinus Headache can enhance the effect of other drugs that depress the CNS, such as barbiturates, tranquilizers, sleeping medications, and alcohol (present in many OTC preparations). If you are taking other depressant drugs, check with your doctor before taking these products. Avoid drinking alcohol if you are taking Benadryl Allergy Sinus Headache.

• The antihistamine ingredient in Benadryl Allergy Sinus Headache can affect the results of skin and blood tests. Notify your health care professional before scheduling these tests if you are taking Benadryl Allergy Sinus Headache.

• Benadryl Allergy Sinus Headache should not be used at the same time as a monoamine oxidase inhibitor (MAOI) or within 2 weeks of stopping treatment with an MAOI. MAOIs are used to treat depression, other psychiatric or emotional conditions, and Parkinson's disease. If you are not sure whether you are or have been taking an MAOI, check with your doctor or pharmacist before you use Benadryl Allergy Sinus Headache.

• Taking Benadryl Allergy Sinus Headache along with another decongestant can increase the risk of adverse effects and toxicity; if you are taking another decongestant, do not use Benadryl Allergy Sinus Headache without first asking your doctor.

• The effects of the decongestant in Benadryl Allergy Sinus Headache may combine with those of caffeine, a CNS stimulant found in many prescription and OTC drugs. This combination can cause disorientation, delirium, and other side effects.

• The effect of the acetaminophen in Benadryl Allergy Sinus Headache may be reduced by long-term use or large doses of barbiturate drugs; the anticonvulsants carbamazepine and phenytoin (and other similar drugs); rifampin, used to treat tuberculosis (TB), and sulfinpyrazone, used to treat gout. These drugs may also increase the chances of liver toxicity if taken with acetaminophen. Chronically taking large doses of acetaminophen with isoniazid (used to treat TB) may also increase the risk of liver damage.

• If Benadryl Allergy Sinus Headache is taken with an anticoagulant such as warfarin, the acetaminophen in it may increase the blood-thinning effect of the anticoagulant agent. This does not occur with occasional use.

• People with AIDS and AIDS-related complex who are taking zidovudine (AZT) may experience increased suppression of bone marrow production if they also take products that contain acetaminophen, such as Benadryl Allergy Sinus Headache. However, studies have not shown that short-term use (less than 7 days) of acetaminophen increases the risk of bone marrow suppression or causes a decrease in white blood cells in people taking AZT. Contact your doctor for proper monitoring of the AZT and acetaminophen interaction.

• Avoid alcohol while taking Benadryl Allergy Sinus Headache. (Be aware that alcohol is found in many OTC preparations.) Alcohol may contribute to the risk of liver damage associated with acetaminophen; it also increases the sedative effects of antihistamines (see "Cautions and Warnings").

Food Interactions

Decongestants interact adversely with caffeine (see "Drug Interactions"), which is found in many popular beverages, including coffee, tea, and cola, and in chocolate.

Usual Dose

If you are taking Benadryl Allergy Sinus Headache for allergies, it is best to take it on a schedule rather than as needed because histamine is released almost continuously.

Each caplet contains 12.5 mg diphenhydramine, 30 mg of pseudoephedrine, and 500 mg of acetaminophen.

Adult and Child (age 12 and over): 2 caplets every 6 hours. Do not take more than 8 caplets in a 24-hour period.

Child (under age 12): Consult your doctor.

You may minimize the inconvenience of the sedative effects of Benadryl Allergy Sinus Headache by taking a full dose at bedtime and by using the smallest recommended dose during the day. You can establish the lowest dose necessary for effective relief by starting with the lowest dose when you begin taking the drug, and gradually increasing the dosage over several days as needed.

If you forget to take a dose of Benadryl Allergy Sinus Headache, do so as soon as you remember. If it is almost time for your next dose, skip the one you forgot and continue with your regular schedule. Do not take a double dose.

Overdosage

Symptoms of overdose include nausea, vomiting, abdominal pain, low blood pressure, fever, flushed face, dry mouth, dilated pupils, loss of muscle coordination, confusion, excitability, hallucinations, drowsiness, coma, seizures, yellowing of the skin and eyes, and liver damage. Symptoms may develop within 30 minutes, but may not be seen for as long as 2 days after the overdose.

Even if the victim is not displaying any of the symptoms listed above, do the following in case of accidental overdose: If the victim is unconscious or having convulsions, call for an ambulance immediately. If you take the victim to an emergency room, be sure to bring the bottle or container with you. If the victim is conscious, call your local poison control center or a health care professional. The poison control center may suggest inducing vomiting with ipecac syrup (available without a prescription at any pharmacy). DO NOT induce vomiting unless specifically instructed to do so.

Special Populations

Pregnancy/Breast-feeding

Antihistamines are not recommended for use during pregnancy unless directed by your doctor. Antihistamines, decongestants, and acetaminophen are known to pass into the breast milk of nursing mothers and may cause side effects in infants. Check with your doctor before taking Benadryl Allergy Sinus Headache if you are or might be pregnant, or if you are breast-feeding.

Infants/Children

Children may be more susceptible to the side effects of Benadryl Allergy Sinus Headache. They are also more susceptible to accidental antihistamine overdose. Do not give Benadryl Allergy Sinus Headache to a child under age 12 unless directed by your doctor.

Seniors

Older persons may be more sensitive to the side effects of Benadryl Allergy Sinus Headache. They may experience nervousness, irritability, and restlessness. Dizziness, sedation, and low blood pressure may also occur. Older men may experience difficulty in urinating. Most mild reactions may be handled by either lowering your dose or trying another antihistamine/decongestant combination. However, persons over age 80 and those with acute physical disorders or dementia may be at risk of developing delirium from even small doses of diphenhydramine.

Seniors taking Benadryl Allergy/Sinus Headache should be especially cautious about the amount of caffeine they ingest (see "Drug Interactions").

Benadryl Dye-Free Allergy Liqui-Gels (BEN-uh-drill)

*see **Diphenhydramine,** page 796*

Brand Name

Drixoral Allergy Sinus (dricks-OR-al)

Generic Ingredients

Acetaminophen
Dexbrompheniramine maleate
Pseudoephedrine

Type of drug

Antihistamine, decongestant, and analgesic (pain reliever).

Used for

Temporary relief of runny nose, sneezing, nasal and sinus congestion, itchy and watery eyes, itching of the nose and throat, headache, and minor pains associated with colds and allergies.

General Information

Some OTC products use a combination of drugs to relieve symptoms that can accompany colds and allergies. Drixoral Allergy Sinus contains an antihistamine, a decongestant, and an analgesic.

The antihistamine ingredient in Drixoral is dexbrompheniramine maleate. Antihistamines block the release of histamine in the body, relieving the sneezing and itching that often occurs with colds and allergies. They can also aid in stopping a runny nose by reducing the secretions caused by histamine release.

Because histamine is only one of several substances released by the body during an allergic reaction, antihistamines can only reduce about 40% to 60% of allergic symptoms.

The decongestant ingredient in Drixoral is pseudoephedrine, an oral decongestant. Decongestants relieve congestion by narrowing or constricting blood vessels. This relieves the swelling of the mucous membranes of the nose and sinuses. Unlike topical decongestants (decongestant nasal sprays) that act on local blood vessels, oral decongestants may constrict blood vessels throughout the body.

Acetaminophen, the analgesic ingredient in Drixoral, relieves pain and headache.

Drixoral will not cure or prevent colds or allergies. The best you can hope for is symptomatic relief. Colds will usually go away in 1 to 2 weeks whether they are treated or not.

Cautions and Warnings

Do not take Drixoral for more than 7 days continuously, or 3 days continuously in the presence of fever. If symptoms do not improve, see your doctor.

Do not exceed the recommended daily dosage of Drixoral.

Drixoral should be used with caution if you have a condition that causes breathing problems, such as emphysema, chronic bronchitis, or asthma. Its antihistamine ingredient dries the mucous membranes. This in turn can inhibit the ability of the lungs to move or get rid of the excess secretions that these conditions produce.

Drixoral should be used with caution by people with glaucoma, hyperthyroidism, heart disease, high blood pressure, diabetes, or an enlarged prostate. If you have any of these conditions, consult your doctor before using Drixoral.

The antihistamine ingredient in Drixoral acts as a depressant on the central nervous system (CNS), and can cause sleepiness or grogginess and interfere with the ability to concentrate. Your ability to perform activities that require your full alertness and coordination, such as driving a motor vehicle or operating machinery, may be affected. Refrain from drinking alcohol while you are taking Drixoral, because alcohol aggravates these effects.

In doses of more than 4 grams per day, acetaminophen, one of the active ingredients in Drixoral, is potentially toxic to the liver. Use Drixoral with caution if you have kidney or liver disease or viral infections of the liver. Studies have shown that the risk of liver damage with acetaminophen is associated with fasting and alcohol use. People with liver disease who are taking other drugs that are potentially damaging to the liver, people who do not eat regularly, or who drink alcohol (even moderately) are especially at risk. If you take Drixoral regularly, avoid drinking alcohol and/or fasting.

Possible Side Effects

- ▼ Most common: restlessness, nervousness, sleeplessness or drowsiness, sedation, excitability, dizziness, lightheadedness, poor coordination, headache, and upset stomach.
- ▼ Less common: dry eyes, nose, and mouth; blurred vision; difficulty urinating; irritability (at high doses); increased blood pressure; increased or irregular heart rate; and heart palpitations.
- ▼ Rare: extreme fatigue; rash, itching, or hives; sore throat or fever; unexplained bleeding or bruising; anemia; yellowing of the skin or eyes; blood in the urine; painful or frequent urination; decreased output of urine volume; anxiety, tremor, hallucinations, seizures, breathing difficulty, and cardiovascular collapse.

Drug Interactions

• The antihistamine ingredient in Drixoral can enhance the effect of other drugs that depress the CNS, such as barbiturates, tranquilizers, sleeping medications, and alcohol (present in many OTC preparations). If you are taking other depressant drugs, check with your doctor before taking these products. Avoid drinking alcohol if you are taking Drixoral.

• Antihistamines can also affect the results of skin and blood tests. Notify your health care professional before scheduling these tests if you are taking Drixoral.

• Drixoral should not be used at the same time as a monoamine oxidase inhibitor (MAOI) or within 2 weeks of stopping treatment with an MAOI. MAOIs are used to treat depression, other psychiatric or emotional conditions, and Parkinson's disease. If you are not sure whether you are or have been taking an MAOI, check with your doctor or pharmacist before you use Drixoral.

• The effects of pseudoephedrine, the decongestant in Drixoral, may combine with those of caffeine, a CNS stimulant found in many prescription and OTC drugs. This combination can cause disorientation, delirium, and other side effects.

• Taking Drixoral along with another decongestant can increase the risk of adverse effects and toxicity; if you are taking another decongestant, do not use Drixoral without first asking your doctor.

• The effect of the acetaminophen in Drixoral may be reduced by long-term use or large doses of barbiturate drugs; the anticonvulsants carbamazepine and phenytoin (and other similar drugs); rifampin, used to treat tuberculosis (TB) and sulfinpyrazone, used to treat gout. These drugs may also increase the chances of liver toxicity if taken with acetaminophen. Chronically taking large doses of acetaminophen with isoniazid (used to treat TB) may increase the risk of liver damage.

• If Drixoral is taken with an anticoagulant such as warfarin, the acetaminophen in it may increase the blood-thinning effect of the anticoagulant agent. This does not occur with occasional use.

• Avoid alcohol while taking Drixoral. (Be aware that alcohol is found in many OTC preparations.) Alcohol may contribute to the risk of liver damage associated with acetaminophen; it also increases the sedative effects of antihistamines (see "Cautions and Warnings").

Food Interactions

Decongestants interact adversely with caffeine (see "Drug Interactions"), which is found in many popular beverages, including coffee, tea, and cola, and in chocolate.

Usual Dose

If you are taking Drixoral for allergies, it is best to take it on a schedule rather than as needed because histamine is released almost continuously.

Each tablet contains 3 mg dexbrompheniramine, 60 mg of pseudoephedrine, and 500 mg of acetaminophen.

Adult and Child (age 12 and over): 2 tablets every 12 hours. Do not take more than 4 caplets in a 24-hour period.

Child (under age 12): Consult your doctor.

Drixoral tablets should be swallowed whole—never chewed, crushed, or dissolved.

If you forget to take a dose of Drixoral, do so as soon as you remember. If it is almost time for your next dose, skip the one you forgot and continue with your regular schedule. Do not take a double dose.

Overdosage

Symptoms of overdose include nausea, vomiting, abdominal pain, low blood pressure, fever, flushed face, dry mouth, dilated pupils, loss of muscle coordination, confusion, excitability, hallucinations, drowsiness, coma, seizures, yellowing of the skin and eyes, and liver damage. Symptoms may develop within 30 minutes, but may not be seen for as long as 2 days after the overdose.

Even if the victim is not displaying any of the symptoms listed above, do the following in case of accidental overdose: If the victim is unconscious or having convulsions, call for an ambulance immediately. If you take the victim to an emergency room, be sure to bring the bottle or container with you. If the victim is conscious, call your local poison control center or a health care professional. The poison control center may suggest inducing vomiting with ipecac syrup (available without a prescription at any pharmacy). DO NOT induce vomiting unless specifically instructed to do so.

Special Populations

Pregnancy/Breast-feeding

Antihistamines are not recommended for use during pregnancy unless directed by your doctor. Antihistamines, decongestants, and acetaminophen are known to pass into the breast milk of nursing mothers and may cause side effects in infants. Check with your doctor before taking Drixoral if you are or might be pregnant, or if you are breast-feeding.

Infants/Children

Children may be more susceptible to the side effects of Drixoral. They are also more susceptible to accidental antihistamine overdose. Do not give Drixoral to a child under age 12 unless directed by your doctor.

Seniors

Seniors should not take Drixoral, which is an extended-release preparation, until they have first tried a short-acting product containing pseudoephedrine and experienced no ill effects.

Older persons may be more sensitive to the side effects of Drixoral. They may experience nervousness, irritability, and restlessness. Dizziness, sedation, and low blood pressure may also occur. Older men may experience difficulty in urinating. Most mild reactions may be handled by either lowering your dose or trying another antihistamine/decongestant combination.

Seniors taking Drixoral should be especially cautious about the amount of caffeine they ingest (see "Drug Interactions").

Efidac/24 (EFF-ih-dak)

*see **Pseudoephedrine,** page 1002*

Brand Name

4-Way Fast Acting Nasal Spray

Generic Ingredients

Naphazoline hydrochloride
Phenylephrine hydrochloride
Pyrilamine maleate

Type of Drug

Topical antihistamine and decongestant.

Used for

Temporary relief of nasal congestion associated with colds and allergies.

General Information

Some OTC products use a combination of drugs to relieve symptoms that accompany colds and allergies. 4-Way Fast Acting Nasal Spray contains an antihistamine and 2 decongestants.

The antihistamine in 4-Way Fast Acting Nasal Spray is pyrilamine maleate. Antihistamines block the release of histamine in the body, relieving the sneezing and itching that often occur with colds and allergies. They can also aid in stopping a runny nose by reducing the secretions caused by histamine release.

Because histamine is only one of several substances released by the body during an allergic reaction, antihistamines can only reduce about 40% to 60% of allergic symptoms.

4-Way Nasal Spray contains 2 topical decongestants which are applied directly in the nose: naphazoline hydrochloride and phenylephrine hydrochloride. Decongestants work by narrowing or constricting the blood vessels. This relieves the swelling of nasal mucous membranes.

4-Way Nasal Spray will not cure or prevent colds or allergies. The best you can hope for is symptomatic relief. Colds will usually go away in 1 to 2 weeks whether they are treated or not.

Cautions and Warnings

Do not use 4-Way Nasal Spray for more than 3 consecutive days. If symptoms do not improve, or if the spray seems to be losing its effectiveness, call your doctor.

Do not exceed the recommended daily dosage of 4-Way Nasal Spray.

Frequent or prolonged use of 4-Way Nasal Spray may cause nasal congestion to recur or worsen. You may experience rebound congestion; that is, you may still have a stuffy nose even though you have been using 4-Way Nasal Spray for several days. The lining of your nose may swell and turn red, giving the appearance of allergic rhinitis. If this happens, stop using 4-Way Nasal Spray and call your doctor. The signs of rebound congestion will usually go away within 7 days of not using the drug. If you have persistent seasonal allergies, you should consult your doctor before using 4-Way Nasal Spray because of the risk of rebound congestion.

Although it is less likely to occur with a topical product, the antihistamine ingredient in 4-Way Nasal Spray can act as a depressant on the central nervous system (CNS), and can cause sleepiness or grogginess and interfere with the ability to concentrate. Your ability to perform activities that require your full alertness and coordination, such as driving a motor vehicle or operating machinery, may be affected.

4-Way Nasal Spray should be used with caution if you have a condition that causes breathing problems, such as emphysema, chronic bronchitis, or asthma. Its antihistamine ingredient acts to dry the mucous membranes. This in turn can inhibit the ability of the lungs to move or get rid of the excess secretions that these conditions produce.

4-Way Nasal Spray should be used with caution by people with glaucoma, hyperthyroidism, heart disease, high blood pressure, diabetes, or an enlarged prostate, because it can worsen these conditions. If you have any of these conditions, consult your doctor before using 4-Way Nasal Spray.

To prevent the spread of infection, a single bottle of 4-Way Nasal Spray should not be used by more than 1 person.

Possible Side Effects

▼ Local: stinging, burning, itching, drying, or an increase in nasal discharge, especially when recommended doses are exceeded. Rebound congestion may also occur (see "Cautions and Warnings").

▼ Systemic (whole-body): restlessness, nervousness, sleeplessness or drowsiness, dizziness, excitability, poor muscle coordination, headache, upset stomach, dry eyes or mouth, blurred vision, difficulty urinating, irritability, increased blood pressure, increased or irregular heart rate, and heart palpitations.

Drug Interactions

• The antihistamine ingredient in 4-Way Nasal Spray can enhance the effect of other drugs that depress the CNS, such as barbiturates, tranquilizers, sleeping medications, and alcohol (present in many OTC preparations). If you are taking other depressant drugs or if you drink alcohol, check with your doctor before using 4-Way Nasal Spray.

• 4-Way Nasal Spray should not be used at the same time as a monoamine oxidase inhibitor (MAOI) or within 2 weeks of stopping treatment with an MAOI. MAOIs are used to treat depression, other psychiatric or emotional conditions, and Parkinson's disease. If you are not sure whether you are or have been taking an MAOI, check with your doctor or pharmacist before you use 4-Way Nasal Spray.

Food Interactions

None known.

Usual Dose

4-Way Nasal Spray contains 0.2% pyrilamine, 0.05% naphazoline, and 0.5% phenylephrine.

Adult and Child (age 12 and over): 2 sprays in each nostril every 6 hours. Do not exceed 4 doses in a 24-hour period.

Child (under age 12): Consult your doctor.

Overdosage

Symptoms of overdose in children include dilated pupils, flushed face, dry mouth, fever, excitation, hallucinations, loss of muscle coordination, and seizures.

In adults, severe overdose can cause drowsiness or coma, which may be followed by excitability or seizures. Eventually fluid can build up in the brain; the kidneys may fail, and the heart and lungs may stop working, resulting in death. Symptoms may develop within 30 minutes to 2 hours following an overdose, and death may occur within 18 hours.

Even if the victim is not displaying any of the symptoms listed above, do the following in case of accidental ingestion or overdose: If the victim is unconscious or having convulsions, call for an ambulance immediately. If you take the victim to an emergency room, be sure to bring the bottle or container with you. If the victim is conscious, call your local poison control center or a health care professional. The poison control center may suggest inducing vomiting with ipecac syrup (available without a prescription at any pharmacy). DO NOT induce vomiting unless specifically instructed to do so.

Special Populations

Pregnancy/Breast-feeding

Antihistamines are not recommended for use during pregnancy unless directed by your doctor. Antihistamines and decongestants are known to pass into the breast milk of nursing mothers and may cause side effects in infants. Check with your doctor before using 4-Way Nasal Spray if you are or might be pregnant, or if you are breast-feeding.

Infants/Children

Children may be more susceptible to the side effects of 4-Way Nasal Spray, especially if it is swallowed. They are also more susceptible to accidental antihistamine overdose. Do not give 4-Way Nasal Spray to a child under age 12 unless recommended by your doctor.

Seniors

Seniors may be more sensitive to the side effects of 4-Way Nasal Spray. They may experience nervousness, irritability, restlessness, dizziness, sedation, hallucinations, seizures, and low blood pressure. Most mild reactions may be handled by either lowering the dose or by switching to another product.

Brand Name

Motrin IB Sinus (MOE-trin)

Generic Ingredients

Ibuprofen
Pseudoephedrine

Type of Drug

Decongestant, nonsteroidal anti-inflammatory drug (NSAID), analgesic (pain reliever), and antipyretic (fever reducer).

Used for

Relief of nasal and sinus congestion, headache, body aches, pains, and fever associated with colds.

General Information

Some OTC products use a combination of drugs to treat the symptoms of colds and allergies. Motrin IB Sinus contains a decongestant to relieve stuffy sinuses and an NSAID/analgesic/antipyretic to reduce pain and fever.

The decongestant in Motrin IB Sinus is pseudophedrine, an oral decongestant. Decongestants work by narrowing or constricting the blood vessels. This relieves the swelling of mucous membranes of the nose and sinuses. Unlike topical decongestants (decongestant nasal sprays), which act on local blood vessels, oral decongestants may constrict blood vessels throughout the body.

The NSAID in Motrin IB Sinus is ibuprofen. NSAIDs appear to work by inhibiting the body's production of a hormone called prostaglandin. This hormone increases the sensitivity of nerves to pain. NSAIDs are also effective in reducing fever.

Motrin IB Sinus will not cure or prevent allergies or colds. The best you can hope for is symptomatic relief. Colds will usually go away in 1 to 2 weeks whether they are treated or not.

Cautions and Warnings

Do not take Motrin IB Sinus for more than 7 consecutive days or more than 3 consecutive days in the presence of fever. If symptoms do not improve, see your doctor.

Do not exceed the recommended daily dosage of Motrin IB Sinus.

Pseudoephedrine and ibuprofen, the ingredients in Motrin IB Sinus, can worsen other medical conditions, such as hyperthyroidism, heart disease, high blood pressure, diabetes, enlarged prostate, and ulcers. If you have any of these conditions, or if you use diuretics, take Motrin IB Sinus only upon the advice of a physician.

Bronchospastic symptoms may worsen in people with asthma who take ibuprofen, the NSAID ingredient in Motrin IB Sinus.

Ibuprofen use can damage the kidneys. It may increase blood levels of urea nitrogen and serum creatinine and may also lead to sodium and water retention. This effect is especially dangerous in patients with kidney damage or congestive heart failure.

In rare instances, severe effects on the liver, including jaundice and hepatitis, have been seen in people taking ibuprofen. If any signs or symptoms of liver damage occur (darkened urine, yellowed eyes), stop taking Motrin IB Sinus and contact your doctor.

Drinking alcoholic beverages has been shown to increase the prolongation of bleeding time associated with ibuprofen. Avoid alcohol when you are taking Motrin IB Sinus.

Ibuprofen can make you drowsy. Be careful when driving a motor vehicle or operating heavy machinery after taking Motrin IB Sinus.

If you develop any severe gastrointestinal (GI) effects, blurred vision, or a rash while taking Motrin IB Sinus, call your doctor.

Don't lie down for 15 to 30 minutes after you take Motrin IB Sinus.

Possible Side Effects

- ▼ Most common: restlessness, nervousness, sleeplessness or drowsiness, dizziness, excitability, poor muscle coordination, headache, and GI problems (e.g., indigestion, heartburn, nausea, diarrhea, stomach irritation).
- ▼ Less common: dry eyes, nose, and mouth; blurred vision; irritability (at high doses); increased blood pressure; increased or irregular heart rate; heart palpitations; stomach ulcers; GI bleeding; loss of appetite; hepatitis; gallbladder attacks; difficult or painful urination; poor kidney function or kidney inflammation; blood in the urine; dizziness; and fainting.
- ▼ Rare: severe allergic reactions, including closing of the throat, fever, chills, changes in liver function, jaundice, kidney failure, and ringing in the ears; anxiety, tremor, hallucinations, seizures, breathing difficulty, and cardiovascular collapse.

Drug Interactions

• Motrin IB Sinus should not be used at the same time as a monoamine oxidase inhibitor (MAOI) or within 2 weeks of stopping treatment with an MAOI. MAOIs are used to treat depression, other psychiatric or emotional conditions, and Parkinson's disease. If you are not sure whether you are or have been taking an MAOI, check with your doctor or pharmacist before you use Motrin IB Sinus.

• Taking Motrin IB Sinus along with another decongestant can increase the risk of adverse effects and toxicity. If you are taking another decongestant, do not use Motrin IB Sinus without first asking your doctor.

• The effects of pseudoephedrine, the decongestant ingredient in Motrin IB Sinus, may combine with those of caffeine, a central nervous system stimulant found in many prescription and OTC drugs. This combination can cause increased heart rate, nervousness, disorientation, delirium and other side effects.

• If you are currently taking an anticoagulant drug such as warfarin, you should not take Motrin IB Sinus without first consulting your doctor. This product's ibuprofen ingredient can increase the anti-clotting effects of these drugs.

• In individuals taking ibuprofen and digoxin, a drug used to treat congestive heart failure, ibuprofen may increase the concentration of digoxin in the blood. Researchers are not sure of the implications of this effect. Ibuprofen may also increase the levels of phenytoin, a drug taken to control epilepsy, in the blood. If you take either digoxin or phenytoin, consult your doctor before taking Motrin IB Sinus.

• Ibuprofen may work against the effects of drugs taken to lower blood pressure, including diuretics, angiotensin-converting enzyme (ACE) inhibitors, beta blockers, and others. If you are taking any drugs to control high blood pressure, ask your doctor before taking Motrin IB Sinus.

• Taking ibuprofen with the antimanic drug lithium may increase the levels of lithium in the blood and increase its side effects, such as tremor. If you take lithium, do not take Motrin IB Sinus without consulting your doctor.

• Ibuprofen can increase the toxicity of methotrexate, used to treat cancer, severe psoriasis, severe rheumatoid arthritis, and to induce abortion.

• Do not take any product containing acetaminophen, aspirin, or any other NSAID while taking Motrin IB Sinus. This combination can cause increased heart rate, nervousness, disorientation, delirium, and other side effects.

Food Interactions

Pseudoephedrine interacts adversely with caffeine (see "Drug Interactions"), which is found in many popular beverages, including coffee, tea, and cola, and in chocolate.

If ibuprofen upsets your stomach, take Motrin IB Sinus with meals or with milk. You can also take an antacid containing aluminum hydroxide or magnesium hydroxide.

Usual Dose

Adult and Child (age 12 and over): 1 caplet, tablet, or gelcap every 4–6 hours. If symptoms do not respond, 2 caplets or tablets may be used. Do not exceed 6 caplets or tablets in a 24-hour period.

Child (under age 12): Consult your doctor.

Overdosage

Signs of overdose in children include flushed face, dry mouth, fever, excitation, hallucinations, difficulty breathing, uncoordinated muscular movements, fixed, dilated pupils, and seizures, followed by depression.

Overdose in adults usually causes CNS depression with drowsiness or coma, which may be followed by excitement, seizures, and then depression.

Do the following in case of accidental overdose: If the victim is unconscious or having convulsions, call for an ambulance immediately. If you take the victim to an emergency room, be sure to bring the bottle or container with you. If the victim is conscious, call your local poison control center or a health care professional. The poison control center may suggest inducing vomiting with ipecac syrup (available without a prescription at any pharmacy). DO NOT induce vomiting unless specifically instructed to do so.

Special Populations

Allergies

People who are allergic to aspirin or to any other NSAID should not take Motrin IB Sinus.

Pregnancy/Breast-feeding

It is not generally recommended that pregnant women take

any drugs, particularly during the first 3 months after conception. Ibuprofen may cross into the blood circulation of a developing fetus, and is especially dangerous to take during the last 3 months of pregnancy. If you are or might be pregnant, do not take Motrin IB Sinus without your doctor's approval.

Small amounts of decongestants such as pseudoephedrine have been shown to pass into breast milk. Ibuprofen has not been proved to pass into breast milk; however, it is not recommended that nursing mothers use this drug, because there is a risk of affecting the baby's heart or cardiovascular system. If you must take Motrin IB Sinus, bottle-feed your baby with formula.

Infants/Children

Motrin IB Sinus should not be taken by children under 12 unless directed by a doctor.

Seniors

Older persons may be more sensitive to the side effects of Motrin IB Sinus. They may experience nervousness, irritability, restlessness, dizziness, sedation, hallucinations, seizures, and low blood pressure. Most mild reactions may be handled by either lowering your dose or trying another product.

Seniors taking Motrin IB Sinus should be especially cautious about the amount of caffeine they ingest (see "Drug Interactions").

Brand Name

Nasalcrom (NAY-zul-krom)

Generic Ingredient

Cromolyn sodium (KROME-uh-lin SOE-dee-um)

Type of Drug

Allergy preventative.

Used for

Prevention and treatment of seasonal or chronic allergies.

General Information

During an allergic reaction, certain cells in the body, known as mast cells, release a variety of potent chemicals that irritate the nerves in the nose and cause congestion, runny nose, sneezing, and itching. Cromolyn sodium, the active ingredient in Nasalcrom, fights against allergic reactions by inhibiting the release of histamine (and other chemicals that cause these reactions). It became available OTC in 1997. Nasalcrom works on a preventative basis and also provides relief from established allergy symptoms, such as nasal congestion, sneezing, and postnasal drip. If you have seasonal allergies, you should start using Nasalcrom before your allergy season begins and continue to take it regularly until the season ends. Nasalcrom must be used on a regular basis to be effective.

In treating chronic allergies, relief of allergy symptoms may not be apparent until after 2 weeks of continuous Nasalcrom use. You may also need to use topical nasal decongestants or oral antihistamines to relieve symptoms until Nasalcrom starts to work.

Nasalcrom is not considered to work as well as corticosteroids for people with severe allergies, but it does not cause the same systemic (whole-body) side effects as corticosteroids.

Nasalcrom is available as a nasal spray.

Cautions and Warnings

If your condition worsens or does not improve, consult your doctor.

Do not exceed the recommended daily dosage of Nasalcrom.

Nasalcrom should never be used to treat an acute allergy attack.

Call your doctor if you develop wheezing, coughing, or skin rash, or if you experience other severe or bothersome side effects.

Nasalcrom does not work in people with rhinitis (nasal inflammation) if it is caused by anything other than allergies (e.g., a cold), neither does it relieve eye or throat irritation. Nasalcrom is unlikely to be effective in people with nasal polyps.

Because Nasalcrom is eliminated from the body via bile and urine, people with impaired liver or kidney function may need to take reduced dosages or avoid this drug.

Possible Side Effects

- ▼ Most common: sneezing, a burning or stinging sensation in the nose, and nasal irritation.
- ▼ Less common: headache and an unpleasant taste in the mouth.
- ▼ Rare: nosebleed, postnasal drip, and rash. Ulcerations in the nose, swelling of the tongue and mouth, and coughing and wheezing have also been reported when used.

Drug Interactions

None known.

Food Interactions

None known.

Usual Dose

Nasalcrom contains 4% cromolyn sodium.

Because histamine is released continuously, it is best to take Nasalcrom on a regular schedule rather than as needed.

Adult and Child (age 6 and over): First blow your nose; then spray once into each nostril and inhale. This may be repeated 3-4 times a day at regular intervals. When necessary, dosage may be increased to 1 spray in each nostril 6 times a day.

Child (under age 6): not recommended unless directed by your doctor.

If you forget to take a dose of Nasalcrom, do so as soon as you remember. If it is almost time for your next dose, skip the one you forgot and continue with your regular schedule. Do not take a double dose.

Overdosage

Do the following in case of accidental ingestion or overdose: If the victim is unconscious or having convulsions, call for an ambulance immediately. If you take the victim to an emergency room, be sure to bring the bottle or container with you. If the victim is conscious, call your local poison control center or a health care professional. The poison control center may suggest inducing vomiting with ipecac syrup (available without a prescription at any pharmacy). DO NOT induce vomiting unless specifically instructed to do so.

Storage Instructions

Nasalcrom must be protected from direct sunlight.

Special Populations

Pregnancy/Breast-feeding

Do not use Nasalcrom if you are pregnant unless it is directed by your doctor.

It is not known if cromolyn sodium passes into breast milk. Check with your doctor before self-medicating with Nasalcrom if you are breast-feeding.

Infants/Children

Nasalcrom is not recommended for children under age 6 unless directed by your doctor.

Seniors

Seniors may be more likely to have impaired liver or kidney function compared with younger adults; therefore, their dosage of Nasalcrom may need to be adjusted (see "Cautions and Warnings").

Brand Names

Sine-Aid (SYE-nade)
Sine-Off No Drowsiness
Sudafed Sinus (SOO-dah-fed)
Tylenol Sinus (TYE-leh-nol)

Generic Ingredients

Acetaminophen
Pseudoephedrine

Type of Drug

Decongestant and analgesic (pain reliever).

Used for

Relief of nasal and sinus congestion, and sinus pain and headache associated with cold and allergy.

General Information

Some OTC products use a combination of drugs to relieve the many symptoms that can accompany colds and allergies. Sine-Aid, Sine-Off No Drowsiness, Sudafed Sinus, and Tylenol Sinus contain a decongestant and an analgesic.

The decongestant in these products is pseudoephedrine oral decongestant. Decongestants work by narrowing or constricting the blood vessels. This relieves the swelling of mucous membranes of the nose and sinuses. Unlike topical decongestants (decongestant nasal sprays) which act on local blood vessels, oral decongestants may constrict blood vessels throughout the body.

Acetaminophen, the analgesic ingredient in these products, relieves the pain and headache associated with cold and allergy.

These products will not cure or prevent allergies or colds. The best you can hope for is symptomatic relief. Colds will usually go away in 1 to 2 weeks whether they are treated or not.

Cautions and Warnings

Do not take Sine-Aid, Sine-Off No Drowsiness, Sudafed Sinus or Tylenol Sinus for more than 7 consecutive days or, in the presence of fever, for more than 3 days, unless directed by your doctor. If symptoms do not improve, or if they worsen or recur, see your doctor.

Do not exceed the recommended daily dosage of these products.

The decongestant ingredient in these products can worsen other medical conditions, such as hyperthyroidism, heart disease, high blood pressure, diabetes, and an enlarged prostate. If you have any of these conditions, take these products only upon the advice of a physician.

The acetaminophen ingredient in these products is potentially toxic to the liver in doses of more than 4 grams per day. Use these products with caution if you have kidney or liver disease or viral infections of the liver. Studies have shown that the risk of liver damage with acetaminophen is associated with fasting and alcohol use. People with liver disease who are taking other drugs that are potentially damaging to the liver, who do not eat regularly, or who drink alcohol (even moderately) are especially at risk. If you take Sine-Aid, Sine-Off, Sudafed Sinus, or Tylenol Sinus regularly, avoid drinking alcoholic beverages and/or fasting.

Possible Side Effects

▼ Most common: restlessness, nervousness, sleeplessness or drowsiness, dizziness, lightheadedness, and headache.

▼ Less common: increased blood pressure; increased or irregular heart rate; and heart palpitations.

▼ Rare: extreme fatigue; rash, itching, or hives; sore throat or fever; unexplained bleeding or bruising; anemia; yellowing of the skin or eyes; blood in urine; painful or frequent urination; decreased output of urine, difficulty breathing, anxiety, tremors, hallucinations, seizures, and cardiovascular collapse.

Drug Interactions

• These products should not be used at the same time as a monoamine oxidase inhibitor (MAOI) or within 2 weeks of stopping treatment with an MAOI. MAOIs are used to treat depression, other psychiatric or emotional conditions, and Parkinson's disease. If you are not sure whether you are or have been taking an MAOI, check with your doctor or pharmacist before you use Sine-Aid, Sine-Off, Sudafed Sinus or Tylenol Sinus.

• The effects of pseudoephedrine, the decongestant in these products, may combine with those of caffeine, a central nervous system stimulant found in many prescription and OTC drugs. This combination can cause disorientation, delirium, and other side effects.

• Taking these products along with another decongestant can increase the risk of adverse effects and toxicity. If you are taking another decongestant, do not take Sine-Aid, Sine-Off No Drowsiness, Sudafed Sinus, or Tylenol Sinus without first asking your doctor.

• The effects of the acetaminophen in these products may be reduced by long-term use or large doses of barbiturate drugs; carbamazepine, an anticonvulsant; phenytoin (and other similar drugs), used to treat epilepsy; rifampin, an antitubercular drug; and sulfinpyrazone, an antigout medication. These drugs may also increase the chances of liver toxicity if taken with Sine-Aid, Sine-Off No Drowsiness, Sudafed Sinus, or Tylenol Sinus. Taking these products with the antitubercular drug isoniazid may also increase the risk of liver damage.

• If these products are taken with an anticoagulant such as warfarin, they may increase the blood-thinning effect of the anticoagulant agent. This does not occur with occasional use.

• Avoid alcohol while taking these products. (Be aware that alcohol is found in many OTC preparations.) Alcohol may contribute to the risk of liver damage associated with acetaminophen. (see "Cautions and Warnings").

Food Interactions

Decongestants interact adversely with caffeine (see "Drug Interactions"), which is found in many popular beverages, including coffee, tea, and cola, and in chocolate.

Usual Dose

If you are taking these products for allergies, it is best to take them on a schedule rather than as needed because histamine is released almost continuously.

Sine-Aid
Each caplet, gelcap, or tablet contains 30 mg of pseudoephedrine and 500 mg of acetaminophen.

Adult and Child (age 12 and over): 2 caplets, gelcaps, or tablets every 4–6 hours. Do not take more than 8 caplets, gelcaps, or tablets in a 24-hour period.

Child (under age 12): not recommended unless directed by your doctor.

Sine-Off No Drowsiness
Each caplet contains 30 mg of pseudoephedrine and 500 mg of acetaminophen.

Adult and Child (age 12 and over): 2 caplets every 6 hours. Do not take more than 8 caplets in a 24-hour period.

Child (under age 12): not recommended unless directed by your doctor.

Sudafed Sinus
Each caplet or tablet contains 30 mg of pseudoephedrine and 500 mg of acetaminophen.

Adult and Child (age 12 and over): 2 caplets or tablets every 6 hours. Do not take more than 8 caplets or tablets in a 24-hour period.

Child (under age 12): not recommended unless directed by your doctor.

Tylenol Sinus
Each caplet, gelcap, geltab, or tablet contains 30 mg of pseudoephedrine and 500 mg of acetaminophen.

Adult and Child (age 12 and over): 2 caplets, gelcaps, geltabs, or tablets every 4–6 hours. Do not take more than 8 caplets, gelcaps, geltabs, or tablets in a 24-hour period.

Child (under age 12): not recommended unless directed by your doctor.

You may minimize the inconvenience of the sedative effects of these products by taking a full dose at bedtime or using the smallest recommended doses during the day. You can establish the lowest dose necessary for effective relief by starting with the lowest dose when you begin taking the drug, and gradually increasing the dosage over several days as needed.

If you forget to take a dose of these products, do so as soon as you remember. If it is almost time for your next dose, skip the one you forgot and continue with your regular schedule. Do not take a double dose.

Overdosage

Symptoms of overdose include nausea, vomiting, abdominal pain, low blood pressure, fever, flushed face, dry mouth, dilated pupils, loss of muscle coordination, confusion, excitability, hallucinations, drowsiness, coma, seizures, yellowing of the skin and eyes, and liver damage. Symptoms may develop within 30 minutes, but may not be seen for as long as 2 days after the overdose.

Even if the victim is not displaying any of the symptoms listed above, do the following in case of accidental overdose: If the victim is unconscious or having convulsions, call for an ambulance immediately. If you take the victim to an emergency room, be sure to bring the bottle or container with you. If the victim is conscious, call your local poison control center or a health care professional. The poison control center may suggest inducing vomiting with ipecac syrup (available without a prescription at any pharmacy). DO NOT induce vomiting unless specifically instructed to do so.

Special Populations

Pregnancy/Breast-feeding

Unless directed by your doctor, Sine-Aid, Sine-Off No Drowsiness, Sudafed Sinus, or Tylenol Sinus are not recommended for use during pregnancy. Decongestants and acetaminophen have been shown to pass into the breast milk of nursing mothers and may cause side effects in infants. Check with your doctor before taking Sine-Aid, Sine-Off, Sudafed Sinus, or Tylenol Sinus if you are or might be pregnant, or if you are breast-feeding.

Infants/Children

Children may be more susceptible to the side effects of Sine-Aid, Sine-Off, Sudafed Sinus, or Tylenol Sinus. Do not give these products to a child under age 12 unless directed by your doctor.

Seniors

Older persons may be more sensitive to the side effects of Sine-Aid, Sine-Off, Sudafed Sinus, or Tylenol Sinus, and may experience nervousness, irritability, restlessness, dizziness, sedation, hallucinations, seizures, and low blood pressure. Most mild reactions may be handled by either lowering the dose or trying another product.

Seniors taking these products should be especially cautious about the amount of caffeine they ingest (see "Drug Interactions").

Brand Names

Sine-Off Sinus
Tylenol Allergy Sinus (TYE-leh-nol)

Generic Ingredients

Acetaminophen
Chlorpheniramine maleate
Pseudoephedrine

Type of Drug

Antihistamine, decongestant, and analgesic (pain reliever).

Used for

Relief of sneezing, runny nose, itchy and watery eyes, itching of the nose or throat, nasal and sinus congestion, and sinus pain and headache associated with allergy.

General Information

Some OTC products use a combination of drugs to relieve the many symptoms that can accompany allergies. Tylenol Allergy Sinus and Sine-Off Sinus contain an antihistamine, a decongestant, and an analgesic.

The antihistamine in these products is chlorpheniramine maleate. Antihistamines block the release of histamine in the body, relieving the sneezing and itching that often occur with allergies. They can also aid in stopping a runny nose by reducing the secretions caused by histamine release.

Since histamine is only one of several substances released by the body during an allergic reaction, antihistamines can only reduce about 40% to 60% of allergic symptoms.

The decongestant in these products is pseudoephedrine, an oral decongestant. Decongestants work by narrowing or constricting the blood vessels. This relieves the swelling of mucous membranes of the nose and sinuses. Unlike topical decongestants (decongestant nasal sprays), which act on local blood vessels, oral decongestants may constrict blood vessels throughout the body.

Acetaminophen, the analgesic ingredient in these products, relieves sinus pain and headache.

Tylenol Allergy Sinus or Sine-Off Sinus will not cure or prevent allergies. The best you can hope for is symptomatic relief.

Cautions and Warnings

Do not take Tylenol Allergy Sinus or Sine-Off Sinus for more than 7 consecutive days, or in the presence of fever, for more than 3 days. If symptoms do not improve, see your doctor.

Do not exceed the recommended daily dosage of these products.

These products should be used with caution if you have a condition that causes breathing problems, such as emphysema, chronic bronchitis, or asthma. Its antihistamine ingredient acts to dry the mucous membranes. This in turn can inhibit the ability of the lungs to move or get rid of the excess secretions that these conditions produce.

Antihistamines also act as a depressant on the central nervous system (CNS), and can cause sleepiness or grogginess and interfere with the ability to concentrate. Your ability to perform activities that require your full alertness and coordination, such as driving a motor vehicle or operating machinery, may be affected. Refrain from drinking alcohol while you are taking these products because alcohol aggravates these effects.

These products should be used with caution by people with glaucoma, hyperthyroidism, heart disease, high blood pressure, diabetes, or an enlarged prostate, because it can worsen these conditions. If you have any of these conditions, take Tylenol Allergy Sinus or Sine-Off Sinus only upon the advice of a physician.

The acetaminophen ingredient in these products is potentially toxic to the liver in doses of more than 4 grams per day. Use these products with caution if you have kidney or liver disease or viral infections of the liver. Studies have shown that the risk of liver damage with acetaminophen is associated with fasting and alcohol use. People with liver disease who are taking other drugs that are potentially damaging to the liver, who do not eat regularly, or who drink alcohol (even moderately) are especially at risk. If you take Tylenol Allergy Sinus or Sine-Off Sinus regularly, avoid drinking alcoholic beverages and/or fasting.

Possible Side Effects

- ▼ Most common: restlessness, nervousness, sleeplessness or drowsiness, dizziness, lightheadedness, excitability, poor muscle coordination, headache, and upset stomach.
- ▼ Less common: dry eyes, nose, and mouth; blurred vision; difficulty urinating; irritability (at high doses); increased blood pressure; increased or irregular heart rate; and heart palpitations.
- ▼ Rare: extreme fatigue, rash, itching, or hives; sore throat or fever; unexplained bleeding or bruising; anemia; yellowing of the skin or eyes; blood in the urine; painful or frequent urination; decreased output of urine; anxiety; tremors; hallucinations; seizures; breathing difficulty; and cardiovascular collapse.

Drug Interactions

• The antihistamine ingredient in these products can enhance the effect of other drugs that depress the CNS, such as barbiturates, tranquilizers, sleeping medications, and alcohol (present in many OTC preparations). If you are taking other depressant drugs, check with your doctor before you take Tylenol Allergy Sinus or Sine-Off Sinus.

• Antihistamines can also affect the results of skin and blood tests. Notify your health care professional before scheduling these tests if you are taking these products.

• These products should not be used at the same time as a monoamine oxidase inhibitor (MAOI) or within 2 weeks of stopping treatment with an MAOI. MAOIs are used to treat depression, other psychiatric or emotional conditions, and Parkinson's disease. If you are not sure whether you are or have been taking an MAOI, check with your doctor or pharmacist before you use Tylenol Allergy Sinus or Sine-Off Sinus.

• The effects of the decongestant ingredient in these products may combine with those of caffeine, a CNS stimulant found in many prescription and OTC drugs. This combination can cause disorientation, delirium, and other side effects.

• Taking these products along with another decongestant can increase the risk of adverse effects and toxicity. If you are taking another decongestant, do not take Tylenol Allergy Sinus or Sine-Off Sinus without first asking your doctor.

• The effects of the acetaminophen in these products may be reduced by long-term use or large doses of barbiturate drugs; carbamazepine, an anticonvulsant; phenytoin (and other similar drugs), used to treat epilepsy; rifampin, an antitubercular drug; and sulfinpyrazone, an antigout medication. These drugs may also increase the chances of liver toxicity if taken with Tylenol Allergy Sinus or Sine-Off Sinus. Taking Tylenol Allergy Sinus or Sine-Off Sinus with the antitubercular drug isoniazid may also increase the risk of liver damage.

• If these products are taken with an anticoagulant such as warfarin, it may increase the blood-thinning effect of the anticoagulant agent. This does not occur with occasional use.

• Avoid alcohol while taking Tylenol Allergy Sinus or Sine-Off Sinus. (Be aware that alcohol is found in many OTC preparations.) Alcohol may contribute to the risk of liver damage associated with acetaminophen; alcohol also increases the sedative effects of antihistamines (see "Cautions and Warnings").

Food Interactions

Decongestants interact adversely with caffeine (see "Drug Interactions"), which is found in many popular beverages, including coffee, tea, and cola, and in chocolate.

Usual Dose

To relieve the symptoms of allergy, it is best to take Tylenol Allergy Sinus or Sine-Off Sinus on a schedule rather than as needed because histamine is released almost continuously.

Tylenol Allergy Sinus
Each caplet, gelcap, or geltab contains 2 mg of chlorpheniramine, 30 mg of pseudoephedrine, and 500 mg of acetaminophen.

Adult and Child (age 12 and over): Take 2 caplets, gelcaps, or geltabs every 6 hours. Do not exceed 8 caplets, gelcaps, or geltabs in a 24-hour period.

Child (under age 12): not recommended unless directed by your doctor.

Sine-Off Sinus
Each caplet contains 2 mg of chlorpheniramine, 30 mg of pseudoephedrine, and 500 mg of acetaminophen.

Adult and Child (age 12 and over): 2 caplets every 6 hours. Do not exceed 8 caplets in a 24-hour period.

Child (under age 12): Consult your doctor.

You may minimize the inconvenience of the sedative effects of these products by taking a full dose at bedtime or using the smallest recommended doses during the day. You can establish the lowest dose necessary for effective relief by starting with the lowest dose when you begin taking the drug, and gradually increasing the dosage over several days, as needed.

If you forget to take a dose of these products, do so as soon as you remember. If it is almost time for your next dose, skip the one you forgot and continue with your regular schedule. Do not take a double dose.

Overdosage

Symptoms of overdose include nausea, vomiting, abdominal pain, low blood pressure, fever, flushed face, dry mouth, dilated pupils, loss of muscle coordination, confusion, excitability, hallucinations, drowsiness, coma, seizures, yellowing of the skin and eyes, and liver damage. Symptoms may develop within 30 minutes, but may not be seen for as long as 2 days after the overdose.

Even if the victim is not displaying any of the symptoms listed above, do the following in case of accidental overdose: If the victim is unconscious or having convulsions, call for an ambulance immediately. If you take the victim to an emergency room, be sure to bring the bottle or container with you. If the victim is conscious, call your local poison control center or a health care professional. The poison control center may suggest inducing vomiting with ipecac syrup (available without a prescription at any pharmacy). DO NOT induce vomiting unless specifically instructed to do so.

Special Populations

Pregnancy/Breast-feeding

Antihistamines are not recommended for use during pregnancy unless directed by your doctor. Antihistamines, decongestants, and acetaminophen are known to pass into the breast milk of nursing mothers and may cause side effects in infants. Check with your doctor before taking Tylenol Allergy Sinus or Sine-Off Sinus if you are or might be pregnant, or if you are breast-feeding.

Infants/Children

Children may be more susceptible to the side effects of these products. They are also more susceptible to accidental overdose. Do not give Tylenol Allergy Sinus or Sine-Off Sinus to a child under age 12 except on the advice of a physician.

Seniors

Older persons may be more sensitive to the side effects of antihistamines and decongestants. They may experience nervousness, irritability, blurred vision, constipation, urinary retention, confusion, restlessness, dizziness, sedation, hallucinations, seizures, and low blood pressure. Most mild reactions may be handled by either lowering the dose or by switching to another product.

Seniors taking Tylenol Allergy Sinus or Sine-Off Sinus should be especially cautious about the amount of caffeine they ingest (see "Drug Interactions").

Brand Name

Sudafed Cold & Allergy (SOO-dah-fed)

Generic Ingredients

Chlorpheniramine maleate
Pseudoephedrine

Type of Drug

Antihistamine and decongestant.

Used for

Relief of nasal congestion, itchy and watery eyes, itching of the nose and throat, runny nose, and sneezing associated with colds and allergies.

General Information

Some OTC products use a combination of drugs to relieve the many symptoms that can accompany colds and allergies. Sudafed Cold & Allergy contains an antihistamine plus a decongestant.

The antihistamine in Sudafed Cold & Allergy is chlorpheniramine maleate. Antihistamines block the release of histamine in the body, relieving the sneezing and itching that often occurs with colds and allergies. They can also aid in stopping a runny nose by reducing the secretions caused by histamine release.

Since histamine is only one of several substances released by the body during an allergic reaction, antihistamines can reduce only about 40% to 60% of allergic symptoms.

The decongestant in Sudafed Cold & Allergy, and the ingredient from which it gets its name, is pseudoephedrine, an oral decongestant. Decongestants work by narrowing or constricting the blood vessels. This relieves the swelling of mucous membranes of the nose and sinuses. Unlike topical decongestants (decongestant nasal sprays), which act on local blood vessels, oral decongestants may constrict blood vessels throughout the body.

Sudafed Cold & Allergy will not cure or prevent allergies or colds. The best you can hope for is symptomatic relief. Colds will usually go away in 1 to 2 weeks whether they are treated or not.

Cautions and Warnings

Do not take Sudafed Cold & Allergy for more than 7 consecutive days unless directed by your doctor.

Do not exceed the recommended daily dosage of Sudafed Cold & Allergy.

Sudafed Cold & Allergy should be used with caution if you have a condition that causes breathing problems, such as emphysema, chronic bronchitis, or asthma. Its antihistamine ingredient, chlorpheniramine, acts to dry the mucous membranes. This in turn can inhibit the ability of the lungs to move or get rid of the excess secretions that these conditions produce.

Sudafed Cold & Allergy should be used with caution by people with glaucoma, hyperthyroidism, heart disease, high blood pressure, diabetes, or an enlarged prostate. If you have any of these conditions, take Sudafed Cold & Allergy only on the advice of your doctor.

Antihistamines act as a depressant on the central nervous system (CNS), and can cause sleepiness or grogginess and interfere with the ability to concentrate. Your ability to perform activities that require your full alertness and coordination, such as driving a motor vehicle or operating machinery, may be affected. Refrain from drinking alcohol while you are taking Sudafed Cold & Allergy because alcohol aggravates these effects.

Possible Side Effects

▼ Most common: restlessness, nervousness, sleeplessness or drowsiness, dizziness, excitability, poor muscle coordination, headache, and upset stomach.

Possible Side Effects ***(continued)***

▼ Less common: dry eyes, nose, and mouth; blurred vision; difficulty urinating; irritability (at high doses); increased blood pressure; increased or irregular heart rate; and heart palpitations.

▼ Rare: anxiety, tremor, hallucinations, seizures, breathing difficulty, and cardiovascular collapse.

Drug Interactions

• Antihistamines can enhance the effect of other drugs that depress the CNS, such as barbiturates, tranquilizers, sleep medications, and alcohol (present in many OTC preparations). If you are taking other depressant drugs, check with your doctor before taking Sudafed Cold & Allergy. Avoid drinking alcohol if you are taking Sudafed Cold & Allergy.

• Antihistamines can affect the results of skin and blood tests. Notify your health care professional before scheduling these tests if you are taking Sudafed Cold & Allergy.

• Sudafed Cold & Allergy should not be used at the same time as a monoamine oxidase inhibitor (MAOI) or within 2 weeks of stopping treatment with an MAOI. MAOIs are used to treat depression, other psychiatric or emotional conditions, and Parkinson's disease. If you are not sure whether you are or have been taking an MAOI, check with your doctor or pharmacist before you use Sudafed Cold & Allergy.

• Taking Sudafed Cold & Allergy along with another decongestant can increase the risk of adverse effects and toxicity. If you are taking another decongestant, do not take Sudafed Cold & Allergy without first asking your doctor.

• The effects of the decongestant in Sudafed Cold & Allergy may also combine with those of caffeine, a CNS stimulant found in many prescription and OTC drugs. This combination can cause disorientation, delirium, and other side effects.

Food Interactions

Decongestants interact adversely with caffeine (see "Drug Interactions"), which is found in many popular beverages, including coffee, tea, and cola, and in chocolate.

Usual Dose

If you are taking Sudafed Cold & Allergy for allergies, it is best to take it on a schedule rather than as needed because histamine is released almost continuously.

Each tablet of Sudafed Cold & Allergy contains 4 mg of chlorpheniramine and 60 mg of pseudoephedrine.

Adult and Child (age 12 and over): 1 tablet every 4 to 6 hours. Do not exceed 4 doses in a 24-hour period.

Child (age 6–11): 1/2 tablet every 4 to 6 hours. Do not exceed 4 doses in a 24-hour period.

Child (under age 6): Consult your doctor.

You may minimize the inconvenience of the sedative effects of Sudafed Cold & Allergy by taking a full dose at bedtime and using the smallest recommended doses during the day. You can establish the lowest dose necessary for effective relief by starting with the lowest dose when you begin taking the drug, and gradually increasing the dosage over several days, as needed.

If you forget to take a dose of Sudafed Cold & Allergy, do so as soon as you remember. If it is almost time for your next dose, skip the one you forgot and continue with your regular schedule. Do not take a double dose.

Overdosage

Symptoms of overdose in children include dilated pupils, flushed face, dry mouth, fever, excitability, hallucinations, loss of muscle coordination, and seizures.

In adults, severe overdose can cause drowsiness or coma, which may be followed by excitability or seizures. Eventually fluid can build up in the brain; the kidneys may fail, and the heart and lungs may stop working, resulting in death. Symptoms may develop within 30 minutes to 2 hours following an overdose, and death may occur within 18 hours.

Even if the victim is not displaying any of the symptoms listed above, do the following in case of accidental overdose: If the victim is unconscious or having convulsions, call for an ambulance immediately. If you take the victim to an emergency room, be sure to bring the bottle or container with you. If the victim is conscious, call your local poison control center or a health care professional. The poison control center may suggest inducing vomiting with ipecac syrup (available without a prescription at any pharmacy). DO NOT induce vomiting unless specifically instructed to do so.

Special Populations

Pregnancy/Breast-feeding

Antihistamines are not recommended for use during pregnancy unless directed by your doctor. Antihistamines and decongestants are known to pass into the breast milk of nursing mothers and may cause side effects in infants. Check with your doctor before taking Sudafed Cold & Allergy if you are or might be pregnant, or if you are breast-feeding.

Infants/Children

Children are more susceptible to the side effects of Sudafed Cold & Allergy. They are also more susceptible to accidental antihistamine overdose. Do not give Sudafed Cold & Allergy to a child under 6 unless directed by your doctor.

Seniors

Older persons may be more sensitive to the side effects of antihistamines and decongestants. They may experience nervousness, irritability, restlessness, dizziness, sedation, hallucinations, seizures, and low blood pressure. Most mild reactions may be handled by either lowering the dose or by switching to another product.

Seniors taking Sudafed Cold & Allergy should be especially cautious about the amount of caffeine they ingest (see "Drug Interactions").

Sudafed Sinus (SOO-dah-fed)

*see **Sine-Aid,** page 460*

Sudafed 12 Hour Caplets (SOO-dah-fed)

*see **Pseudophedrine,** page 1002*

Brand Name

Tavist-D (TAV-ist)

Generic Ingredients

Clemastine fumarate (CLEM-us-teen FOO-muh-rate)
Phenylpropanolamine

Type of Drug

Antihistamine and decongestant.

Used for

Relief of runny nose, sneezing, nasal congestion, itchy and watery eyes, and itching of the nose or throat associated with allergies.

General Information

Some OTC products use a combination of drugs to relieve the many symptoms that can accompany colds and allergies. Tavist-D contains an antihistamine and a decongestant.

The antihistamine in Tavist-D is clemastine fumarate. Antihistamines block the release of histamine in the body, relieving the sneezing and itching that often occurs with colds and allergies. They can also aid in stopping a runny nose by reducing the secretions caused by histamine release.

Since histamine is only one of several substances released by the body during an allergic reaction, antihistamines can only reduce about 40% to 60% of allergic symptoms.

The decongestant in Tavist-D is phenylpropanolamine, an oral decongestant. Decongestants work by narrowing or constricting the blood vessels. This relieves the swelling of mucous membranes of the nose and sinuses. Unlike topical decongestants (decongestant nasal sprays), which act on local blood vessels, oral decongestants may constrict blood vessels throughout the body.

Tavist-D will not cure or prevent allergies or colds. The best you can hope for is symptomatic relief. Colds will usually go away in 1 to 2 weeks whether they are treated or not.

Cautions and Warnings

Do not take Tavist-D for more than 7 days continuously. If symptoms do not improve, or fever is present, see a doctor.

Do not exceed the recommended daily dosage of Tavist-D.

Tavist-D should be used with caution if you have a condition that causes breathing problems, such as emphysema, chronic bronchitis, or asthma. Its antihistamine ingredient acts to dry the mucous membranes. This in turn can inhibit the ability of the lungs to move or get rid of the excess secretions that these conditions produce.

Tavist-D should be used with caution by people with glaucoma, hyperthyroidism, heart disease, high blood pressure, diabetes, or an enlarged prostate. If you have any of these conditions, take Tavist-D only on the advice of your doctor.

Antihistamines act as a depressant on the central nervous system (CNS), and can cause sleepiness or grogginess and interfere with the ability to concentrate. Your ability to perform activities that require your full alertness and coordination, such as driving a motor vehicle or operating machinery, may be affected. Refrain from drinking alcohol while you are taking Tavist-D because alcohol aggravates these effects.

Possible Side Effects

▼ Most common: restlessness, nervousness, sleeplessness or drowsiness, dizziness, excitability, poor muscle coordination, headache, and upset stomach.

▼ Less common: dry eyes, nose, and mouth; blurred vision; difficulty urinating; irritability (at high doses); increased blood pressure; increased or irregular heart rate; heart palpitations; and loss of appetite.

▼ Rare: severe headache, feelings of tightness in the chest, greatly elevated blood pressure, rapid heartbeat, and heart palpitations.

Drug Interactions

• Antihistamines can enhance the effect of other drugs that depress the CNS, such as barbiturates, tranquilizers, sleeping medications, and alcohol (present in many OTC preparations). If you are taking other depressant drugs, check with your doctor before you take Tavist-D. Avoid drinking alcohol if you are taking Tavist-D.

• Antihistamines can also affect the results of skin and blood tests. Notify your health care professional before scheduling these tests if you are taking Tavist-D.

• Tavist-D should not be used at the same time as a monoamine oxidase inhibitor (MAOI) or within 2 weeks of stopping treatment with an MAOI. MAOIs are used to treat depression, other psychiatric or emotional conditions, and Parkinson's disease. If you are not sure whether you are or have been taking an MAOI, check with your doctor or pharmacist before you use Tavist-D.

• The effects of phenylpropanolamine, the decongestant in Tavist-D, may combine with those of caffeine, a CNS stimulant found in many prescription and OTC drugs. This combination can cause disorientation, delirium, and other side effects.

• Taking Tavist-D along with another decongestant can increase the risk of adverse effects and toxicity. If you are taking another decongestant, do not take Tavist-D without first asking your doctor.

Food Interactions

Decongestants interact adversely with caffeine (see "Drug Interactions"), which is found in many popular beverages, including coffee, tea, and cola, and in chocolate.

Usual Dose

Each tablet contains 1.34 mg of clemastine and 75 mg of phenylpropanolamine. Because histamine is released almost continuously, it is best to take Tavist-D on a schedule rather than as needed.

Adult and Child (age 12 and over): 1 tablet every 12 hours, not to exceed 2 tablets in 24 hours.

Child (under age 12): Consult your doctor.

If you forget to take a dose of Tavist-D, do so as soon as you remember. If it is almost time for your next dose, skip the one you forgot and continue with your regular schedule.

Tavist-D tablets should be swallowed whole with fluid—never chewed, crushed, or dissolved.

Overdosage

Symptoms of overdose in children include dilated pupils, flushed face, dry mouth, fever, excitability, hallucinations, loss of muscle coordination, and seizures.

In adults, severe overdose can cause drowsiness or coma, which may be followed by excitability or seizures. Eventually fluid can build up in the brain; the kidneys may fail, and the heart and lungs may stop working, resulting in death. Symptoms may develop within 30 minutes to 2 hours following an overdose, and death may occur within 18 hours.

Even if the victim is not displaying any of the symptoms listed above, do the following in case of accidental overdose: If the victim is unconscious or having convulsions, call for an ambulance immediately. If you take the victim to an emergency room, be sure to bring the bottle or container with you. If the victim is conscious, call your local poison control center or a health care professional. The poison control center may suggest inducing vomiting with ipecac syrup (available without a prescription at any pharmacy). DO NOT induce vomiting unless specifically instructed to do so.

Special Populations

Pregnancy/Breast-feeding

Antihistamines are not recommended for use during pregnancy unless directed by your doctor. Antihistamines and decongestants are known to pass into the breast milk of nursing mothers and may cause side effects in infants. Check with your doctor before taking Tavist-D if you are or might be pregnant, or if you are breast-feeding.

Infants/Children

Children may be more susceptible to the side effects of Tavist-D. They are also more susceptible to accidental antihistamine overdose. Do not give Tavist-D to a child under 12 unless directed by your doctor.

Seniors

Older individuals should not take Tavist-D, which is an extended-release preparation, until they have first tried a short-acting product containing the decongestant phenylpropanolamine and experienced no ill effects.

Older persons may be more sensitive to the side effects of antihistamines and decongestants. They may experience nervousness, irritability, restlessness, dizziness, sedation, hallucinations, seizures, and low blood pressure. Most mild reactions may be handled by either lowering the dose or switching to another product.

Seniors taking Tavist-D should be especially cautious about the amount of caffeine they ingest (see "Food Interactions").

Brand Name

Tavist-1 (TAV-ist)

Generic Ingredient

Clemastine fumarate (CLEM-us-teen FOO-muh-rate)

Type of Drug

Antihistamine.

Used for

Temporary relief of runny nose, itching of the nose or throat, sneezing, and itchy and watery eyes associated with allergies.

General Information

Histamine is one of the substances released by the body during an allergic reaction. When it is released, the body reacts with a variety of symptoms, including itching and sneezing. Antihistamines work by competitively inhibiting the pharmacological action of histamine, which makes them very effective in relieving the symptoms of allergic reactions. Antihistamines may also help relieve a runny nose. The antihistamine in Tavist-1 is clemastine fumarate.

Because antihistamines do not work against the other substances released by the body during an allergic reaction, they can reduce only about 40% to 60% of allergic symptoms. They are also not effective in clearing up a stuffy nose.

If you have seasonal allergies, antihistamines work best

if you begin treatment before the allergy season starts. Once these allergies begin, the body releases histamine continuously. Thus the best method of controlling histamine release is to keep taking antihistamines on a continuous schedule once you start. This helps the antihistamine keep up with the constant release of histamine. People who experience allergies year round (e.g., allergies to pet hair or dust mites) may need to take antihistamines throughout the year.

Tavist-1 will not cure or prevent allergies. The best you can hope for is temporary relief of some symptoms.

Cautions and Warnings

Do not exceed the recommended daily dosage of Tavist-1.

Unless directed by a doctor, Tavist-1 should not be used by people with asthma, emphysema, or chronic bronchitis.

Tavist-1 should be used with caution by people with hyperthyroidism, heart disease, hypertension, glaucoma, or difficulty urinating due to a prostate problem. If you have any of these conditions, consult your doctor before taking Tavist-1.

Antihistamines act as a depressant on the central nervous system (CNS), and can cause sleepiness or grogginess and interfere with the ability to concentrate. Your ability to perform activities that require your full alertness and coordination, such as driving a motor vehicle or operating machinery, may be affected. Refrain from drinking alcohol while you are taking Tavist-1 because alcohol aggravates these effects.

Possible Side Effects

- ▼ Most common: restlessness, nervousness, sleeplessness or drowsiness, poor muscle coordination, dizziness, excitability, and upset stomach.
- ▼ Least common: dry eyes, nose, and mouth; blurred vision; constipation; difficulty urinating; irritability (at high doses); increased or irregular heart rate; and heart palpitations.

Drug Interactions

• Antihistamines can enhance the effect of other drugs that depress the CNS, such as barbiturates, tranquilizers, sleeping medications, and alcohol (present in many OTC preparations). If you are taking other depressant drugs, check with your doctor before you take Tavist-1. Avoid drinking alcohol if you are taking Tavist-1.

• Tavist-1 should not be used at the same time as a monoamine oxidase inhibitor (MAOI) or within 2 weeks of stopping treatment with an MAOI. MAOIs are used to treat depression, other psychiatric or emotional conditions, and Parkinson's disease. If you are not sure whether you are or have been taking an MAOI, check with your doctor or pharmacist before you use Tavist-1.

• Antihistamines can affect the results of skin and blood tests. Notify your health care professional before scheduling these tests if you are taking Tavist-1.

Food Interactions

None known.

Usual Dose

During an allergic reaction, histamine release occurs continuously; therefore Tavist-1 should be taken at scheduled times (every 12 hours) rather than on an as-needed basis.

Adult and Child (age 12 and over): One tablet twice daily. Do not exceed 2 tablets in a 24-hour period.

Child (under age 12): Consult your doctor.

If you forget to take a dose of Tavist-1, do so as soon as you remember. If it is almost time for your next dose, skip the one you forgot and continue with your regular schedule. Do not take a double dose.

Tavist-1 tablets should be swallowed whole with fluid—never chewed, crushed, or dissolved.

Overdosage

Symptoms of antihistamine overdose in children include dilated pupils, flushed face, dry mouth, fever, excitability, hallucinations, loss of muscle coordination, and seizures.

In adults, severe overdose can cause drowsiness or coma, which may be followed by excitability or seizures. Eventually fluid can build up in the brain; the kidneys may fail, and the heart and lungs may stop working, resulting in death. Symptoms may develop within 30 minutes to 2 hours following an overdose, and death may occur within 18 hours.

Even if the victim is not displaying any of the symptoms listed above, do the following in case of accidental overdose: If the victim is unconscious or having convulsions, call for an ambulance immediately. If you take the victim to an emergency room, be sure to bring the bottle or container with you. If the victim is conscious, call your local poison control center or a health care professional. The poison control center may suggest inducing vomiting with ipecac syrup (available without a prescription at any pharmacy). DO NOT induce vomiting unless specifically instructed to do so.

Special Populations

Pregnancy/Breast-feeding

Antihistamines are not recommended for use during pregnancy unless directed by your doctor. Antihistamines are known to pass into the breast milk of nursing mothers and may cause side effects in infants. Check with your doctor before taking Tavist-1 if you are or might be pregnant, or if you are breast-feeding.

Infants/Children

Children may be more susceptible to the side effects of Tavist-1. They are also more susceptible to accidental antihistamine overdose. Do not give Tavist-1 to a child under 12 unless directed by your doctor.

Seniors

Older individuals are more sensitive to antihistamines than younger adults and can experience nervousness, irritability, and restlessness when taking one of these drugs. Seniors may also be more sensitive to the anticholinergic side effects (dry eyes, nose, or mouth; blurred vision; constipation; difficult urination) of Tavist-1. Most mild reactions may be handled by either lowering your dose or trying another antihistamine.

Brand Names

Teldrin (TELL-drin)
Triaminic Syrup (TRYE-uh-MIN-ick)

Generic Ingredients

Chlorpheniramine maleate
Phenylpropanolamine

Type of Drug

Antihistamine and decongestant.

Used for

Relief of runny nose, sneezing, nasal congestion, itchy and watery eyes, and itching of the nose or throat associated with colds and allergies.

General Information

Some OTC products use a combination of drugs to relieve the many symptoms that can accompany colds and allergies. Teldrin and Triaminic Syrup contain an antihistamine and a decongestant.

The antihistamine in these products is chlorpheniramine maleate. Antihistamines block the release of histamine in the body, relieving the sneezing and itching that often occurs with colds and allergies. They can also aid in stopping a runny nose by reducing the secretions caused by histamine release.

Since histamine is only one of several substances released by the body during an allergic reaction, antihistamines can only reduce about 40% to 60% of allergic symptoms.

The decongestant in these products is phenylpropanolamine, an oral decongestant. Decongestants work by narrowing or constricting the blood vessels. This relieves the swelling of the mucous membranes of the nose and sinuses. Unlike topical decongestants (decongestant nasal sprays), which act on local blood vessels, oral decongestants may constrict blood vessels throughout the body.

Teldrin or Triaminic Syrup will not cure or prevent allergies or colds. The best you can hope for is symptomatic relief. Colds will usually go away in 1 to 2 weeks whether they are treated or not.

Cautions and Warnings

Do not take Teldrin or Triaminic Syrup for more than 7 days continuously. If symptoms do not improve, or fever is present, see a doctor.

Do not exceed the recommended daily dosage of these products.

Teldrin should be used with caution if you have a condition that causes breathing problems, such as emphysema, chronic bronchitis, or asthma. Its antihistamine ingredient acts to dry the mucous membranes. This in turn can inhibit the ability of the lungs to move or get rid of the excess secretions that these conditions produce.

Teldrin should be used with caution by people with glaucoma, hyperthyroidism, heart disease, high blood pressure, diabetes, or an enlarged prostate, because it can worsen these conditions. If you have any of these conditions, consult your doctor before taking Teldrin or Triaminic Syrup.

Antihistamines act as a depressant on the central nervous system (CNS), and can cause sleepiness or grogginess and interfere with the ability to concentrate. Your ability to perform activities that require your full alertness and coordination, such as driving a motor vehicle or operating machinery, may be affected. Refrain from drinking alcohol while you are taking these products because alcohol aggravates these effects.

Possible Side Effects

- ▼ Most common: restlessness, nervousness, sleeplessness or drowsiness, dizziness, excitability, poor muscle coordination, headache, and upset stomach.
- ▼ Less common: dry eyes, nose, and mouth; blurred vision; difficulty urinating; irritability (at high doses); increased blood pressure; increased or irregular heart rate; heart palpitations; and loss of appetite.
- ▼ Rare: severe headache, feelings of tightness in the chest, greatly elevated blood pressure, rapid heartbeat, and heart palpitations.

Drug Interactions

• Antihistamines can enhance the effect of other drugs that depress the CNS, such as barbiturates, tranquilizers, sleeping medications, and alcohol (present in many OTC preparations). If you are taking other depressant drugs, check with your doctor before taking Teldrin or Triaminic Syrup. Avoid drinking alcohol if you are taking Teldrin or Triaminic Syrup.

• Antihistamines can also affect the results of skin and blood tests. Notify your health care professional before scheduling these tests if you are taking these products.

• These products should not be used at the same time as a monoamine oxidase inhibitor (MAOI) or within 2 weeks of stopping treatment with an MAOI. MAOIs are used to treat depression, other psychiatric or emotional conditions, and Parkinson's disease. If you are not sure whether you are or have been taking an MAOI, check with your doctor or pharmacist before you use Teldrin or Triaminic Syrup.

• The effects of phenylpropanolamine, the decongestant in these products, may combine with those of caffeine, a CNS stimulant found in many prescription and OTC drugs. This combination can cause disorientation, delirium, and other side effects.

• Taking these products along with another decongestant can increase the risk of adverse effects and toxicity. If you are taking another decongestant, do not take Teldrin or Triaminic Syrup without first asking your doctor.

Food Interactions

Decongestants interact adversely with caffeine (see "Drug Interactions"), which is found in many popular beverages including coffee, tea, and cola, and in chocolate.

Usual Dose

If you are taking Teldrin or Triaminic Syrup for allergies, it is best to take them on a schedule rather than as needed because histamine is released almost continuously.

Teldrin

Each capsule contains 75 mg of phenylpropanolamine and 8 mg of chlorpheniramine.

Adult and Child (age 12 and over): 1 capsule every 12 hours. Do not exceed 2 capsules in 24 hours.

Child (under age 12): Consult your doctor.

Teldrin is a timed-release formulation. The active drugs are contained within a substance that releases the medication slowly over 12 hours. The capsules should be swallowed whole with fluid. Do not crush, chew, or dissolve the tablets. Breaking the timed-release coating causes the medications to be released too quickly, increasing the risk of side effects.

Triaminic
Each 5 ml (1 tsp.) contains 1 mg of chlorpheniramine and 6.25 mg of phenylpropanolamine.

Adult and Child (age 12 and over): 3 tsp. every 4–6 hours. Do not exceed 6 doses in a 24-hour period.

Child (age 6–11): 2 tsp. every 4–6 hours. Do not exceed 6 doses in a 24-hour period.

Child (under age 6): Consult your doctor.

You may minimize the inconvenience of the sedative effects of these products by taking a full dose at bedtime or using the smallest recommended doses during the day. You can establish the lowest dose necessary for effective relief by starting with the lowest dose when you begin taking the drug, and gradually increasing the dosage over several days, as needed.

If you forget to take a dose of these products, do so as soon as you remember. If it is almost time for your next dose, skip the one you forgot and continue with your regular schedule. Do not take a double dose.

Overdosage

Symptoms of overdose in children include dilated pupils, flushed face, dry mouth, fever, excitability, hallucinations, loss of muscle coordination, and seizures.

In adults, severe overdose can cause drowsiness or coma, which may be followed by excitability or seizures. Eventually fluid can build up in the brain; the kidneys may fail, and the heart and lungs may stop working, resulting in death. Symptoms may develop within 30 minutes to 2 hours following an overdose, and death may occur within 18 hours.

Even if the victim is not displaying any of the symptoms listed above, do the following in case of accidental overdose: If the victim is unconscious or having convulsions, call for an ambulance immediately. If you take the victim to an emergency room, be sure to bring the bottle or container with you. If the victim is conscious, call your local poison control center or a health care professional. The poison control center may suggest inducing vomiting with ipecac syrup (available without a prescription at any pharmacy). DO NOT induce vomiting unless specifically instructed to do so.

Special Populations

Pregnancy/Breast-feeding
Antihistamines are not recommended for use during pregnancy unless directed by your doctor. Antihistamines and decongestants are known to pass into the breast milk of nursing mothers and may cause side effects in infants. Check with your doctor before taking Teldrin or Triaminic Syrup if you are or might be pregnant, or if you are breast-feeding.

Infants/Children
Children may be more susceptible to the side effects of Teldrin. They are also more susceptible to accidental antihistamine overdose. Unless directed by your doctor, do not give Teldrin to a child under age 12 or Triaminic Syrup to a child under age 6.

Seniors
Older individuals should not take Teldrin, which is an extended-release preparation, until they have first tried a short-acting product containing the decongestant phenylpropanolamine and experienced no ill effects.

Older persons may be more sensitive to the side effects of these products. They may experience nervousness, irritability, restlessness, dizziness, sedation, hallucinations, seizures, and low blood pressure. Most mild reactions may be handled by either lowering the dose or switching to another product.

Seniors taking these products should be especially cautious about the amount of caffeine they ingest (see "Drug Interactions").

Tylenol Allergy Sinus (TYE-leh-nol)

*see **Sine-Off Sinus,** page 465*

Tylenol Sinus (TYE-leh-nol)

*see **Sine-Aid,** page 460*

Chapter 8: Eye, Ear, and Mouth Care

Eye Problems

Our eyes are delicate structures, vulnerable to many kinds of injuries and infections. Fortunately, they are also able to protect themselves in a number of ways: Eyelids create a physical barrier that blocks out particles; eyelashes act like nets to trap debris before it reaches the eye; and tear glands produce a complex fluid that washes across the eye to lubricate the surface and remove particles. The fluid also contains antimicrobial enzymes that help destroy potential infectious agents. When we blink, the eyelids force the tears to flow toward a canal, through which they drain into the nose. The cornea (the surface of the eye) is a clear layer that acts as a shield to protect the rest of the eyeball. The blink reflex protects our eyes from any potential threat of injury.

Certain eye problems can be safely and easily treated at home. Others, however, need the attention of health care professionals. Vision is too precious to risk.

Eye Problems

Corneal Swelling

Swelling (edema) can occur if fluid becomes trapped between the layers that make up the cornea. The swelling distorts the surface, causing optical distortions, halos or starbursts around lights, and reduction of vision. A number of factors can contribute to the problem, including wearing contact lenses longer than indicated, infection, trauma, surgical damage, or inherited problems.

Dry Eye

Dryness can arise due to the normal process of aging. It can also be a side effect of various medications, including antihistamines, antidepressants, and diuretics, or it may result from medical conditions such as rheumatoid arthritis. Symptoms include a mild redness and the feeling of sand or grit under the eyelid. In many cases, people with dry eye produce tears that do not supply adequate lubrication or moisture. The eye then tries to secrete more fluid to counteract the problem. Thus, despite the name, dry eye can often involve watery, runny eyes.

Eyelid Infection

Blepharitis (eyelid infection), a common and chronic complaint, is usually caused by staphylococcus, although it may also be a complication of seborrheic dermatitis (see Chapter 5). Symptoms include redness and thickening of the eyelids, crusting or scaling, itching and burning, and loss of eyelashes.

Inflammation

Different parts of the eye can develop inflammation. Inflammation of the cornea is known as keratitis; inflammation of the iris (the colored part of the eye) and uvea (the iris and other nearby tissues) is iritis or uveitis. All these conditions cause redness, blurred vision, sensitivity to light, and pain, and possibly excess tear production. In some cases self-treatment may improve the problem, but as a rule you should see a doctor.

Pinkeye

Conjunctivitis (pinkeye) is a general name for inflammation of either the membrane along the inner surface of the eyelids or that which covers the sclera (the white of the eye). The problem can result from allergy or from an infection caused by a virus, bacteria, or chlamydia. Symptoms of pinkeye vary depending on the cause, but they generally include redness, watery discharge, crusting and sticking together of the eyelids on waking, and an annoying feeling that an object has become lodged under the eyelid. Infectious pinkeye might involve minor fever and swollen lymph nodes, while allergic pinkeye usually causes itching.

Stye

A hordeolum (stye) is a raised, tender nodule resulting from an inflammation of glands in the eye. In severe cases, the eyelid can swell almost shut. Styes are caused by the same staphylococcal germs that cause eyelid infection.

Seek medical attention if any of the following applies to you

- Blurred vision
- Decreased light perception (compared to normal)
- Chemical burns
- Eye problems resulting from head injury
- Eye problems that persist for longer than 3 days despite self-treatment with lubricants or decongestants
- Flash burns or other thermal (heat) injuries
- Foreign object lodged in the eyé, especially metal particles from high-speed grinding
- Infection of the tear ducts
- Injury from a blunt object
- Light sensitivity
- Mucus discharge
- Wounds or ulcers (tears) on the cornea
- Corneal abrasions (scrapes)
- Blunt trauma

Treatment for Eye Problems

OTC products for the eye must be sterile in their original container. They also must have preservative added to maintain sterility while the product is being used. Eye products must also have their pH adjusted to ensure compatibility with the tissue of the eye.

Lubricants

Human tears serve to lubricate, moisten, and cleanse the eye. Various OTC preparations are intended to duplicate one or more of these functions.

If tears are too watery, they flow across the eye and out the drainage canal too rapidly to be effective. This is the problem in conditions such as dry eye. Lubricants are ingredients that help make the tears more viscous (stickier). The tears thus remain on the surface of the eye, allowing the eyelid to close more easily and the eye to move more easily in the socket.

There are 2 main types of lubricants: demulcents (artificial tears and nonmedicated emollients (ointments).

Artificial tears come in drops and liquid solutions. The active ingredient in artificial tears helps stabilize the tear film and slow down its evaporation. Examples of such ingredients include cellulose ethers, polyvinyl alcohol, and povidone, which are used alone or in combination. Each of these works in a similar way and is safe to use, even as often as every hour. In addition to increasing viscosity, povidone helps to enhance the amount of water contained within the cells of the cornea. People who wear contact lenses might want to avoid lubricants containing polyvinyl alcohol because there is some chance that polyvinyl alcohol may interact with the products used for cleaning the lenses.

Emollients, which are oil-based, help increase the stickiness of tears. Examples include petrolatum, mineral oil, and lanolin. Generally, emollients remain in the eye longer than the artificial tear solutions. These products are usually applied once or twice a day, but can be used every few hours if needed. Because they are long lasting, they are often used at bedtime for relief throughout the night. One drawback of daytime use is that ointments can cause minor temporary blurring of vision. Another disadvantage is that while the emollient ingredient does not irritate the eye, sometimes the preservative contained in the product can have this effect. If treatment is likely to continue for several days, an emollient without preservatives may be a better choice. However, these are intended for single-dose use and should be discarded after they are used. Read the label; if you still have questions, ask your pharmacist.

Decongestants

Decongestants work by reducing swollen blood vessels, thus shrinking the nearby tissues and relieving irritation. As eyedrops, they can relieve swollen membranes in the eyelid and the eyeball. Decongestants also relieve swollen nasal passages, because the medication drains through a canal from the eye into the nose.

Most OTC decongestant products contain either phenylephrine or one of a group of medications called imidazolines, which include naphazoline, tetrahydrozoline, and oxymetazoline. In high, prescription-strength concentrations (up to 20%), phenylephrine is used by doctors to dilate the pupils for eye exams. The concentrations available in OTC products are quite low (around 0.12%).

The imidazolines work to shrink membranes and have only a minimal effect on other blood vessels in the white of the eye. Generally, even in low concentrations naphazoline seems be more effective than the other imidazolines. People with blue or green eyes are more likely to experience pupil dilation when using this decongestant. Tetrahydrozoline, often used to treat conjunctivitis, does not alter pupil size. Its effects usually last up to 4 hours, but some people may experience mild temporary stinging after application. Oxymetazoline may be effective for up to 6 hours, and is usually used for relief of burning, itching, tearing, and the sensation of a foreign body in the eye.

Prolonged use of these products may cause side effects, including dryness. When decongestants are used more than 3 or 4 times a day for more than 3 or 4 days they can have a rebound effect, causing even more congestion between doses. Naphazoline and tetrahydrozoline are less likely to cause rebound congestion and so are probably the best choices. Still, decongestants should not be used for more than 3 days. If symptoms persist beyond that point, see a physician.

Antihistamines

The action of antihistamine drugs is described in detail in Chapter 7. Briefly, these medications counteract the effects of histamine, a chemical that cells release in response to the presence of an irritant or allergen (a substance that triggers an allergic response). Histamine causes irritation, itching, and increased mucus production. Like decongestants, antihistamines administered through the eyes work in part because they drain into the nasal passages, where histamine does most of its damage.

The 2 antihistamines available in OTC products are pheniramine and antazoline. Both are indicated for relief of pinkeye resulting from allergies. The usual dosage is 1 or 2 drops applied to each eye up to 4 times a day. These products also contain the decongestant naphazoline, described above, which helps increase the effects of the antihistamine. Pheniramine appears to be less likely to cause stinging than antazoline. Otherwise, the medications are about the same in terms of safety and efficacy.

Irrigants
An irrigant is a product—basically saltwater—used to cleanse the eye and help preserve moisture. Although generally very harmless, irrigants should be used only for short periods, not on a regular basis. They are often used as emergency eyewashes in cases of chemical injuries to the eye, but people exposed to chemicals, especially acids or alkalis, should see a physician as soon as possible.

Hyperosmotics
Eye care products classified as hyperosmotics are intended to increase the fluidity of tears, thus helping them to wash across the eyeball more efficiently. Because they draw water out of cells in the cornea, these products can reduce swelling. Despite the fancy name, the only active ingredient in OTC hyperosmotics is good old sodium chloride—salt. These products are available in ointments and solutions. Generally, ointments with a 5% concentration of sodium chloride are the most effective, but a 2% concentration is better for long-term use. Do not use these products if the cornea is scratched or torn.

Antiseptics
Since pinkeye and other eye problems can arise from bacterial infection, use of antiseptics may provide some relief in mild cases. As a rule, though, the products available for use in the eyes have not been proven to be of much value. Many OTC eye care products contain weak antiseptics along with other active ingredients. Examples of these include silver protein, boric acid, and zinc sulfate. These are not effective in treating existing eye infections.

Eyelid Scrubs
These products contain mild detergents to facilitate removal of oil, debris, or dead skin cells from the eyelids. They are primarily used to treat cases of eyelid infection. The eyelid should first be treated with a hot water compress, applied for 15 to 20 minutes 4 times a day. Then the lid scrub should be applied with a soft cloth or gauze pad, using gentle side-to-side strokes. In many cases, a baby shampoo works just as well, but there is a somewhat greater risk of stinging or burning with shampoo than with a specially formulated scrub. If symptoms do not improve, treatment with a prescription antibacterial agent may be needed.

Tips for Using Eyedrops

All eye care products intended for multiple-dose use contain preservatives and sometimes antioxidants. Take care when using these products to ensure that tears or other fluids are not drawn back up into the container, which would dilute the effects of the preservative. Discard any eye medication that has turned cloudy or has separated in the bottle. Pay close attention to the expiration date—do not use after the expiration date.

1. Wash hands.
2. Tilt head back.
3. Grasp the lower eyelid and pull it forward, creating a pouch.
4. Position the dropper above the eye and look straight at it.
5. Look upward as far as possible and squeeze the dropper.
6. After applying the drop, look down for a few seconds.
7. Slowly release the eyelid.
8. Close eyes for a few minutes. Resist the urge to blink or squeeze the eyes.
9. Press gently on the tear duct area (inner corner of the eye); this prevents the medication from draining too rapidly.
10. With a tissue, blot away any excess fluid.

OTC Products for Eye Problems

Lubricants
- Artificial tear solutions
- Nonmedicated ointments

Decongestants

Antihistamines

Irrigants

Hyperosmotics

Antiseptics

Eyelid scrubs

Ear Problems

The ears are channels through which sound travels. Inside the ear is a membrane called the eardrum, which vibrates when sound waves hit it. The vibrations move the 3 tiniest bones in the body (called the hammer, the anvil, and the stirrup). The motions of these bones in turn stimulate the auditory nerve, which converts the vibrations to electrical impulses and speeds them to the brain.

Because the ears are exposed to the outside world, they are vulnerable to damage. However, like the eyes, the ears have their own set of defenses. The outer part of the ear canal is lined with hairs that trap foreign bodies such as dust particles, preventing them from penetrating further. The skin of the ear also contains large numbers of glands that secrete an oily yellow-brown material called cerumen, more commonly known as earwax. Cerumen is the ear's self-cleaning system; it works to trap dirt, bacteria, and other particles. Usually, the wax hardens and falls out, swept along by the movement of the hairs, and a fresh layer takes its place.

Ear problems are common. The outer shell of the ear can suffer injury. The inner canal can become infected. As is the case everywhere in the body, swellings and nodules can develop on the skin. The delicate eardrum can rupture; the fragile neighboring bones can break. Even earwax, normally a protective substance, can build up and cause pain or hearing loss. The ear canals are located near the jaw, and the eustachian, or auditory, tubes drain from the ears to the throat. Because of their proximity, problems in those parts of the head and neck can also cause trouble in the ears.

For the most part, ear conditions should be treated by physicians. Conditions for which OTC remedies are of use include wax buildup and boils. In some cases, other OTC products may soothe minor inflammation.

Wax buildup results from a number of factors. For example, the glands may produce wax at too fast a rate, or the hairs may lose their ability to push the cerumen out.

Boils are infections that develop in hair follicles. The skin erupts into a pus-filled swelling that becomes red, irritated, and painful.

Minor inflammation usually results from a small-scale infection. Sometimes water gets trapped in one of the ear's many cul-de-sacs. Like a tiny stagnant pond, the water can serve as a breeding ground for bacteria and fungi. This condition is commonly known as swimmer's ear.

Seek medical attention if any of the following applies to you

- Severe pain
- Swollen lymph glands
- Discharge from the ear
- Fever
- Hearing loss
- Recurrent ear infections that do not respond to treatment
- Foreign object lodged in the ear
- Constant ringing, humming, or other noise in the ear
- A spinning sensation when you move your head

Treatment for Ear Problems

Earwax Removal

Certain chemicals act to soften earwax and loosen it, making it somewhat easier to remove through careful rinsing. It is a bad idea to use devices such as cotton swabs, tweezers, or bobby pins to try and remove the wax. Poking can damage your eardrum or make the wax form a thick ball, which might then block the passage. If your ears are plugged with cerumen, your physician can flush it out using a special kind of squirt gun.

The main ingredient in OTC earwax products is hydrogen peroxide. When applied, this simple chemical releases oxygen in the form of bubbles, which dissolve the wax and scrub away debris. Another ingredient is a softening agent such as glycerin or mineral oil. These oily substances make the wax more slippery. A gentle jet of warm water can then rinse away the material. Earwax removal products are typically used twice a day for up to 4 days (see box).

Steps for Earwax Removal

1. Wash hands.
2. Tilt the head so the affected ear is up.
3. Position the medication bottle just above (not in) the ear opening.
4. Apply the drops as directed.
5. Keep the medication in place for at least 15 minutes. Keep the head tilted or insert a cotton plug.
6. Repeat in the other ear if needed.
7. Flush using tepid (not hot or cold) water from a rubber syringe.
8. Repeat in each ear if necessary.
9. If the problem persists after 4 days, see a physician.

Boils

If the boil is small, hot compresses—soft cloths soaked in hot saltwater, pressed against the area—usually relieve the pain. An antibiotic ointment can be applied to the boil and the surrounding area. There are dozens of OTC antibiotic products (see chapter 4 for more information). Large or recurring boils should be treated by a doctor.

Minor Inflammation

There is little scientific evidence to show that medications available without a prescription are very effective in treating inflammation of the outer ear. Still, use of these eardrops may help some people. OTC products available to treat swimmer's ear contain a combination of ingredients. Some work by increasing the acid level inside the ear, making it harder for bacteria to grow there. Astringents (drying agents) such as alcohol or aluminum acetate can relieve inflammation and itching, and softening agents, described earlier, help break up earwax. A homemade solution for treatment of swimmer's ear can be made using distilled household vinegar mixed with equal parts of either water, glycerin, or rubbing alcohol. In more serious cases, where infection is involved, prior use of eardrops to clean the area can make topical anti-infective therapy, prescribed by a doctor, more effective.

OTC Products for Ear Problems

Earwax & wax softener (glycerin, oil products)
Hydrogen peroxide
Topical antibiotic products
Topical ear products

Canker Sores

Canker sores are small, painful ulcers that develop in the mouth. The technical term for these annoying growths is aphthous ulcers or aphthous stomatitis. They often emerge where the lips and gums meet, but can also develop on the tongue, soft palate, or the inside of the lips or cheeks. They do not usually affect the gums. The sores can appear individually, or they can develop in groups.

About 1 person in 5 has a canker sore at any given time. They most commonly affect people between ages 10 and 40, although sometimes they emerge in children as young as age 2. They occur in women somewhat more often than in men. Usually canker sores vanish on their own after a week or 10 days. Most people have only 1 or 2 episodes of sores a year. In more serious cases, however, they can recur so often that they are present almost constantly. Severe cankers can interfere with drinking or swallowing, and they can leave scars after they heal.

The exact cause of canker sores is unknown, but there are a number of possibilities (see box). The sores, about the size of a small pea, are round or oval-shaped, gray in the center, and surrounded by a ring of inflammation. Many people notice a tingling or painful sensation shortly before the cankers emerge. The sores usually rupture within a day after they form. Because they are open sores, they can produce constant pain, and can cause sharp stabbing pain if touched or when they come into contact with acidic foods or other irritating substances.

Possible Causes of Canker Sores

- Stress
- Hypersensitivity to components of common mouth bacteria
- Sensitivity to spicy or acidic foods, such as tomatoes or fruit juice
- Genetic predisposition
- Hormonal changes (such as during menstrual periods or pregnancy)
- Hypersensitivity to the presence of bacteria or bacterial secretions
- Mouth acids and digestive enzymes
- Nutritional deficiency (e.g., lack of iron, vitamin B12, folic acid)
- Disease (e.g., colds or allergies)
- Injury: chemical irritation, needle injection, mouth scrapes caused by toothbrushing or braces or by chewing hard abrasive foods
- Biting or nibbling on inside of cheek or lip
- Immune system activity

Because they are not caused by an infectious agent, canker sores are not contagious. They are different from cold sores, which are infectious and which usually appear outside the mouth (see below).

Seek medical attention if any of the following applies to you

- Clusters of canker sores on the back of the throat
- Fever or swollen lymph glands
- Symptoms that persist for longer than 14 days

Strategies for Relieving or Avoiding Canker Sores

- Use chewable antacids.
- Rinse the mouth with lukewarm water 3 to 4 times a day.
- Suck on anesthetic lozenges or cold or frozen foods (such as ice pops).
- Avoid irritating foods, such as nuts, chocolates, and citrus fruit.
- Use manual (not electric) toothbrushes.
- Replace old, worn toothbrushes.

Treatment for Canker Sores

Most canker sores are not serious and will heal by themselves within a week or so. However, if the sores are very painful and make eating difficult or interfere with oral hygiene, they should be treated.

The first strategy is to identify what may be causing the sores and then avoiding that factor. Obviously, if you find that your morning orange juice promotes cankers, switch to another beverage.

Saltwater rinses (1 to 3 teaspoons of salt in 4 to 8 ounces of water) can be soothing and can be used to cleanse area prior to application of a topical medication.

OTC products that contain benzoin tincture coat the sore with a protective layer, thus reducing irritation and friction.

Local anesthetics or analgesics (pain relievers) applied to the area in pastes or gels can reduce the discomfort of the sores. Examples of these active ingredients include benzocaine, benzyl alcohol, and butacaine.

Oral rinses that produce foam (such as hydrogen peroxide) can soothe the area and help keep it clean. Do not use such rinses for longer than 7 days. They should be diluted with an equal amount of water before use.

Nonsteroidal anti-inflammatory drugs (NSAIDs) taken orally can help relieve pain and discomfort. Placing an aspirin tablet directly on the sore is unsafe because aspirin can burn or destroy the tissue.

If a nutritional deficiency is clearly involved, dietary supplements may be a good idea to restore adequate supplies of missing vitamins or minerals.

Topical products containing such ingredients as camphor, menthol, or phenol should not be used. These can make the inflammation worse and can damage the tissue.

OTC Products for Canker Sores

Protectants

Topical local anesthetics or analgesics

Oral hygiene rinses

NSAIDs

Cold Sores

Cold sores are infectious lesions caused by the herpes simplex virus. These painful blisters usually erupt on the outside of the mouth and lips, especially in the corners of the mouth where the mucous membrane meets the skin, or along the outside edge of the nostrils. In rare cases, outbreaks occur inside the mouth, particularly on the gums or the roof of the mouth. Because the lesions often erupt following onset of a fever, cold sores are also known as fever blisters.

Most people carry the herpes virus, but not all of them develop blisters. Still, about 8 out of 10 people have cold sores at some time in their lives. Infection usually occurs early in life, before age 10. The first infection typically does not lead to cold sore symptoms. Instead, the virus lies dormant inside the body until some event, such as an infectious disease or stress, causes it to become active. Once infection occurs, it cannot be eradicated or cured. As people reach middle age, the severity and frequency of outbreaks tend to decline.

A number of factors may trigger a bout of blistering. As noted, fevers or infectious ailments such as colds can often cause an outbreak. Exposure to sunlight or wind, menstruation, emotional excitement or stress, fatigue, or injury to the face may be involved.

People who get cold sores often feel a burning, itching, tingling, or numbness around the mouth that indicates an outbreak is imminent. The blisters first emerge as small, red vesicles (fluid-filled blisters) 1 to 3 days later. There may be several distinct blisters in the area. As they grow, they may merge into one irregularly shaped patch. The blisters ooze fluid, which forms a yellowish crust as it dries.

In most cases, the lesions heal and disappear within 10 to 14 days. They do not usually produce scarring. Cold sores are usually recurrent; people may experience several outbreaks during the course of a year. Exposure to the sun may cause recurrence in some people. The time between episodes is unpredictable. Some people have outbreaks every few weeks, while others may suffer only once a year. Often, outbreaks recur on the same part of the body, but they can erupt in different places each time.

The herpes virus can be transmitted through direct contact, such as kissing. To minimize the risk of transmission wash hands frequently and do not kiss other people, especially in the early days of the outbreak. The form of the virus most often involved in mouth sores is herpes simplex type 1. A related virus, herpes simplex type 2, produces lesions on the genitals but can also cause blisters on the facial area. In about 10% of cases, such infections result from hand-to-mouth transfer of the virus or from oral sex with an infected person.

Seek medical attention if

- Pus-filled blisters form underneath the crust of a cold sore.

Strategies for Relieving Cold Sores

- Keep the area moist and clean to prevent bacterial infections.
- Eat soft, bland foods to avoid irritating mouth lesions.
- Avoid touching the sores.
- Wear lip balm with sunscreen to protect vulnerable areas from exposure.
- Minimize stress or emotional tension.
- Do not pick, squeeze, or pinch blisters.

Treatment for Cold Sores

Herpes infection cannot be eliminated or cured. If you suffer from cold sores, the best you can hope for from OTC treatment is some relief of pain and discomfort.

An important strategy is to keep the blisters clean and moist. If they become dry and cracked, there is an increased risk that they will develop a secondary bacterial infection, which will delay healing and make the symptoms worse.

OTC medications known as oral discomfort products can ease some of the symptoms of cold sores. These products contain one or more ingredients that relieve pain (for example, acetaminophen) or that act as mild anesthetics (such as benzocaine or benzyl alcohol). The anesthetics often help by relieving the itch that can accompany blisters. Some of these products also contain protectants such as allantoin, petrolatum, or cocoa butter to relieve dryness and keep the blisters soft. The products are available in a variety of forms, including liquids, gels, lotions, ointments, creams, and aerosol sprays.

As is true of canker sore treatment, products used in treating cold sores should be free of ingredients such as camphor or menthol since these can stimulate nerves and increase irritation; nor should astringents be used. Cold sores do not respond to topical corticosteroids.

If the lesions become infected, it may be a good idea to use a triple antibiotic ointment such as Mycitracin or Neosporin. More severe cases may require use of oral antibiotics, which are available only with a prescription. Aspirin or other NSAIDs can help ease pain and reduce inflammation.

OTC Products for Cold Sores

Oral discomfort products containing
- Analgesics
- Anesthetics
- Protectants

Topical antibiotics
Systemic analgesics

Minor Mouth Pain

Because the tissues of the mouth are soft and moist, they are susceptible to various types of injuries. The mouth can be injured by dentures, braces, or tooth plates, and accidental injury such as biting the cheek or biting down on a hard or crisp food at a bad angle. The number of nerves in mouth tissues also makes these tissues sensitive to pain. People who have an irritated taste bud often perceive the injured area to be at least the size of a quarter. Looking in the mirror, though, they are surprised to see that the affected bud is only as big as the head of a pin.

Seek medical attention if any of the following applies to you

- Pain due to tooth decay or gum disease
- Fever or swelling
- Tooth sensitivity
- A fractured, chipped, or damaged tooth
- Risk for oral cancer
  - Use of smoked or smokeless tobacco
  - High consumption of alcohol
  - High exposure to sunlight
- Persistent pain despite up to 7 days of self-treatment

Treatment for Minor Mouth Pain

The various OTC products available to help relieve the suffering from mouth injury or irritation are the same ones described in the preceding sections on canker and cold sores. None of these products is formulated to actually heal the wound; they work only to relieve symptoms. There is no OTC product approved by the FDA for use as an oral antiseptic to prevent infection following mouth injury.

Common Sense About Mouth Pain

Many people are afraid to see a dentist. They often try to treat themselves for mouth problems using products available in drugstores. But often this approach can do more harm than good. If a tooth is cracked or decayed, simply using a toothpaste formulated for sensitive teeth or applying a protectant to the surface will not heal the damage, and may even make it worse. Similarly, mouthwashes or plaque removers may not be enough, in themselves, to treat gum disease. Serious mouth infections, such as a fungal infection called candidiasis, may require the use of medications only a doctor can prescribe.

If you experience pain or injury in the mouth that does not improve after a few days of self-treatment, see a dentist or other health care professional.

OTC Products for Minor Mouth Pain

Topical anesthetics
Topical analgesics
Systemic (whole-body) analgesics
Astringents
Protectants
Wound cleansers

Dry Mouth

Glands inside the mouth and cheeks produce saliva. This complex fluid contains water, salts, and other components. Saliva serves a number of important functions. It keeps the mouth moist and lubricated. An enzyme in saliva, amylase (also called ptyalin), mixes with food and helps break down carbohydrates (starch), thus facilitating digestion. Saliva also makes chewed food easier to swallow. Without saliva to dissolve food, the tongue would not be able to taste. By constantly washing the oral cavity, saliva limits the growth of bacteria, thus reducing the risk of tooth decay and other oral infections. Minerals in saliva can penetrate the enamel on teeth, thus helping repair cavities.

Xerostomia (dry mouth) is a condition in which the glands do not secrete enough saliva. In some cases, dry mouth can cause tremendous discomfort. People may complain of a dry or burning sensation. They may be unable to eat, or they may not be able to taste food. Swallowing may become extremely difficult, and it may be hard to talk. Dry mouth can cause the lips and corners of the mouth to become painfully dry, chapped, and cracked. Without the protective benefits of saliva, people with dry mouth are at greater risk of serious oral infections and extensive tooth decay. Bad breath is a common consequence. In severe cases, the surface of the tongue may change, and painful sores can develop on the gums and inside the cheeks. People with dentures who suffer from dry mouth may resist wearing their dentures, which can contribute to a poor diet or social embarrassment.

The problem of dry mouth is more common among seniors and women, affecting perhaps 1 person in 5. In some cases, dry mouth is a symptom of an underlying disease such as diabetes or rheumatoid arthritis. A condition called Sjögren's syndrome, in which the immune system begins to destroy the glands that lubricate mucous membranes, causes dryness in various tissues of the body, including the eyes, mouth, and vagina. Over 400 prescription medications list dry mouth as a potential side effect; examples include antidepressants, diuretics, and antihypertensive (blood-pressure-lowering) drugs. Sometimes personal habits such as smoking, breathing through the mouth, or excess intake of calcium contribute to the problem. So can anxiety or stress. People who undergo radiation therapy of the head and neck can experience dry mouth as a side effect.

Seek medical attention if any of the following applies to you

- Persistent dryness
- A history of serious tooth decay

Treatment for Dry Mouth

There are a number of simple strategies you can follow to help relieve dry mouth (see box).

Strategies for Relieving Dry Mouth

- Take frequent sips of water, especially when speaking.
- Consume beverages without sugar.
- Avoid drinks with alcohol or caffeine; these chemicals act to remove water from the body.
- Keep water beside the bed at night and sip it as often as needed.
- Chew sugarless gum for a few minutes at a time to help stimulate saliva production.
- Suck on sugarless cinnamon or mint candies.
- Do not smoke.
- Resist spicy, salty, or acidic foods.
- Use a humidifier to keep air moist, especially in the bedroom at night.

Just as there are artificial tears to relieve dry eyes, there are artificial salivas to relieve dry mouth. These products are formulated to recreate the complex mix of ingredients found in natural saliva. Thus, for many people, they offer a more complete approach to restoring moisture in the mouth than frequent rinsing with water or mouthwashes can offer. Keep in mind, however, that use of artificial saliva is for relief of symptoms. It does not cure the underlying problem that is causing dryness in the first place.

Most artificial salivas contain an ingredient to increase their viscosity (stickiness), so that they remain in the mouth for an appropriate period of time. The primary ingredient for this purpose is a form of cellulose. Artificial salivas also contain mineral salts such as calcium, potassium, sodium, and magnesium, which help maintain the natural chemical balance inside the mouth.

To make artificial saliva products more acceptable and pleasant, they are made with flavorings and sweeteners. Artificial salivas also contain preservatives, such as propylparaben. People who are sensitive to these preservatives may experience redness or irritation. Sterile aerosol formulations do not contain preservatives. Other forms of artificial saliva are pump sprays, liquids, and swabs. These products are considered very safe and effective and can be used as often as needed.

People with dry mouth should use toothbrushes with soft bristles and should avoid use of mouthwashes that contain alcohol.

OTC Product for Dry Mouth

Artificial saliva

Bad Breath

Many people worry that their breath carries an offensive odor. Bad breath, or halitosis, can result from eating certain foods. Garlic and onions, for example, are notorious for their lingering smell. The presence of bacteria acting to break down food particles trapped between teeth can also contribute to the problem. Bad breath on waking, or morning mouth, a nearly universal complaint, also results from the activity of oral bacteria. Other common contributors include tobacco smoking, dry mouth (see previous section in this chapter), the use of certain prescription medications, and chronic gum, sinus, or lung infections.

In most cases, good oral hygiene—effective brushing, using dental floss, frequent mouth rinsing, and brushing or scraping the tongue—will alleviate the problem. While there are many OTC products available for treatment or prevention of bad breath, some of these contain ingredients such as alcohol or sodium dodecyl sulfate, which can actually harm the soft tissues of the mouth. Alcohol, for example, is a drying agent that can make dry mouth, and the accompanying bad breath, worse.

Sometimes, though, bad breath is a sign of a more serious medical condition. It may result from decaying teeth or from gum disease. Trench mouth is an infection of the gums or throat involving lesions that produce an unpleasant odor. Some cases of bad breath result from a medical condition elsewhere in the body. Lung infections, tonsillitis, sinus or nasal infections, and liver disease may lie at the root of the problem. Infections may involve types of bacteria that produce sulfurous gas as a by-product. As you probably know, the smell of sulfur is often compared to that of rotten eggs. Because of their severely disturbed metabolisms, people with severe diabetes or alcoholism often have an unpleasant breath odor. There is also a rare genetic condition, trimethylaminuria, a symptom of which is fishy-smelling breath. Constipation and indigestion do not cause halitosis.

If you have persistent bad breath that does not improve with brushing and rinsing and good dental care, see your doctor.

Strategies for Avoiding Bad Breath

- Keep the mouth moist. Increase saliva flow by chewing gum for a few minutes or sucking on lozenges (preferably sugarless).
- Drink 8 glasses of water a day.
- Rinse the mouth often when drinking water. Hold the water in the mouth for at least 20 seconds and swish it around. Using water is about as effective as using commercial mouthwashes.
- You can also rinse with a solution of equal parts hydrogen peroxide and water. Peroxide releases oxygen bubbles and helps destroy bacteria. Retain the solution in the mouth for at least 1 minute so the bubbles have time to work.
- For snacks, chew on carrots or celery, which can help scrub the teeth and prevent plaque.
- Stop smoking.
- Brush teeth and tongue using a paste made from baking soda.
- Brush after every meal. Floss twice daily.
- Ask your dentist whether you should use an oral irrigating system (e.g., WaterPik).
- Some experts believe vitamin C supplements can help freshen breath.

Artificial Tears

KEY:
carb = carboxymethylcellulose sodium
Dextran = Dextran
glycerin = glycerin
hyd cel = hydroxethyl cellulose
lanolin = lanolin
met = methylcellulose or hydroxypropyl methylcellulose/methylcellulose
mineral = mineral oil
petrol = petrolatum or white petrolatum
poly g = polyethylene glycol
polyv = polyvinyl alcohol
pov = povidone
prop = propylene glycol

BRAND NAME	VISCOSITY AGENTS											
	carb	Dextran	glycerin	hyd cel	lanolin	met	mineral	petrol	poly g	polyv	pov	prop
20/20 Tears										1.4%		
Adsorbotear				0.41%							1.67%	
Akwa Tears (drops)										1.4%		
Akwa Tears (ointment)					x		x	x				
AquaSite		0.1%										
Bion Tears		0.1%				0.3%						
Celluvisc	1%											
Comfort Tears				x								
Dry Eye Therapy			0.3%									
Duolube							20%	80%				
DuraTears Naturale					x		x	x				
GenTeal Lubricant						x						
Hypotears (drops)									x	1%		
Hypotears (ointment)							x	x				
Hypotears PF									x	1%		
Isopto Alkaline						1%						
Isopto Tears						0.5%						
Lacri-Lube N.P.					x		42.5%	57.3%				
Lacri-Lube S.O.P.					x		42.5%	56.8%				

BRAND NAME	VISCOSITY AGENTS											
	carb	Dextran	glycerin	hyd cel	lanolin	met	mineral	petrol	poly g	polyv	pov	prop
Liquifilm Tears										1.4%		
Moisture Drops			0.2%			0.5%					0.1%	
Murine Tears Lubricant										0.5%	0.6%	
Murocel Lubricant Ophthalmic						1%			x			x
Ocucoat Lubricating		0.1%				0.8%						
Ocucoat PF Lubricating		0.1%				0.8%						
Puralube Tears									1%	1%		
Refresh										1.4%	0.6%	
Refresh P.M.					x		41.5%	56.8%				
Refresh Plus CelluFresh Formula	0.5%											
Stye Sterile Lubricant							32%	55%				
Teargen II		0.1%				0.3%						
Tearisol						0.5%						
Tears Naturale		0.1%				0.3%						
Tears Natural II		0.1%				0.3%						
Tears Naturale free		0.1%				0.3%						
Tears Plus										1.4%	0.6%	
Tears Renewed (drops)		x				0.3%						
Tears Renewed (ointment)							x	x				
Ultra Tears						1%						
Visine Lubricating			0.2%			0.2%						

Ophthalmic Decongestants

KEY:

Viscosity Agents
Dextran = Dextran
glycerin = glycerin
hyd cel = hydroxyethyl cellulose
hyd met = hydroxypropyl methylcellulose
pol gly = polyethylene glycol
polyv alc = polyvinyl alcohol
pov = povidone

Vasoconstrictors
naph = naphazoline HCl
oxy = oxymetazoline
phen = phenylephrine
tet = tetrahydrozoline

BRAND NAME	VISCOSITY AGENT							VASOCONSTRICTOR			
	Dextran	glycerin	hyd cel	hyd met	pol gly	polyv alc	pov	naph	oxy	phen	tet
20/20 Drops		0.4%						0.012%			
AK-Nefrin						1.4%				0.12%	
Allerest Eye Drops								0.012%			
Clear Eyes ACR		0.2%						0.012%			
Clear Eyes Lubricant Eye Redness Reliever		0.2%						0.012%			
Collyrium Fresh		1%									0.05%
Comfort Eye Drops								0.03%			
Degest 2			x				x	0.012%			
Estivin II	0.1%			0.3%				0.012%			
Eye-Sed											0.05%
EyeSine											0.05%
Geneye											0.05%
Isopto-Frin				0.5%						0.12%	
Murine Plus Lubricant Eye Redness Reliever						0.5%	0.6%				0.5%
Naphcon								0.012%			
Naphcon-A								0.025%			
Ocu Clear									0.025%		
OcuHist								0.025%			
Opcon-A				0.5%				0.027%			

BRAND NAME	VISCOSITY AGENT							VASOCONSTRICTOR			
	Dextran	glycerin	hyd cel	hyd met	pol gly	polyv alc	pov	naph	oxy	phen	tet
Optigene											0.05%
Prefrin Liquifilm						1.4%				0.12%	
Relief						1.4%				0.12%	
Sensitive Eyes Redness Reliever Lubricant					0.2%			0.012%			
Sensitive Eyes Redness Reliever Lubricant Maximum Strength				0.5%				0.03%			
Soothe					x	1.67%					0.05%
Vaso Clear						x		0.02%			
Vaso Clear A						0.25%		0.02%			
Vasocon A								0.05%			
Visine Allergy Relief											0.05%
Visine L.R.									0.025%		
Visine Moisturizing					1%						0.05%
Visine Original Formula											0.05%
Zincfrin										0.12%	

Other Eye Care Products

CATEGORY	BRAND NAMES
Eyelid Scrubs	Eye-Scrub
	Lid Wipes-SPF
Hyperosmotics	Adsorbonac
	AK-NaCl (ointment)
	AK-NaCl (solution)
	Muro 128 (ointment)
	Muro 128 (solution)

Irrigants	Blinx
	Collyrium for Fresh Eyes
	Dacriose
	Eye-Stream
	Eye Wash
	Lavoptic Eye Wash
	Optigene

Ear Care Products

BRAND NAME	ANTI-INFECTIVE AGENT				GLYCERIN	OTHER
	alcohol	boric acid	carbamide peroxide	isopropyl alcohol		
Auro			6.5%			
Aurocaine			x		x	
Aurocaine 2		2.75%		x		
Auro-Dri				97.25%		
Debrox			6.5%		x	
Dent's Ear Wax Drops			x		x	
Dri-Ear				95%	5%	
E.R.O.			6.5%		x	
Ear-Dry				95%	5%	
Earsol-HC	x					hydrocortisone 1%
Moline			6.5%		x	
Murine Ear Wax Removal System	6.3%		6.5%		x	
Swim-Ear				95%	5%	

Oral Discomfort Products

BRAND NAME	ANESTHETIC/ANALGESIC											CLEANSER
	acetaminophen	benzocaine	benzyl alcohol	camphor	dyclonine HCl	eugenol	lidocaine	menthol	phenol	salicylic acid	pramoxine HCl	
Amosan [A]												sodium peroxyborate
Anbesol (gel)		6.3%							0.5%			
Anbesol (liquid)		6.4%							0.5%			
Anbesol Baby [A]		7.5%										
Anbesol Maximum Strength		20%										
Babee Teething		2.5%		x				x				
Benzodent Denture Analgesic		20%										
Blistex Lip Medex				1%				1%	0.5%			
Blistex Medicated				0.5%				0.6%	0.5%			
Campho-phenique [A]				10.8%					4.7%			
Cankaid												carbamide peroxide 10%
Carmex Lip Balm				x				x	x	x		
ChapStick Medicated Lip Balm				1%				0.6%	0.5%			
Curasore											1%	
Dent's 3 in 1 Toothache Relief (drops)		20%										
Dent's 3 in 1 Toothache Relief (gel)		5%										
Dent's Double Action Kit (tablet)	325mg											
Dent's Double-Action Kit (drops)		20%										
Dent's Extra Strength Toothache Gum		20%										
Dent-Zel-Ite Oral Mucosal Analgesic		5%		x								
Dent-Zel-Ite Temporary Dental Filling				x								
Dent-Zel-Ite Toothache Relief				x		85%						

Gly-Oxide							carbamide peroxide 10%
HDA Toothache Gel	6.5%						
Hurricaine [A]	20%						
Kanka-A Professional Strength	20%	x					
Little Teethers Oral Pain Relief [A] [S]	7.5%						
Lotion-Jel	5%						
Medadyne	10%	x	x		x		
Numzident Adult Strength	10%						
Numzit Teething (gel)	7.5%						
Numzit Teething (lotion)	0.2%						
Orabase	15%						
Orabase Baby [A]	7.5%						
Orabase Lip Cream [A]	5%		x		0.5%	x	
Orabase-B with Benzocaine [A]	20%						
Oragesic		2%			x		
Orajel Baby [A]	7.5%						
Orajel Baby Nighttime Formula [A]	10%						
Orajel CoverMed				1.0%			
Orajel Denture	10%						
Orajel Maximum Strength	20%						
Orajel Mouth-Aid (gel)	20%						
Orajel Mouth-Aid (liquid)	20%					0.5%	
Orajel Perioseptic							carbamide peroxide 15%
Orajel Regular Strength	10%						
Orasol	6.3%					0.5%	

BRAND NAME	ANESTHETIC/ANALGESIC											CLEANSER
	acetamin-ophen	benzo-caine	benzyl alcohol	cam-phor	dyclonine HCl	eugenol	lido-caine	menthol	phenol	salicylic acid	pramoxine HCl	
Peroxyl Hygienic Dental Rinse												hydrogen peroxide 1.5%
Peroxyl Oral Spot Treatment												hydrogen peroxide 1.5%
Red Cross Canker Sore Medication		20%							x			
Red Cross Toothache Medication						85%						
Rid-a-Pain Dental Drops		6.3%							0.5%			
SensoGARD [A]		20%										
Tanac (liquid)		10%										
Tanac (stick)		7.5%										
Tanac Medicated					1.0%							
Tanac Roll-On		5%										
Vaseline Lip Therapy				0.8%				0.8%	0.5%			
Zilactin B		10%										
Zilactin Medicated			10%									
Zilactin-L							2.5%					

Artificial Saliva Products

BRAND NAME	VISCOSITY AGENT		
	carboxymethylcellulose	hydroxyethyl cellulose	sodium carboxymethylcellulose
Entertainer's Secret Throat Relief			x
Glandosane Mouth Moisturizer			0.51g
Moi-Stir Mouth Moistening	x		
Moi-Stir Oral Swabsticks	x		
Optimoist		x	

Brand Names

Naphcon A (NAFF-con)
Ocuhist (OCK-yew-hist)
Opcon A (OP-kon)
Vasocon A (VAZE-uh-kon)

Generic Ingredients

Naphazoline hydrochloride
Pheniramine maleate or antazoline phosphate

Type of Drug

Decongestant and antihistamine eyedrop.

Used for

Relief of congestion, itching, irritation, and redness of the eye.

General Information

Decongestants work by narrowing or constricting the blood vessels throughout the body, reducing the blood supply, and decreasing the swelling in mucous membranes. However, decongestants do not work against histamine or any other substance that is released by the body tissues during allergic reactions. To treat allergy symptoms, they are usually given in combination with antihistamines, which do block the body's release of histamine.

Naphcon A, Ocuhist, Opcon-A, and Vasocon A, which are available only in eyedrop form, are combinations of the decongestant naphazoline hydrochloride and an antihistamine. The antihistamine in Naphcon A, Ocuhist, and Opcon-A is pheniramine maleate and the antihistamine in Vascon A is antazoline phosphate. The naphazoline ingredient constricts the eye's blood vessels to clear up redness and also helps to reduce tearing and pain, while the pheniramine ingredient works to prevent any further allergic reaction.

Cautions and Warnings

Naphcon A, Ocuhist, Opcon-A, and Vasocon A should not be used for longer than 3 to 4 days unless directed by a doctor.

Do not exceed the recommended daily dosage of these products.

If you experience eye pain or changes in your vision, continued redness or irritation, worsening or persistence of the condition for more than 48 hours, or signs of systemic (whole-body) absorption, such as headache, nausea, or decreased body temperature, stop taking these products and call your doctor.

If you have hyperthyroidism, heart disease, high blood pressure, diabetes, or difficulty urinating because of an enlarged prostate, you should use these products only under the supervision of a doctor, because the drug can aggravate these conditions.

Do not use these products if you have narrow-angle glaucoma, except under a doctor's supervision.

These products may cause enlarged pupils; individuals with light-colored eyes (blue or green) may be more sensitive to this effect.

A problem common to all forms of topical decongestants is rebound congestion; that is, you may still have red eyes even though you have been using these products for several days, and your eyes may become more inflamed each time you apply the drug. If this happens, stop using these products and contact your doctor. The signs of rebound congestion will usually go away in about a week after you stop using the drug.

These products may cause the pupils to become abnormally dilated, a condition known as mydriasis. This may be more likely to occur in people with light-colored irises or those who have had prior damage to the cornea. In some people, mydriasis can lead to angle-closure glaucoma.

Always check the expiration date before using these products. If the product is discolored or cloudy, do not use it.

To reduce the risk of spreading infection, the container should not be used by more than 1 person. Do not touch the tip of the container to any surface. Replace the cap after use.

Possible Side Effects

▼ Most common: blurred vision, mild temporary stinging and irritation, enlarged pupils, increased or decreased pressure within the eye.

Possible Side Effects ***(continued)***

▼ Less common: loss of sense of smell, headache, high blood pressure, heart irregularities, nervousness, nausea, dizziness, weakness, and sweating. If you develop any of these effects while using Naphcon A, Ocuhist, Opcon-A, or Vasocon A, stop taking the drug immediately and contact your doctor.

Drug Interactions

• Naphcon A, Ocuhist, Opcon-A, and Vasocon A should not be used at the same time as a monoamine oxidase inhibitor (MAOI) or within 2 weeks of stopping an MAOI. MAOIs are used to treat depression, other psychiatric or emotional conditions, and Parkinson's disease. If you are not sure whether you are taking or took an MAOI, check with your doctor before you use these products.

• The effects of these products may be increased if the drug is taken with a tricyclic antidepressant (e.g., imipramine or desipramine) or with the tetracyclic antidepressant maprotiline.

Usual Dose

Naphcon A and Ocuhist each contain pheniramine maleate 0.3% and naphazoline hydrochloride 0.025%.

Opcon-A contains pheniramine maleate 0.315% and naphazoline hydrochloride 0.027%.

Vasocon A contains antazoline phosphate 0.5% and naphazoline hydrochloride 0.05%.

Adult and Child (age 6 and over): Apply 1–2 drops in the affected eye(s) up to 4 times daily.

Child (under age 6): not recommended except under the supervision of a doctor.

Overdosage

Accidental ingestion of Naphcon A, Ocuhist, Opcon-A, or Vasocon A by infants and children can lead to drowsiness, drastically lowered body temperature, slowed heartbeat, low blood pressure (giving the appearance of shock), and coma.

Even if the victim is not displaying any of the symptoms listed above, do the following in case of accidental ingestion: If the victim is unconscious or having convulsions, call for an ambulance immediately. If you take the victim to an emergency room, be sure to bring the bottle or container with you. If the victim is conscious, call your local poison control center or a health care professional. The poison control center may suggest inducing vomiting with ipecac syrup (available without a prescription at any pharmacy). DO NOT induce vomiting unless specifically instructed to do so.

Special Populations

Pregnancy/Breast-feeding

Antihistamines are not recommended for use during pregnancy unless directed by your doctor. Antihistamines and decongestants are known to pass into the breast milk of nursing mothers and may cause side effects in infants. Check with your doctor before using Naphcon A, Ocuhist, Opcon-A, or Vasocon A if you are or might be pregnant, or if you are breast-feeding.

Infants/Children

Children may be more susceptible to the side effects of Naphcon A, Ocuhist, Opcon-A, or Vasocon A. They are also more susceptible to accidental antihistamine and decongestant overdose. Do not give these products to a child under 6 unless directed by your doctor

Seniors

Naphcon A, Ocuhist, Opcon-A, or Vasocon A may cause bits of the pigment that color the iris to loosen and float free in the eye. This may be more likely to occur in seniors.

Brand Name

Visine Allergy Relief (VYE-zeen)

Generic Ingredients

Tetrahydrozoline hydrochloride
Zinc sulfate

Type of Drug

Decongestant and astringent/antiseptic.

Used for

Temporary relief of discomfort and redness associated with minor eye irritation.

General Information

Visine Allergy Relief uses a combination of 2 drugs to treat minor eye irritation. It contains a decongestant and an astringent/antiseptic.

The decongestant in Visine Allergy Relief is tetrahydrozoline hydrochloride. Decongestants relieve congestion by narrowing or constricting the blood vessels. Administered as eyedrops, tetrahydrozoline is considered effective in relieving the surface discomfort of itchy, red eyes, without unduly affecting the underlying blood vessels of the eye structure.

Visine Allergy Relief also contains zinc sulfate, an astringent and antiseptic used to relieve minor eye irritation.

Cautions and Warnings

Do not use Visine Allergy Relief for longer than 3 days continuously unless directed by a doctor.

Do not exceed the recommended daily dosage of Visine Allergy Relief.

Stop using Visine Allergy Relief if you experience visual disturbances, pain, or increased redness. If your condition worsens over a 72-hour period, discontinue use and contact your doctor.

Excessive use of tetrahydrozoline should be avoided, especially in children (see "Special Populations").

Tetrahydrozoline is less likely to cause the pupils to alter in size than other ophthalmic decongestants. This prevents the symptom of light sensitivity during use of a product containing tetrahydrozoline. However, some individuals may experience a mild, temporary stinging sensation immediately after using one of these products.

These products are not to be taken internally.

If you have hyperthyroidism, heart disease, high blood pressure, or diabetes, you should consult your doctor before using Visine Allergy Relief, because there is a slight risk that it could aggravate these conditions.

A problem common to all forms of topical decongestants is rebound congestion; that is, you may still have red eyes even though you have been using tetrahydrozoline for several days. Your eyes may become more inflamed each time you apply the drug. If this happens while you are using Visine Allergy Relief, stop using Visine Allergy Relief and contact your doctor. The signs of rebound congestion will usually go away about a week after you stop using the drug.

Visine Allergy Relief should not be used by people with glaucoma or other serious eye diseases except under a doctor's supervision.

To reduce the risk of spreading infection, eye drops should not be used by more than one person. Rinse dropper and bottle tips with hot water after use. Be careful not to let hot water into the bottle. Do not let the bottle tip come into contact with any surface.

Possible Side Effects

Excessive use of Visine Allergy Relief can irritate tissues.

Upon application, some people may experience temporary burning, stinging, and a feeling of surface dryness. Blurred vision and dilation of the pupils may occur.

Drug Interactions

None known.

Food Interactions

None known.

Usual Dose

Visine Allergy Relief contains tetrahydrozoline hydrochloride 0.05% and zinc sulfate 0.25%.

Adult and Child (age 12 and over): 1–2 drops up to 4 times daily.

Child (age 6–11): Consult your doctor for the appropriate dose for children in this age group. Do not overuse (see "Special Populations").

Child (under age 6): not recommended.

Overdosage

Overdose can cause central nervous system depression, drowsiness, lowered body temperature, slowed heartbeat, lowered blood pressure, shortness of breath, and eventually, coma.

Even if the victim is not displaying any of the symptoms listed above, do the following in case of accidental ingestion: If the victim is unconscious or having convulsions, call for an ambulance immediately. If you take the victim to an emergency room, be sure to bring the bottle or container with you. If the victim is conscious, call your local poison control center or a health care professional. The poison control center may suggest inducing vomiting with ipecac syrup (available without a prescription at any pharmacy). DO NOT induce vomiting unless specifically instructed to do so.

Special Populations

Pregnancy/Breast-feeding

It is not generally recommended that pregnant women take any drugs, particularly during the first 3 months after conception. Check with your doctor if you are or might be pregnant before using Visine Allergy Relief.

It is not known if tetrahydrozoline passes into breast milk. If you must use Visine Allergy Relief, bottle-feed your baby with formula.

Infants/Children

Excessive use of tetrahydrozoline in children can cause systemic complications, including severe drowsiness and profuse sweating. Consult your doctor for the appropriate use of Visine Allergy Relief in children under age 12. Do not use Visine Allergy Relief in children under age 6.

Seniors

In some older individuals, use of tetrahydrozoline, especially in high doses, may cause tiny fragments of the iris (colored portion of the eye) to become detached. If this happens, call your doctor.

Chapter 9: Hemorrhoid Relief

Hemorrhoids (also called piles) are bulges of the veins supplying blood to the skin and membranes of the anal region. There are 3 main types of hemorrhoids, depending on their location (see box).

Types of Hemorrhoids

Internal hemorrhoids arise above the anus, along the inside lining of the lower rectum.

External hemorrhoids arise on the tissue around the outside rim of the anus.

Prolapsed hemorrhoids are internal hemorrhoids that grow until they protrude (prolapse) outside the anal opening.

Causes of Hemorrhoids

A number of factors can contribute to the formation of hemorrhoids, but the basic cause is stress or pressure on anal tissues. Straining during bowel movements, due sometimes to constipation or difficulty passing hard dry stools, can engorge blood vessels and weaken the surrounding support tissues. Sitting for prolonged periods—for example, at work or on the toilet—can increase the risk of hemorrhoids, as can frequent heavy lifting. Reading while going to the bathroom, in particular, is not a good idea if it prolongs the time spent on the toilet significantly. Pregnant women are especially prone to hemorrhoids because the increased weight of the swelling uterus constantly presses on rectal tissues. The strain of labor can cause hemorrhoids or can make existing hemorrhoids worse. Tumors in the pelvic region can press on the lower bowel and trigger hemorrhoid formation. Some people may be born with a predisposition to develop hemorrhoids. People of all ages can be afflicted by the condition, but hemorrhoids are most common in those between ages 20 and 50.

Symptoms of Hemorrhoids

- Pain
- Bleeding (bright red blood)
- Discomfort
- Itching
- Prolapse
- Burning
- Inflammation

The extent and severity of symptoms depend on the location and type of the hemorrhoid. External hemorrhoids do not usually cause pain unless a thrombosis (blood clot) forms or unless the tissue develops an ulcer (open sore). Nor as a rule do external hemorrhoids bleed unless a vein breaks or becomes blocked.

Internal hemorrhoids often bleed, especially following a bowel movement. The blood is usually bright red and may be noticed on toilet tissue or in the toilet bowl, although sometimes the bleeding may occur between bowel movements as a mild persistent oozing. There is a slight chance that bleeding from hemorrhoids may persist for a long time, posing a risk of iron deficiency and anemia. Anyone who experiences rectal bleeding (especially if over age 30) should see a doctor to make sure that some other more serious disease, such as cancer, is not the cause.

Often an internal hemorrhoid can become prolapsed. This usually occurs after defecation, after standing for a long time, or after physical exertion. Such hemorrhoids may secrete a fluid that can cause itching. It is often possible to reduce discomfort by gently pushing the hemorrhoid back into the rectum.

Because the internal rectum does not have many nerve endings, internal hemorrhoids are not always painful. However, there is a risk that prolapsed hemorrhoids can thrombose (develop blood clots), which can block the flow of blood. Sometimes, too, the hemorrhoid becomes strangulated, which means the ring of the anus squeezes the hemorrhoidal tissue like the neck of a balloon and prevents the hemorrhoid from returning to its internal position. The pain from a thrombosed or strangulated hemorrhoid can range from mild to severe.

Inflammation can result when the pouch of a hemorrhoid becomes swollen, causing the skin and tissues to stretch beyond their normal limits. This swelling causes the cells to release substances that irritate the tissues, causing burning and irritation.

Seek medical attention if any of the following applies to you

- Seepage (involuntary passing of material from the anus)
- Prolapse
- Blood in the stool
- Persistent or severe itching
- Persistent or severe pain
- A change in your normal bowel habits

Treatment for Hemorrhoids

Good eating and bowel habits can prevent hemorrhoids or reduce their severity. Drinking plenty of fluids and consuming adequate bulk and fiber in the diet can reduce constipation and improve the consistency of stools. Some people may want to ask their doctors or pharmacists about the use of bulk-forming or emollient laxatives. It's a good idea to avoid straining during bowel movements and not to sit on the toilet for longer than necessary. Use soft, unscented toilet tissue. Cleaning the area with mild soap and water after a bowel movement can prevent irritation and itching. Use lubricated pads to blot or pat the area clean; avoid strenuous wiping. Sitting in a bathtub full of warm water (110 to 115°F) or using a sitz bath (available at most drugstores) can be soothing. Some people benefit from using special pillows or doughnut-shaped cushions when sitting to avoid pressure on affected areas.

There are a number of OTC products available that contain different ingredients to relieve the common symptoms of hemorrhoids (see box). These preparations are available in ointments or creams for external use and in suppositories for internal use.

Local anesthetics work by blocking nerves from transmitting pain signals. Generally, products with a local anesthetic are intended for topical use—that is, for use on external tissues. An anesthetic is not usually effective for internal hemorrhoids, since these arise in rectal tissue that contains few nerve cells. The most common local anesthetics are benzocaine, benzyl alcohol, dibucaine, cyclonine, lidocaine, pramoxine, and tetracaine. Depending on their concentration, these compounds may be safely applied between 3 and 6 times a day.

Vasoconstrictors cause blood vessels to shrink in diameter and therefore reduce swelling, itching, and discomfort. However, vasoconstrictors do not prevent or control bleeding. The vasoconstrictive ingredients found in OTC hemorrhoid preparations include epinephrine base, epinephrine hydrochloride, ephedrine sulfate, and phenylephrine hydrochloride. Each of these may be found in topical products, and the latter 2 are also approved for treatment of internal hemorrhoids.

Protectants form a protective barrier over the skin or tissue to reduce or prevent irritation, itching, burning, discomfort, and loss of water. Examples of protectants found in hemorrhoid preparations include aluminum hydroxide gel, cocoa butter, glycerin, kaolin, lanolin, mineral oil, and petrolatum. With the exception of glycerin, which is for external use only, all are approved for both external and internal use.

Astringents (drying agents) cause shrinkage by preventing tissues from absorbing water. Promoting dryness in turn relieves irritation, itching, and burning. Common astringents found in hemorrhoid preparations include calamine, zinc oxide, and witch hazel.

Not all cases of hemorrhoids can be treated effectively with OTC products. Often the problem can be treated by a physician using an outpatient technique called rubber band ligation, in which tight bands are placed around the neck of an internal hemorrhoid. The tissue withers and falls off in a few days. Large and prolapsed hemorrhoids may require hemorrhoidectomy (surgical removal) or use of electrical or freezing probes to destroy the tissue. Since hemorrhoids cause pain and are associated with inflammation, the use of oral nonsteroidal anti-inflammatory drugs (NSAIDs) such as ibuprofen, taken regularly for several days, can sometimes bring significant relief.

OTC Products for Hemorrhoids

- Local anesthetics
- Vasoconstrictors
- Protectants
- Astringents
- NSAIDS to reduce pain and inflammation

Hemorrhoid Relief

BRAND NAME	ANESTHETIC					ASTRINGENT		PROTECTANTS	VASOCONSTRICTOR	
	benzo-caine	benzyl alcohol	cam-phor	dibu-caine	pramo-xine	witch hazel	zinc oxide		ephedrine sulfate	phenyle-phrine HCl
Americaine Hemorrhoidal	20%									
Anusert								hard fat		0.25%
Anusol (ointment)					1%		12.5%	mineral oil cocoa butter		
Anusol (suppository)		x						topical starch		
Balneol								lanolin oil mineral oil		
Calmol 4							10%	cocoa butter		
Fleet Medicated Wipes						50%		glycerin		
Fleet Pain-Relief					1%			glycerin		
Hemorid for Women					1%			mineral oil petrolatum		0.25%
Hemorid for Women (suppository)							231mg	hard fat		0.25%
Hem-Prep (ointment)							11%	petrolatum		0.25%
Hem-Prep (suppository)							11%	hard fat		0.25%
Hydrosal Hemorrhoidal		1.4%					5%	lanolin mineral oil petrolatum	0.2%	
Lanacane Creme	6%									
Medicone (ointment)	20%							mineral oil petrolatum		
Medicone (suppository)								hard fat		0.25%
Nupercainal (ointment)				1%						

Nupercainal (suppository)					0.25g	cocoa butter		
Pazo (ointment)		2%			5%	lanolin petrolatum	0.2%	
Pazo (suppository)					5%		0.2%	
Preparation H (cream)						glycerin petrolatum shark liver oil		0.25%
Preparation H (ointment)						mineral oil petrolatum shark liver oil		0.25%
Preparation H (suppository)						cocoa butter shark liver oil		
Procto Foam			1%					
Prompt Relief (ointment)						petrolatum shark liver oil		
Prompt Relief (suppository)						cocoa butter shark liver oil		
Sani				50%		glycerin		
Sooth-It				50%		glycerin		
Sooth-It Plus			1%	21%		glycerin		
Tronolane (cream)			1%		x	glycerin		
Tronolane (suppository)					5%	hard fat		
Tronothane Hydrochloride			1%			glycerin		
Tucks				50%		glycerin		
Tucks Clear	x			50%		glycerin		
Vaseline Pure Petroleum Jelly						petrolatum		
Wyanoids Relief Factor						cocoa butter glycerin shark liver oil		

Brand Name

Anusol Suppositories (AN-yew-sol)

Generic Ingredients

Benzyl alcohol
Topical starch

Type of Drug

Topical anesthetic, skin protectant.

Used for

Temporary relief of pain and burning sensation of hemorrhoids and other anorectal disorders.

General Information

Hemorrhoids are swellings in the anal area. These swellings develop due to many factors, such as heredity, posture, prolonged standing or sitting, inadequate dietary bulk intake, constipation, heavy lifting, and pregnancy. They are formed either by inflamed connective tissue under the skin surface or by blood clots in veins.

Anusol Suppositories combine a topical anesthetic, benzyl alcohol, and a skin protectant, topical starch. Benzyl alcohol is a clear, colorless, oily liquid used as a topical anesthetic for various minor skin problems. It is available in concentrations of 5% to 25% for relief of pain caused by hemorrhoids.

Topical starch is used as a protectant in Anusol. It guards against irritation of the skin and prevents dehydration of the tissues by forming a physical barrier on the skin surface. This provides temporary relief from the itching, burning, and discomfort of hemorrhoids and other anorectal disorders, and it helps promote healing.

Cautions and Warnings

Do not use Anusol for more than 7 consecutive days.

Do not exceed the recommended daily dosage of Anusol. If your condition worsens or does not improve within 7 days, stop using Anusol and consult your doctor.

In case of bleeding from the rectal area, discontinue using Anusol and contact your doctor immediately. The presence of blood can be an indication of a more serious condition, such as cancer of the colon or rectum.

Possible Side Effects

Adverse reactions are rare; however, discontinue using Anusol if you suspect an allergic reaction.

Drug Interactions

None known.

Usual Dose

Anusol contains topical starch 51%.

Adult and Child (age 12 and over): Cleanse the affected area with medicated pads or mild soap and warm water. Rinse thoroughly. Gently dry the affected area by patting or blotting with toilet tissue or soft cloth before using Anusol.

Detach 1 suppository from the strip of suppositories and remove the wrapper. Insert 1 suppository rectally up to 6 times daily or after each bowel movement. If the suppository seems soft, before removing the foil hold it under cold water for 2 or 3 minutes. Carefully separate the foil covering and peel it down evenly on both sides, exposing the suppository. Avoid excessive handling of the suppository, as it is designed to melt at body temperature.

Child (under age 12): Consult a doctor for the appropriate use of Anusol for children in this age group.

Overdosage

Do the following in case of accidental ingestion: If the victim is unconscious or having convulsions, call for an ambulance immediately. If you take the victim to an emergency room, be sure to bring the bottle or container with you. If the victim is conscious, call your local poison control center or a health care professional. The poison control center may suggest inducing vomiting with ipecac syrup (available without a prescription at any pharmacy). DO NOT induce vomiting unless specifically instructed to do so.

Storage Instructions

Store Anusol in a cool place. They may melt at temperatures above 86°.

Special Populations:

Pregnancy/Breast Feeding

It is not generally recommended that pregnant women take any drugs, particularly during the first 3 months after conception. Check with your doctor before using Anusol if you are or might be pregnant, or if you are breast-feeding.

Infants/Children

Do not give Anusol to a child under the age of 12 unless directed by a doctor.

Seniors

Seniors should exercise the same caution as younger adults when using Anusol.

Brand Name

Preparation H Ointment

Generic Ingredients

Mineral oil	Phenylephrine hydrochloride
Petrolatum	Shark liver oil

Type of Drug

Vasoconstrictor, skin protectant, and emollient (softener).

Used for

Temporary shrinking of hemorrhoidal tissue and temporary relief of pain and burning associated with hemorrhoids.

General Information

Hemorrhoids develop due to many factors, such as heredity, posture, prolonged standing or sitting, inadequate dietary bulk intake, constipation, heavy lifting, and pregnancy. They are formed either by inflamed connective tissue under the skin surface, or by blood clots in veins.

Preparation H Ointment combines a vasoconstrictor, phenylephrine hydrochloride, with petrolatum, mineral oil, and shark liver oil.

Vasoconstrictors work by narrowing blood vessels and reducing blood flow. Phenylephrine is believed to reduce congestion in the anorectal area and to relieve itching caused by hemorrhoids.

Petrolatum (also known as mineral jelly or petroleum jelly), which is derived from petroleum, is commonly used in hemorrhoidal products. It soothes the skin surface, protects it against outside irritants, and prevents the evaporation of moisture.

Liver oils have been used in folk medicine for many years for their healing properties. Shark liver oil, which contains a high concentration of vitamins A and D, has been approved by the FDA as a natural skin protectant.

Mineral oil is used as a lubricant to prevent straining during bowel movements.

Cautions and Warnings

If your condition worsens or does not improve within 7 days of continuous use, discontinue using Preparation H Ointment and consult your doctor.

Do not exceed recommended daily dosage of Preparation H.

In case of bleeding from the rectal area, discontinue using Preparation H and contact your doctor immediately. The presence of blood can be an indication of a more serious condition.

Unless directed by your doctor, do not use Preparation H if you have hyperthyroidism, heart disease, high blood pressure, diabetes, or an enlarged prostate.

Do not apply Preparation H with an applicator if the introduction of the applicator into the rectum causes additional pain. If this occurs, call your doctor.

Possible Side Effects

Adverse reactions are rare; however, discontinue using Preparation H Ointment if you suspect an allergic reaction.

Drug Interactions

• Preparation H Ointment should not be used at the same time as a monoamine oxidase inhibitor (MAOI) or within 3 weeks of stopping an MAOI. MAIOs are used to treat depression, other psychiatric or emotional conditions, and Parkinson's disease. If you are not sure whether you are or have been taking an MAOI, check with your doctor or pharmacist before you use Preparation H.

• Unless directed by your doctor, do not use Preparation H if you are currently taking an antidepressant.

• Do not use Preparation H if you are taking medication for high blood pressure.

Usual Dose

Preparation H Ointment contains petrolatum 71.9%, mineral oil 14%, shark liver oil 3%, and phenylephrine 0.25%.

Adult and Child (age 12 and over): Cleanse the affected area with medicated pads or mild soap and warm water. Rinse thoroughly. Gently dry the affected area by patting or blotting with toilet tissue or soft cloth before using Preparation H Ointment.

Apply, either externally to the affected area or intrarectally using the enclosed applicator, especially at night, in the morning, or after a bowel movement. Do not exceed 4 doses in a 24-hour period.

Child (under age 12): Consult your doctor.

Overdosage

Do the following in case of accidental ingestion: If the victim is unconscious or having convulsions, call for an ambulance immediately. If you take the victim to an emergency room, be sure to bring the bottle or container with you. If the victim is conscious, call your local poison control center or a health care professional. The poison control center may suggest inducing vomiting with ipecac syrup (available without a prescription at any pharmacy). DO NOT induce vomiting unless specifically instructed to do so.

Special Populations

Pregnancy/Breast-feeding

Is is not generally recommended that pregnant women take any drugs, particularly during the first three months after conception. Check with your doctor before using Preparation H Ointment if you are or might be pregnant, or if you are breast-feeding.

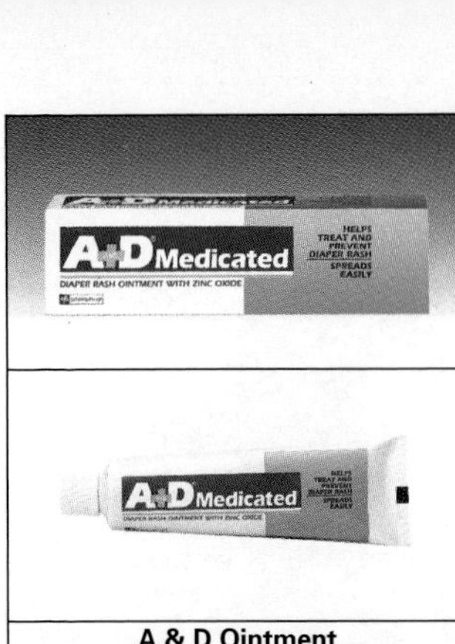

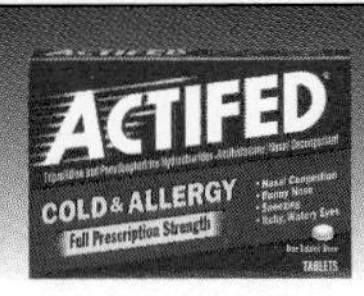

A & D Ointment
p. 641

Actifed Tablets
p. 428

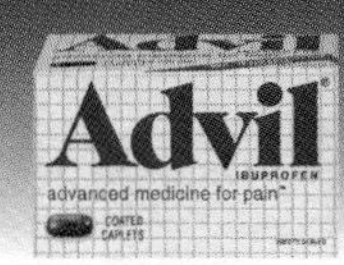

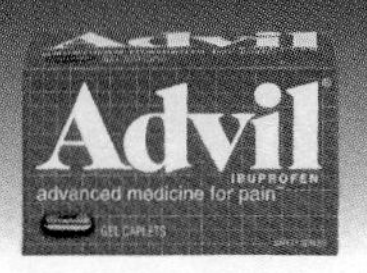

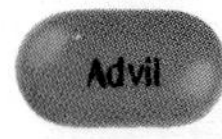

Advil

Advil Caplets
p. 39

Advil Gel Caplets
p. 39

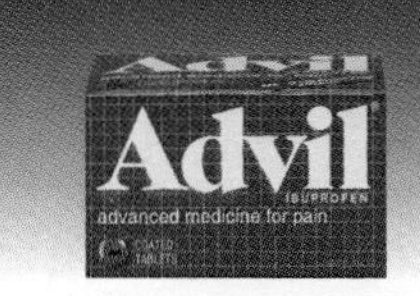

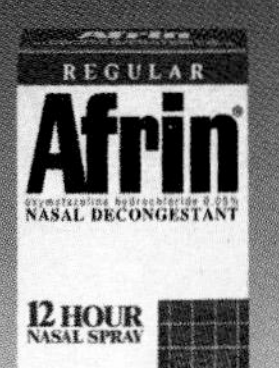

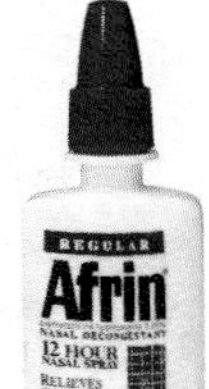

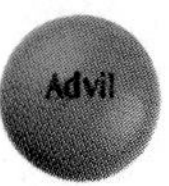

Advil Coated Tablets
p. 39

Afrin Nasal Spray
p. 432

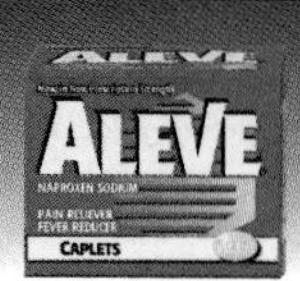

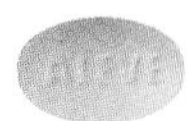

Aleve Caplets
p. 39

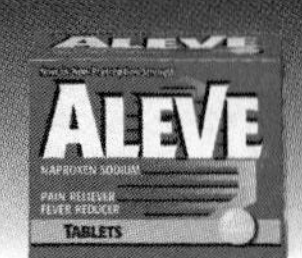

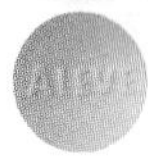

Aleve Tablets
p. 39

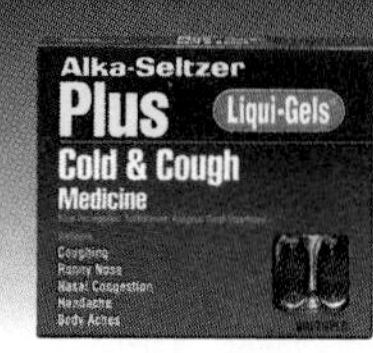

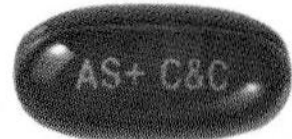

Alka-Seltzer Plus Cold & Cough Liqui-Gels p. 117

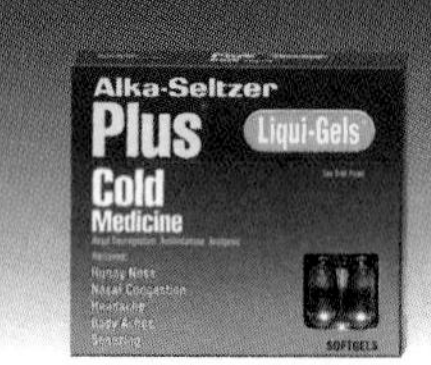

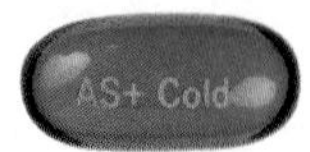

Alka-Seltzer Plus Cold Liqui-Gels p. 130

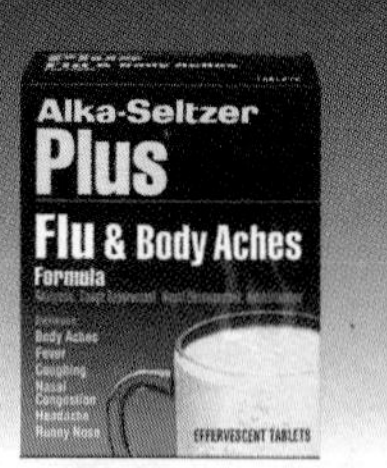

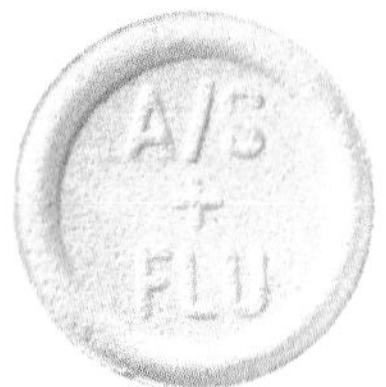

Alka-Seltzer Plus Flu Effervescent Tablets
p. 136

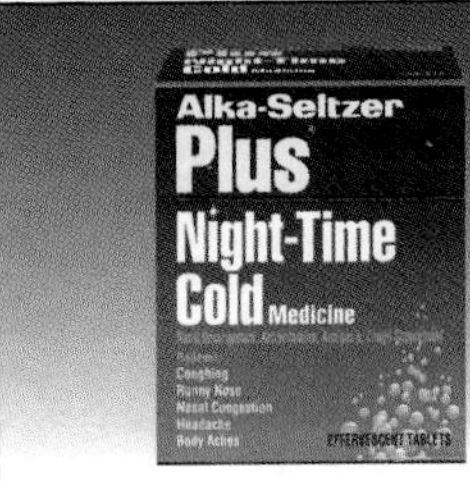

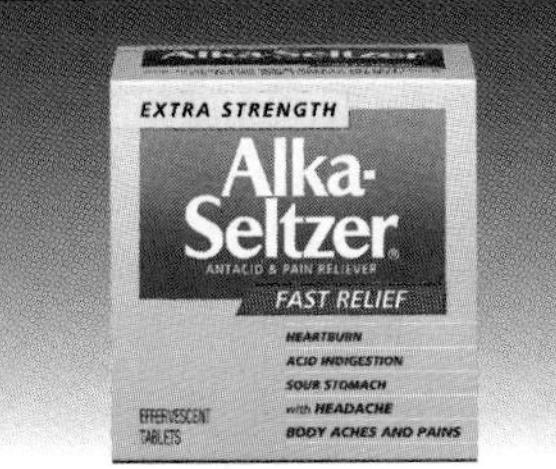

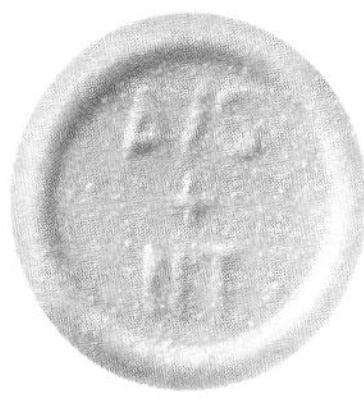

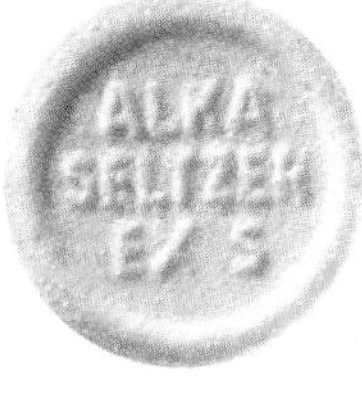

Alka-Seltzer Plus Night Time Cold Effervescent Tablets p. 148

Alka-Seltzer Extra Strength Effervescent Tablets p. 43

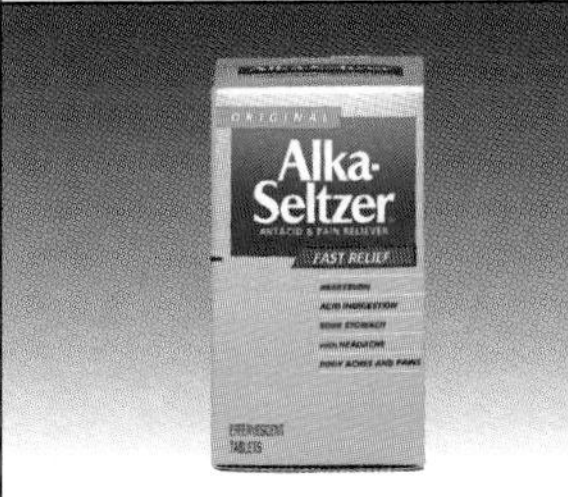

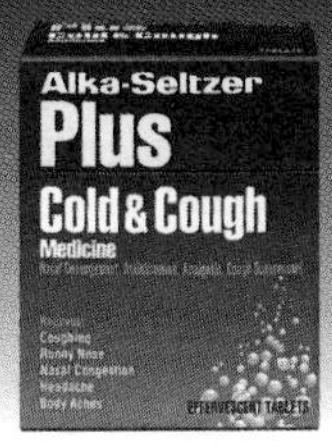

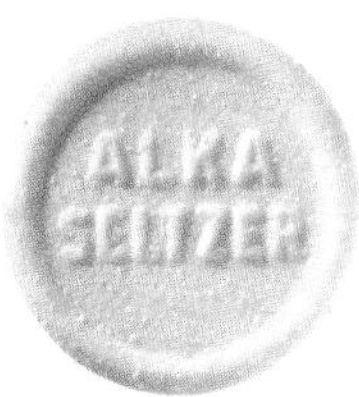

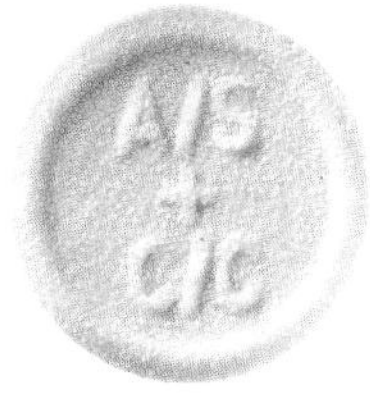

Alka-Seltzer Original Effervescent Tablets p. 43

Alka-Seltzer Plus Cold & Cough Effervescent Tablets p. 110

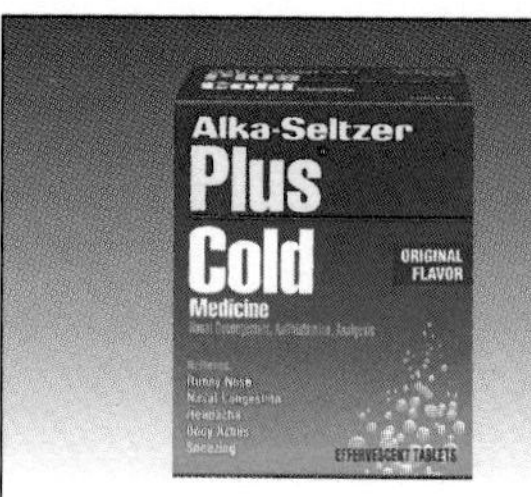

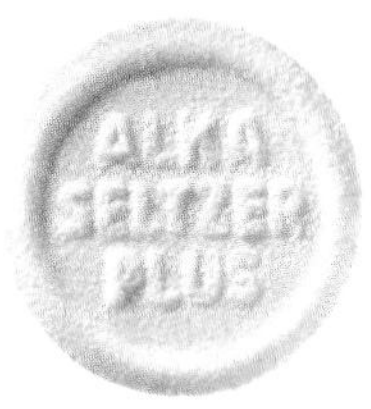

Alka-Seltzer Plus Cold Medicine Effervescent Tablets
p. 124

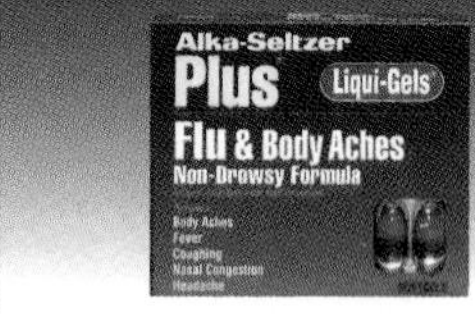

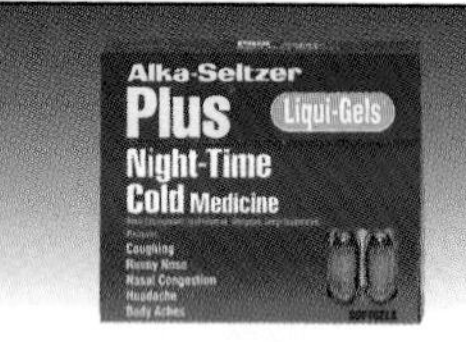

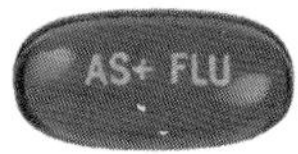

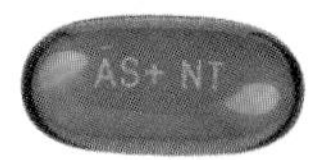

Alka-Seltzer Plus Flu Liqui-Gels
p. 142

Alka-Seltzer Plus Night Time Cold Liqui-Gels p. 155

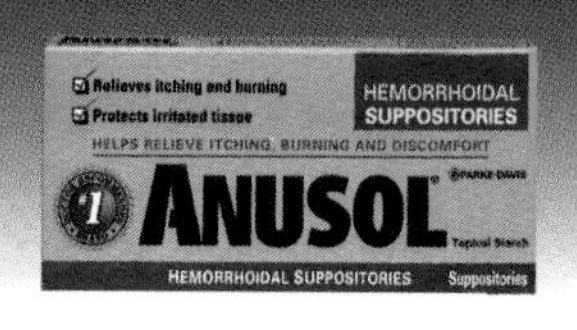

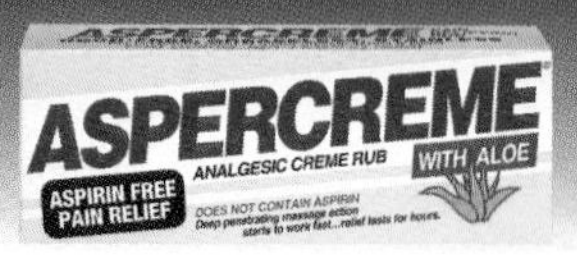

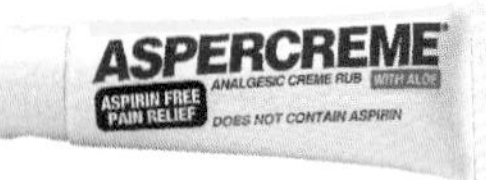

Anusol Suppositories
p. 534

Aspercreme Creme Rub
p. 54

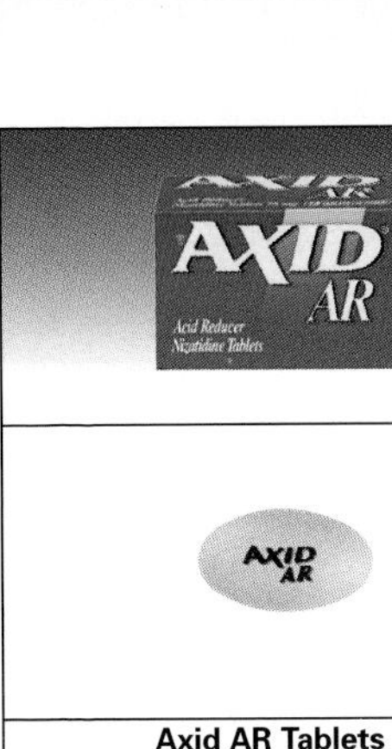

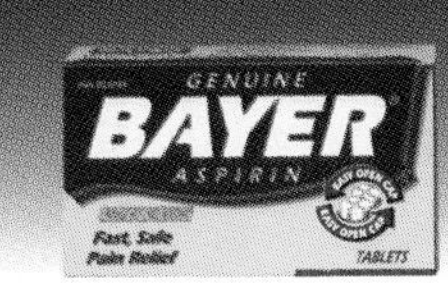

Axid AR Tablets
p. 259

Bayer Tablets
p. 57

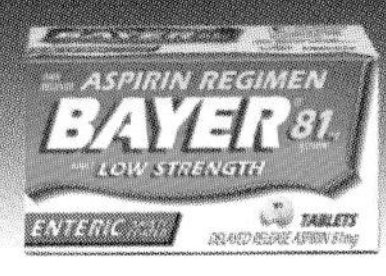

Bayer Enteric Low Strength Tablets p. 57

Bayer Enteric Caplets
p. 57

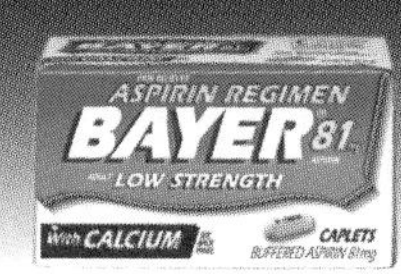

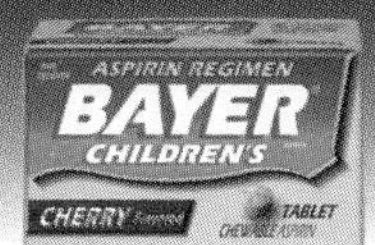

Bayer Low Strength With Calcium Caplets p. 57

Bayer Children's Chewable Cherry Tablets p. 57

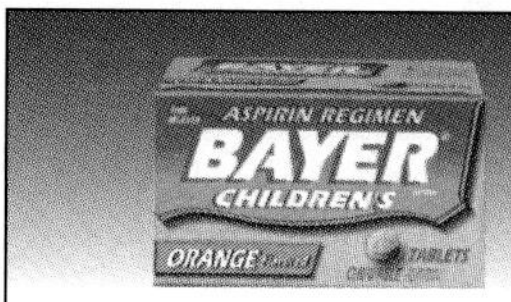

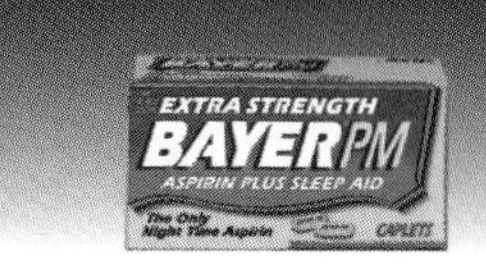

BAYER PM

Bayer Children's Chewable Orange Tablets p. 57

Bayer PM Caplets p. 404

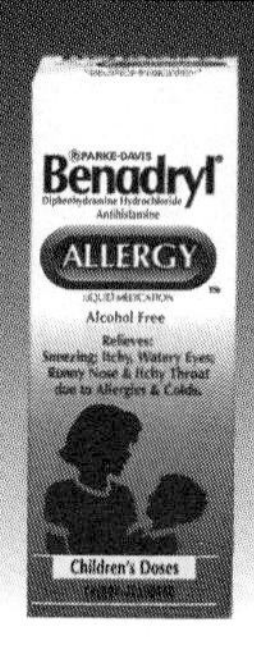

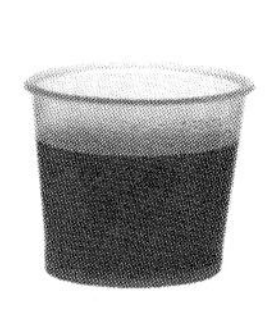

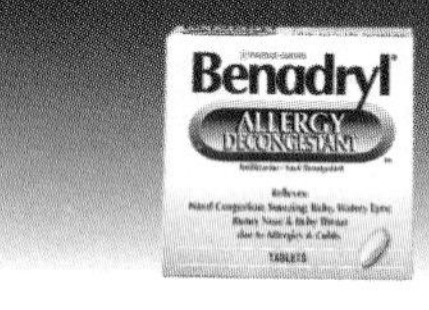

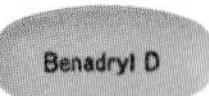

Benadryl Allergy Liquid p. 432

Benadryl Allergy Decongestant Tablets p. 432

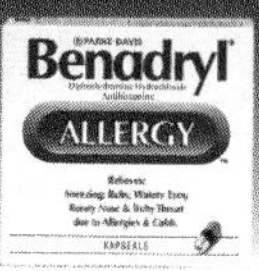

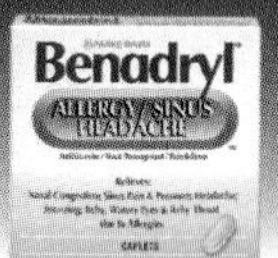

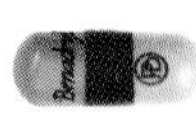

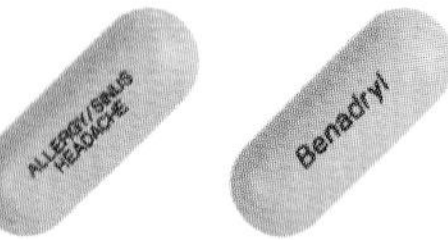

Benadryl Allergy Kapseals p. 432

Benadryl Allergy/Sinus Headache Caplets p. 437

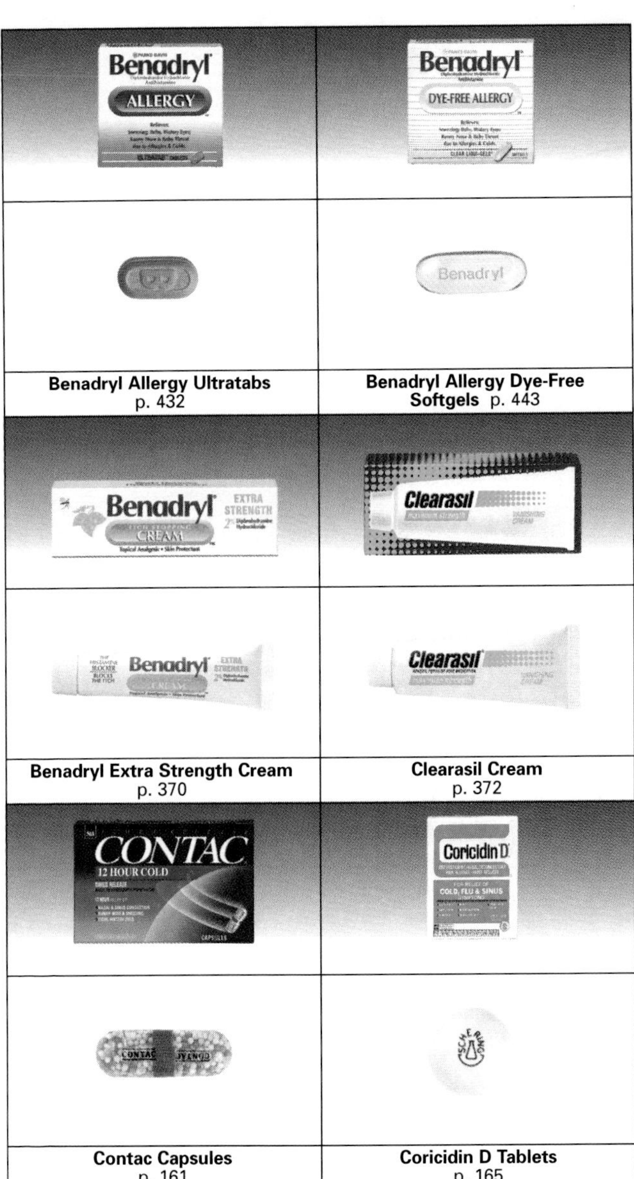

Benadryl Allergy Ultratabs
p. 432

Benadryl Allergy Dye-Free Softgels p. 443

Benadryl Extra Strength Cream
p. 370

Clearasil Cream
p. 372

Contac Capsules
p. 161

Coricidin D Tablets
p. 165

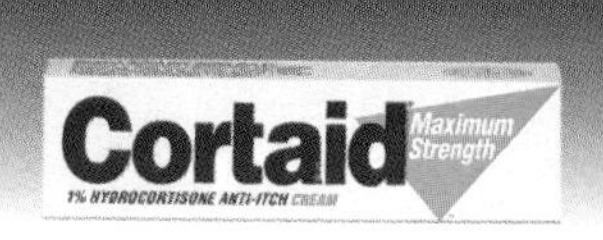

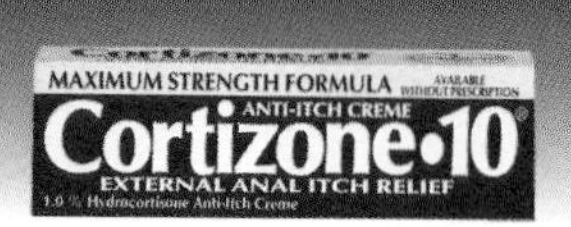

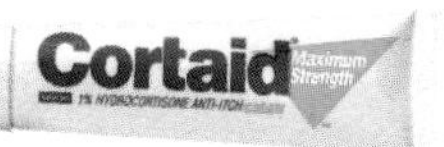

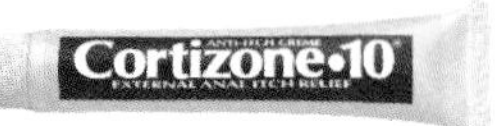

Cortaid Cream
p. 372

Cortizone 10 Creme
p. 372

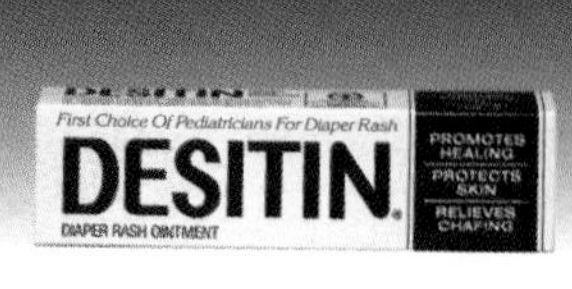

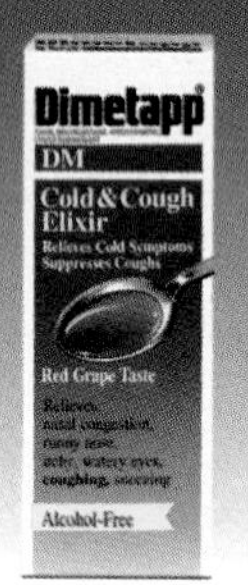

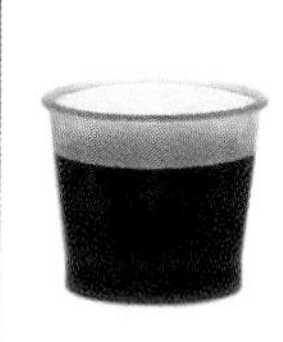

Desitin Ointment
p. 643

Dimetapp DM Cold & Cough Elixir p. 170

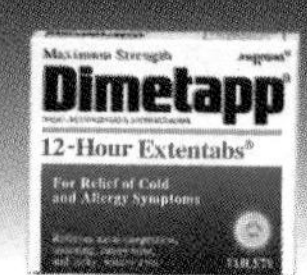

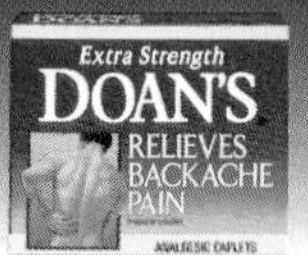

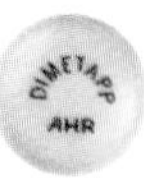

Dimetapp Extentabs
p. 175

Doan's Caplets
p. 57

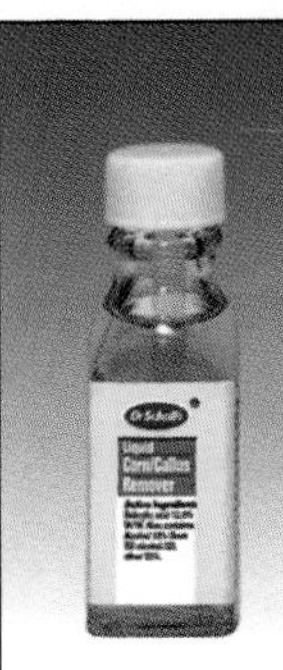

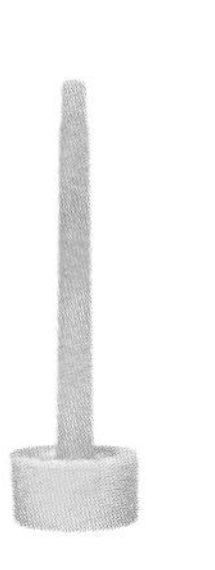

Dr. Scholl's Liquid
p. 373

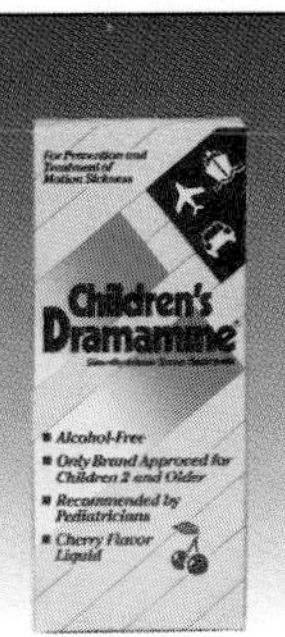

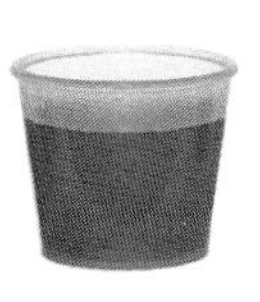

Dramamine Children's Liquid
p. 621

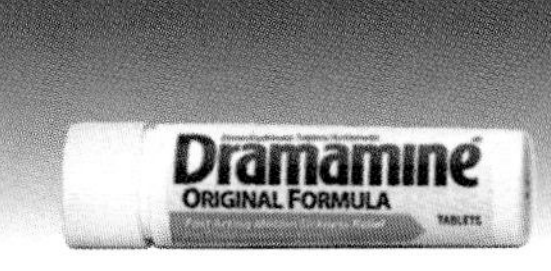

Dramamine Tablets
p. 621

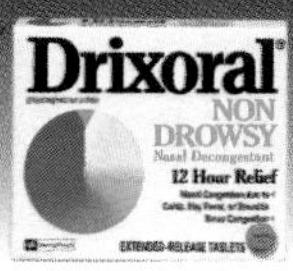

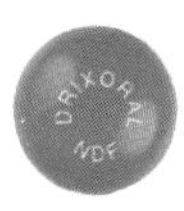

Drixoral Tablets
p. 179

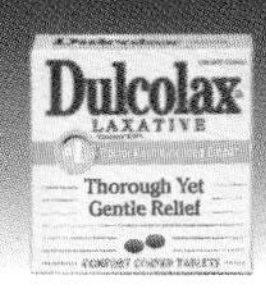

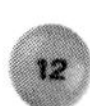

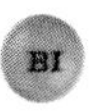

Dulcolax Tablets
p. 269

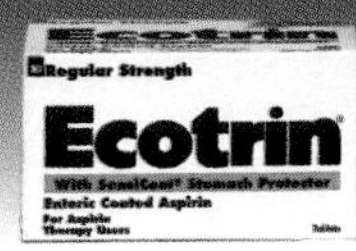

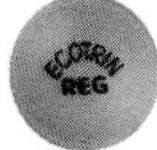

Ecotrin Tablets
p. 60

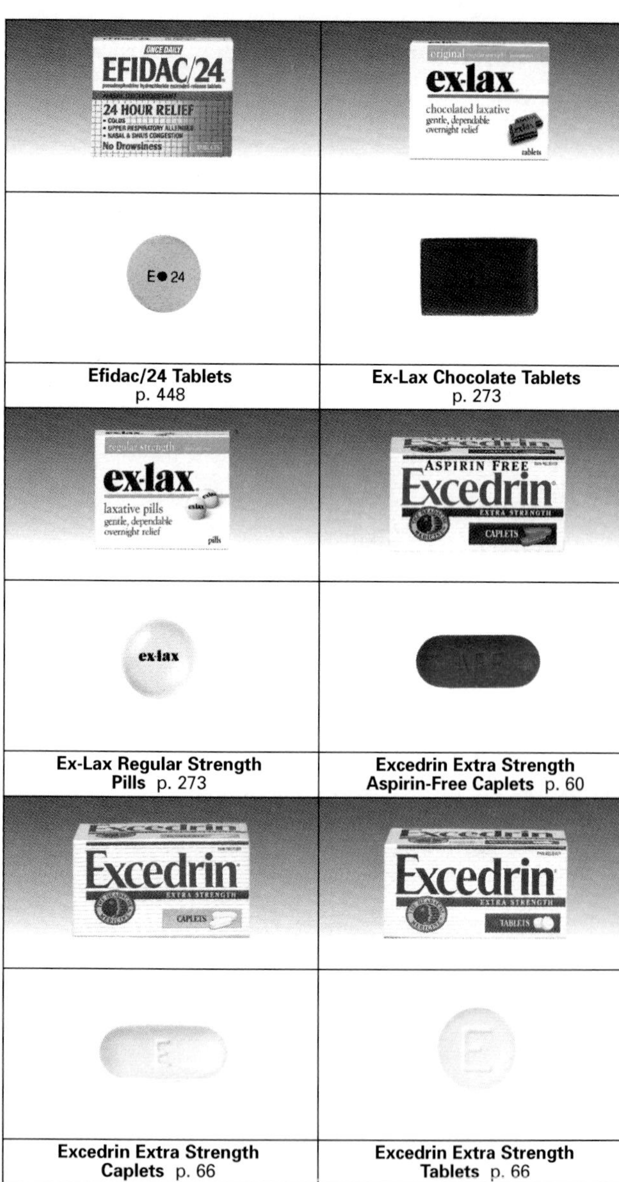

Efidac/24 Tablets
p. 448

Ex-Lax Chocolate Tablets
p. 273

Ex-Lax Regular Strength Pills p. 273

Excedrin Extra Strength Aspirin-Free Caplets p. 60

Excedrin Extra Strength Caplets p. 66

Excedrin Extra Strength Tablets p. 66

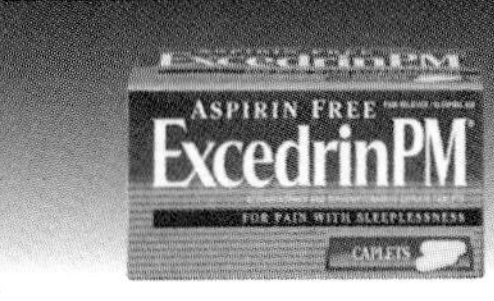

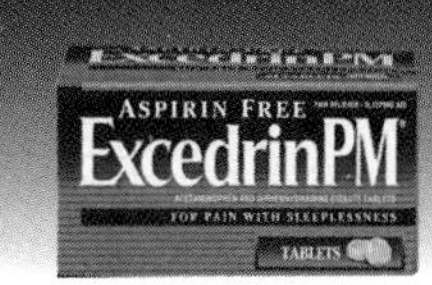

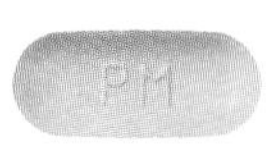

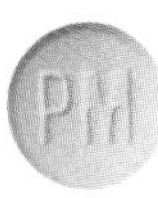

Excedrin PM Caplets
p. 409

Excedrin PM Aspirin-Free Tablets p. 409

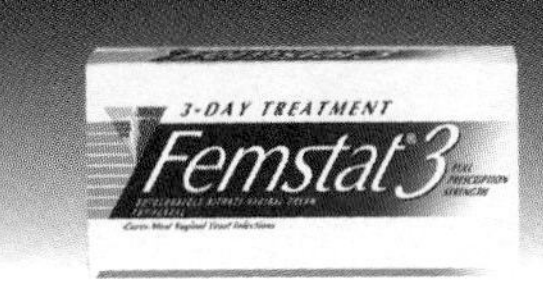

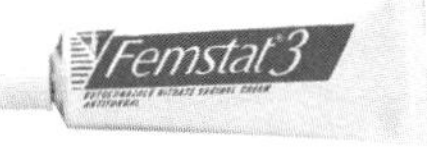

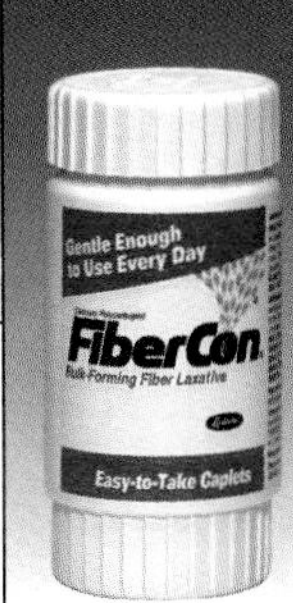

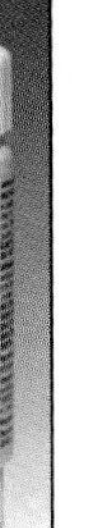

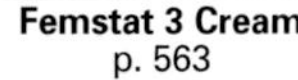

Femstat 3 Cream
p. 563

FiberCon Caplets
p. 273

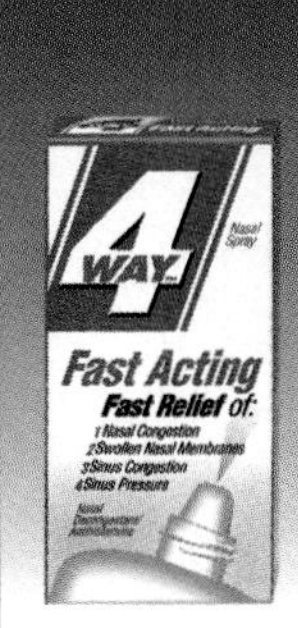

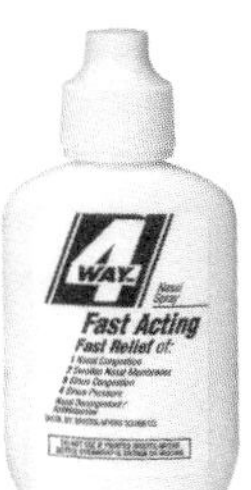

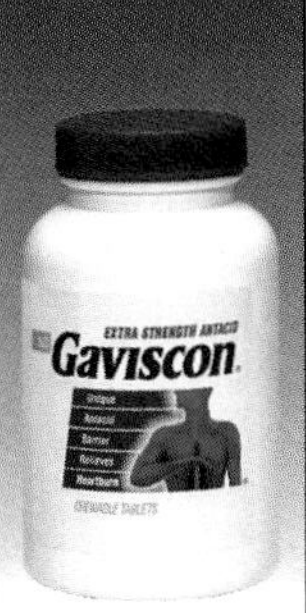

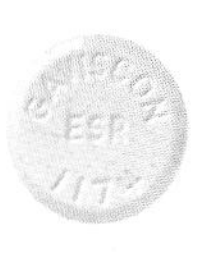

4-Way Nasal Spray
p. 448

Gaviscon Tablets
p. 273

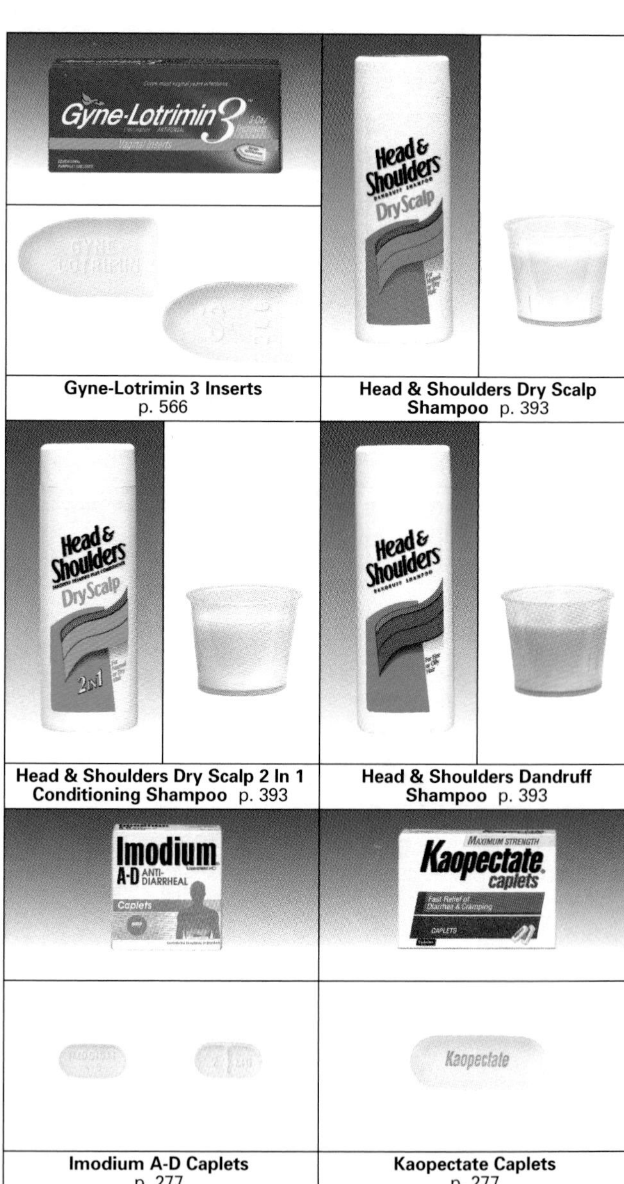

Gyne-Lotrimin 3 Inserts
p. 566

Head & Shoulders Dry Scalp Shampoo p. 393

Head & Shoulders Dry Scalp 2 In 1 Conditioning Shampoo p. 393

Head & Shoulders Dandruff Shampoo p. 393

Imodium A-D Caplets
p. 277

Kaopectate Caplets
p. 277

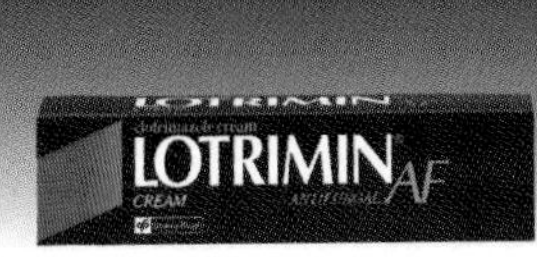

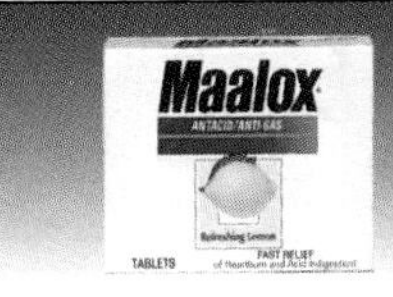

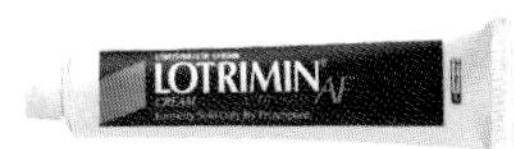

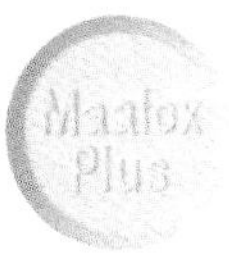

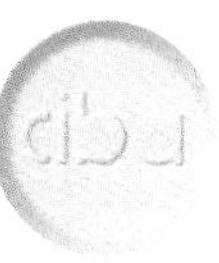

Lotrimin AF Cream
p. 375

Maalox Tablets
p. 281

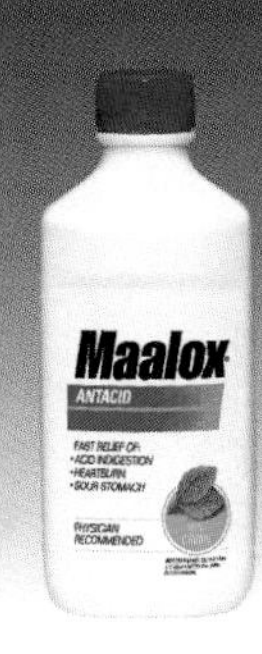

Maalox Liquid
p. 277

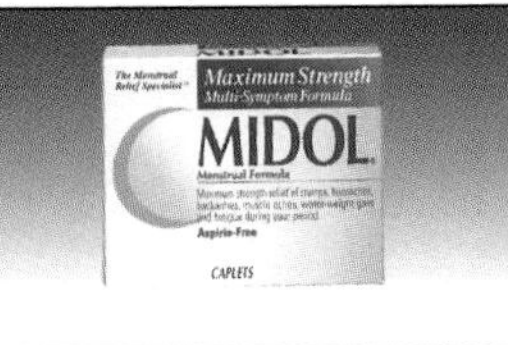

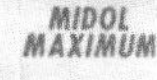

Midol Multi-Symptom Caplets p. 566

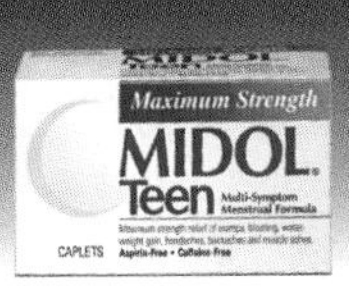

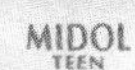

Midol Multi-Symptom Teen Caplets p. 578

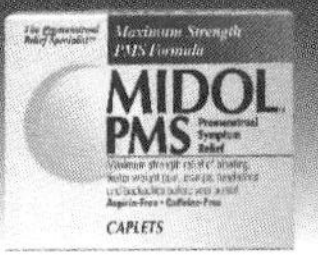

Midol PMS Multi-Symptom Caplets p. 573

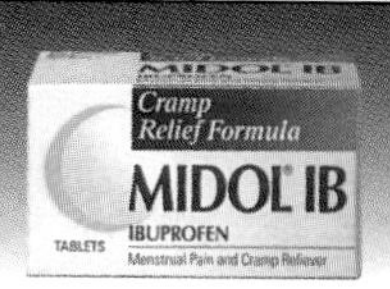

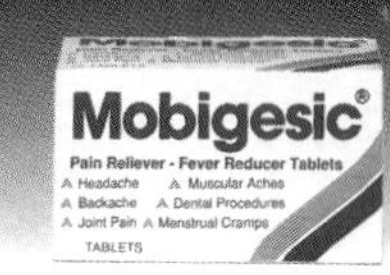

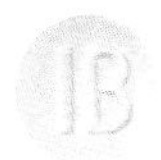
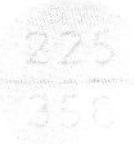

Midol IB Tablets
p. 566

Mobigesic Tablets
p. 72

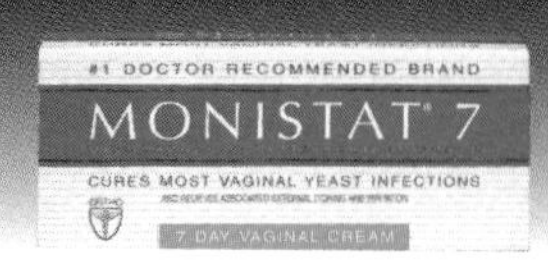

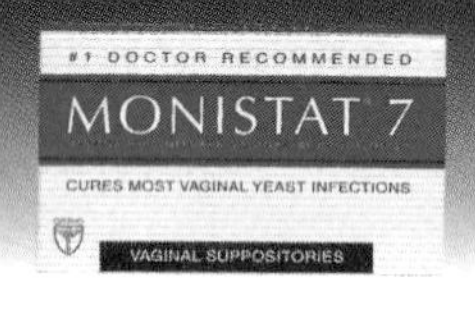

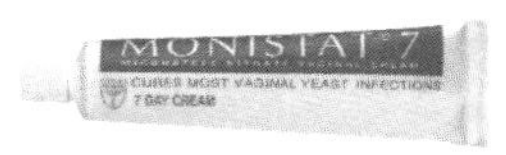

Monistat 7 Cream
p. 581

Monistat 7 Suppositories
p. 584

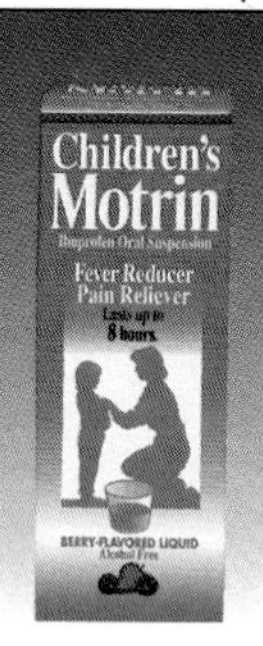

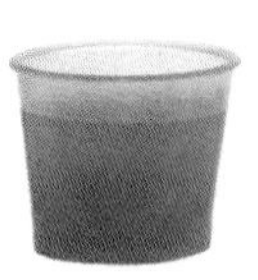

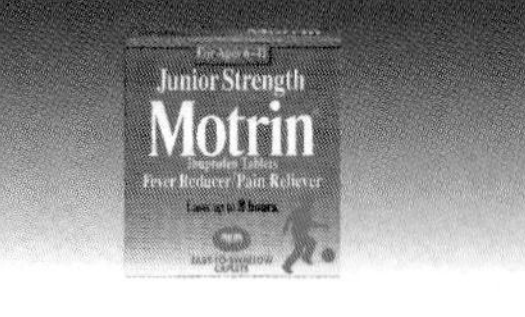

Motrin Children's Liquid
p. 76

Motrin Junior Caplets
p. 76

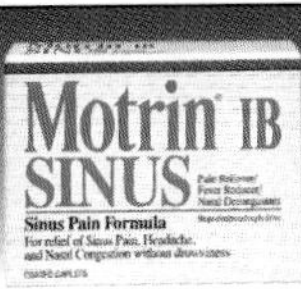

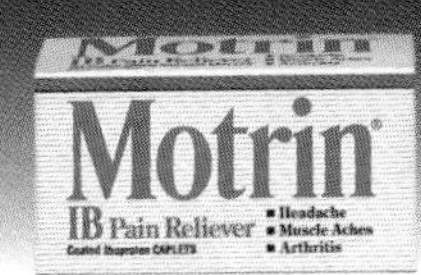

Motrin IB Sinus Caplets
p. 452

Motrin IB Caplets
p. 76

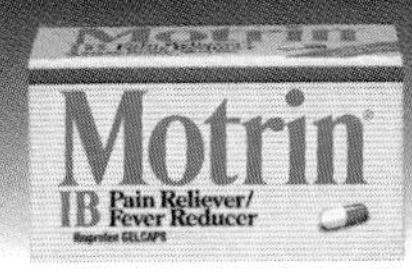

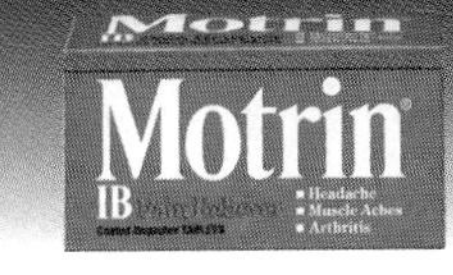

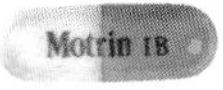

Motrin IB Gelcaps
p. 76

Motrin IB Tablets
p. 76

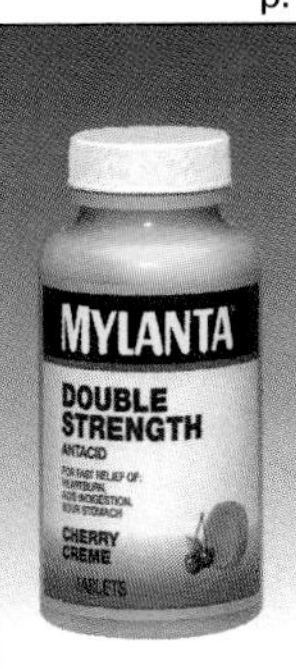

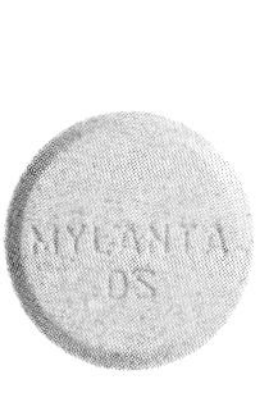

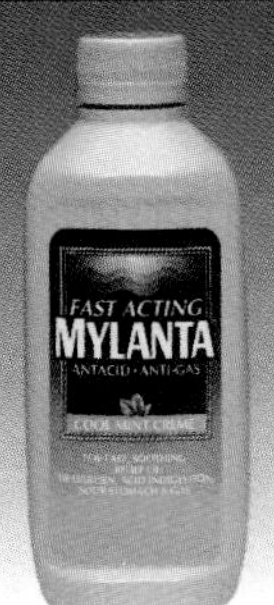

Mylanta Tablets
p. 289

Mylanta Mint Liquid
p. 281

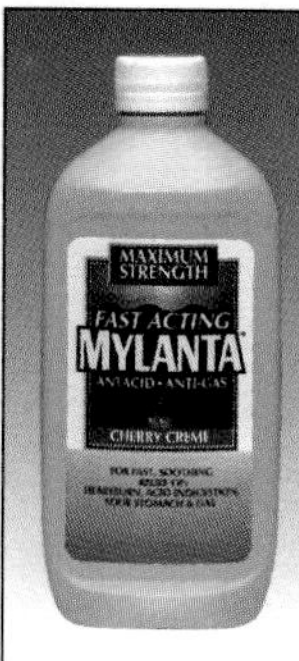

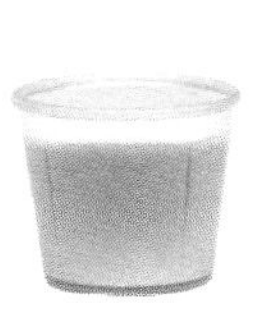
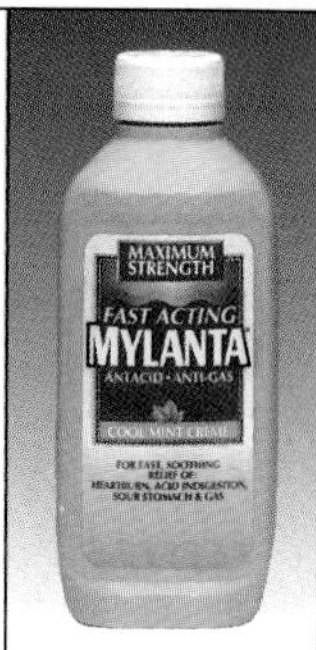

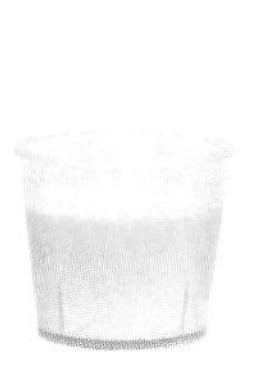

Mylanta Maximum Strength Cherry Liquid p. 281

Mylanta Maximum Strength Mint Liquid p. 281

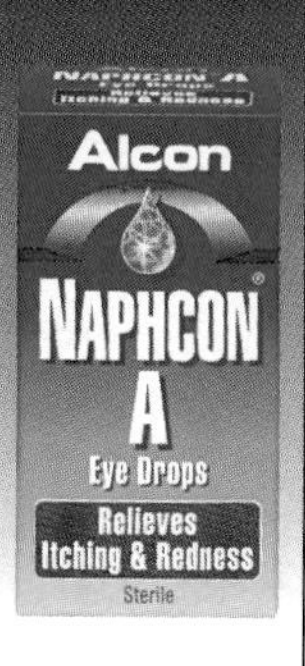

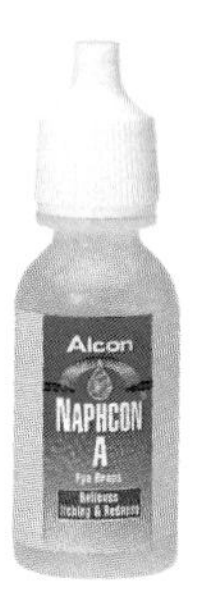

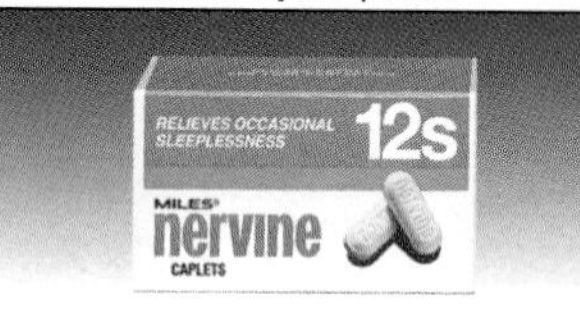

Naphcon A Eyedrops p. 519

Nervine Caplets p. 413

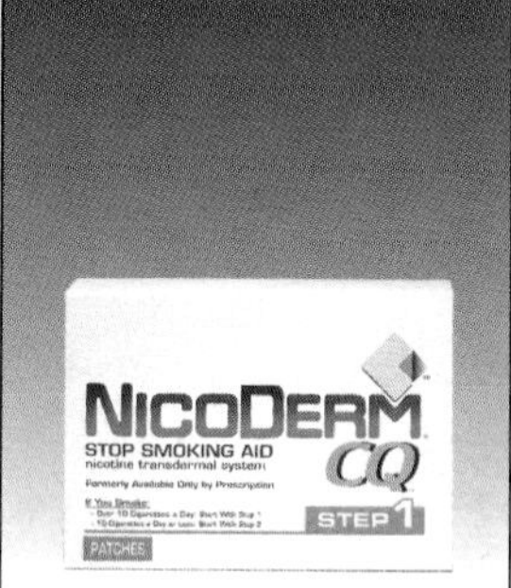

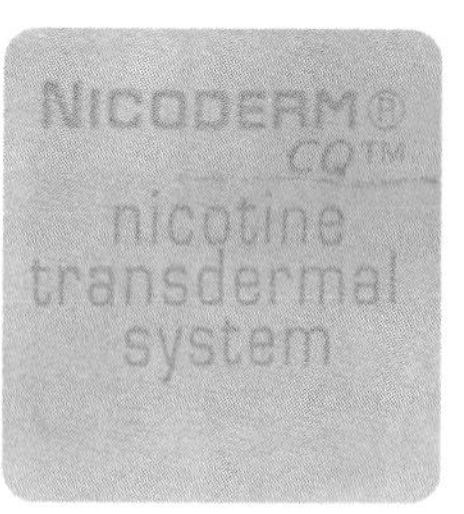

NicoDerm CQ Step 1 Patches p. 602

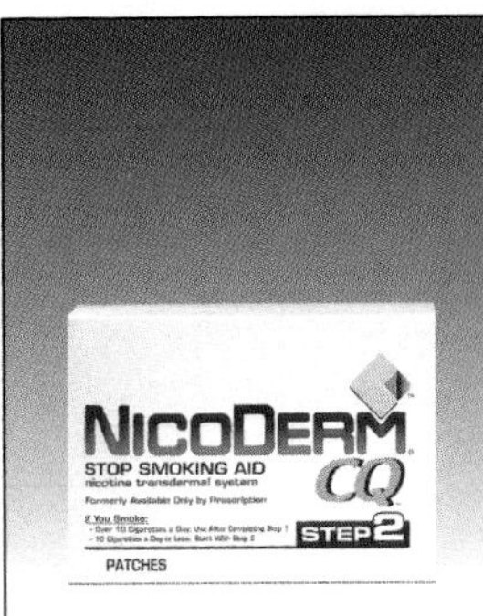

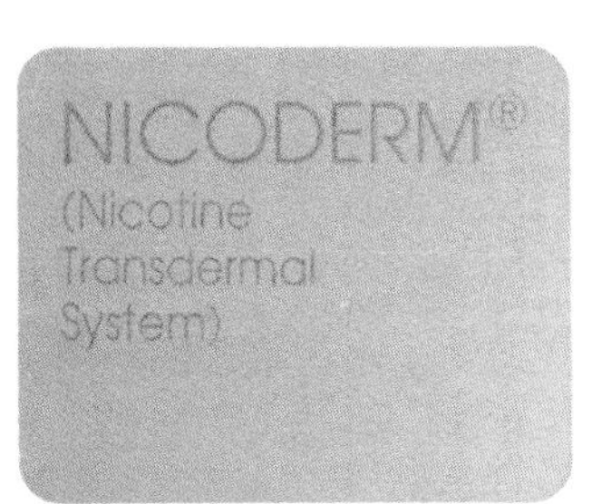

NicoDerm CQ Step 2 Patches
p. 602

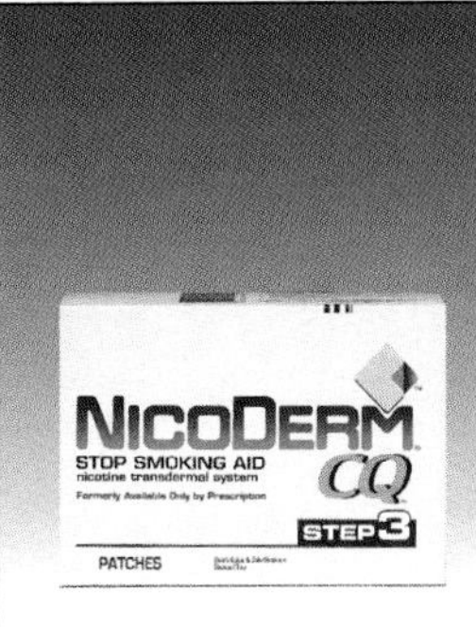

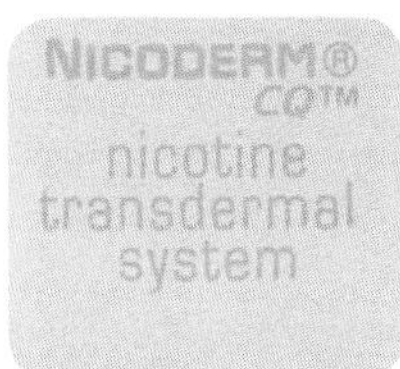

NicoDerm CQ Step 3 Patches
p. 602

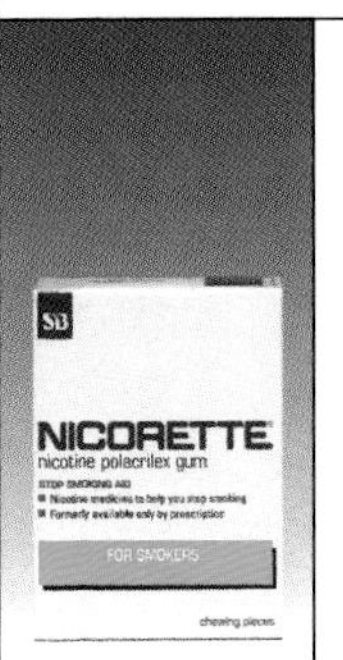

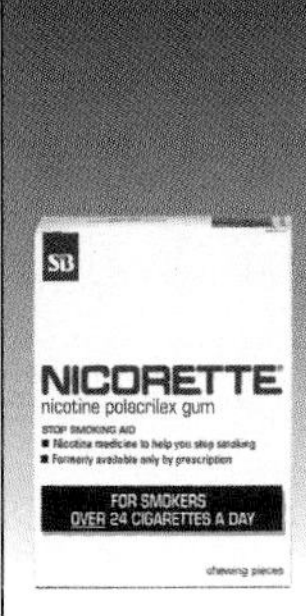

Nicorette 2 mg Gum
p. 608

Nicorette 4 mg Gum
p. 608

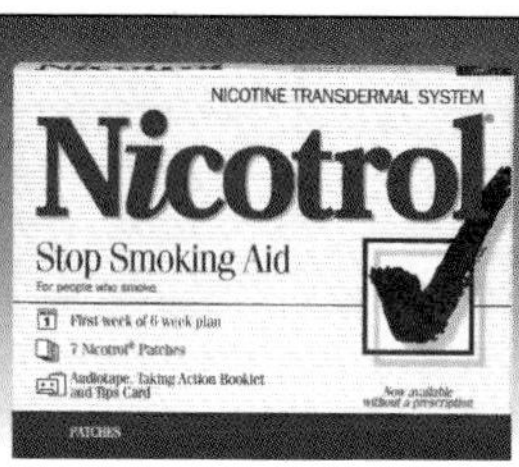

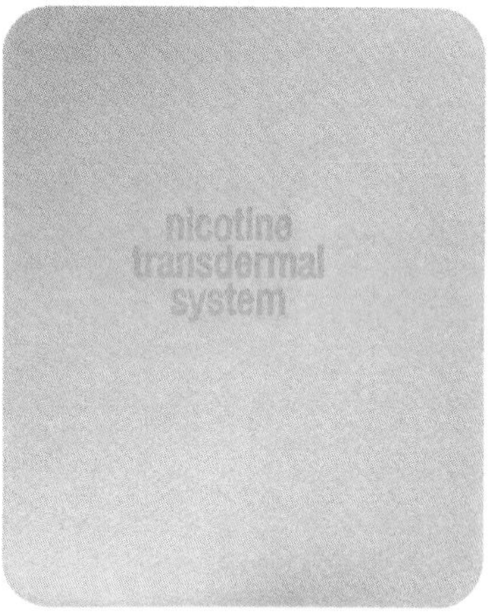

Nicotrol Patches
p. 602

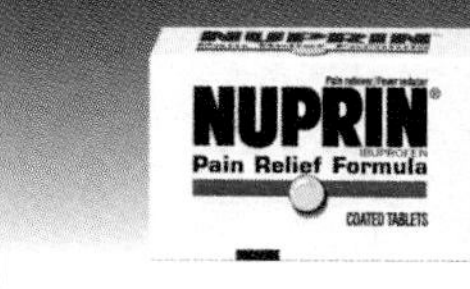

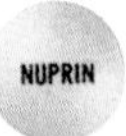

Nuprin Tablets
p. 76

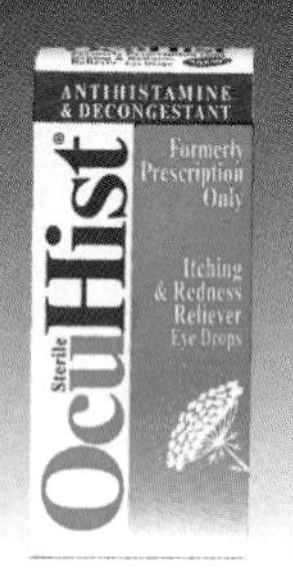

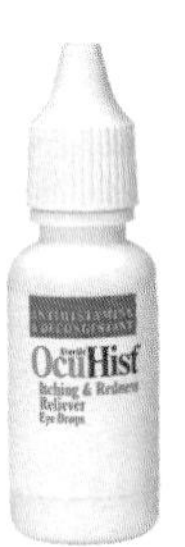

OcuHist Eye Drops
p. 519

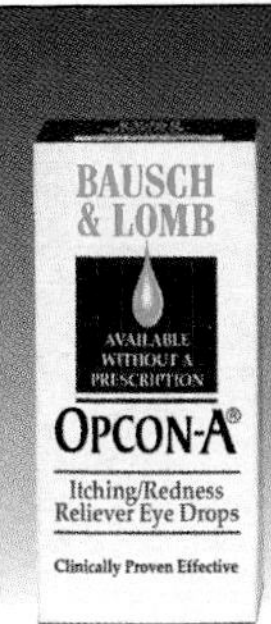

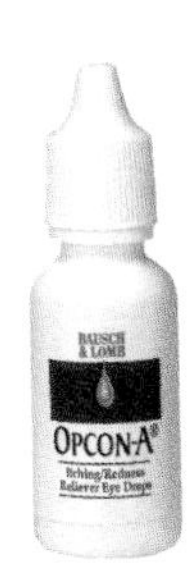

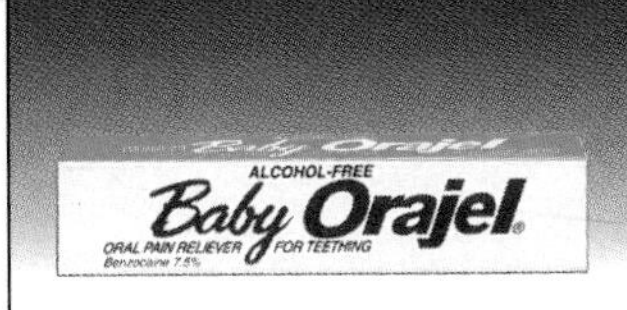

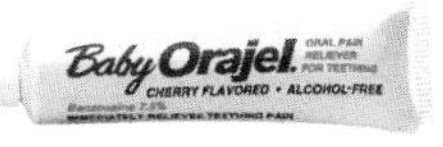

Opcon-A Eye Drops
p. 519

Orajel Baby Gel
p. 646

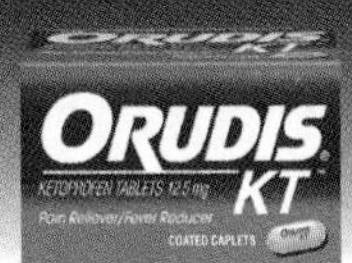

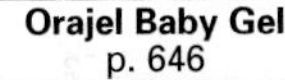

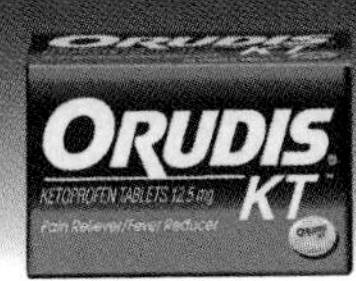

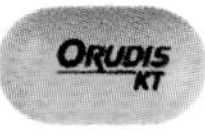

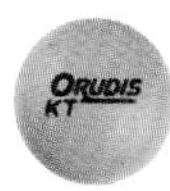

Orudis KT Caplets
p. 76

Orudis KT Tablets
p. 76

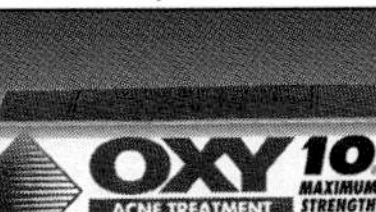

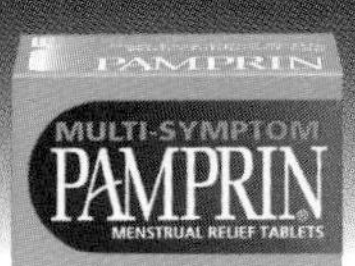

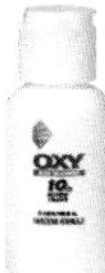

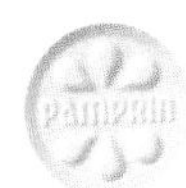

Oxy 10 Gel
p. 375

Pamprin Tablets
p. 585

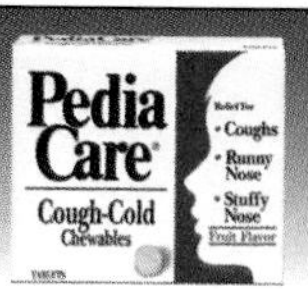

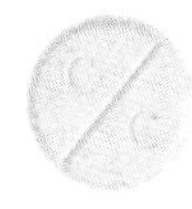

PediaCare Tablets
p. 180

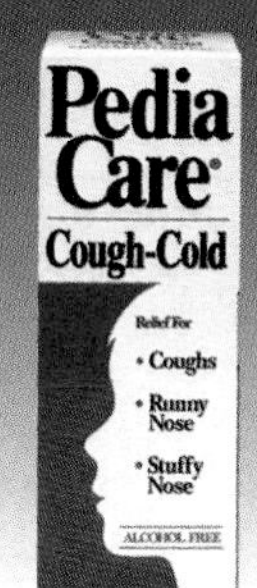

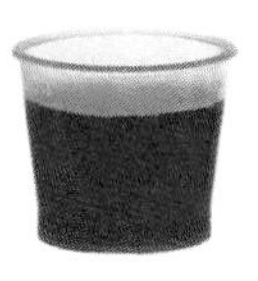

PediaCare Liquid
p. 180

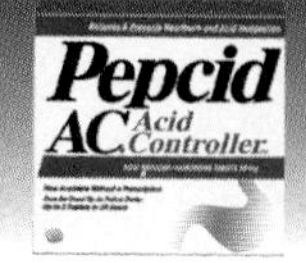

Pepcid AC Tablets
p. 285

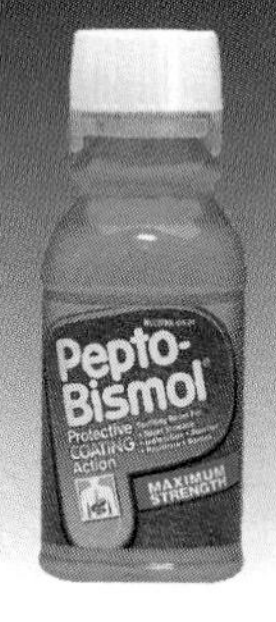

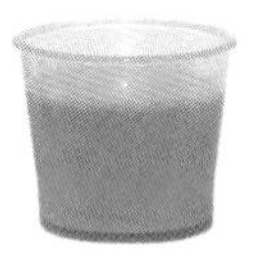

Pepto-Bismol Maximum Strength Liquid p. 293

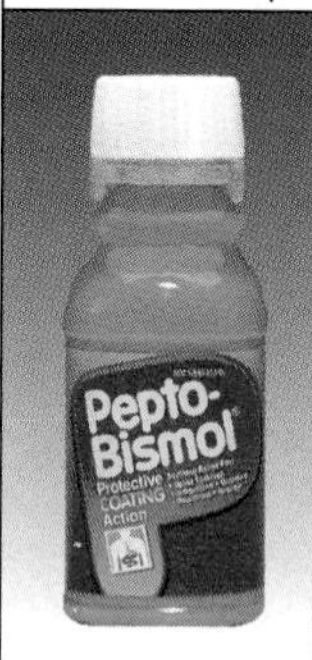

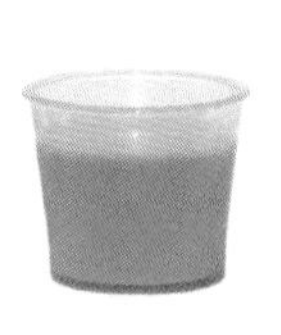

Pepto-Bismol Liquid
p. 293

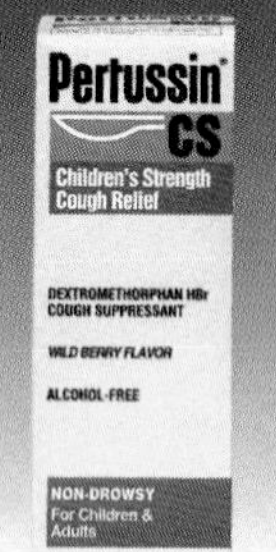

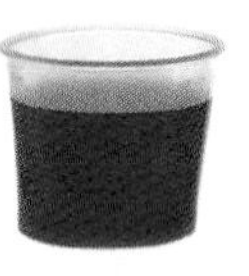

Pertussin CS Liquid
p. 185

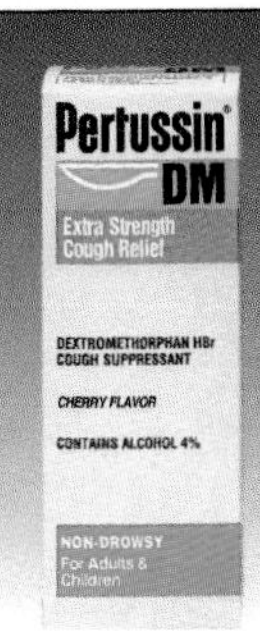

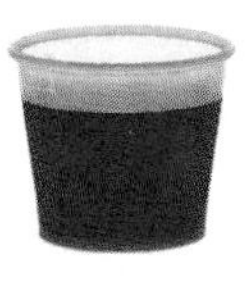

Pertussin DM Liquid
p. 185

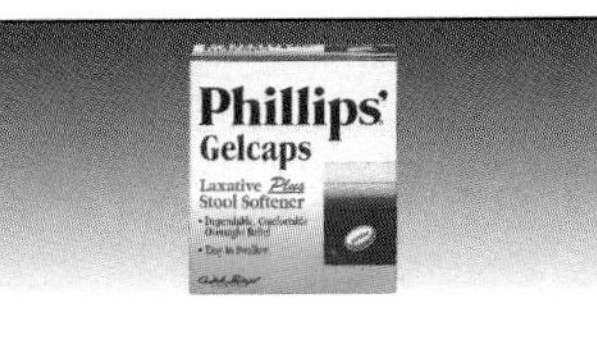

Phillips' Gelcaps
p. 293

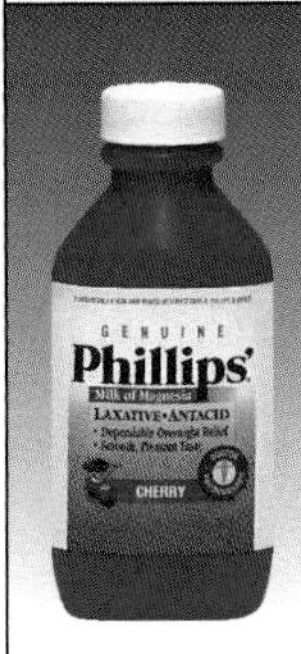

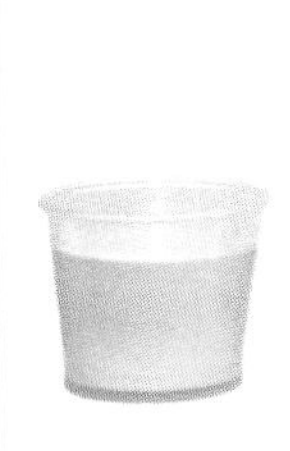

Phillips' Cherry Liquid
p. 298

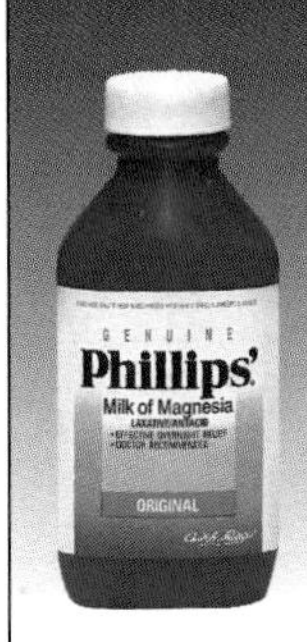

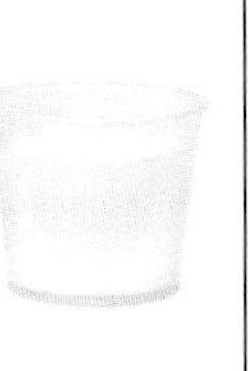

Phillips' Original Liquid
p. 298

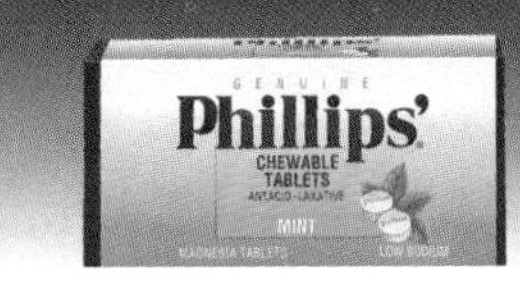

Phillips' Tablets
p. 298

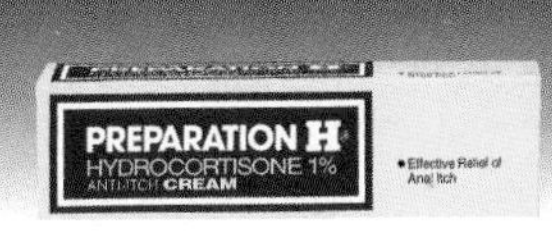

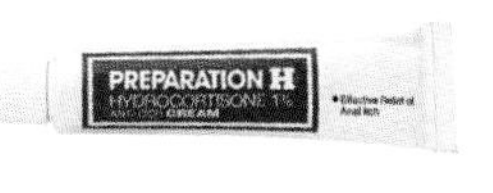

Preparation H Cream
p. 375

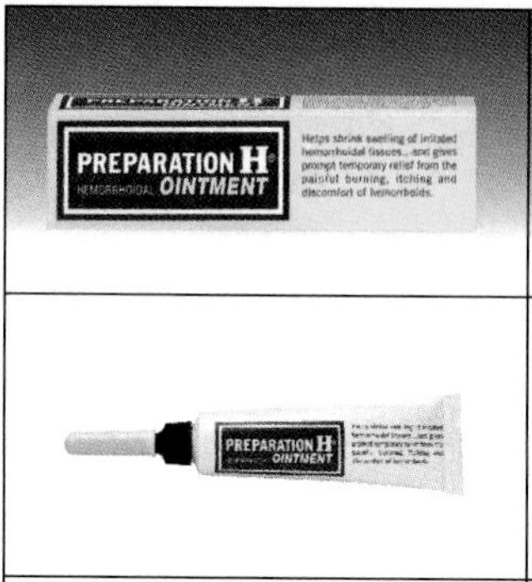

Preparation H Ointment
p. 536

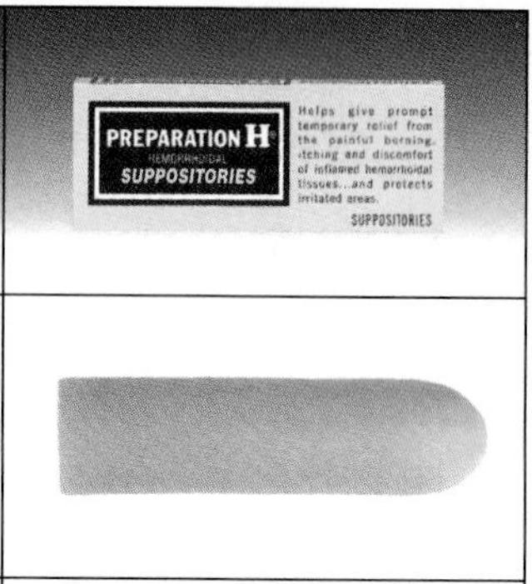

Preparation H Suppositories
p. 539

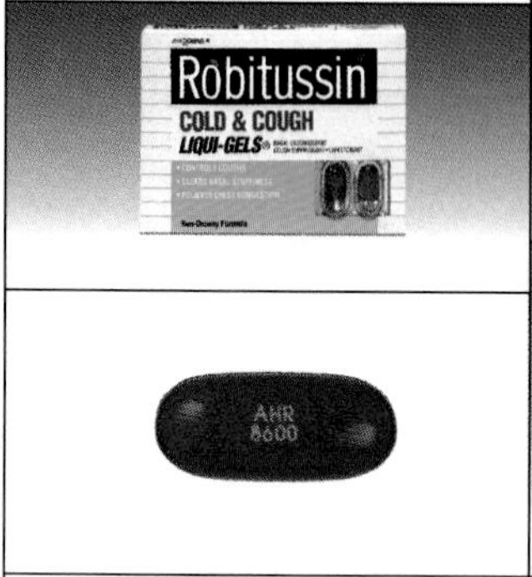

Robitussin Cold & Cough Liqui-Gels p. 189

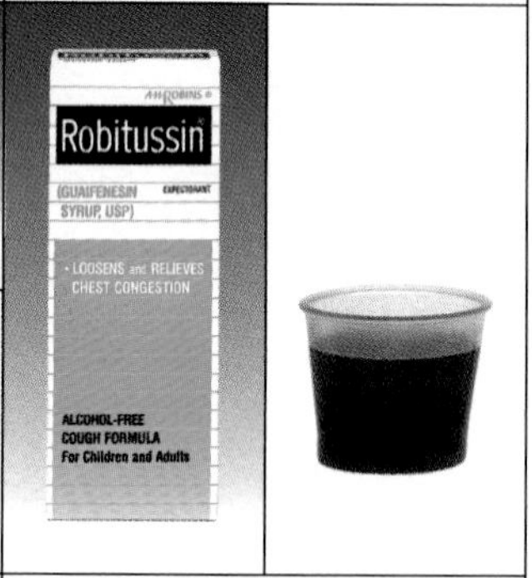

Robitussin Expectorant Liquid
p. 185

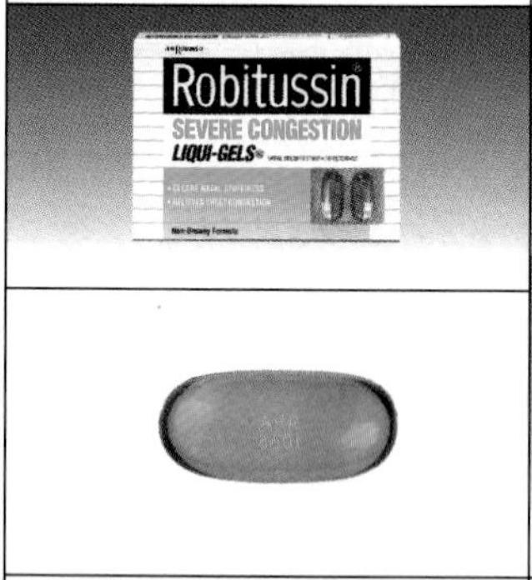

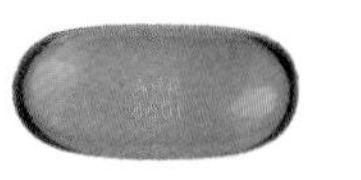

Robitussin Severe Congestion Liqui-Gels p. 197

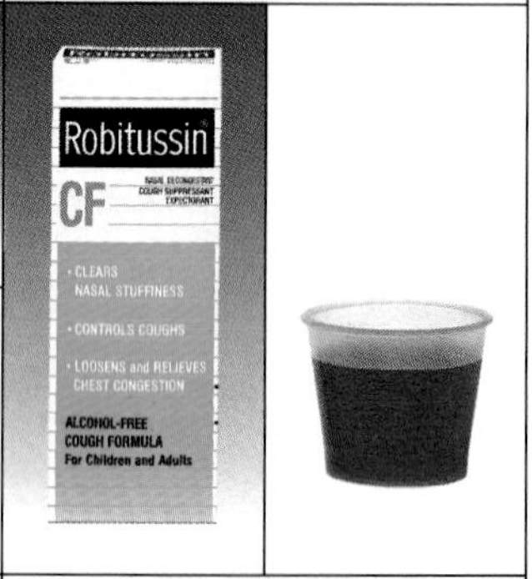

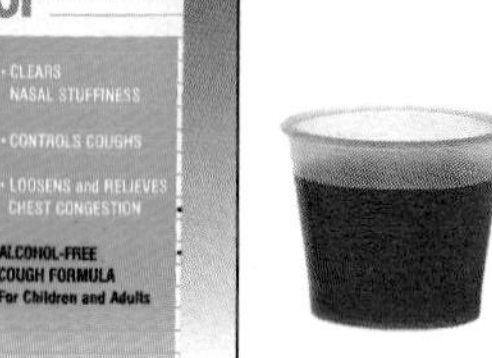

Robitussin CF Liquid
p. 185

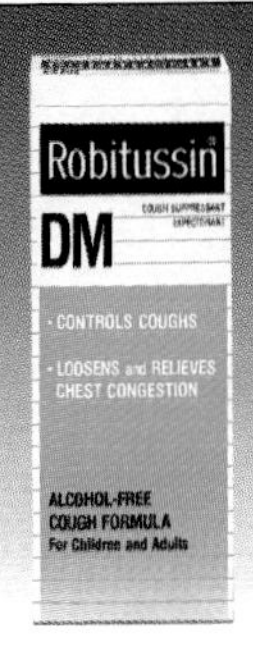

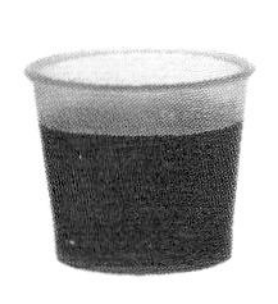

Robitussin DM Liquid
p. 193

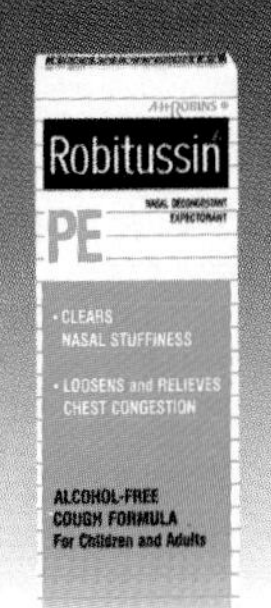

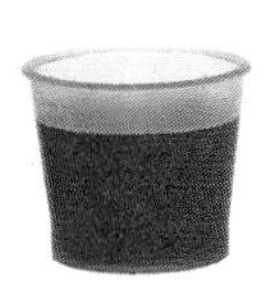

Robitussin PE Liquid
p. 197

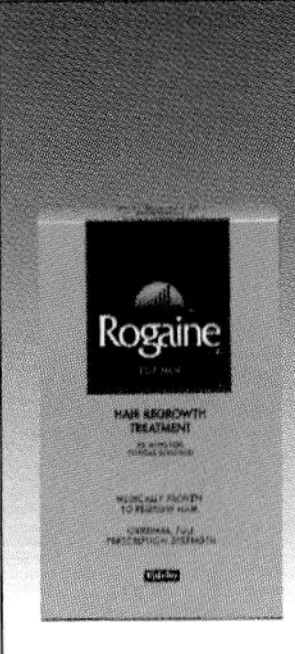

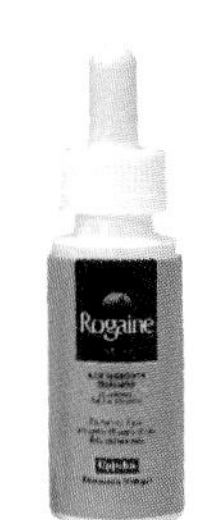

Rogaine For Men Solution
p. 393

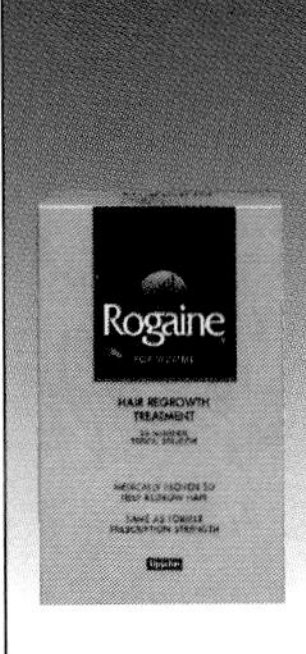

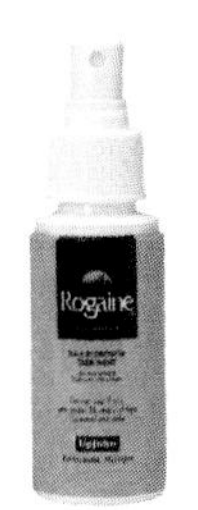

Rogaine For Women Solution
p. 393

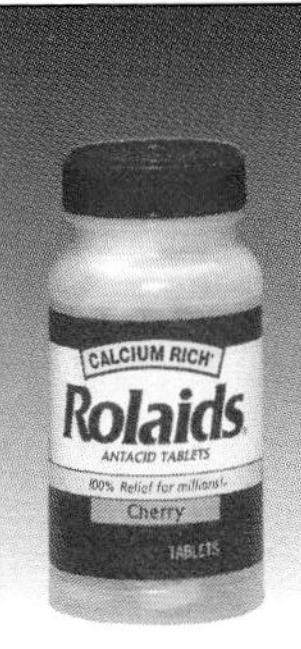

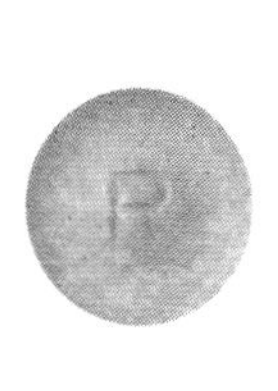

Rolaids Tablets
p. 289

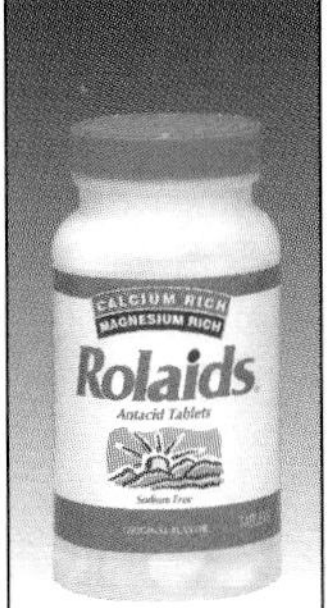

Rolaids Calcium Rich/Sodium Free Tablets p. 298

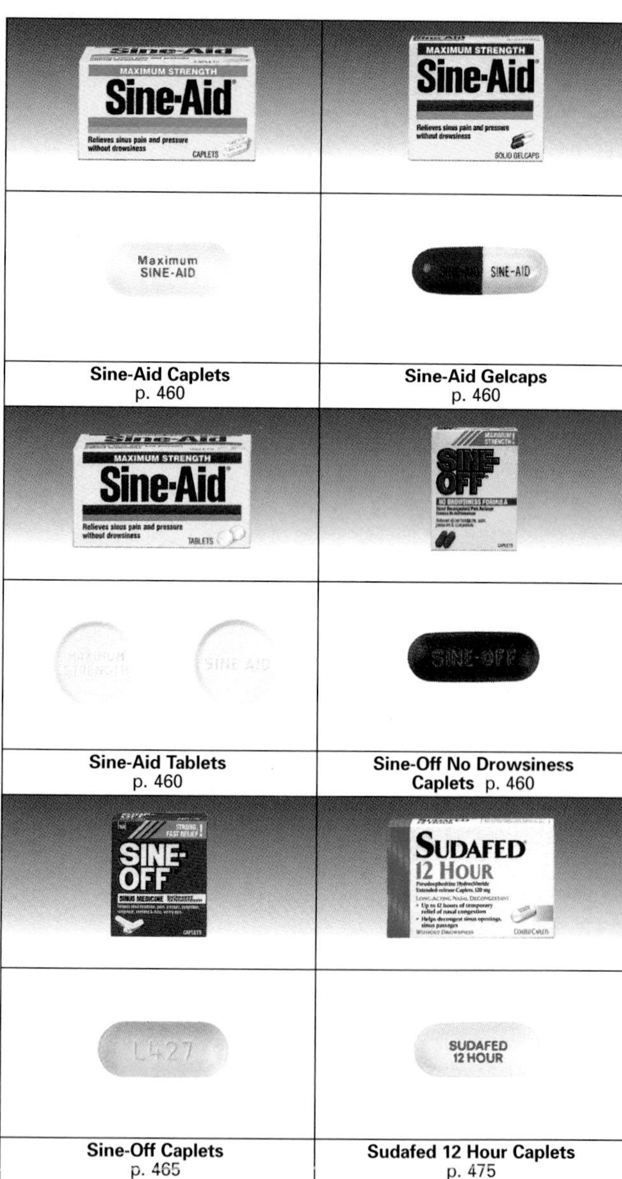

Sine-Aid Caplets
p. 460

Sine-Aid Gelcaps
p. 460

Sine-Aid Tablets
p. 460

Sine-Off No Drowsiness Caplets p. 460

Sine-Off Caplets
p. 465

Sudafed 12 Hour Caplets
p. 475

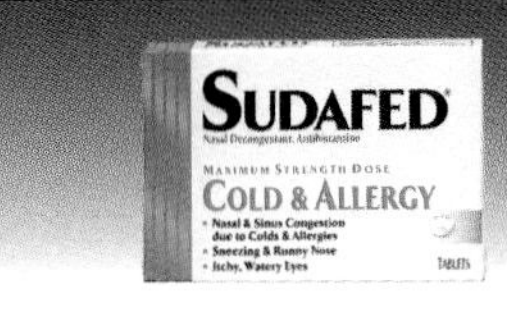

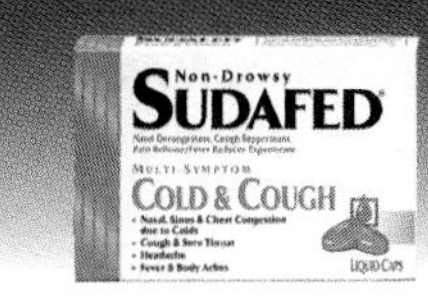

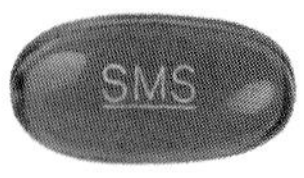

Sudafed Plus Cold & Allergy Tablets p. 471

Sudafed Cold & Cough Liquid-Caps p. 201

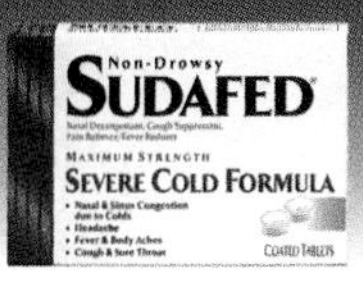

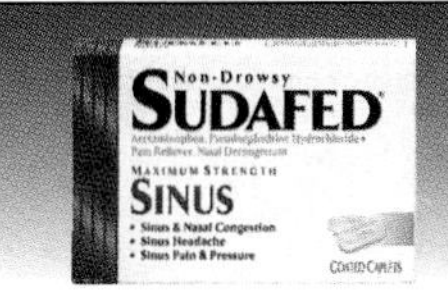

Sudafed Cold Tablets p. 142

Sudafed Sinus Caplets p. 460

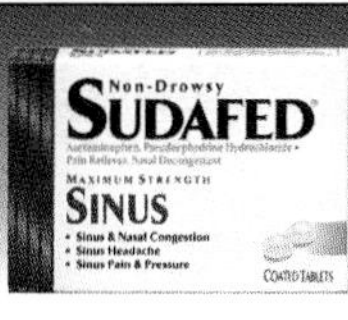

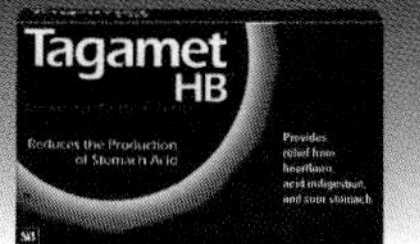

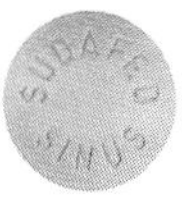

Sudafed Sinus Tablets p. 460

Tagamet HB Tablets p. 298

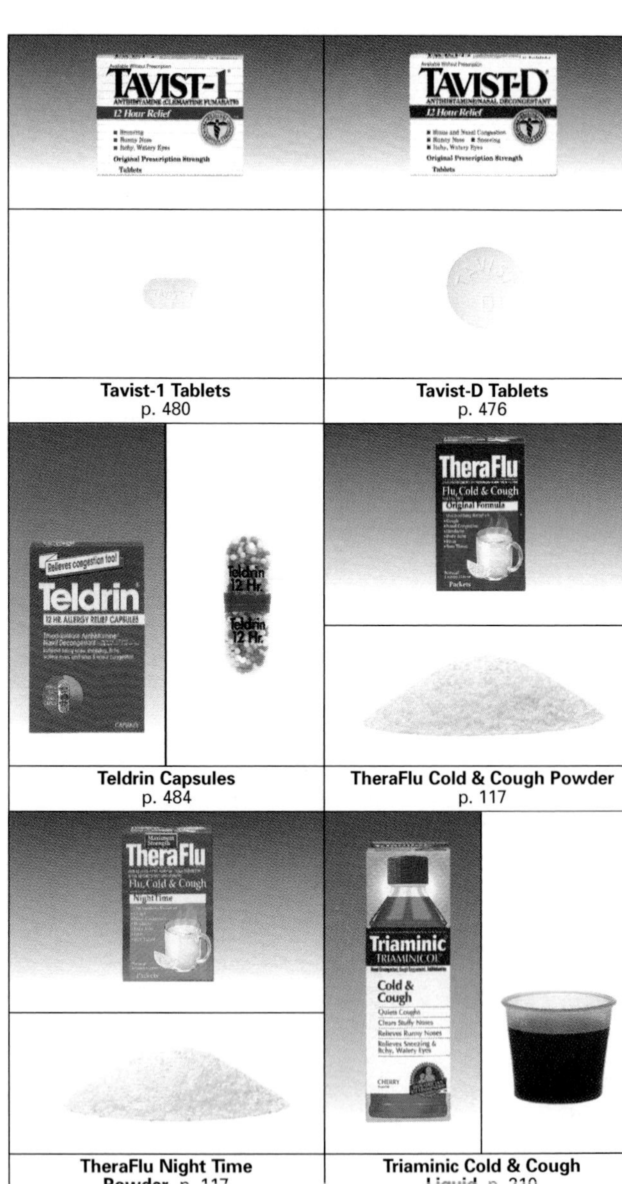

Tavist-1 Tablets
p. 480

Tavist-D Tablets
p. 476

Teldrin Capsules
p. 484

TheraFlu Cold & Cough Powder
p. 117

TheraFlu Night Time Powder p. 117

Triaminic Cold & Cough Liquid p. 210

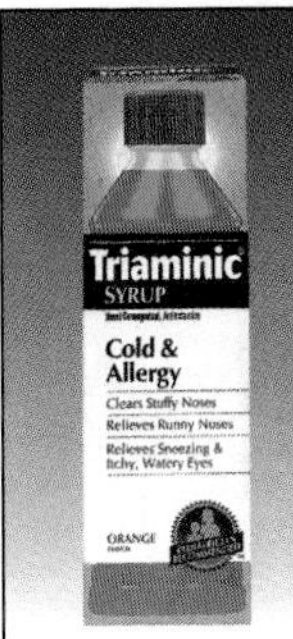

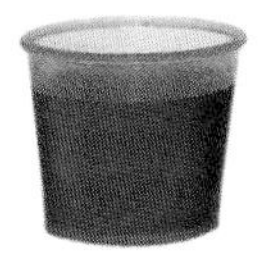

Triaminic Cold & Allergy Syrup p. 484

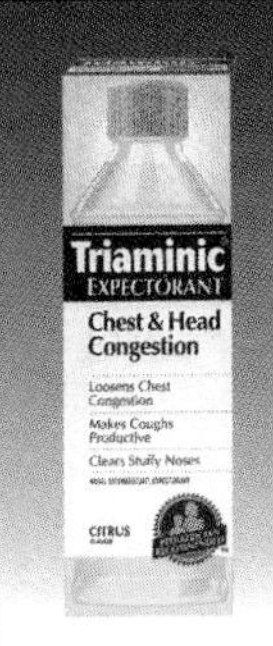

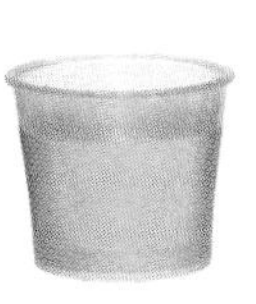

Triaminic Expectorant Liquid p. 207

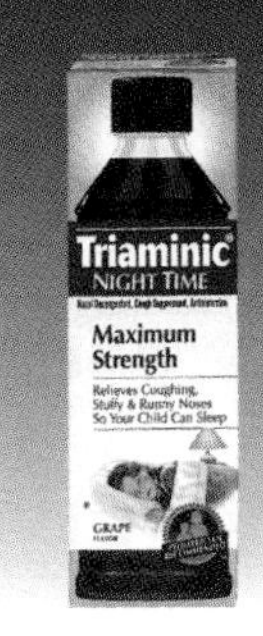

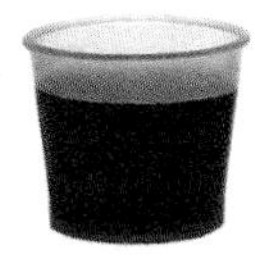

Triaminic Night Time Maximum Strength Children's Liquid p. 180

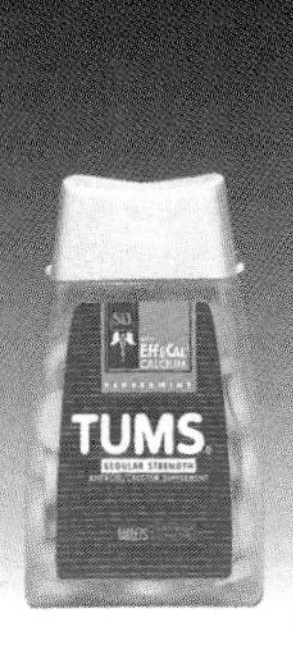

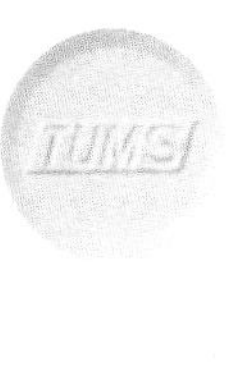

Tums Tablets p. 302

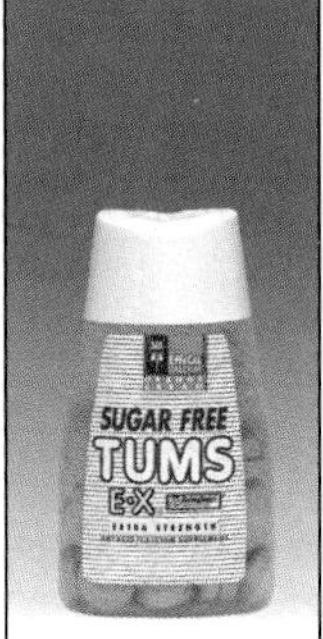

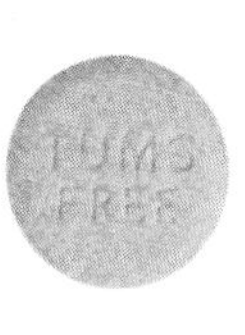

Tums Sugar Free Tablets p. 302

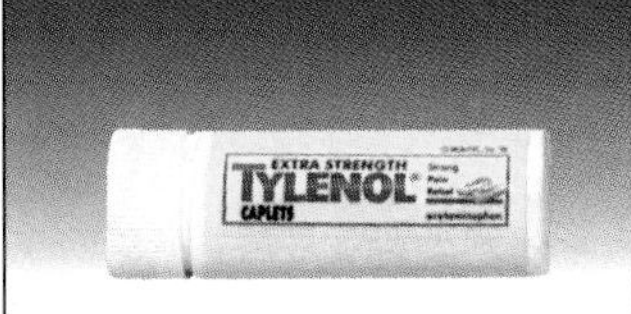

Tylenol Extra Strength Caplets p. 76

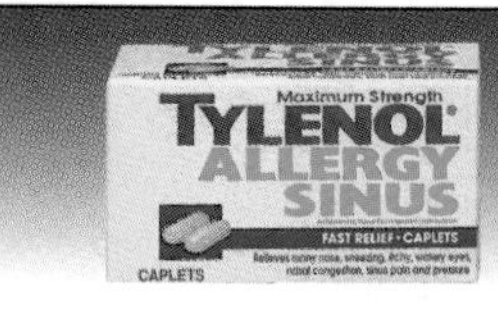

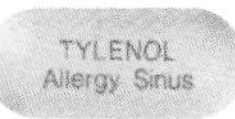

Tylenol Allergy Sinus Caplets p. 465

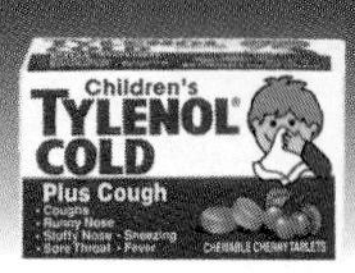

Tylenol Children's Cold Plus Cough Chewable Cherry Tablets p. 117

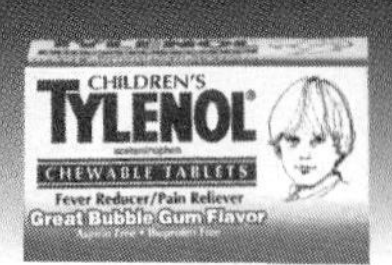

Tylenol Children's Chewable Tablets p. 76

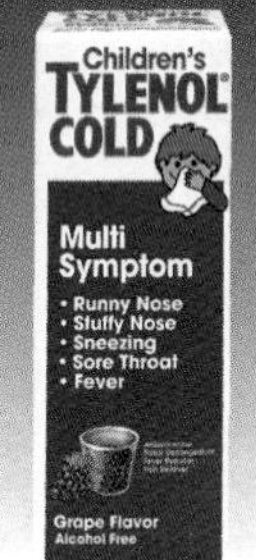

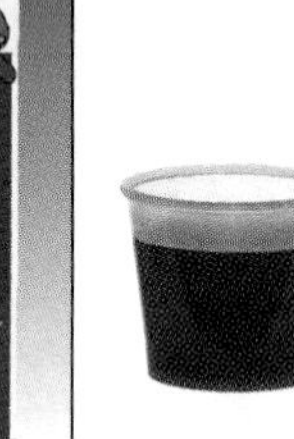

Tylenol Cold Children's Liquid p. 130

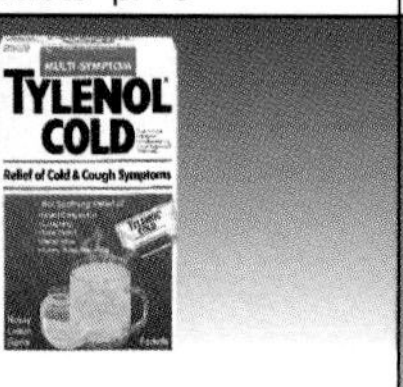

Tylenol Cold Multi Symptom Powder p. 117

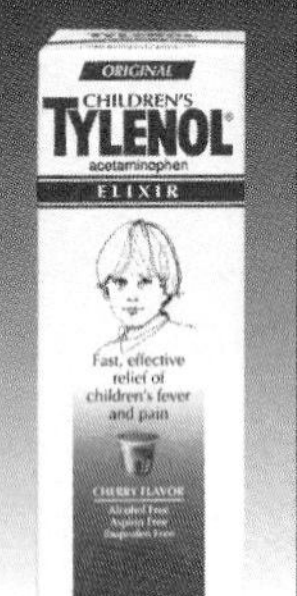

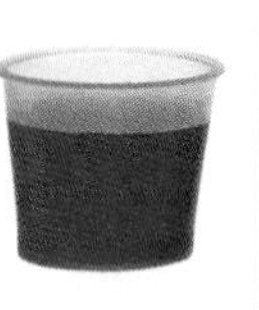

Tylenol Children's Elixir p. 76

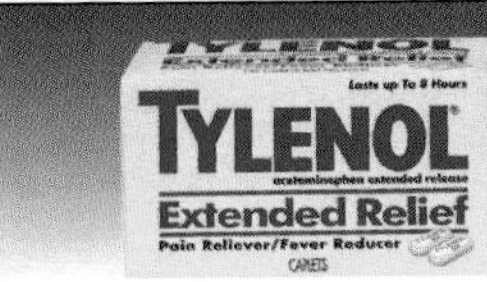

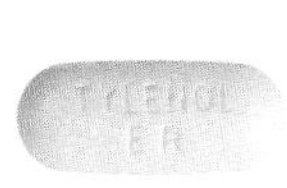

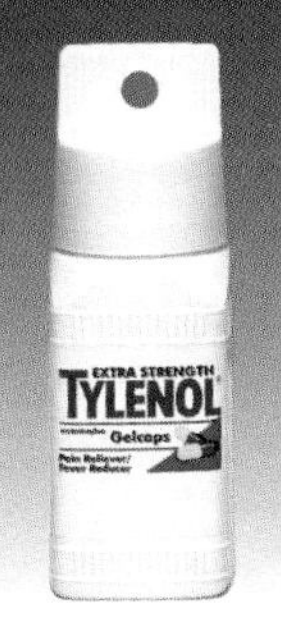

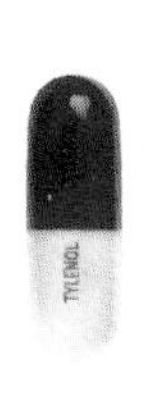

Tylenol Extended Relief Caplets
p. 76

Tylenol Extra Strength Gelcaps
p. 76

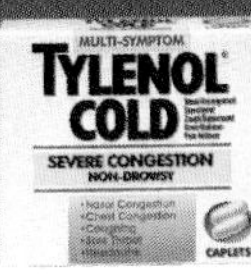

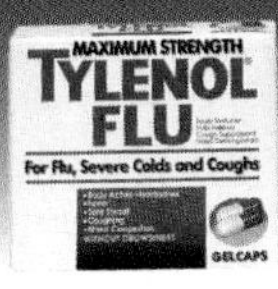

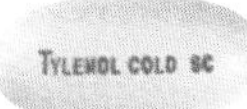

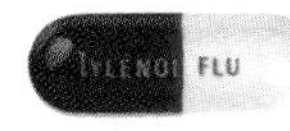

Tylenol Cold Non Drowsy Caplets
p. 201

Tylenol Flu Gelcaps
p. 142

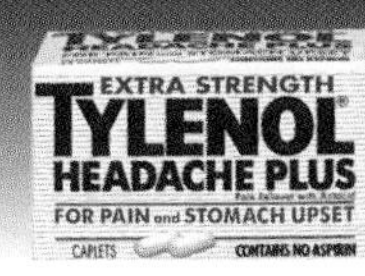

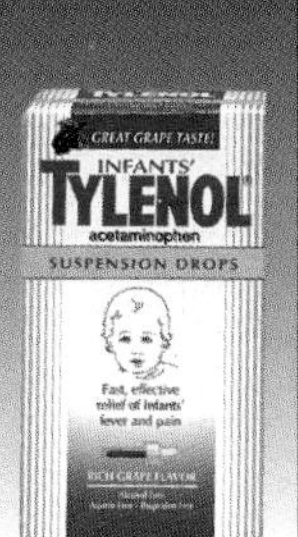

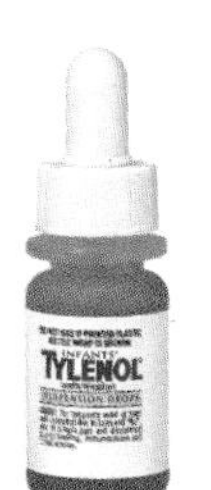

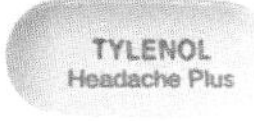

Tylenol Headache Plus Caplets p. 303

Tylenol Infant's Drops
p. 646

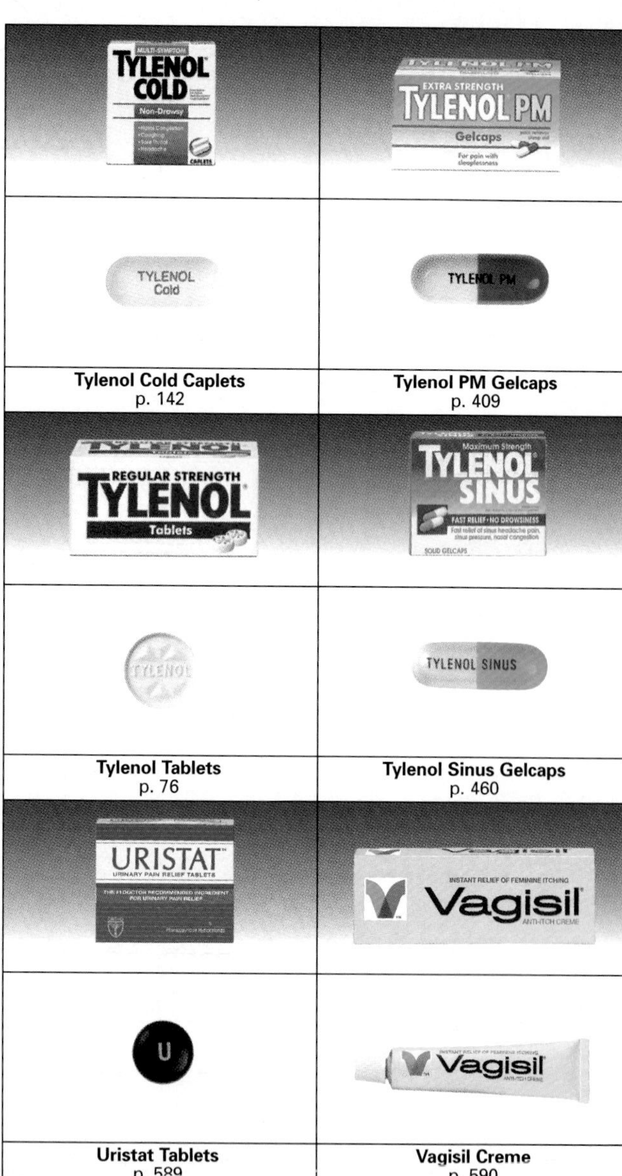

Tylenol Cold Caplets p. 142	Tylenol PM Gelcaps p. 409
Tylenol Tablets p. 76	Tylenol Sinus Gelcaps p. 460
Uristat Tablets p. 589	Vagisil Creme p. 590

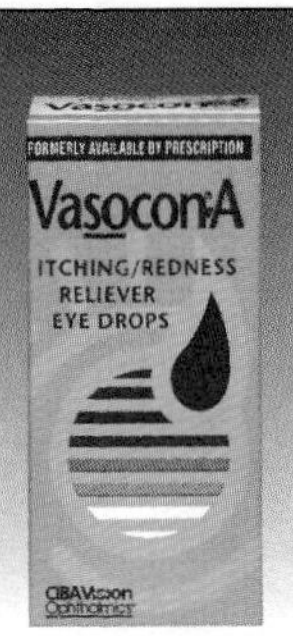

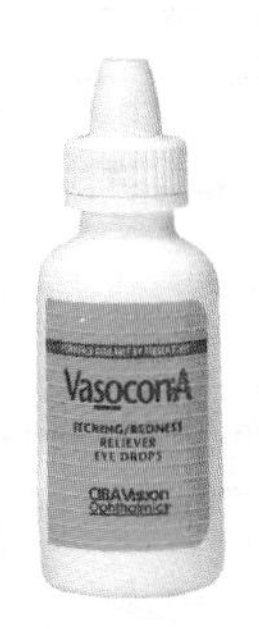

Vasocon A Eye Drops
p. 519

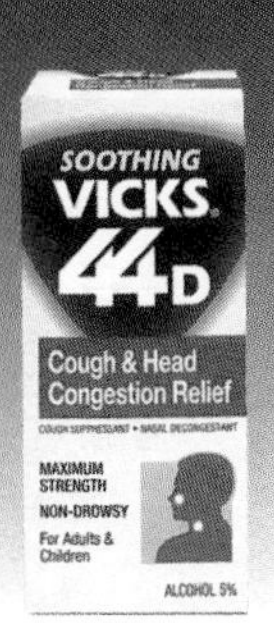

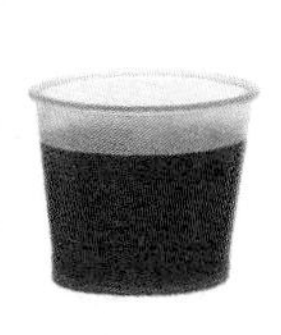

Vicks 44D Liquid
p. 216

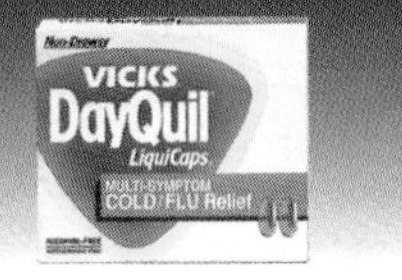

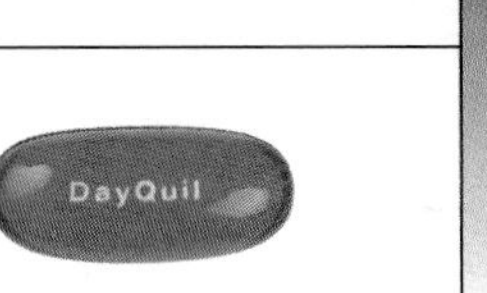

Vicks Dayquil LiquiCaps
p. 201

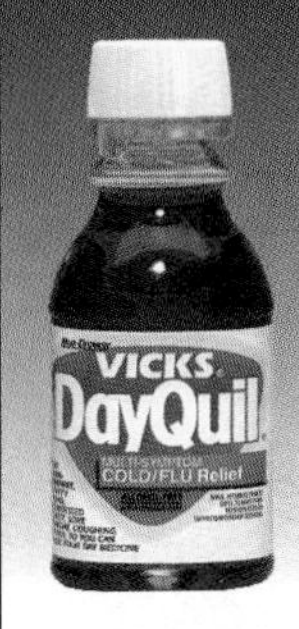

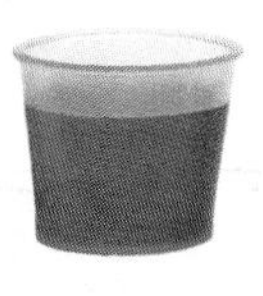

Vicks Dayquil Liquid
p. 201

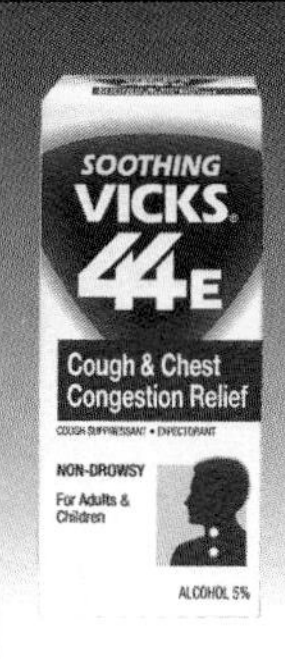

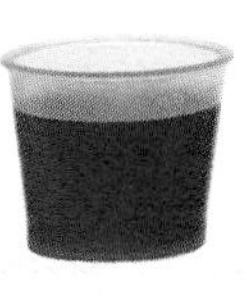

Vicks 44E Liquid
p. 193

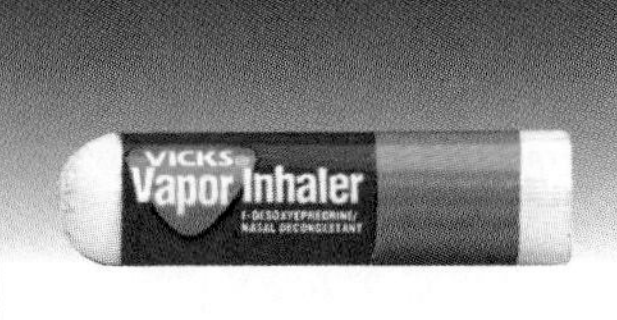

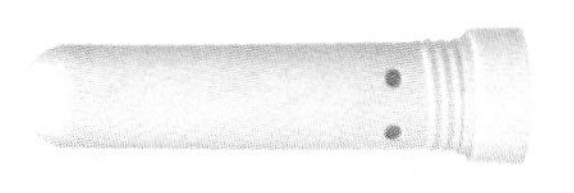

Vicks Inhaler
p. 220

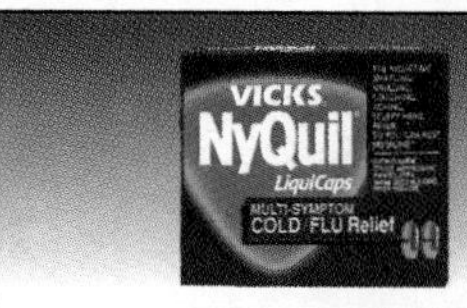

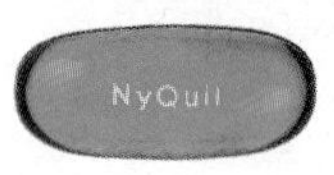

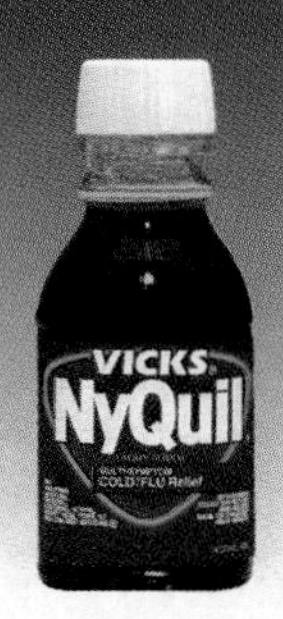

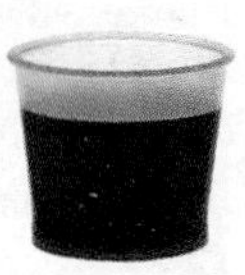

Vicks NyQuil LiquiCaps
p. 155

Vicks Nyquil Liquid
p. 155

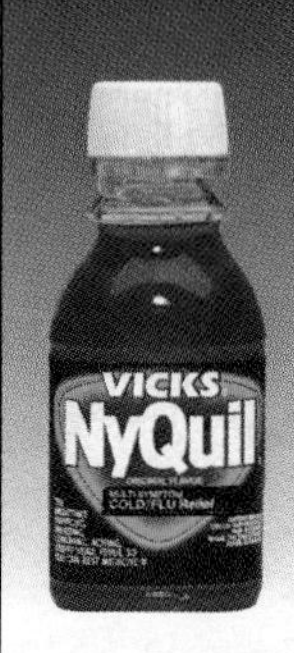

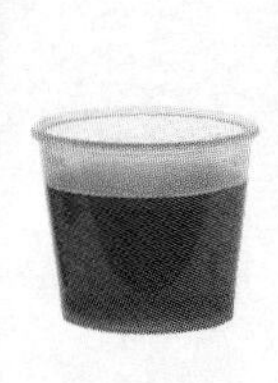
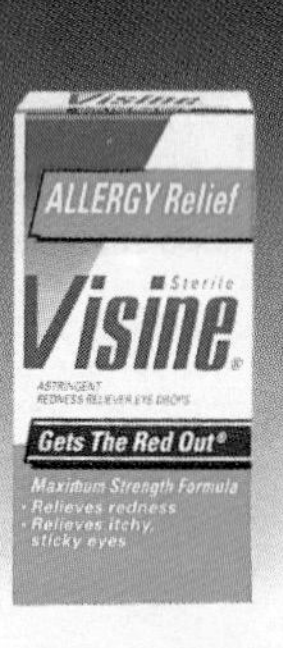

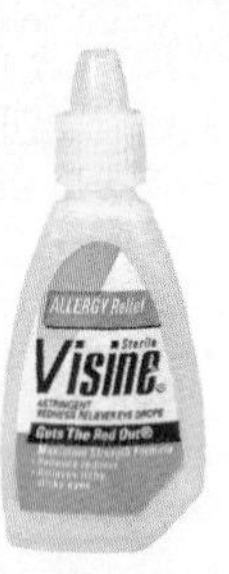

Vicks Nyquil Multi-Symptom Liquid p. 155

Visine Eye Drops
p. 522

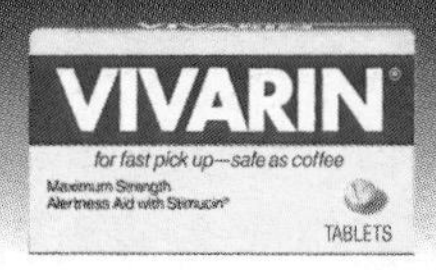

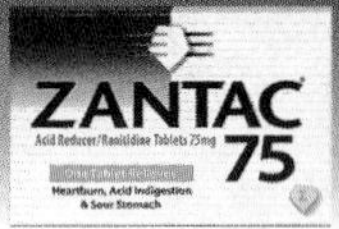

Vivarin Tablets
p. 414

Zantac 75 Tablets
p. 308

Infants/Children

Do not give Preparation H to a child under age 12 unless directed by your doctor.

Seniors

Seniors should exercise the same caution as younger adults when using Preparation H.

Brand Name

Preparation H Suppositories

Generic Ingredients

Cocoa butter
Shark liver oil

Type of Drug

Skin protectant and emollient (softener).

Used for

Temporary relief of pain and burning sensation of hemorrhoids.

General Information

Hemorrhoids develop due to many factors, such as heredity, posture, prolonged standing or sitting, inadequate dietary bulk intake, constipation, heavy lifting, and pregnancy. They are formed either by inflamed connective tissue under the skin surface, or by blood clots in veins.

Liver oils have been used in folk medicine for many years for their healing properties. Shark liver oil, which contains a high concentration of vitamins A and D, has been approved by the FDA as a natural skin protectant and softener.

Cocoa butter is another skin protectant and softener used in Preparation H Suppositories. Cocoa butter provides an oleaginous (oily) base for the shark liver oil. It melts rapidly, allowing the shark liver oil to be released quickly. Preparation H guards against irritation of the skin and prevent dehydration of the tissues by forming a physical barrier on the skin's surface. This provides temporary relief from the itching, burning, and discomfort of hemorrhoids and promotes healing of the skin.

Cautions and Warnings

Do not use Preparation H Suppositories for more than 7 consecutive days.

If your condition worsens or does not improve within 7 days, stop using Preparation H and consult your doctor.

Do not exceed recommended daily dosage of Preparation H.

In case of bleeding from the rectal area, discontinue using Preparation H and contact your doctor immediately. The presence of blood can be an indication of a more serious condition.

Possible Side Effects

Adverse reactions are rare; however, discontinue using Preparation H Suppositories if you suspect an allergic reaction.

Drug Interactions

None Known.

Usual Dose

Preparation H Suppositories contain cocoa butter 79% and shark liver oil 3%.

Adult and Child (age 12 and over): Cleanse the affected area with medicated pads or mild soap and warm water. Rinse thoroughly. Gently dry the affected area by patting or blotting with toilet tissue or soft cloth before using Preparation H Suppositories.

Detach 1 suppository from the strip of suppositories and remove the wrapper. If the suppository seems soft, before removing the foil hold it under cold water for 2 or 3 minutes. Carefully separate the foil covering and peel it down evenly on both sides, exposing the suppository. Avoid excessive handling of the suppository, which is designed to melt at body temperature.

Insert 1 suppository rectally up to 6 times daily or after each bowel movement.

Child (under age 12): Consult your doctor.

Overdosage

Do the following in case of accidental ingestion: If the victim is unconscious or having convulsions, call for an ambulance immediately. If you take the victim to an emergency room, be sure to bring the bottle or container with you. If the victim is conscious, call your local poison control center or a health care professional. The poison control center may suggest inducing vomiting with ipecac syrup (available without a prescription at any pharmacy). DO NOT induce vomiting unless specifically instructed to do so.

Storage Instructions

Store Preparation H Suppositories in a cool place. They may melt at temperatures above 86° F.

Special Populations

Pregnancy/Breast-feeding

Is is not generally recommended that pregnant women take any drugs, particularly during the first 3 months after conception. Check with your doctor before using Preparation H Suppositories if you are or might be pregnant, or if you are breast-feeding.

Infants/Children

Do not give Preparation H to a child under age 12, unless directed by your doctor.

Seniors

Seniors should exercise the same caution as younger adults when using Preparation H.

Chapter 10: Sex

In the last 15 years, the publicity concerning AIDS has increased public awareness of the importance of preventing the spread of sexually transmitted diseases (STDs). Contraceptive methods once used primarily for preventing unwanted pregnancies are now used as the first lines of defense against these illnesses. This chapter describes the contraceptive options available to both men and women. Other conditions covered here are vaginal yeast infections, vaginal dryness, menstrual pain, and urinary tract infections (UTIs).

Contraception

Condoms

A condom, also called a rubber, is a sheath or sleeve usually made out of latex (synthetic rubber). It fits over the man's erect penis and should be applied prior to the start of sexual intercourse. Condoms are sold without a prescription in drugstores, supermarkets, and convenience stores.

Like diaphragms, condoms are classified as a barrier form of contraception (birth control) because they prevent sperm from entering the woman's vagina during ejaculation. The other main approaches to contraception are medical and surgical. Medical contraception—the birth control pill or hormonal implants—is available only with a prescription. Barrier and medical methods are considered reversible, because pregnancy can occur if their use is stopped. Surgical strategies for contraception—vasectomy (cutting the tubes that carry sperm from the man's testicles) and tubal ligation (cutting or tying the tubes that carry eggs from the ovary into the woman's uterus)—are generally irreversible.

In addition to reducing unwanted pregnancies, condoms are an effective method for preventing STDs. These infections can involve various microorganisms, including bacteria, viruses, and fungi. The infectious agent may be carried on the skin or other surfaces, or may be present in the blood or semen. The infection enters the other person's body through an orifice (vagina, mouth, anus, or the urethral opening) or through small wounds or tears in the skin or mucous membranes. Either infected partner can pass an STD on to the other.

Proper Condom Use

1. Open the package carefully to avoid tearing the condom.
2. Apply the condom before the penis comes into contact with the vagina, mouth, or anus.
3. Do not unroll the condom (or test it for leaks) before applying.
4. If you add a spermicide, place a small amount inside the reservoir at the tip.
5. If the man is uncircumcised, pull back the foreskin.
6. Place the unrolled condom on the tip of the erect penis.
7. Squeeze air out of the reservoir (or leave a half-inch space at the top of a condom without a reservoir).
8. Unroll the condom completely. Smooth out any air bubbles.
9. Apply a water-based lubricant if desired. Do not use an oil-based lubricant, such as petroleum jelly, mineral oil, or hand cream, which can weaken or damage the latex.
10. Apply spermicide to the outside of the condom. The spermicide may also be inserted into the vagina.
11. If the condom breaks or slips during intercourse, withdraw the penis and the condom immediately.
12. After ejaculation, and before the erection is lost, grip the condom rim around the base of the penis to prevent leakage of the semen. Withdraw the penis.
13. Remove the condom and check it for tears or leaks.
14. If a tear occurs during vaginal intercourse, a spermicidal foam, cream, or jelly should be used.
15. Wash the genital area thoroughly before engaging in any further sexual activity. Use a fresh condom each time intercourse takes place.

Properly used (see box), condoms can help prevent pregnancy or disease. But they are not 100% effective. Although most condoms are tested for safety by their manufacturers, some can develop leaks or tears, especially if they are old, have been stored in warm places (such as wallets or glove compartments), or have been exposed to air. They can also tear or slip off during intercourse. Studies show that, on average, pregnancy can result from improper use of condoms or from faulty condoms as much as 12% of the time during the first year of use. Even when condoms are used correctly, pregnancy can occur 2% of the time.

Condoms come in different varieties. Some contain a lubricant to make insertion easier. A water-based lubricant can be applied separately to unlubricated condoms. Using a lubricant reduces the risk that the condom will break during use and can prevent irritation. Most condoms contain a reservoir at the tip for trapping and holding semen. Others may be designed with added textures (ribbing) or shapes to enhance pleasure.

To increase their effectiveness as contraceptives, some condoms contain a spermicide, a chemical that kills sperm cells. Spermicides can also be applied separately to nonmedicated condoms. Many experts advise using additional spermicide even if the condom already contains one. A spermicide called nonoxynol-9 also appears to kill germs, which can increase the disease-preventing ability of the condom. Spermicides are available as jellies, creams, or foams. Do not use spermicide if you plan to engage in oral sex. Another strategy for improving the effectiveness of condoms is for both partners to use some form of protection. For example, a woman can use a vaginal contraceptive, such as a foam or cream.

Some people have allergic reactions to latex. Condoms made from plastic or animal tissue are available. However, these products are less effective against STDs, especially those carried by viruses such as the human immunodeficiency virus (HIV), which causes AIDS.

OTC Products for Men

Condoms
Spermicides

Seek medical attention if

- You desire to have a vasectomy or other permanent form of birth control

The safest approach to contraception and prevention of STDs is for both partners to share responsibility. The only OTC form of protection for men is the condom. Women have more choices available (see box).

Vaginal Contraceptives

Vaginal contraceptives available over the counter kill sperm after it has entered the vaginal tract. The main chemical in these products is nonoxynol-9, the same spermicide used in male condoms.

Spermicides are available in a number of formulations, including creams and jellies (applied through an applicator tube), foams (applied through a nozzle), and suppositories (inserted with finger pressure). Creams may offer more lubrication and may spread more easily, but jellies are usually less messy. Vaginal foams usually are distributed well throughout the vagina after application, and so may be more effective, but some women find that they cause dryness and reduced lubrication. Suppositories supply spermicide in a solid form. The product takes about 15 minutes to dissolve and spread. Generally, these are not as effective or as easy to use as the other formulations. A contraceptive film is also available. The material comes in 2-inch squares that are inserted with the finger. Within 5 minutes, the film dissolves in the heat and moisture of the vagina, releasing the spermicide.

Spermicide concentrations range from 2% to 12.5% in creams, jellies, and foams and 28% in film. Women who do not use an additional method of contraception, such as a diaphragm or an intrauterine device (IUD), should select a product with a higher concentration of the active ingredient. Creams and jellies may be used with a diaphragm or cervical cap; they should be placed in the center of the device and spread around the entire rim prior to insertion. The product should be applied at least 10 minutes but no more than an hour prior to intercourse. The spermicide is effective for at least 6 hours, but the dose should be repeated each time intercourse takes place. Women should not douche until at least 8 hours after sex.

Another approach is the female condom, a lubricated pouchlike lining made of polyurethane that is inserted into the vagina. The innermost end contains a ring that fits over the cervix. An outer ring extends outside the vagina and covers the external genitals. Like its male counterpart, the female condom should be used only once and then discarded. Additional lubricant can be applied if desired. This approach is not foolproof; pregnancy can still occur, and there may be some risk of disease transmission. Some couples find the device awkward or unpleasant to use—much the same as with latex condoms.

Vaginal spermicides are easily available, inexpensive, and generally effective. As is true of male condoms, however, they do not by themselves provide perfect protection. The success rate improves if these products are used in combination with a barrier method, such as condoms or diaphragms. Even if they do not use this approach regularly, women should have a vaginal spermicide available for use in case the condom breaks or slips or in case they forget to take their birth control pill. Women accustomed to using tampons will be able to use contraceptive suppositories or the female condom easily. Those who prefer not to touch their genitals may wish to select other formulations.

OTC Products for Women

- Vaginal contraceptives
  - Creams
  - Jellies
  - Foams
  - Suppository capsules
  - Films
- Vaginal pouches (female condoms)

Vaginal Infections

The vagina is the natural home to a number of microorganisms that do not pose a threat to health in normal numbers. They actually play a protective role by maintaining the proper acidity and preventing harmful pathogens from gaining a foothold. If something happens to disrupt the balance of fluids or acidity within the vagina, or the normal bacteria are killed when an antibiotic is taken, overgrowth of either bacteria or fungi can occur and cause infections.

There are 3 main types of vaginal infections. Bacterial vaginosis is the most common, accounting for between 30% and 50% of cases. It is usually not a serious condition. In fact, often a bacterial infection may go unnoticed and may clear up on its own. If symptoms exist, they include a vaginal discharge with a characteristic fishy odor, especially following intercourse. The problem is more common in women who use an IUD, are breast-feeding, or who have multiple sexual partners. Frequent bacterial infections may increase the risk of pelvic inflammatory disease or urinary tract infections.

About 1 in 5 vaginal infections involves trichomoniasis, which is caused by a tiny parasite and usually occurs in women under age 30. In over half of the cases, symptoms include a copious foamy and smelly discharge that is yellow, gray, or green in color. Some women experience vaginal itching or lower abdominal pain. However, many women do not notice any symptoms at all.

The third main form of vaginal infection—and the only one that can be treated with OTC products—is candida vulvovaginitis, more commonly known as a vaginal yeast infection. About 33% of vaginal infections are yeast infections. Perhaps 3 of 4 women of childbearing years and 4 out of 10 women after menopause will experience this problem at least once. The main culprit, responsible for nearly 90% of cases of yeast infections, is a fungus called *Candida albicans.* The fungus is normally found in the vagina and other places in the body, including the mouth and the intestinal tract. However, if the population increases, symptoms can develop. A number of factors can contribute to the illness (see box).

Factors that Increase Risk of Vaginal Yeast Infection

- Use of antibiotics
- Use of other medications such as systemic corticosteroids or cancer drugs
- Excess sugar levels, such as those that occur in people with diabetes, severe infections, or other diseases
- Hormonal fluctuations due to pregnancy, menstruation, or use of oral contraceptives
- Stress and fatigue
- Wearing constricting clothing made of dense fibers (such as pantyhose, swimsuits, or sportswear)
- Use of feminine pads
- Increased heat and humidity
- Any disease that causes the suppression of the body's immune function (including AIDS)

The most common symptoms of yeast infections are itching, burning, and redness in the vagina and the vulva (outer genital tissues). Some women also have a thick, white, odorless discharge that resembles cottage cheese. When the infection is present, intercourse can cause pain or a burning sensation. In some cases, painful urination can occur.

Because the symptoms of different vaginal infections can be similar, it can be difficult to determine which type of infection you have. Knowing the cause is important, however, since use of a product designed to kill yeast will have no effect on an infection produced by bacteria. If you have not had a yeast infection before, or if a current infection seems different than past infections, see a doctor before treating the condition yourself (see box).

OTC Treatment for Vaginal Yeast Infection Might be an Option if

- You have no more than 3 vaginal infections a year.
- You have had no infection within the last 2 months.
- Your yeast infection was previously diagnosed by a physician.
- Current symptoms are the same as for those previous infections.
- You do not have painful urination.

Seek medical attention if any of the following applies to you

- No previous yeast infections
- Frequent vaginal yeast infections (every 2 to 3 months)
- An infection that has not cleared up after treatment
- Fever
- Pregnancy (confirmed or suspected) or breast-feeding
- Under age 12
- Pain in the lower abdomen, back, or shoulder
- Taking systemic corticosteroids or other drugs
- Diabetes or HIV infection

Treatment for Vaginal Yeast Infection

In the past few years, a number of antifungal products have been approved for OTC use. Each contains a drug known to be effective in killing or controlling the spread of fungal growth. Examples of these drugs include clotrimazole, butoconazole, miconazole, and tioconazole. Most of these products are creams, but tablets and suppositories are also available. Creams are the treatment of choice if symptoms occur on the vulva, as cream may be applied directly to the vulva in addition to insertion into the vagina. Typically, results begin to be noticed within 24 hours, but to cure the condition and to minimize the risk of recurrence, some products must be used for a full week.

Use of an antifungal cream can damage condoms or diaphragms, causing them to leak and increasing the risk of pregnancy.

There is not a lot of risk involved in using a vaginal antifungal agent. Some people may notice burning, itching, or irritation at first, but these problems tend to disappear with use. If abdominal cramping, headache, or rash develops, or if symptoms do not improve or get worse in 3 days, discontinue use and contact a physician.

In about 1 case in 20, the yeast infection does not respond to the medication and must be treated by a stronger prescription product. If you experience frequent infections, or if the problem returns within 2 months, see a doctor. Delaying treatment with more effective prescription products can increase the risk of other, more serious problems.

There are other OTC products that are promoted as treatments for vaginal itching, such as Vagisil and Yeast-Gard. These agents contain a local anesthetic and an antiseptic, but they do not kill the *Candida* fungus.

OTC Products for Vaginal Yeast Infection
Antifungal agents

Vaginal Dryness

The mucous membranes inside the vagina secrete fluid that bathes the tissue and keeps it moist. These secretions increase at times, such as during moments of sexual arousal or heightened stress. However, a number of factors can reduce the amount of vaginal secretions or alter their composition, resulting in vaginal dryness. Symptoms include irritation, burning, itching, increased susceptibility to infection, and painful intercourse.

Vaginal dryness is a common complaint among women after menopause. During this time, the body produces significantly lower amounts of estrogen, a hormone that the membranes need to maintain their thickness and to produce sufficient fluid. Breast-feeding can also contribute to dryness. A condition known as Sjögren's syndrome causes dryness in various tissues, including the vagina and the mouth.

Seek medical attention if any of the following applies to you

- Severe vaginal dryness
- Pain during intercourse

Treatment for Vaginal Dryness

There are several OTC products available that are formulated to lubricate vaginal tissues or to replace moisture (see box). Water-soluble lubricants generally contain glycerin, water, and other ingredients. Some also contain mineral oil or silicone oil to provide additional lubrication. These products can be used on internal as well as external tissues. Up to 2 tablespoons should be applied at first; the dose can be adjusted depending on results. If the lubricant is intended for use in relieving painful intercourse, the product should be applied to both the vagina and the penis for maximum effect.

Petroleum jelly products such as Vaseline are not recommended as moisturizing agents, nor are common home remedies such as butter or baby oil. Such treatments can actually make the problem worse. Only water-soluble lubricants without mineral or silicone oil should be used in conjunction with condoms or diaphragms, since oil-based products can damage the latex and cause leaks.

In certain cases, hormone replacement therapy with prescription oral or topical estrogen products may offer a more effective or more acceptable solution. Hormone therapy may offer other benefits, such as protection against cardiovascular disease, Alzheimer's disease, and osteoporosis. Ask your physician if this treatment is appropriate for you.

OTC Products for Vaginal Dryness

Topical lubricants
Moisturizing skin lotions

Menstrual Pain

For many women, the days prior to the onset of their menstrual periods are times of pain, cramping, mood changes, weight gain, fatigue, and feelings of bloatedness. These symptoms are collectively known as premenstrual syndrome, (PMS). Although the vast majority of women remain productive and functional during their periods, about 1 in 10 women experiences symptoms serious enough to interfere with work, social life, or family activities.

Treatment for Menstrual Pain

OTC products are available to reduce some of the symptoms of PMS. Basically, these products—available as tablets or capsules—contain a pain reliever (acetaminophen) plus a diuretic, which helps eliminate excess water from the body and thus eases bloating and weight gain.

The 3 nonprescription diuretics approved by the FDA are ammonium chloride, caffeine, and pamabrom. Ammonium chloride should not be taken for longer than 6 consecutive days. In large doses, this chemical can cause digestive problems or nervous system side effects such as dizziness or confusion. Caffeine is safe and effective in doses up to 200 mg every 3 to 4 hours. Side effects include anxiety, restlessness, insomnia, and stomach upset. Women taking a product for PMS that contains caffeine should avoid taking additional caffeine in coffee, tea, cola, or foods. Pamabrom, chemically related to caffeine, is used in doses of up to 200 mg per day (50 mg taken 4 times a day).

In more serious cases, a physician should be consulted. Prescription medications may be needed to address other symptoms of PMS or painful menstrual periods, such as severe anxiety and depression.

OTC Products for Menstrual Pain

Analgesic (acetaminophen) + diuretic
(ammonium chloride, pamabrom, or caffeine)

Urinary Tract Infections

UTIs, sometimes called cystitis or bladder infections, are primarily caused by the introduction of bacteria into the bladder during sexual intercourse. Once there, the bacteria can start to multiply. UTIs are especially common in sexually active women ages 20 to 50. Women who are not sexually active and girls can contract a UTI if bacteria spreads from the anus to the vagina, due to poor hygiene. Males under 50 rarely suffer from UTIs.

Symptoms of UTI

- Frequent and urgent need to urinate
- Burning pain during urination
- Pain in lower abdomen or back
- Blood in urine
- Foul-smelling urine

Treatment for UTIs

Minor cases can clear up without treatment, as the bacteria can be flushed out by urination. However, recurrent and serious infections will need to be treated with prescription antibiotics.

To relieve the pain caused by a UTI, there are several OTC treatments available. Systemic analgesics (whole-body pain-relievers), such as acetaminophen or the nonsteroidal anti-inflammatory drugs (NSAIDs), will ease the pain and discomfort. Phenazopyridine hydrochloride is another OTC analgesic that is specifically targeted at relieving the pain, burning, and urgent and frequent need to urinate caused by a UTI.

Seek medical attention if any of the following applies to you

- Symptoms last for more than 2 days
- Fever
- Chills
- Back pain
- Blood in urine
- Kidney trouble
- Pregnancy
- Breast-feeding
- Child under 12

Strategies for avoiding UTIs

- Drink 6-8 glasses of water every day
- Reduce intake of caffeine and alcohol
- Wipe from front to back after urination
- Urinate every time you feel the need
- Urinate before and after sexual intercourse
- Wear cotton underwear and avoid tight clothing
- Change sanitary pads and tampons frequently during menstruation
- Take showers instead of baths

Condoms

BRAND NAME	Material	Spermicide
Avanti	polyurethane	
Avanti Super Thin	polyurethane	
Class Act Sensitive	latex	
Class Act Sensitive with Spermicide	latex	x
Fourex	animal membrane	
Fourex with Spermicide	animal membrane	nonoxynol-9, 7%
Gold Circle Coin	latex	
Gold Circle Rainbow Coin	latex	
Mentor	latex	
Mentor Plus with Spermicide	latex	x
Naturalamb	lamb cecum	
Naturalamb with Spermicide	lamb cecum	x
Ramses Extra Strength with Spermicide	latex	nonoxynol-9, 8%
Ramses Extra with Spermicide	latex	nonoxynol-9, 5%
Ramses Sensitol	latex	
Ramses Ultra Thin	latex	
Ramses Ultra Thin with Spermicide	latex	nonoxynol-9, 5%
Reality Female Condom	polyurethane	
Saxon Gold Rainbow	latex	
Saxon Gold Ultra Lube, Ribbed, Sensitive	latex	
Saxon Gold Ultra with Spermicide	latex	nonoxynol-9, 6.6%
Sheik Classic	latex	
Sheik Classic with Spermicide	latex	nonoxynol-9, 8%
Sheik Excita Extra with Spermicide	latex	nonoxynol-9, 8%
Sheik Fiesta	latex	

Sheik Super Thin	latex	
Sheik Super Thin with Spermicide	latex	nonoxynol-9, 8%
Sure	latex	
Sure with Spermicide	latex	nonoxynol-9
Touch	latex	
Touch Lubricated	latex	
Touch with Spermicide	latex	nonoxynol-9, 8%
Trojan-Enz	latex	
Trojan-Enz Large	latex	
Trojan-Enz Large with Spermicide	latex	x
Trojan-Enz with Spermicide	latex	x
Trojan Extra Strength	latex	
Trojan Extra Strength with Spermicide	latex	x
Trojan Magnum	latex	
Trojan Magnum with Spermicide	latex	x
Trojan Naturalube	latex	
Trojan Plus	latex	
Trojan Plus 2 with Spermicide	latex	x
Trojan Ribbed	latex	
Trojan Ribbed with Spermicide	latex	x
Trojan Ultra Texture	latex	
Trojan Ultra Texture with Spermicide	latex	x
Trojan Very Sensitive	latex	
Trojan Very Sensitive with Spermicide	latex	x
Trojan Very Thin	latex	
Trojan Very Thin with Spermicide	latex	x
Trojans	latex	

Spermicides

BRAND NAME	SPERMICIDE
Advantage 24	nonoxynol-9, 3.5%
Contraceptrol	nonoxynol-9, 4%
Contraceptrol Inserts	nonoxynol-9, 8.34%
Contraceptrol Prefilled Disposable	nonoxynol-9, 4%
Delfen	nonoxynol-9, 12.5%
Emko	nonoxynol-9, 12%
Encare	nonoxynol-9, 100mg
Gynol II	nonoxynol-9, 2%
Gynol II ES	nonoxynol-9, 3%
Koromex (foam)	nonoxynol-9,12.5%
Koromex (jelly)	nonoxynol-9, 3%
Koromex Crystal Clear	nonoxynol-9, 3%
Koromex Inserts	nonoxynol-9, 125 mg (5%)
K-Y Plus	nonoxynol-9, 2.2%
Ortho-Creme	nonoxynol-9, 2%
Ortho-Gynol	octoxynol-9, 1%
Ramses Personal Spermicidal Lubricant	nonoxynol-9, 3%
Semicid Inserts	nonoxynol-9, 100mg
Shur-Seal	nonoxynol-9, 2%
VCF	nonoxynol-9, 3%
VCF Vaginal Contraceptive Film	nonoxynol-9, 28%

Vaginal Antifungal Products

BRAND NAME	ANTIFUNGAL			ANTISEPTIC	
	butoconazole nitrate	clotrimazole	miconazole nitrate	benzoic acid	povidone
Femizole-7		1%			
Femstat 3	2%				
Gyne-Lotremin		1%			
Gyne-Lotremin Inserts		100mg			x
Monistat 7 (cream)			2%	x	
Monistat 7 (suppository)			100mg		
Monistat 7 Prefilled Applicators			2%	x	
Mycelex-7		1%			
Mycelex-7 Inserts		100mg			x
Yeast-X			2%		

Vaginal Lubricant Products

BRAND NAME	LUBRICANT			PRESERVATIVES
	mineral oil + hydrogenated palm oil glyceride	mineral oil + stearic acid	silicone oil + sodium lauryl sulfate	
Astroglide				glycerin
				propylene glycol
				polyquaternium #5
				methylparaben
				polyparaben

BRAND NAME	LUBRICANT			PRESERVATIVES
	mineral oil + hydrogenated palm oil glyceride	mineral oil + stearic acid	silicone oil + sodium lauryl sulfate	
Feminease		x		glycerin
				propylene glycol
				benzoic acid
				BHT
Gyne-Moistrin Moisturizing				propylene glycol
				methylparaben
				polyparaben
H-R Lubricating				propylene glycol
				polyparaben
				methylparaben
K-Y Jelly				chlorhexidine gluconate
				glycerin
				methylparaben
Lubrin Inserts				glycerin
Maxilube			x	glycerin
				methylparaben
				polyparaben
Moist Again Vaginal Moisturizing				glycerin
				chlorhexidine gluconate
				sodium benzoate
				potassium sorbate
				diazolidinyl urea
				sorbic acid

Replens	x	sorbic acid
		glycerin
Surgel		propylene glycol
		glycerin
Touch Personal Lubricant		propylene glycol
		benzoic acid
Women's Health Institute Lubricating		chlorhexidine gluconate
		methylparaben
		glycerin

Menstrual Pain Products

BRAND NAME	ANALGESIC	DIURETIC	OTHER				
	acetamino-phen	magnesium salicylate	potassium salicylate	salicylamide	caffeine	pamabrom	
Aqua -Ban [C]						50mg	
Backaid Pills [C] [S]	500mg					25mg	
Bayer Select Aspirin-Free Menstrual [C]	500mg					25mg	
Diurex Long Acting	x		x		195mg		
Diurex MPR [C]	500mg					25mg	
Diurex PMS [C]	500mg					25mg	pyrilamine maleate 15mg
Diurex Water Caplet [C] [S]	325mg					50mg	
Diurex Water Pills [C]			x	x	x		
Diurex-2 Water Pills [C]	162.5mg					25mg	

BRAND NAME	ANALGESIC	DIURETIC	OTHER				
	acetamino-phen	magnesium salicylate	potassium salicylate	salicylamide	caffeine	pamabrom	
Fem-1	500mg					25mg	
Lurline PMS [C] [S]	500mg					25mg	pyridoxine HCl 50mg
Midol Menstrual Maximum Strength Multisymptom Formula	500mg				60mg		pyrilamine maleate 15mg
Midol PMS Maximum Strength Multisymptom Formula [C]	500mg					25mg	pyrilamine maleate 15mg
Midol PMS Multisymptom Formula [C]	500mg					25mg	pyrilamine maleate 15mg
Midol Teen Multisymptom Formula [C]	400mg					25mg	
Odrinil Water Pills [C]						25mg	
Pamprin Maximum Pain Relief [C]	250mg	250mg				25mg	
Pamprin MultiSymptom Formula [C]	500mg					25mg	pyrilamine maleate 15mg
Premsyn PMS [C]	500mg					25mg	pyrilamine maleate 15mg

Brand Name

Femstat 3 (FEM-stat)

Generic Ingredient

Butoconazole nitrate (bew-toe-CON-ah-zole NYE-trate)

Type of Drug

Vaginal antifungal agent.

Used for

Treatment of vaginal yeast infection.

General Information

A fungus is an organism that obtains nutrients from other living organisms or from dead organic matter in order to survive. In doing so, fungi cause infections that only an antifungal agent can cure.

Butoconazole is classified as an imidazole; 3 other topical antifungals in the group, clotrimazole, miconazole, and tioconazole, are also available without a prescription. These drugs inhibit the growth of and kill fungi, as well as relieve the symptoms associated with the infection.

Studies have shown that butoconazole, clotrimazole, miconazole, and tioconazole are equally effective in inhibiting the growth of and killing the fungus known as *Candida,* which causes yeast infections. They have an effectiveness rate of about 85% to 90%. All 4 are well tolerated.

Butoconazole is available by brand name in intravaginal cream form.

Cautions and Warnings

Do not take the maximum daily dosage of Femstat 3 for more than 3 days continuously except under a doctor's supervision.

Do not exceed the recommended daily dosage of Femstat 3.

Self-medicate with Femstat 3 *only* if a doctor has previously diagnosed a vaginal yeast infection and you recognize the same symptoms now. If this is the *first* time you have had vaginal itch and discomfort, DO NOT SELF-MEDICATE WITH FEMSTAT 3. Call your doctor and have him or her determine whether you have a yeast infection and not another type of vaginal infection, such as one caused by bacteria, which can't be effectively treated with butoconazole.

Do not use Femstat 3 if you have abdominal or back pain, fever, or foul-smelling discharge. Call your doctor immediately.

If you are taking certain medications (e.g., corticosteroids—drugs that suppress the immune system) or if you have a medical condition such as diabetes or HIV infection, do not use Femstat 3 without first consulting your doctor.

Self-treatment with Femstat 3 is not appropriate for girls under age 12 or women who are pregnant. These individuals should consult a doctor if they experience symptoms of a yeast infection.

Women experiencing recurrent infections (more than 4 in 1 year) should see a physician and avoid using OTC butoconazole unless medically advised to use it.

Stop using Femstat 3 and call your doctor if you develop abdominal cramping, headache, hives, or skin rash.

If you do not get well after 3 days of treatment with Femstat 3, you may have a condition other than a yeast infection or you may require more prolonged therapy with the drug. Call your doctor.

If your symptoms return within 2 months, or if you have infections that do not clear up easily with treatment, call your physician. You could be pregnant, or there could be a serious, underlying medical reason for your infections, such as diabetes or an impaired immune system (such as that associated with HIV infection).

You must use Femstat 3 for 3 consecutive days for it to cure your fungal infection. Do not stop therapy before then, even if your symptoms disappear right away, as often happens.

You may use Femstat 3 during your period, but do not use tampons. If your period begins after you have started your 3-day treatment, do not stop treatment.

It is recommended that you avoid sexual intercourse during your 3-day treatment. Butoconazole can damage condoms, diaphragms, and cervical caps, thus increasing your risk of pregnancy.

Femstat 3 is for external use only. Avoid contact with your eyes. After using the product, wash your hands with soap and water.

Possible Side Effects

▼ Rare: abdominal cramps, headache, burning, itching, irritation, and allergic reactions.

Drug Interactions

None known.

Usual Dose

Femstat 3 contains butoconazole nitrate 2%.

Adult and Child (age 12 and over): 1 full applicator into the vagina at bedtime.

Child (under age 12): not recommended.

Read the package carefully before using Femstat 3.

Wash your entire vaginal area with mild soap and water and dry thoroughly before inserting the cream.

Attach the applicator to the tube and squeeze the tube from the bottom to force the cream into the applicator. Once the applicator is full, remove it from the tube and insert it as far back into the vagina as possible.

Repeat the procedure daily for 3 *consecutive* days even if your symptoms disappear right away.

Be sure to wash the applicator in soap and water and air dry, so that it is clean for use the next day.

It is best to use Femstat 3 at bedtime to avoid the dripping or leaking that occurs when you are standing upright. Since there may still be some leakage, you may want to wear a sanitary pad. Do not use a tampon to prevent leakage.

Overdosage

Do the following in case of accidental ingestion: If the victim is unconscious or having convulsions, call for an ambulance immediately. If you take the victim to an emergency room, be sure to bring the bottle or container with you. If the victim is conscious, call your local poison control center or a health care professional. The poison control center may suggest inducing vomiting with ipecac syrup (available without a prescription at any pharmacy). DO NOT induce vomiting unless specifically instructed to do so.

Special Populations

Pregnancy/Breast-feeding

Do not self-medicate with Femstat 3 if you are or might be pregnant.

It is not known if butoconazole passes into breast milk. Check with your doctor before self-medicating with Femstat 3 if you are breast-feeding.

Infants/Children

Femstat 3 should not be used for self-medication in children under age 12.

Seniors

Seniors should exercise the same caution as younger adults when using Femstat 3.

Gyne-Lotrimin 3 (GUY-nuh-LOE-truh-min)

*see **Clotrimazole,** page 769*

Midol IB (MYE-doll)

*see **Ibuprofen,** page 845*

Brand Name

Midol Maximum Strength Multi-Symptom Formula (MYE-doll)

Generic Ingredients

Acetaminophen
Caffeine
Pyrilamine maleate

Type of Drug

Analgesic (pain reliever), mild diuretic, central nervous system (CNS) stimulant, and antihistamine.

Used for

Relief from abdominal cramping, headaches, backaches, muscle aches, water-weight gain, and fatigue.

General Information

Acetaminophen, one of the active ingredients in Midol Maximum Strength Multi-Symptom Formula, is used to relieve pain associated with simple headache, menstrual cramps, bloating, and minor muscular aches. It has not been clearly established that OTC combination products containing acetaminophen and other drugs are any more effective in reducing pain that acetaminophen alone.

Caffeine, a mild diuretic (related to pamabrom and theophylline) and CNS stimulant, helps remove excess water from the body. This drug is often used in OTC combination products for the treatment of premenstrual syndrome (PMS). The stimulant effect of caffeine may also offset the sleep-inducing properties of pyrilamine, the antihistamine contained in Midol Maximum Strength.

Pyrilamine blocks the release of histamine in the body, decreasing the inflammation in mucous membranes. This action works in conjunction with the diuretic to help relieve the discomfort of fluid retention during the premenstrual cycle.

Cautions and Warnings

Do not take Midol Maximum Strength for more than 10 consecutive days. If pain persists for more than 10 days, consult your doctor.

Do not exceed the recommended daily dosage of Midol Maximum Strength.

In doses of more than 4 grams per day, the acetaminophen in Midol Maximum Strength is potentially toxic to the liver. Use Midol Maximum Strength with caution if you have kidney or liver disease or viral infections of the liver. Studies have shown that the risk of liver damage with acetaminophen is associated with fasting and alcohol use. People with pre-existing liver disease who are taking other drugs that are potentially damaging to the liver, who do not eat regularly, or who drink alcohol (even moderately) are especially at risk. Alcohol can also lead to adverse gastrointestinal (GI) effects if taken with Midol Maximum Strength. If you take Midol Maximum Strength regularly, avoid drinking alcoholic beverages and/or fasting.

The effectiveness of Midol Maximum Strength may be decreased if you smoke, and you may need a higher dose to achieve the desired effect.

Midol Maximum Strength should be used with caution if you have a condition that causes breathing problems, such as emphysema, chronic bronchitis, or asthma. Antihistamines dry out the mucous membranes. This in turn can inhibit the ability of the lungs to move or get rid of the excess secretions that these diseases produce.

Midol Maximum Strength should be used with caution by people with glaucoma, hyperthyroidism, heart disease, high blood pressure, or difficulty in urinating due to an enlarged prostate, because its use can worsen these conditions.

Midol Maximum Strength acts as a depressant on the CNS, which can cause sleepiness or grogginess and can interfere with the ability to concentrate. Your ability to perform activities that require your full alertness and coordination, such as driving a motor vehicle or operating machinery, may be affected. Refrain from drinking alcohol while you are taking Midol Maximum Strength because alcohol aggravates these effects.

Midol Maximum Strength should be used with caution by individuals with a history of peptic ulcer.

Midol Maximum Strength may have the potential to cause cardiac arrhythmia (irregular heartbeats), although this effect is still under investigation. As a precaution, individuals should avoid Midol Maximum Strength if they have symptomatic cardiac arrhythmias and/or palpitations and if they are in the first several days or weeks of recovery after a heart attack.

Other potential effects of Midol Maximum Strength on mood include an increase in aggressive behavior, worsened symptoms in people with anxiety or panic disorder, and worsened symptoms in women with moderate to severe PMS.

Midol Maximum Strength may have adverse effects on the quality of your sleep. You may wake up more frequently during the night or may be awakened more easily by noises or other disturbances.

The prolonged use of Midol Maximum Strength can lead to adverse gastrointestinal (GI) effects if taken with alcohol (see "Drug Interactions").

Possible Side Effects

If you develop nausea, vomiting, drowsiness, confusion, or abdominal pain other than normal menstrual cramping, stop taking Midol and contact your doctor.

- ▼ Most common: restlessness, nervousness, sleeplessness or drowsiness, dizziness, excitability, lightheadedness, tremors, nausea, vomiting, poor muscle coordination, headache, and upset stomach.
- ▼ Less common: dry eyes, nose, and mouth; trembling and pain in lower back or side; blurred vision; difficulty urinating; irritability, increased blood pressure; increased or irregular heart rate; and heart palpitations.
- ▼ Rare: extreme fatigue, rash, itching or hives; sore throat or fever; unexplained bleeding or bruising; anemia; yellowing of the skin or eyes; blood in the urine; painful or frequent urination; and decreased output of urine volume.

Drug Interactions

• Midol Maximum Strength's effects may be reduced by long-term use or large doses of barbiturate drugs; the anticonvulsants carbamazepine and phenytoin (and other similar drugs); rifampin, used to treat tuberculosis (TB); and sulfinpyrazone, used to treat gout. These drugs may also increase the chances of liver toxicity if taken with Midol Maximum Strength.

• Taking chronic, large doses of Midol Maximum Strength with isoniazid (used to treat TB) may also increase the risk of liver damage.

• If Midol Maximum Strength is taken with an anticoagulant such as warfarin, it may increase the blood-thinning effect of the anti-coagulant agent. This does not occur with occasional use.

• Midol Maximum Strength can enhance the effect of other CNS depressants, such as barbiturates, tranquilizers, sleeping medications, and alcohol (present in many OTC preparations). If you are taking other depressant drugs, check with your doctor before using Midol Maximum Strength.

• Alcohol also increases the liver toxicity caused by large doses of acetaminophen, one of the active ingredients in Midol Maximum Strength (see "Cautions and Warnings"). Alcohol can also increase the adverse GI effects of Midol Maximum Strength. If you take Midol Maximum Strength regularly, avoid alcohol.

• Nonsteroidal anti-inflammatory drugs (NSAIDs) and corticosteroids may increase the risk of adverse GI effects in people taking Midol Maximum Strength.

• It has been reported that patients with AIDS and AIDS-related complex taking zidovudine (AZT) with acetaminophen have an increased incidence of bone marrow suppression. However, studies performed to try to determine if a harmful interaction exists have not shown that short-term use of acetaminophen (less than 7 days) increases the risk of bone marrow suppression or causes a decrease in white blood cells in AIDS patients taking AZT. Acetaminophen, when taken on a short-term basis or only as needed, is the recommended OTC pain-relieving drug for these patients.

• Midol Maximum Strength should not be used at the same time as a monamine oxidase inhibitor (MAOI) or within 2 weeks of stopping treatment with an MAOI. MAOIs are used to treat depression, other psychiatric or emotional conditions and Parkinson's disease. If you are not sure whether you are or have been taking an MAOI, check with your doctor or pharmacist before you use Midol Maximum Strength.

• Midol Maximum Strength can affect the results of skin and blood tests. Notify your health care professional before scheduling these tests if you are taking Midol Maximum Strength.

• The body's metabolism of Midol Maximum Strength is inhibited by the following drugs: mexiletine, an antiarrhythmic; cimetidine, used to treat peptic ulcers, heartburn, and acid indigestion; the fluoroquinolone anti-infectives norfloxacin, enoxacin, and ciprofloxacin; and oral contraceptives containing estrogen. This effect is also seen when

Midol Maximum Strength is ingested with alcohol or the drug disulfiram, which is used in the treatment of chronic alcoholism.

• Because Midol Maximum Strength may decrease the body's absorption of iron, iron supplements should be taken 1 hour before or 2 hours after Midol Maximum Strength is consumed.

• Co-administration of Midol Maximum Strength and phenylpropanolamine, a decongestant, may increase blood pressure.

• Midol Maximum Strength may interfere with the therapeutic benefit of drugs given to regulate heart rhythm, such as quinidine, and propranolol. It may also increase the breakdown of phenobarbitol or aspirin, thus decreasing the beneficial effects of these drugs.

• The effects of both the benzodiazepine tranquilizer diazepam and Midol Maximum Strength may either be increased or decreased when these 2 drugs are taken together.

• Midol Maximum Strength may cause false-positive results in tests performed to diagnose pheochromocytoma (tumor of the adrenal gland) or neuroblastoma (tumor of the nervous system), and may also affect readings of uric acid concentrations.

Food Interactions

To avoid the potential danger of caffeine overdose, be aware of your consumption of coffee, tea, cola drinks, chocolate, and other caffeine-containing foods if you are taking Midol Maximum Strength. Check with your doctor about a safe level of caffeine intake for you.

Usual Dose

Each caplet contains 500 mg of acetaminophen, 60 mg of caffeine, and 15 mg of pyrilamine.

Adult and Child (age 12 and over): 2 caplets every 4 hours with water, not to exceed 8 caplets in 24 hours.

Child (under age 12): Consult your doctor.

Overdosage

Symptoms of overdose include nausea, vomiting, abdominal pain, low blood pressure, fever, flushed face, dry mouth, dilated pupils, loss of muscle coordination, nervousness, restlessness, increased heart rate, sleeplessness, frequent urination, flushing, muscle twitching, disordered thoughts and speech, irregular heartbeat, confusion, excitability, hallucinations, drowsiness, coma, seizures, yellowing of the skin and eyes, and liver damage. Symptoms may develop within 30 minutes, but may not be seen for as long as 2 days after the overdose.

Even if the victim is not displaying any of the symptoms listed above, do the following in case of accidental overdose: If the victim is unconscious or having convulsions, call for an ambulance immediately. If the victim is conscious, call your local poison control center or a health care professional. The poison control center may suggest inducing vomiting with ipecac syrup (available without a prescription at any pharmacy). DO NOT induce vomiting unless specifically instructed to do so. If you take the victim to an emergency room, be sure to bring the bottle or container with you.

Special Populations:

Pregnancy/Breast-feeding

It is not generally recommended that pregnant women take any drugs, particularly during the first 3 months after conception. Although taking normal dosages of acetaminophen is considered relatively safe for the expectant mother and her baby, taking continual high doses may cause birth defects or interfere with the baby's development.

Antihistamines are not recommended for use during pregnancy unless directed by your doctor.

Acetaminophen is considered acceptable for use during breast-feeding by the American Academy of Pediatrics. Although acetaminophen does pass into breast milk when taken by nursing mothers, the only side effect reported in infants is a rash that goes away when the mother stops taking the drug.

Antihistamines and acetaminophen are known to pass into the breast milk of nursing mothers and may cause side effects in infants.

Check with your doctor before taking Midol Maximum Strength if you are or might be pregnant, or if you are breast-feeding.

Infants/Children
Children may be more susceptible to the CNS effects of Midol. Don't give Midol to children under age 12 without consulting your doctor.

Seniors
Seniors may be more sensitive to the side effects of antihistamines. They may experience nervousness, irritability, restlessness, dizziness, sedation, hallucinations, seizures, and low blood pressure.

Because acetaminophen may clear the body more slowly in older adults, the effects of Midol Maximum Strength may be more noticeable.

Older people may be more sensitive to caffeine's stimulant effects and may be more liable to have nervousness, anxiety, sleeplessness, and irritability. Be especially cautious about your caffeine intake if you are taking other drugs that stimulate the CNS, such as theophylline, amantadine (used to treat Parkison's disease), tricyclic antidepressants, or appetite suppressants.

Brand Name

Midol PMS Multi-Symptom Formula (MYE-doll)

Generic Ingredients

Acetaminophen
Pamabrom
Pyrilamine maleate

Type of Drug

Analgesic (pain reliever), mild diuretic, and antihistamine.

Used for

Relief from abdominal cramping, headaches, body aches from water retention, and bloating.

General Information

Acetaminophen, one of the active ingredients in Midol PMS Multi-Symptom Formula, is used to relieve pain associated with simple headache, menstrual cramps, bloating, and minor muscular aches. It has not been clearly established that OTC combination products containing acetaminophen and other drugs are any more effective in reducing pain than acetaminophen alone.

Pamabrom, a mild diuretic related to caffeine and theophylline, helps remove excess water from the body. This drug is often used in OTC combination products for the treatment of premenstrual syndrome (PMS).

Pyrilamine blocks the release of histamine in the body, decreasing the inflammation in mucous membranes. This action works in conjunction with the diuretic to help relieve the discomfort of fluid retention during the premenstrual cycle.

Cautions and Warnings

Do not take Midol PMS for more than 10 consecutive days. If pain persists for more than 10 days, consult your doctor.

Do not exceed the recommended daily dosage of Midol PMS.

In doses of more than 4 grams per day, the acetaminophen in Midol PMS is potentially toxic to the liver. Use Midol PMS with caution if you have kidney or liver disease or viral infections of the liver. Studies have shown that the risk of liver damage with acetaminophen is associated with fasting and alcohol use. People with pre-existing liver disease who are taking other drugs that are potentially damaging to the liver, who do not eat regularly, or who drink alcohol (even moderately) are especially at risk. Alcohol can also lead to adverse gastrointestinal (GI) effects if taken with Midol PMS. If you take Midol PMS regularly, avoid drinking alcoholic beverages and/or fasting.

The effectiveness of Midol PMS may be decreased if you smoke, and you may need a higher dose to achieve the desired effect.

Midol PMS should be used with caution if you have a condition that causes breathing problems, such as emphysema, chronic bronchitis, or asthma. Antihistamines dry out the mucous membranes. This in turn can inhibit the ability of the lungs to move or get rid of the excess secretions that these diseases produce.

Midol PMS should be used with caution by people with glaucoma, hyperthyroidism, heart disease, high blood pressure, or difficulty in urinating due to an enlarged prostate, because its use can worsen these conditions.

Midol PMS acts as a depressant on the CNS, which can cause sleepiness or grogginess and can interfere with the ability to concentrate. Your ability to perform activities that require your full alertness and coordination, such as driving a motor vehicle or operating machinery, may be affected. Refrain from drinking alcohol while you are taking Midol PMS because alcohol aggravates these effects.

Possible Side Effects

- ▼ Most common: restlessness, lightheadedness, nervousness, sleeplessness, drowsiness, dizziness, excitability, poor muscle coordination, headache, and upset stomach.
- ▼ Less common: blurred vision, difficulty urinating, irritability (at high doses), increased blood pressure, increased or irregular heart rate, heart palpitations, trembling and pain in lower back or side, and dry eyes, nose, and mouth.
- ▼ Rare: extreme fatigue, rash, itching, or hives, sore throat or fever, unexplained bleeding or bruising, anemia, yellowing of the skin or eyes, blood in urine, painful or frequent urination, and decreased output of urine.

Drug Interactions

• Midol PMS's effects may be reduced by long-term use or large doses of barbiturate drugs; the anticonvulsants carbamazepine and phenytoin (and other similar drugs); rifampin, used to treat tuberculosis (TB); and sulfinpyrazone, used to treat gout. These drugs may also increase the chances of liver toxicity if taken with Midol PMS.

• Taking chronic, large doses of Midol PMS with isoniazid (used to treat TB) may also increase the risk of liver damage.

• If Midol PMS is taken with an anticoagulant such as warfarin, it may increase the blood-thinning effect of the anticoagulant agent. This does not occur with occasional use.

• Midol PMS can enhance the effect of other CNS depressants, such as barbiturates, tranquilizers, sleeping medications, and alcohol (present in many OTC preparations). If you are taking other depressant drugs, check with your doctor before using Midol PMS.

• Alcohol also increases the liver toxicity caused by large doses of acetaminophen, one of the active ingredients in Midol PMS (see "Cautions and Warnings"). Alcohol can also increase the adverse GI effects of Midol PMS. If you take Midol PMS regularly, avoid alcohol.

• Nonsteroidal anti-inflammatory drugs (NSAIDs) and corticosteroids may increase the risk of adverse GI effects in people taking Midol PMS.

• It has been reported that patients with AIDS and AIDS-related complex taking zidovudine (AZT) with acetaminophen have an increased incidence of bone marrow suppression. However, studies performed to try to determine if a harmful interaction exists have not shown that short-term use of acetaminophen (less than 7 days) increases the risk of bone marrow suppression or causes a decrease in white blood cells in AIDS patients taking AZT. Acetaminophen, when taken on a short-term basis or only as needed, is the recommended OTC pain-relieving drug for these patients.

• Midol PMS should not be used at the same time as a monamine oxidase inhibitor (MAOI) or within 2 weeks of stopping treatment with an MAOI. MAOIs are used to treat depression, other psychiatric or emotional conditions, and Parkinson's disease. If you are not sure whether you are or have been taking an MAOI, check with your doctor or pharmacist before you use Midol PMS.

• Midol PMS can affect the results of skin and blood tests. Notify your health care professional before scheduling these tests if you are taking Midol PMS.

Food Interactions

None known.

Usual Dose

Each tablet contains 500 mg of acetaminophen, 25 mg of pamabrom, and 15 mg of pyrilamine.

Adult and Child (age 12 and over): 2 caplets every 4 hours with water, not to exceed 8 caplets in 24 hours.

Child (under age 12): Consult your doctor.

Overdosage

Symptoms of overdose include nausea, vomiting, drowsiness, confusion, abdominal pain, low blood pressure, yellowing of the skin and eyes, liver damage, dilated pupils, flushed face, dry mouth, fever, excitability, hallucinations, loss of muscle coordination, seizures, drowsiness or coma, fluid buildup in the brain, and kidney, heart, and lung failure. Symptoms may develop within 30 minutes, but may not be seen for as long as 2 days after the overdose.

Even if the victim is not displaying any of the symptoms listed above, do the following in case of accidental overdose: If the victim is unconscious or having convulsions, call for an ambulance immediately. If the victim is conscious, call your local poison control center or a health care professional. The poison control center may suggest inducing vomiting with ipecac syrup (available without a prescription at any pharmacy). DO NOT induce vomiting unless specifically instructed to do so. If you take the victim to an emergency room, be sure to bring the bottle or container with you.

Special Populations

Pregnancy/Breast-feeding

It is not generally recommended that pregnant women take any drugs, particularly during the first 3 months after conception. Although taking normal dosages of acetaminophen is considered relatively safe for the expectant mother and her baby, taking continual high doses may cause birth defects or interfere with the baby's development.

Antihistamines are not recommended for use during pregnancy unless directed by your doctor.

Acetaminophen is considered acceptable for use during breast-feeding by the American Academy of Pediatrics. Although acetaminophen does pass into breast milk when taken by nursing mothers, the only side effect reported in infants is a rash that goes away when the mother stops taking the drug.

Antihistamines and acetaminophen are known to pass into the breast milk of nursing mothers and may cause side effects in infants.

Check with your doctor before taking Midol PMS if you are or might be pregnant, or if you are breast-feeding.

Infants/Children
Don't give Midol PMS to children under age 12 without consulting your doctor.

Seniors
Seniors may be more sensitive to the side effects of antihistamines. They may experience nervousness, irritability, restlessness, dizziness, sedation, hallucinations, seizures, and low blood pressure.

Because acetaminophen may clear the body more slowly in older adults, the effects of Midol PMS may be more noticeable.

Brand Name

Midol Teen Maximum Strength Multi-Symptom Formula (MYE-doll)

Generic Ingredients

Acetaminophen
Pamabrom

Type of Drug

Analgesic (pain reliever) and mild diuretic.

Used for

Relief from abdominal cramping, bloating, water-weight gain, headaches, backaches, and muscular aches and pains.

General Information

Acetaminophen, one of the active ingredients in Midol Teen Maximum Strength Multi-Symptom Formula, is used to relieve pain associated with simple headache, menstrual cramps, bloating, and minor muscular aches. It has not been clearly established that OTC combination products containing acetaminophen and other drugs are any more effective in reducing pain than acetaminophen alone.

Pamabrom, a mild diuretic related to caffeine and theophylline, helps remove excess water from the body. This drug is often used in OTC combination products for the treatment of premenstrual syndrome (PMS).

Cautions and Warnings

Do not use Midol Teen for more than 10 days unless directed by your doctor. If pain persists for more than 10 days, consult your doctor.

Do not exceed the recommended daily dosage of Midol Teen Maximum Strength.

In doses of more than 4 grams per day, the acetaminophen in Midol Teen is potentially toxic to the liver. Use Midol Teen with caution if you have kidney or liver disease or viral infections of the liver. Studies have shown that the risk of liver damage with acetaminophen is associated with fasting and alcohol use. People with pre-existing liver disease who are taking other drugs that are potential damaging to the liver, who do not eat regularly, or who drink alcohol (even moderately) are especially at risk. If you take Midol Teen regularly, avoid drinking alcoholic beverages and/or fasting.

The effectiveness of taking Midol Teen may be decreased if you smoke, and you may need a higher dose to achieve the desired effect.

Possible Side Effects

- ▼ Most common: lightheadedness.
- ▼ Less common: trembling and pain in lower back or side.
- ▼ Rare: extreme fatigue, rash, itching, or hives; sore throat or fever; unexplained bleeding or bruising; anemia; yellowing of the skin or eyes; blood in urine; painful or frequent urination; and decreased output of urine.

Drug Interactions

• Midol Teen Maximum Strength's effects may be reduced by long-term use or large doses of barbiturate drugs; the anticonvulsants carbamazepine and phenytoin (and other similar drugs); rifampin, used to treat tuberculosis (TB); and sulfinpyrazone, used to treat gout. These drugs may also increase the chances of liver toxicity if taken with Midol Teen.

• Taking chronic, large doses of Midol Teen with isoniazid (used to treat TB) may increase the risk of liver damage.

• If Midol Teen taken with an anticoagulant such as warfarin, it may increase the blood-thinning effect of the anticoagulant agent. This does not occur with occasional use.

• Alcohol increases the liver toxicity caused by large doses of acetaminophen (see "Cautions and Warnings"). If you take Midol Teen regularly, avoid alcohol.

• It has been reported that patients with AIDS and AIDS-related complex taking zidovudine (AZT) with acetaminophen have an increased incidence of bone marrow suppression. However, studies performed to try to determine if a harmful interaction exists have not shown that short-term use of acetaminophen (less than 7 days) increases the risk of bone marrow suppression or causes a decrease in white blood cells in AIDS patients taking AZT. Acetaminophen, when taken on a short-term basis or only as needed, is the recommended OTC pain-relieving drug for these patients.

Food Interactions

None known.

Usual Dose

Each caplet contains 500 mg of acetaminophen and 25 mg of pamabrom.

Adult and Child (age 12 and over): 2 caplets every 4 hours with water, not to exceed 8 caplets in 24 hours.

Child (under age 12): Consult your doctor.

Overdosage

Symptoms of overdose include nausea, vomiting, drowsiness, confusion, abdominal pain, low blood pressure, yellowing of the skin and eyes, and liver damage. These symptoms usually occur within 2 to 3 hours but may not be seen for as long as 2 days after the overdose is taken.

Even if the victim is not displaying any of the symptoms listed above, do the following in case of accidental overdose: If the victim is unconscious or having convulsions, call for an ambulance immediately. If you take the victim to an emergency room, be sure to bring the bottle or container with you. If the victim is conscious, call your local poison control center or a health care professional. The poison control center may suggest inducing vomiting with ipecac syrup (available without a prescription at any pharmacy). DO NOT induce vomiting unless specifically instructed to do so.

Special Populations:

Pregnancy/Breast-feeding

It is not generally recommended that pregnant women take any drugs, particularly during the first 3 months after conception. Although taking normal dosages of acetaminophen is considered relatively safe for the expectant mother and her baby, taking continual high doses may cause birth defects or interfere with the baby's development.

Antihistamines are not recommended for use during pregnancy unless directed by your doctor.

Acetaminophen is considered acceptable for use during breast-feeding by the American Academy of Pediatrics. Although acetaminophen does pass into breast milk when taken by nursing mothers, the only side effect reported in infants is a rash that goes away when the mother stops taking the drug.

Check with your doctor before taking Midol Teen if you are or might be pregnant, or if you are breast-feeding.

Infants/Children

Midol Teen should not be given to children under age 12 without consulting your doctor.

Seniors

Because acetaminophen may clear the body more slowly in older adults, the effects of Midol Teen may be more noticeable.

Brand Name

Monistat 7 Creme (MON-ih-stat)

Generic Ingredients

Benzoic acid
Miconazole nitrate

Type of Drug

Vaginal antifungal agent and antimicrobial.

Used for

Treating vaginal yeast infection.

General Information

A fungus is an organism that obtains nutrients from other living organisms or from dead organic matter in order to survive. In doing so, fungi cause infections that only an antifungal agent can cure.

Monistat 7 Creme combines the antifungal drug miconazole and the antifungal/antiseptic benzoic acid.

Miconazole is one of the antifungal agents known as imidazoles. Imidazoles inhibit the growth of and kill fungi and also relieve the symptoms of the infection caused by the fungi.

Imidazoles are effective in inhibiting the growth of and killing the fungus known as *Candida,* which causes yeast infections. They have an effectiveness rate of about 85% to 90%. Miconazole must be taken for 7 days to cure a vaginal yeast infection.

Benzoic acid works against fungal infections by damaging the cell walls of the fungus, thus killing the cell and stopping the fungus from spreading. Besides deterring fungal growth, benzoic acid acts as a mild antiseptic.

Cautions and Warnings

If you do not improve after 3 days of treatment with Monistat 7 or if you do not get well in 7 days, you may have a condition other than a yeast infection. Call your doctor.

Do not exceed the recommended daily dosage of Monistat 7.

Self-medicate with a miconazole vaginal product only if you have had a doctor diagnose a vaginal yeast infection previously and you recognize the same symptoms now. If this is the first time you have had vaginal itch and discomfort, DO NOT SELF-MEDICATE WITH MONISTAT 7. Call your doctor, and have him or her determine whether what you have is truly a yeast infection and not another type of vaginal infection, such as one caused by bacteria, which can't be effectively treated with Monistat 7.

Do not use Monistat 7 if you have abdominal pain, fever, or foul-smelling discharge. Call your doctor immediately.

Stop using Monistat 7 and call your doctor if you develop abdominal cramping, headache, hives, or skin rash.

If your symptoms return within 2 months or if you have infections that do not clear up easily with treatment, call your physician. You could be pregnant, or there could be a serious underlying medical reason for your infections, such as diabetes or an impaired immune system (such as that associated with HIV infection).

You must use Monistat 7 for 7 consecutive days for them to cure your fungal infection. Do not stop therapy before then even if your symptoms disappear right away, as often happens.

You may use Monistat 7 during your period, but do not use tampons. If your period begins after you have started your 7-day treatment, do not stop treatment.

It is recommended that you avoid sexual intercourse during your 7-day treatment. Be aware that miconazole can damage condoms, diaphragms, and cervical caps, thus increasing your risk of pregnancy.

Monistat 7 is for external use only. Avoid contact with your eyes. After use, wash your hands with soap and water.

Possible Side Effects

Burning, itching, and irritation have been seen in a small percentage of individuals using miconazole vaginally. Benzoic acid may also cause irritation, stinging, and inflammation. These effects usually occur after the first application. This kind of irritation should stop after the first few applications. If is does not, stop using Monistat 7 and contact your doctor.

▼ Rare: abdominal cramps, headache, and allergic reactions.

Drug Interactions

None known.

Usual Dose

Adult and Child (age 12 and over): Read the package carefully before using Monistat 7.

Wash your entire vaginal area with mild soap and water and dry thoroughly before applying the cream or suppository.

If you are using the cream, attach the applicator to the tube and squeeze the tube from the bottom to force the cream into the applicator. (Monistat 7 is available in prefilled applicator form.) Once the applicator is full, remove it from the tube and insert it as far back into the vagina as possible.

Repeat either procedure daily for 7 consecutive days.

Be sure to wash the applicator in soap and water and air-dry it so that it is clean for use the next day.

It is best to use these products at bedtime to avoid the dripping or leaking that occurs when you are upright. There may still be some leakage; you may want to wear a sanitary pad but do not use a tampon to prevent leakage.

Child (under age 12): not recommended.

Overdosage

Do the following in case of accidental ingestion: If the victim is unconscious or having convulsions, call for an ambulance immediately. If you take the victim to an emergency room, be sure to bring the bottle or container with you. If the victim is conscious, call your local poison control center or a health care professional. The poison control center may suggest inducing vomiting with ipecac syrup (available without a prescription at any pharmacy). DO NOT induce vomiting unless specifically instructed to do so.

Special Populations

Pregnancy/Breast-feeding

Do not use Monistat 7 during pregnancy except under the advice and supervision of your doctor.

It is not known if miconazole passes into breast milk. Check with your doctor before using Monistat 7 if you are breast-feeding.

Infants/Children

Children under 12 should not be treated with Monistat 7.

Seniors

Seniors should exercise the same caution as younger adults when using Monistat 7.

Brand Name

Monistat 7 Suppositories (MON-ih-stat)

*see **Miconazole Nitrate,** page 920*

Brand Name

Pamprin Multi-Symptom (PAM-prin)

Generic Ingredients

Acetaminophen
Pamabrom
Pyrilamine maleate

Type of Drug

Analgesic (pain reliever), mild diuretic, and antihistamine.

Used for

Relief from abdominal cramping, headaches, body aches from water retention, and bloating.

General Information

Acetaminophen, one of the active ingredients in Pamprin Multi-Symptom, is used to relieve pain associated with simple headache, menstrual cramps, bloating, and minor muscular aches. It has not been clearly established that OTC combination products containing acetaminophen and other drugs are any more effective than acetaminophen alone.

Pamabrom, a mild diuretic related to caffeine and theophylline, helps remove excess water from the body. This drug is often used in OTC combination products for the treatment of premenstrual syndrome (PMS).

Pyrilamine, the antihistamine in Pamprin, blocks the release of histamine in the body, decreasing the inflammation in mucous membranes. This action works in conjunction with the diuretic to help relieve the discomfort of fluid retention during the premenstrual cycle.

Pamprin is available in tablet form.

Cautions and Warnings

Do not use Pamprin for more than 10 days unless directed by your doctor.

Do not exceed the recommended daily dosage of Pamprin. In doses of more than 4 grams per day, the acetaminophen in Pamprin is potentially toxic to the liver. Use Pamprin with caution if you have kidney or liver disease or viral infections of the liver. Studies have shown that the risk of liver damage with acetaminophen is associated with fasting and alcohol use. People with pre-existing liver disease who are taking other drugs that are potentially damaging to the liver, who do not eat regularly, or who drink alcohol (even moderately) are especially at risk. If you take Pamprin regularly, avoid drinking alcoholic beverages and/or fasting.

The effectiveness of Pamprin may be decreased if you smoke, and you may need a higher dose to achieve the desired effect.

Pamprin should be used with caution if you have a condition that causes breathing problems, such as emphysema, chronic bronchitis, or asthma. Antihistamines like pyrilamine dry out the mucous membranes. This in turn can inhibit the ability of the lungs to move or get rid of the excess secretions that these diseases produce.

Pamprin should be used with caution by people with glaucoma, hyperthyroidism, heart disease, hypertension (high blood pressure), or who have difficulty urinating due to an enlarged prostate, because its use can worsen these conditions.

Pamprin acts as a depressant on the central nervous system (CNS), which can cause sleepiness or grogginess and can interfere with the ability to concentrate. Your ability to perform activities that require your full alertness and coordination, such as driving a motor vehicle or operating machinery, may be affected. Refrain from drinking alcohol while you are taking Pamprin because alcohol aggravates these effects.

Possible Side Effects

If you develop nausea, vomiting, drowsiness, confusion, or abdominal pain other than normal menstrual cramping, stop taking Pamprin and contact your doctor.

▼ Most common: lightheadedness, restlessness, nervousness, sleeplessness or drowsiness, dizziness, excitability, poor muscle coordination, headache, and upset stomach.

Possible Side Effects ***(continued)***

- ▼ Less common: trembling and pain in lower back or side, blurred vision, difficulty urinating, irritability (at high doses), increased blood pressure, increased or irregular heart rate, heart palpitations, and dry eyes, nose, and mouth.
- ▼ Rare: extreme fatigue, rash, itching, or hives; sore throat or fever; unexplained bleeding or bruising; anemia; yellowing of the skin or eyes; blood in urine; painful or frequent urination; and decreased output of urine.

Drug Interactions

• Pamprin's effects may be reduced by long-term use or large doses of barbiturate drugs; the anticonvulsants carbamazepine and phenytoin (and other similar drugs); rifampin, used to treat tuberculosis (TB); and sulfinpyrazone, used to treat gout. These drugs may also increase the chances of liver toxicity if taken with Pamprin.

• Taking chronic, large doses of Pamprin with isoniazid (used to treat TB) may also increase the risk of liver damage.

• If Pamprin is taken with an anticoagulant such as warfarin, it may increase the blood-thinning effect of the anticoagulant agent. This does not occur with occasional use.

• Alcohol increases the liver toxicity caused by large doses of acetaminophen (see "Cautions and Warnings"). If you take Pamprin regularly, avoid alcohol.

• It has been reported that patients with AIDS and AIDS-related complex taking zidovudine (AZT) with acetaminophen have an increased incidence of bone marrow suppression. However, studies performed to try to determine if a harmful interaction exists have not shown that short-term use of acetaminophen (less than 7 days) in creases the risk of bone marrow suppression or causes a decrease in white blood cells in AIDS patients taking AZT. Acetaminophen, when taken on a short-term basis or only as needed, is the recommended OTC pain-relieving drug for these patients.

• Pamprin can enhance the effect of other CNS depressants, such as barbiturates, tranquilizers, sleeping medications, and alcohol (present in many OTC preparations). If you are taking other depressant drugs, check with your doctor before using Pamprin or any other antihistamine.

• Pamprin should not be used at the same time as a monoamine oxidase inhibitor (MAOI) or within 2 weeks of stopping treatment with an MAOI. MAOIs are used to treat depression, other psychiatric or emotional conditions, and Parkinson's disease. If you are not sure whether you are or have been taking an MAOI, check with your doctor or pharmacist before you use Pamprin.

• Do not use Pamprin if you are taking medication for high blood pressure.

• Pamprin can affect the results of skin and blood tests. Notify your health care professional before scheduling these tests if you are taking Pamprin.

Food Interactions

None known.

Usual Dose

Each tablet contains 500 mg of acetaminophen, 25 mg of pamabrom, and 15 mg of pyrilamine.

Adult and Child (age 12 and over): 2 caplets every 4 hours with water, not to exceed 8 caplets in 24 hours.

Child (under age 12): Consult your doctor.

Overdosage

Symptoms of overdose include nausea, vomiting, abdominal pain, low blood pressure, fever, flushed face, dry mouth, dilated pupils, loss of muscle coordination, confusion, excitability, hallucinations, drowsiness, coma, seizures, yellowing of the skin and eyes, and liver damage. Symptoms may develop within 30 minutes, but may not be seen for as long as 2 days after the overdose.

Even if the victim is not displaying any of the symptoms listed above, do the following in case of accidental overdose: If the victim is unconscious or having convulsions, call for an ambulance immediately. If you take the victim to an emergency room, be sure to bring the bottle or container with you. If the victim is conscious, call your local poison control center or a health care professional. The poison control center may suggest inducing vomiting with ipecac syrup (available without a prescription at any pharmacy). DO NOT induce vomiting unless specifically instructed to do so.

Special Populations

Pregnancy/Breast-feeding

It is not generally recommended that pregnant women take any drugs, particularly during the first 3 months after conception. Although taking normal dosages of acetaminophen is considered relatively safe for the expectant mother and her baby, taking continual high doses may cause birth defects or interfere with the baby's development.

Antihistamines are not recommended for use during pregnancy unless directed by your doctor.

Acetaminophen is considered acceptable for use during breast-feeding by the American Academy of Pediatrics. Although acetaminophen does pass into breast milk when taken by nursing mothers, the only side effect reported in infants is a rash that goes away when the mother stops taking the drug.

Antihistamines like pyrilamine are known to pass into the breast milk of nursing mothers and may cause side effects in infants.

Check with your doctor before taking Pamprin if you are or might be pregnant, or if you are breast-feeding.

Infants/Children

Pamprin should not be given to children under age 12 without consulting your doctor.

Seniors

Seniors may be more sensitive to the side effects of antihistamines. They may experience nervousness, irritability, restlessness, dizziness, sedation, hallucinations, seizures, and low blood pressure.

Because acetaminophen may clear the body more slowly in older adults, the side effects of Pamprin may be more noticeable.

Uristat (YUR-ih-stat)

see ***Phenazopyridine Hydrochloride,*** *page 959*

Brand Name

Vagisil Anti-Itch Creme (VAJ-i-sil)

Generic Ingredients

Benzocaine
Resorcinol

Type of Drug

Topical anesthetic, antipruritic, and antimicrobial.

Used for

Temporary relief of itching and discomfort from vaginal infections.

General Information

A fungus is an organism that obtains nutrients from other living organisms or from dead organic matter in order to survive. In doing so, fungi cause infections that only an antifungal agent can cure.

Most vaginal infections are caused by either the fungus *candida albicans* (yeast infections) or the parasite *trichomonas vaginalis* (trichomoniasis). While a parasitic infection requires prescription medication, some yeast infections can be treated effectively with the aid of topical OTC products such as Vagisil Anti-Itch Creme.

When applied to the skin, the benzocaine in Vagisil temporarily numbs itching by blocking pain signals in the skin and keeping them from traveling along the nerves to the brain. Because the sensation of itching is produced by the nerve fibers that carry pain impulses, benzocaine relieves itching at the same time as it reduces pain.

Resorcinol is used as an antimicrobial agent in Vagisil. The FDA considers resorcinol to be of limited or questionable value as an antimicrobial agent.

Cautions and Warnings

If your condition worsens, or symptoms last for more than 7 days or clear up and recur within a few days, discontinue the use of Vagisil and consult your doctor. You may need treatment with an OTC medication that contains butoconazole, clotrimazole, or miconazole.

Do not exceed the recommended daily dose of Vagisil.

Vagisil is for external use only.

If this is your first vaginal infection, do not use Vagisil without first consulting your doctor. Vaginal disorders and infections have many different possible causes, and Vagisil may mask the symptoms of a more serious condition.

To avoid irritation or accidental ingestion, do not allow Vagisil to come into contact with the area near your eyes or mouth.

Vagisil should not be used over a large area of skin. If the itching and inflammation cover more than the immediate genital area, consult your doctor. If you experience recurrent infections (more than 4 in a year), consult your doctor. Do not use Vagisil if you have abdominal or back pain, fever, or foul-smelling discharge. Call your doctor immediately.

Products containing benzocaine should not be used by individuals with known or suspected hypersensitivity to it or to other ester-type local anesthetics (e.g., proparacaine hydrochloride or tetracaine). Individuals with methemoglobinemia (a rare blood disorder) should not use benzocaine products.

Possible Side Effects

In about 1% of people, the benzocaine in Vagisil can cause a hypersensitivity reaction leading to allergic contact dermatitis (rash). This reaction will not be apparent the first time you use benzocaine; an initial sensitizing exposure is necessary. If you develop sensitivity to benzocaine, the next time you use it, you will notice an itchy, possibly oozing, rash that can appear minutes to hours after exposure. If this occurs, stop using benzocaine immediately. Wash the area gently to remove any traces of benzocaine and apply compresses of cool tap water if the area is oozing. Calamine lotion, colloidal oatmeal baths, and hydrocortisone cream may help relieve the itching and inflammation. Call your doctor if you have a severe reaction, if the reaction covers a large area of your body, or if the rash does not begin to improve in a few days or worsens.

▼ Common: rash and irritation.

Drug Interactions

• Vagisil can cross-react with the chemicals in hair dyes and with sunscreens containing para-aminobenzoic acid (PABA) and cause allergic contact dermatitis.

Usual Dose

Vagisil contains benzocaine 5.0% and resorcinol 2.0%.

Adult and Child (age 2 and over): Apply to the affected area not more than 3–4 times daily.

Child (under age 2): Consult your doctor.

Overdosage

Do the following in case of accidental ingestion: If the victim is unconscious or having convulsions, call for an ambulance immediately. If you take the victim to an emergency room, be sure to bring the bottle or container with you. If the victim is conscious, call your local poison control center or a health care professional. The poison control center may suggest inducing vomiting with ipecac syrup (available without a prescription at any pharmacy). DO NOT induce vomiting unless specifically instructed to do so.

Special Populations

Pregnancy/Breast-feeding

It is not generally recommended that pregnant women take any drugs, particularly during the first 3 months after conception. Check with your doctor if you are or might be pregnant, or if you are breast-feeding.

Infants/Children

Vaginal infections and disorders have many forms and causes. If this is your child's first episode, consult your doctor for a positive diagnosis before using Vagisil. Do not use Vagisil in children under age 2 without consulting your doctor.

Seniors

Seniors should exercise the same caution as younger adults when using Vagisil.

Brand Name

Vagistat-1 (VAJ-i-stat)

Generic Ingredient

Tioconazole (TYE-oh-CON-uh-zole)

Type of Drug

Vaginal antifungal agent.

Used for

Treatment of vaginal yeast infection.

General Information

A fungus is an organism that obtains nutrients from other living organisms or from dead organic matter in order to survive. In doing so, fungi cause infections that only an antifungal agent can cure.

Tioconazole is classified as an imidazole; 3 other topical antifungals in the group, butoconazole, clotrimazole, and miconazole are also available without a prescription. These drugs kill fungi and inhibit their growth, as well as relieving the symptoms associated with the infection.

Studies have shown that butoconazole, clotrimazole, miconazole, and tioconazole are equally effective in inhibiting the growth of and killing the fungus known as *Candida,* which causes yeast infections. They have an effectiveness rate of about 85% to 90%. All 4 are well tolerated. One advantage of tioconazole is that it is only taken for 1 day; butoconazole is taken for 3 days and both clotrimazole and miconazole must be taken for 7 days to cure a vaginal yeast infection.

Tioconazole is available by brand name in intravaginal cream form.

Cautions and Warnings

Do not take the maximum daily dosage of Vagistat-1 for more than 1 day, except under a doctor's supervision.

Do not exceed the recommended daily dosage of Vagistat-1.

Self-medicate with Vagistat-1 *only* if a doctor has previously diagnosed a vaginal yeast infection, and you recognize the same symptoms now. If this is the *first* time you have had vaginal itch and discomfort, DO NOT SELF-MEDICATE WITH VAGISTAT-1. Call your doctor and have him or her determine whether you have a yeast infection or another type of vaginal infection, such as one caused by bacteria, which can't be effectively treated with tioconazole.

Do not use Vagistat-1 if you have abdominal or back pain, fever, or foul-smelling discharge. Call your doctor immediately.

If you are taking certain medications (e.g., corticosteroids, drugs that suppress the immune system) or if you have a medical condition such as diabetes or HIV infection, do not use Vagistat-1 without first consulting your doctor.

Self-treatment with Vagistat-1 is not appropriate for girls under age 12 or women who are pregnant. These individuals should consult a doctor if they experience symptoms of a yeast infection.

Women experiencing recurrent infections (more than 4 in 1 year) should see a physician and avoid using OTC tioconazole, unless advised by a physician.

Stop using Vagistat-1 and call your doctor if you develop abdominal cramping, headache, hives, or skin rash.

If your symptoms do not improve after 1 day of treatment with Vagistat-1, you may have a condition other than a yeast infection or you may require more prolonged therapy with the drug. Call your doctor.

If your symptoms return within 2 months, or if you have infections that do not clear up easily with treatment, call your physician. You could be pregnant; or there could be a serious, underlying medical reason for your infections, such as diabetes or an impaired immune system (such as that associated with HIV infection).

You may use Vagistat-1 during your period, but do not use tampons.

It is recommended that you avoid sexual intercourse for 3 days following treatment. Butoconazole can damage condoms, diaphragms, and cervical caps, thus increasing your risk of pregnancy.

Vagistat-1 is for external use only. Avoid contact with your eyes. After using the product, wash your hands with soap and water.

Possible Side Effects

- ▼ Most common: vaginal burning, itching, or irritation.
- ▼ Less common: vaginal discharge, swelling of the vulva, vaginal pain; painful urination, nighttime urination, vaginal dryness, and pain during intercourse.

Drug Interactions

None known.

Usual Dose

Adult and Child (age 12 and over): 1 full applicator into the vagina at bedtime.

Child (under age 12): not recommended.

Read the package carefully before using Vagistat-1.

Wash your entire vaginal area with mild soap and water and dry thoroughly before using Vagistat-1.

Insert the applicator as high into the vagina as possible.

It is best to use Vagistat-1 at bedtime to avoid the dripping or leaking that occurs when you are standing upright. Since there may still be some leakage, you may want to wear a sanitary pad. Do not use a tampon to prevent leakage.

Overdosage

Do the following in case of accidental ingestion: If the victim is unconscious or having convulsions, call for an ambulance immediately. If you take the victim to an emergency room, be sure to bring the bottle or container with you. If the victim is conscious, call your local poison control center or a health care professional. The poison control center may suggest inducing vomiting with ipecac syrup (available without a prescription at any pharmacy). DO NOT induce vomiting unless specifically instructed to do so.

Special Populations

Pregnancy/Breast-feeding

Do not self-medicate with Vagistat-1 if you are or might be pregnant.

It is not known if tioconazole passes into breast milk. However, because of the possibility of tioconazole passing into breast milk, nursing should be discontinued while tioconazole is being used. If you must use tioconazole, bottle-feed your baby with formula.

Infants/Children

Vagistat-1 should not be used for self-medication in children under age 12.

Seniors

Seniors should exercise the same caution as younger adults when using Vagistat-1.

Chapter 11: Smoking Cessation

The dangers of tobacco use are well known. Smoking is directly responsible for at least 75% of all cases of lung cancer. Cigarettes and other forms of tobacco (including chewing tobacco) cause 30% of all other types of cancer, including cancers of the mouth and throat. Smoking also contributes to emphysema, coronary heart disease, and other serious and debilitating illnesses. Smoke in the environment (secondhand smoke) can be inhaled by other people, increasing their risk of health problems. About 16% of all deaths, and about half of all premature deaths, are linked to tobacco. Lung cancer due to smoking is the leading cause of cancer-related deaths among men; it is second only to breast cancer as a killer of women.

Tobacco contains hundreds of toxic chemicals. Among these is a highly addictive drug called nicotine. By itself, nicotine is used as an agricultural pesticide. When nicotine is inhaled into the lungs, swallowed, or absorbed through the mucous membranes of the mouth or nose, it quickly enters the bloodstream, where it circulates to the brain. There it acts as a stimulant that speeds up heart rate, constricts the blood vessels (thus raising blood pressure), increases alertness and concentration, and reduces fatigue.

Like other addictive drugs, nicotine triggers the reward reflex in the brain. In other words, nicotine stimulates pleasurable feelings. In response, the brain seeks to repeat the behavior that produced those feelings. This results in the cravings that smokers feel when they go too long between cigarettes. Eventually, though, the body becomes tolerant to the dose of nicotine. In time, higher and higher doses of the drug must be inhaled to produce the same effect. The more smoke that enters the body and the longer smoking continues, the higher the risk of disease and death.

The cravings nicotine produces and nicotine's impact on the reward reflex reinforce the desire to keep smoking. And often smoking simply becomes a habit (a psychological addiction). Smokers may get used to lighting up after a meal or when drinking coffee or reading a book. Any time they engage in those activities, they instinctively reach for a cigarette.

Many people who try to quit smoking find it very hard to do so. Very few are able to stop permanently on their first attempt. Of the 17 million people who try to quit smoking each year, only a little more than 1 million succeed. One reason is that, as with many other addictive drugs, cessation of nicotine use can cause a range of unpleasant sensations known as withdrawal symptoms (see box). Even if they do eventually quit and remain nonsmokers for long periods, many people still notice cravings for cigarettes years later.

Nicotine Withdrawal Symptoms

- Cravings
- Frustration
- Anxiety
- Depression
- Restlessness
- Increased appetite
- Irritability
- Anger
- Difficulty concentrating
- Fatigue
- Decreased heart rate
- Weight gain

Seek medical attention if you are thinking about using nicotine replacement therapy and any of the following applies to you

- Pregnancy (or you are contemplating getting pregnant)
- Under age 18
- Heart disease
- Irregular heartbeat
- Recent heart attack
- High blood pressure not controlled by medication
- Current or past history of esophagitis or peptic ulcer disease
- Taking insulin for diabetes
- Taking prescription medications for depression or asthma
- Unable to quit on your own
- Using nicotine replacement therapy and experience:
  - Mouth, teeth, or jaw problems
  - Irregular or rapid heartbeat or palpitations
  - Nausea
  - Vomiting
  - Dizziness
  - Weakness

Treatment for Smoking Cessation

Nicotine replacement therapy is an effective method of diminishing a person's dependence on tobacco. The idea behind this strategy is to gradually reduce the amount of nicotine in the body supplied by tobacco with a controlled amount (a pharmacological dose). OTC products for nicotine replacement are available in 2 forms: gum and skin patches.

Nicotine replacement products became available in nonprescription form in 1996. The gum is available in 2-mg and 4-mg doses. The higher doses are intended for use by people who smoke more than 24 cigarettes (more than a pack) a day. It is important to stop smoking before using any nicotine replacement therapy; otherwise, between the 2 sources of nicotine, there is a risk of overdose.

To get the maximum benefit from nicotine gum, you should follow directions closely (see box).

Tips for Using Nicotine Gum

- Because food and drink can interfere with nicotine absorption, do not eat just before using the gum or while you are chewing it.
- Chew the gum very slowly. This increases the release of nicotine and helps minimize the risk of side effects.
- After a minute or so, you may notice a peppery taste or tingling in the mouth. This means it's time to park the gum in your cheek. When the taste is gone, you can chew again. Repeat this cycle as often as needed for about 30 minutes, at which time all the nicotine has been released from the gum.
- You should start to chew a piece of nicotine gum whenever you first feel a craving for a cigarette.
- For the first 6 weeks, use 1 piece no more than every 1 to 2 hours (no more than 24 pieces in a day).
- In the next 3 weeks, reduce the dose to 1 piece every 2 to 4 hours, and in the 3 weeks after that, cut down to once every 4 to 8 hours.
- If you feel like continuing this treatment beyond 12 weeks, speak to your health care provider first.

With nicotine gum, the patient controls the amount of nicotine consumed. Transdermal nicotine (nicotine patch) allows a controlled daily dose to enter the bloodstream. The patch looks like a square bandage. The medication is contained in a fabric underneath the protective outer covering. Nicotine is easily absorbed through the skin and is released in steady amounts. To reduce the risk of skin irritation, the patch should be applied to different places on the body. (If irritation does occur, hydrocortisone cream, available over the counter, can be used for relief.) As with the gum, the dose of nicotine is decreased over the next 8 to 16 weeks. People who have heart disease, who weigh under 100 pounds, or who smoke less than half a pack a day typically begin with low doses.

Some brands of the patch are meant to be worn 24 hours a day, while others are intended for use only while awake. Using the daytime-only patch may have an advantage. Nicotine is a stimulant, and even smokers take a break while they sleep. Receiving a nicotine dose around-the-clock can sometimes cause sleep disturbances, including vivid dreams.

Even with these treatments, however, quitting smoking requires determination and dedication. For one thing, although nicotine replacement reduces cravings and helps minimize withdrawal symptoms, the dose from OTC products does not produce the same effects on the body as nicotine from cigarettes. Many smokers notice a difference and consequently still feel a strong urge to smoke. Also, these products are not supposed to be used for longer than 6 months, and it may take longer than that to overcome the addiction built up by years of smoking. That's especially true in people who smoked more than a pack of cigarettes a day. Other forms of treatment may be needed to make smoking cessation permanent (see box).

Half the Battle

Smoking cessation programs have a better chance of succeeding if they help people change their behaviors relating to the use of tobacco. Among the strategies available are aversion therapy, education, group therapy, and hypnosis. Learning behavioral techniques—such as going for a walk after dinner instead of lighting up a cigarette—can be helpful. If use of nicotine replacement therapy is not enough to help you quit smoking, talk to your health care provider about other approaches.

OTC Products for Smoking Cessation

Nicotine gum
Nicotine skin patch

Smoking Cessation Products

DOSAGE FORM	BRAND	NICOTINE
GUM	Nicorette	2mg
	Nicorette DS	2mg
TRANSDERMAL PATCH	Habitrol	21, 14, 7mg
	Nicoderm	21, 14, 7mg
	Nicotrol	15, 10, 5mg
	Prostep	22, 11mg

Brand Names

Nicoderm CQ (NIK-uh-derm)
Nicotrol (NIK-uh-trol)

Generic Name

Nicotine (NIK-uh-teen)

Type of Drug

Smoking cessation product.

Used for

Ending smoking habit through nicotine replacement therapy.

General Information

There are more than 500,000 smoking-related deaths in the U.S. each year, accounting for 16% of all deaths. Smoking is linked to cardiovascular disease, pulmonary disease, and cancer.

To quit smoking it is necessary to beat the addiction to nicotine, an ingredient in tobacco. One obstacle is overcoming nicotine withdrawal symptoms, including irritability, impatience, anxiety, confusion, depression, hunger, awakening at night, impaired concentration, and/or restlessness. Research has shown that, because of the nature of nicotine addiction, some individuals take up smoking again years after quitting. Few people are able to quit permanently on their first try.

There are several behavioral therapies designed to aid smokers in quitting, including group therapy and hypnosis. When such therapies fail, a smoker desiring to quit may turn to nicotine replacement therapy. Nicotine replacement therapy entails taking nicotine in a pharmacological form in which the nicotine dose is tapered over a period of time in order to decrease withdrawal symptoms and lessen the craving for nicotine.

In the early 1990s, nicotine became available by prescription in the form of nicotine transdermal systems, or patches.

In 1996, the patch became available without a prescription. The patch consists of a backing layer, a drug-containing reservoir, an adhesive layer, and a removable protective liner. It is generally applied to the hip, abdomen, upper torso, or upper arm, and the nicotine is absorbed through the skin.

Cigarettes deliver nicotine to the brain rapidly, which can cause stimulatory and/or euphoric feelings that only increase an individual's dependency on nicotine. The patch, which is applied once a day, provides low, relatively constant levels of nicotine, and thus does not cause these habit-forming feelings.

Patches are available in either a 16-hour (Nicotrol) or a 24-hour (Nicoderm CQ) delivery system. The Nicoderm theoretically minimizes morning withdrawal symptoms, while the Nicotrol, which is worn only during waking hours, is intended to reduce adverse effects such as insomnia. Overall, they appear to be equally effective.

There is insufficient data to support recommending the nicotine patch over nicotine polacrilex gum (Nicorette), which also became available OTC in 1996. The gum has one perceived advantage over the patch: It serves as a substitute oral activity—although it does not provide the same rapid satisfaction that smoking a cigarette does. The patch has several advantages: It reduces symptoms of craving, it is more convenient than the gum, it has no oral adverse effects, and it has fewer gastrointestinal (GI) adverse effects. Some individuals also object to the gum's taste, which is deliberately unlike that of normal chewing gum.

Studies have shown that nicotine replacement therapy is effective in helping smokers overcome withdrawal symptoms, but there are many other factors, both behavioral and environmental, that make it difficult to quit smoking. Counseling can help you deal with these factors. Through counseling, for example, you can learn how to combat stress without lighting up a cigarette, or break the habit of smoking immediately after a meal by going for a walk instead. Ask your pharmacist about counseling.

Above all, for smoking cessation to be successful, the individual must truly wish to stop smoking.

Cautions and Warnings

Do not use Nicoderm CQ for longer than 12 weeks, or Nicotrol for longer than 20 weeks. It is possible for nicotine addiction to pass from cigarettes to the patch, or for the addiction to worsen. Some clinicians believe that a total of 6 to 8 weeks of therapy is sufficient.

Do not use the same patch for more than 24 hours.

Do not continue to smoke while undergoing nicotine replacement therapy. You may experience adverse effects or overdose from receiving too much nicotine. There have also been reports of individuals with stable coronary artery disease who experienced cardiac complications because they continued to smoke during therapy.

Do not use the patch if you are currently using nicotine polacrilex gum (Nicorette).

Stop using the patch if you have irregular heartbeat or palpitations, or if you have symptoms of overdose, such as nausea, dizziness, weakness, and/or rapid heartbeat (see "Overdosage"). Call your doctor.

Do not use these products if you are recovering from a recent heart attack, or if you have angina or severe abnormal heart rhythms.

These products should be used with caution by individuals with coronary artery disease, serious cardiac arrhythmia, vasospastic disease, high blood pressure, an overactive thyroid, insulin-dependent diabetes mellitus, or an ulcer. Speak to your physician, who can help you weigh the possible benefits of nicotine replacement therapy against the possible risks.

Call your doctor if you develop a severe or persistent skin reaction at the site of application.

There is the possibility that impaired liver function may reduce the elimination of nicotine from the body, but this has not been sufficiently studied.

Follow directions carefully for handling and applying these products (see "Usual Dose").

Be sure to store your patches and discard used ones out of the reach of children and pets. The amount of nicotine in a used patch can be fatal if applied or swallowed by a child or pet.

Possible Side Effects

Nicoderm CQ and Nicotrol appear to be well tolerated. Adverse effects are generally dose-related. They do not usually require stopping of therapy. It should be noted that many of the side effects potentially caused by excessive intake of nicotine are indistinguishable from nicotine withdrawal symptoms.

▼ Most common: temporary irritation, itching, or redness at the site of application; weakness (particularly during the first 6 days of treatment); headache; elevated heart rate; and increased appetite.

▼ Less common: nausea and vomiting, diarrhea rash, dyspepsia, abdominal pain, dry mouth, insomnia and abnormal dreams, somnolence, dizziness and vertigo, nervousness, impaired concentration, depression, fatigue, and muscle pain.

Drug Interactions

• Heavy smokers who suddenly stop smoking may experience an increase in the effects of a variety of drugs whose breakdown is known to be stimulated by cigarettes. If you are taking any of the following medications, your dosage may need to be reduced: theophylline, used to treat bronchical asthma; imipramine, a tricyclic antidepressant; pentazocine, a narcotic analgesic; oxazepam, a benzodiazepine tranquilizer; and the analgesics acetaminophen and propoxyphene hydrochloride.

• Smoking increases the rate at which your body breaks down caffeine. Stopping your intake of nicotine may make you more sensitive to the effects of caffeine in coffee, tea, or cola drinks.

• Smoking reduces the absorption of glutethimide, used to treat insomnia. Stopping smoking may reverse this effect, and you may have to have your dosage adjusted.

• Any drug that affects the central nervous system (CNS) (e.g., stimulants) may be affected by nicotine. Your doctor may have to adjust your dosage while you undergo nicotine replacement therapy.

• Smoking may reduce the effect of furosemide, a diuretic, and alter the effect of the beta blocker propranolol, used to treat high blood pressure. Stopping smoking may reverse these effects, and you may have to have your dosages adjusted accordingly.

Food Interactions

None known.

Usual Dose

Each Nicoderm CQ patch contains 21 mg (Step 1), 14 mg (Step 2), or 7 mg (Step 3) of nicotine.

Each Nicotrol patch contains 15 mg of nicotine.

Read the package carefully before beginning therapy.

Patches are applied once daily. Nicotrol is applied every morning after awakening and removed before going to sleep. Do not use the same patch for more than 24 hours.

Apply the patch promptly after removal from its protective pouch, or the nicotine may evaporate.

The patch should be applied to clean, dry, hairless areas of the skin on the trunk, hip, or the upper outer arm. Do not apply the patch to oily, damaged, or irritated skin, and do not shave the application site.

Press the patch firmly in place to make sure that it sticks. If it accidentally comes off, apply a new patch.

Use different application sites to avoid skin irritation.

After handling a patch, wash your hands with water alone, because soap may enhance absorption of the drug. Do not touch your eyes before washing your hands.

Overdosage

Nicotine toxicity is characterized by nausea, increased salivation, abdominal pain, vomiting, diarrhea, sweating, headache, dizziness, hearing and visual disturbances, mental confusion, and marked weakness. Death may occur within a few minutes after severe overdosage, due to paralysis of respiratory muscles.

Even if the victim is not displaying any of the symptoms listed above, do the following in case of accidental ingestion or overdose: If the victim is unconscious or having convulsions, call for an ambulance immediately. If you take the victim to an emergency room, be sure to bring the packaging with you. If the victim is conscious, call your local poison control center or a health care professional. The poison control center may suggest inducing vomiting with ipecac syrup (available without a prescription at any pharmacy). DO NOT induce vomiting unless specifically instructed to do so.

Storage Instructions

Nicotine is very sensitive to heat and must be stored at room temperature. Nicotine turns brown if exposed to light or air; this does not affect its potency or effectiveness.

Special Populations

Pregnancy/Breast-feeding

Nicotine may cause harm to the fetus. Cigarette smoking has also been associated with miscarriage and with low birth weight. Some clinicians maintain that the risk to the fetus is less with nicotine replacement therapy than with cigarette smoking, but it is recommended that behavioral and educational smoking cessation therapies be considered first by pregnant women who want to quit smoking. Talk to your doctor to discuss possible hazards to your unborn baby if you undergo nicotine replacement therapy.

Nicotine passes into breast milk. Talk to your doctor to weigh the possible risks associated with continued cigarette smoking against those associated with Nicoderm CQ and Nicotrol.

Infants/Children

The safety of these products in children or teenagers (under age 18) who smoke has not been established, and its use is not recommended.

Seniors

According to limited evidence, these products appear to be as effective in seniors as in younger adults. However, there have been no studies specifically geared toward older individuals. For now, seniors should exercise the same caution as younger adults when undergoing nicotine replacement therapy.

Brand Name

Nicorette (NIH-kor-et)

Generic Name

Nicotine polacrilex (NIK-uh-teen POL-uh-cril-eks)

Type of Drug

Smoking cessation product.

Used for

Ending smoking habit through nicotine replacement therapy.

General Information

There are more than 500,000 smoking-related deaths in the U.S. each year, accounting for 16% of all deaths. Smoking is linked to cardiovascular disease, pulmonary disease, and cancer.

To quit smoking it is necessary to beat the addiction to nicotine, an ingredient in tobacco. One obstacle is overcoming nicotine withdrawal symptoms, including irritability, impatience, anxiety, confusion, depression, hunger, awakening at night, impaired concentration, and restlessness. Research has shown that, because of the nature of nicotine addiction, some individuals take up smoking again years after quitting. In addition, few people are able to quit permanently on their first try.

There are several behavioral therapies designed to aid smokers in quitting, including group therapy and hypnosis. When such therapies fail, a smoker desiring to quit may supplement behavioral modification with nicotine replacement therapy, which entails taking nicotine in a pharmacological form. The nicotine dose is gradually decreased over a period of about 3 months; the individual is thus weaned from nicotine. Any nicotine withdrawal symptoms are much less severe than they would be if the smoker were to quit cold turkey and the craving for nicotine is also lessened. However, be aware that nicotine taken in pharmacological doses does not reduce these symptoms to the degree that smoked nicotine does.

In 1984 nicotine polacrilex resin became available by prescription in the form of gum. In 1996 the gum became available without a prescription. The gum comes in either a 2-mg or a 4-mg dose; the latter is for individuals who smoke more than 24 cigarettes a day. Unlike the nicotine patch, which is applied once a day, Nicorette must be chewed throughout the day (see "Usual Dose").

There are insufficient data to support recommending nicotine gum over the patch. The gum has 1 perceived advantage over the patch: It serves as a substitute oral activity—although it does not provide the same rapid satisfaction that smoking a cigarette does. The patch has several advantages over the gum: It reduces symptoms of craving, it is more convenient, it has no oral adverse effects, and it has fewer gastrointestinal (GI) adverse effects. Some individuals also object to the gum's taste, which is deliberately unlike that of normal chewing gum.

Studies have shown that nicotine replacement therapy is effective in helping smokers overcome withdrawal symptoms, but there are many other factors, both behavioral and environmental, that make it difficult to quit smoking. Counseling can help you deal with these factors. Through counseling, for example, you can learn how to combat stress without lighting up a cigarette, or break the habit of smoking immediately after a meal by going for a walk instead. Ask your pharmacist about counseling.

Above all, for smoking cessation to be successful, the individual must truly wish to stop smoking.

Cautions and Warnings

Do not continue to smoke or chew tobacco while undergoing nicotine replacement therapy. You may experience adverse effects or overdose from receiving too much nicotine. There have also been reports, albeit rare, of individuals with stable coronary artery disease experiencing cardiac complications because they continued to smoke during therapy.

Do not use Nicorette if you are currently using the nicotine patch.

Do not stop using Nicorette until your craving is satisfied by 1 or 2 pieces daily, but do not use it for longer than 12 weeks. In addition, you should not exceed the recommended daily dose of 24 pieces. It is possible for nicotine addiction to pass from cigarettes to the patch or gum, or for your addiction to worsen.

Stop using Nicorette and call your doctor if you have irregular heartbeat or palpitations; if you have symptoms of overdose, such as nausea, dizziness, weakness, and rapid heartbeat; or if you develop mouth, teeth, or jaw problems.

Do not use Nicorette if you are recovering from a recent heart attack, or if you have angina (chest pain) or severe abnormal heart rhythms.

Nicorette should be used with caution by individuals with coronary artery disease, serious cardiac arrhythmia, vasospastic disease, high blood pressure, an overactive thyroid, insulin-dependent diabetes mellitus, an ulcer, or esophagitis. Speak to your physician, who can help you weigh the possible benefits of nicotine replacement therapy against the possible risks.

There is the possibility that impaired liver function may reduce the elimination of nicotine from the body, but this has not been sufficiently studied.

Do not chew Nicorette too rapidly or you may experience light-headedness, nausea, irritation of the throat and mouth, hiccups, and indigestion.

Do not swallow Nicorette.

Do not chew more than 1 piece at a time.

Nicorette is gooier than normal chewing gum and may stick to dentures or loosen inlays or fillings. If you experience this consistently, you may need to stop therapy and see a dentist.

Keep this product out of the reach of children and pets.

Possible Side Effects

Adverse effects associated with Nicorette are generally mild and temporary, and are mainly related to the physical effects of gum chewing.

▼ Most common oral effects: injury to the oral mucosa and/or teeth, irritation and/or tingling of the tongue, ulceration of the oral mucosa, aching jaw muscle, belching from swallowing too much air, gum sticking

Possible Side Effects ***(continued)***

to teeth, and unpleasant taste. Most of these effects go away after the first few days of therapy.

▼ Most common GI effects: indigestion and nausea, caused in part by excessive chewing that releases the nicotine too rapidly causing excess saliva and accidental swallowing of the gum. These adverse effects generally occur within the first week of therapy and may be reduced by modifying chewing technique.

▼ Other common effects: dry mouth, loss of appetite, diarrhea, constipation, flatulence, dizziness, light-headedness, headache, insomnia, irritability, and hiccups.

Drug Interactions

• Heavy smokers who suddenly stop smoking may experience an increase in the effects of a variety of drugs whose breakdown is known to be stimulated by cigarettes. If you are taking any of the following medications, your dosage may have to be reduced: theophylline, used to treat bronchial asthma; imipramine, a tricyclic antidepressant; pentazocine, a narcotic analgesic; oxazepam, a benzodiazepine tranquilizer; and the analgesics acetaminophen and propoxyphene hydrochloride.

• Smoking increases the rate at which your body breaks down caffeine. Stopping your intake of nicotine may make you more sensitive to the effects of caffeine in coffee, tea, or cola drinks.

• Smoking increases the absorption of glutethimide, used to treat insomnia. Stopping smoking may reverse this effect, and you may have to have your dosage adjusted.

• Any drug that affects the central nervous system (CNS) (e.g., stimulants) may be affected by nicotine. Your doctor may have to adjust your dosage of the drug while you undergo nicotine replacement therapy.

• Smoking may reduce the effect of furosemide, a diuretic, and alter the effect of the beta blocker propranolol, used to treat high blood pressure. Stopping smoking may reverse these effects, and you may have to have your dosages adjusted accordingly.

Food Interactions

Do not eat or drink coffee, juice, wine, or a soft drink for 15 minutes before chewing Nicorette or while chewing. Food and certain drinks may interfere with the absorption of the nicotine. After eating or drinking, rinse your mouth out with water before chewing Nicorette.

Usual Dose

Nicorette is available in either a 2-mg or a 4-mg dose; the latter is for individuals who smoke more than 24 cigarettes a day.

Read package carefully before beginning therapy.

Do not chew Nicorette on an as-needed basis. Follow this schedule:

Weeks 1–6: 1 piece every 1–2 hours.
Weeks 7–9: 1 piece every 2–4 hours.
Weeks 10–12: 1 piece every 4–8 hours.

Chew Nicorette very slowly until you taste nicotine (a peppery taste) or feel a slight tingling in your mouth. Stop chewing until the tingling is almost gone (about 1 minute), then repeat the process intermittently for about 30 minutes. This takes advantage of Nicorette's slow-release formula.

If you forget to take a dose of Nicorette, do so as soon as you remember. If it is almost time for your next dose, skip the one you forgot and continue with your regular schedule. Do not take a double dose.

Do not chew Nicorette too rapidly or swallow it.

Do not use Nicorette for longer than 12 weeks. Do not chew more than 24 pieces a day.

Nicorette may be combined with normal, sugar-free chewing gum to make it softer and easier to chew.

Overdosage

Overdose with Nicorette can occur if many pieces of the gum are chewed simultaneously or in rapid succession. Nicotine toxicity is characterized by nausea, excess salivation, abdominal pain, vomiting, diarrhea, perspiration, headache, dizziness, hearing and visual disturbances, mental confusion, and marked weakness. Death due to paralysis of respiratory muscles may occur within a few minutes after severe overdose.

Even if the victim is not displaying any of the symptoms listed above, do the following in case of accidental overdose: If the victim is unconscious or having convulsions, call for an ambulance immediately. If you take the victim to an emergency room, be sure to bring the bottle or container with you. If the victim is conscious, call your local poison control center or a health care professional. The poison control center may suggest inducing vomiting with ipecac syrup (available without a prescription at any pharmacy). DO NOT induce vomiting unless specifically instructed to do so.

Assuming proper dosing guidelines have been followed, accidentally swallowing the gum may cause adverse effects, but does not cause overdose.

Storage Instructions

Nicotine is very sensitive to heat and must be stored at room temperature. Nicotine turns brown if exposed to light or air; this does not affect its potency or effectiveness.

Special Populations

Pregnancy/Breast-feeding

Nicotine may cause harm to the fetus. Cigarette smoking has also been associated with miscarriage and with decreased birthweight. Some clinicians maintain that the risk to the unborn baby is less with nicotine replacement therapy than with cigarette smoking, but it is recommended that behavioral and educational smoking cessation therapies be tried first by pregnant women who want to quit smoking. Talk to your doctor to discuss possible hazards to your unborn baby before you undergo nicotine replacement therapy.

Nicotine passes into breast milk. Talk to your doctor to weigh the possible risks associated with continued cigarette smoking against those associated with use of Nicorette.

Infants/Children

The safety of Nicorette in children or teenagers (under age 18) who smoke has not been established, and its use is not recommended.

Seniors

According to limited evidence, Nicorette appears to be as effective in seniors as in younger adults. However, there have been no studies specifically geared toward older individuals.

For now, seniors should exercise the same caution as younger adults when undergoing nicotine replacement therapy.

Nicotrol (NIK-uh-trol)

*see **Nicoderm CQ,** page 602*

Chapter 12: Vomiting and Motion Sickness

As unpleasant as it is, vomiting serves a purpose: It is the body's way of getting rid of toxic substances from the stomach. In emergencies, such as accidental poisoning, drugs called emetics are sometimes given to trigger vomiting.

At other times, vomiting can be a symptom of medical illnesses, such as peptic ulcer, appendicitis, or gastroenteritis (viral stomach infection). Usually vomiting is preceded by nausea, a queasy, upset feeling in the stomach. But vomiting can also occur without nausea. This sometimes happens if a brain tumor has developed or a head injury has occurred. Metabolic disorders such as diabetes can sometimes disrupt body function to the point where vomiting occurs. Extreme pain, such as that arising during a migraine headache, can trigger nausea and vomiting. About half of all pregnant women suffer from bouts of morning sickness, which in most cases involves both nausea and vomiting. Emotional stress or feelings of disgust may be so powerful that they induce vomiting. Some people vomit in response to medications such as anesthesia or chemotherapy. Prescription and OTC drugs can also occasionally cause both nausea and vomiting.

Nausea and vomiting can also be triggered by sensations of dizziness or loss of balance. The body's center of balance is located in the inner ear. Structures there (known as the labyrinth and the vestibule) help coordinate signals from the eyes, skin, and joints to let the brain know what position the body is in: whether it is upright or lying down; if it is in motion; and if so, in which direction it is going. Conditions such as ear infections can disrupt the sense of balance. So too can unusual rhythmic movement in different directions, such as that experienced in a boat or a carnival ride. These movements cause dizziness because they overstimulate the inner ear and make it hard for the brain to remain oriented to a fixed point in space. The brain needs an accurate and stable orienting image to process information properly. Usually that image is a stationary object on the near horizon.

Motion sickness refers to the nausea and vomiting that occur during travel. Carsickness, airsickness, and seasickness are all forms of motion sickness. (For a select few, space sickness—resulting from the absence of gravity and changes in pressure on the ears—is also a concern.) Everyone is vulnerable to motion sickness if the stimulation is strong enough.

Riding along a winding road in a bouncing car can upset your sense of balance. Passengers in the back seat of a car often do not have a clear view of objects in the distance—objects that remain relatively steady and that help the brain stay oriented. Instead, rear passengers usually look out the side windows, where objects are whizzing by, making it hard to focus. Planes and boats add a vertical dimension to travel and there are usually no fixed points on the horizon to gaze at. Motion sickness can also be triggered by other factors, such as unpleasant odors, emotional stress, fatigue—or that greasy hamburger you wolfed down at the last rest stop.

In mild cases, motion sickness may cause only a vague feeling of uneasiness, tiredness, or headache. As it worsens, the illness can lead to anxiety, sweating, loss of color, rapid breathing, and excessive saliva production. The digestive process basically shuts down. Nausea may develop, which often progresses to vomiting.

Symptoms of motion sickness almost always vanish as soon as you stop riding in the vehicle. Fortunately, during long trips, many people eventually get accustomed to the sensations of travel, and the nausea usually vanishes. However, once people have experienced severe motion sickness, they may become more tense and anxious about traveling again. That anxiety may contribute to future episodes of the problem.

Treatment for Motion Sickness, Nausea, and Vomiting

It is generally easier to prevent motion sickness than to treat it once it develops (see box). Some OTC products are available that reduce the risk of travel-related illness. The main ingredients in these products are antihistamines, which work by reducing the sensitivity of the balance-regulating structures in the inner ear. An antihistamine should be taken 30 to 60 minutes before travel begins, and should be taken as needed for the duration of the trip. The different types of antihistamine work somewhat differently. For example, meclizine (Bonine) and cyclizine (Marezine) are effective for up to 24 hours, while dimenhydrinate

(Dramamine) should be taken every 4 to 6 hours. Be sure and read package directions and follow your pharmacist's recommendations for proper use.

Seek medical attention if any of the following applies to you

- Blood in the vomit
- Abdominal pain or swelling
- An inability to keep down liquids
- Nausea and vomiting that persist for longer than 1 or 2 days
- Projectile vomiting
- Dehydration
- Loss of 5% or more of body weight
- Fever
- Severe headache, especially if worse in the morning
- Suspected poisoning

Tips for Preventing Motion Sickness

- Sit in the middle or front seat of the car if possible.
- Stop the car periodically and get out to stretch your legs.
- Open the car window for fresh air.
- Place a shade over the side window.
- Avoid eating large meals prior to or during a trip.
- Look out the car window and focus on the horizon or on distant sites.
- Avoid reading.
- Minimize exposure to fumes (car exhaust, perfumes, tobacco smoke).
- Take OTC antinausea medications prior to departure.
- If riding in a small boat, try to sit in the center of the vessel. Lean back against a firm surface and keep your eye on the horizon. Avoid moving the neck.
- On a ship, go up on deck and stare at the ocean.

The main side effect of antihistamines is drowsiness. If you take one of these medications, do not drive or operate other vehicles. Avoid drinking alcohol or taking other drugs that act on the central nervous system, such as tranquilizers or sedatives. In high doses, antihistamines can cause blurred vision, dry mouth, and urinary retention.

There is always concern about whether pregnant women should take medications because of potential danger to the developing fetus. The same is true in cases of morning sickness. Generally, the OTC antihistamines available pose a low risk, but if you are pregnant, you should talk to your doctor before taking any medication. Diphenhydramine and dimenhydrinate are among the products approved as safe and effective for treatment of morning sickness.

Phosphorated carbohydrate solution is an option for treating nausea and vomiting associated with intestinal flu, indigestion, or emotional stress. This product is taken in doses of 1 to 2 tablespoons every 15 minutes until vomiting stops.

Bismuth salts (e.g., Pepto-Bismol) can be taken for relief of nausea brought on by overeating or drinking. This medication will not prevent vomiting, nor is it used in treatment of motion sickness.

OTC Products for Motion Sickness, Nausea, and Vomiting

Antihistamines
- Cyclizine
- Dimenhydrinate
- Diphenhydramine
- Meclizine

Other
- Bismuth salts
- Phosphorated carbohydrate solution

Accidental Poisoning or Drug Overdose

Emetics are usually administered in cases of accidental poisoning or drug overdose. Physicians recommend that every household keep an emetic on hand to treat such emergencies. However, emetics should not be used without first calling the doctor or local poison control center.

The main drug for this purpose—in fact, the only one considered safe and effective—is ipecac syrup. Children should be given 1 tablespoon of the medication; the dosage in adolescents and adults is 1 to 2 tablespoons. The person should then drink a glass or 2 of fluid. If possible, the person should try to keep moving around rather than lying still.

Usually the drug works as intended, but if vomiting does not occur within 20 minutes, the dose can be repeated. Ipecac syrup should not be given if the person is unconscious, and it should not be used if the person has swallowed a petroleum product (such as gasoline), strong acids or alkalis, or strychnine. Vomiting up these substances can cause serious damage to the delicate tissues of the esophagus and poses a risk of inhaling them into the lungs. If the person has swallowed these substances (or if vomiting does not occur after ipecac syrup is administered), an ambulance should be called so that treatment in an emergency room can be administered. Side effects of ipecac syrup are not usually a problem, but sometimes diarrhea, stomach upset, and mild mental confusion or dullness may develop.

Another option for treatment of poisoning is the adsorbent, activated charcoal. This substance, also available as an OTC product and classified as a gastric decontaminant, works like a sponge: It soaks up drugs and chemicals to prevent them from being absorbed by the stomach and intestines. Activated charcoal has been shown to prevent poisoning from overdoses or ingestion of acetaminophen, aspirin, kerosene, insecticides, nicotine, strychnine, and a number of other substances. Some forms of charcoal must be mixed with water; others come ready-mixed. Activated charcoal should not be given at the same time as ipecac syrup, because in many cases the charcoal will bind with ipecac and vomiting will not occur. Activated charcoal may be given after vomiting has been induced.

OTC Product for Inducing Vomiting
Ipecac syrup

OTC Product for Counteracting Poison or Drug Overdose
Activated charcoal

Antiemetic Products

BRAND NAME	ANTIEMETIC INGREDIENT					
	cyclizine HCl	dimen-hydrinate	diphen-hydramine	meclizine HCl	phos-phorated carbo-hydrate	phos-phoric acid
Bonine				25mg		
Calm-X		50mg				
Cola						x
Dramamine		50mg				
Dramamine II Less Drowsy Formula				25mg		
Dramamine Original		50mg				
Dramamine, Children's [A]		12.5mg/5ml				
Emetrol						12.5g/5ml
Especol					x	
Marezine	50mg					
Nauzene [S]			25mg			
Triptone		50mg				

Emetics

BRAND NAME	ACTIVE INGREDIENT	OTHER INGREDIENTS
Ipecac	powdered ipecac	alcohol glycerin purified water

Gastric Decontaminants

BRAND NAME	ACTIVATED CHARCOAL
Actidose with Sorbitol	25g/120ml; 50g/240 ml
Actidose-Aqua	15g/72ml; 25g/120ml; 50g/240ml
CharcoAid [S]	30g/120ml
CharcoAid 2000 [S]	50g/240ml
Charcoal Plus DS	250mg
CharcoCaps (caplet)	260mg
CharcoCaps (capsule) [S]	260mg
CharcoCaps (tablet)	250mg
Liqui Char	25g/4oz

Dramamine (DRA-muh-meen)

*see **Dimenhydrinate,** page 791*

Brand Name

Marezine (MARE-eh-zeen)

Generic Ingredient

Cyclizine hydrochloride (SYE-kli-zeen HYE-droe-KLOR-ide)

Type of Drug

Antihistamine used as an antiemetic.

Used for

The prevention and treatment of nausea, vomiting, and dizziness associated with motion sickness.

General Information

Nausea and emesis (vomiting) may be caused by various disorders: some minor, some serious. Various antiemetics are used to treat nausea and vomiting caused by motion sickness; pregnancy; mild infectious disease; radiation therapy; cancer chemotherapy; and metabolic, central nervous system (CNS), gastrointestinal (GI), and endocrine disorders.

Cyclizine is approved only for the prevention and treatment of motion sickness, the nausea and vomiting associated with traveling, a relatively minor, temporary condition.

Cyclizine is one of a group of drugs called antihistamines. Besides having many other uses, including the treatment of colds and allergies, antihistamines are the primary ingredient in OTC antiemetic products. Cyclizine is used only as an antiemetic. Its use as an allergy and cold remedy has not been evaluated.

While it is not known precisely how cyclizine works, certain antihistamines have a depressant effect on overstimulated labyrinthine (inner ear) function, which is what causes motion sickness. Cyclizine is equal in effectiveness to the antihistamine antiemetic dimenhydrinate, but causes drowsiness (a common side effect of antihistamines) less frequently.

Cyclizine is indicated for the prevention as well as the treatment of motion sickness. Motion sickness is much easier to prevent than to treat once it has already begun.

Cyclizine begins working within 1 hour and continues to work for 4 to 6 hours. It has a much shorter duration of action than a similar antihistamine, meclizine, which is usually taken only once a day. However, cyclizine, unlike meclizine, may be safely taken by children under age 12 (although cyclizine is not recommended for children under age 6).

Marezine is available in tablet form.

Cautions and Warnings

Do not use Marezine too frequently or for a prolonged period unless directed by your doctor.

Do not exceed the recommended daily dosage of Marezine.

Cyclizine, like all antihistamines, may cause extreme drowsiness, which may be exacerbated by the concurrent use of alcoholic beverages, sedatives, hypnotics, or tranquilizers (see "Drug Interactions"). If you are taking Marezine, use caution when performing activities that require mental alertness or physical coordination, such as driving a motor vehicle or operating machinery.

Unless recommended by a doctor, Marezine should not be used by people who have a breathing problem, such as emphysema or chronic bronchitis, or by people with asthma.

Marezine should be used with caution by people with glaucoma, hyperthyroidism, heart disease, high blood pressure, an enlarged prostate, or obstructive disease of the GI tract. If you have any of these conditions, take Marezine only on the advice of your doctor.

Nausea and vomiting associated with radiation therapy; cancer chemotherapy; and metabolic, CNS, GI, and endocrine disorders are serious conditions that should not be self-medicated with Marezine. Consult your doctor.

Marezine should not be used for treating nausea and vomiting caused by pregnancy.

Possible Side Effects

▼ Common: drowsiness.

▼ Rare: blurred vision, dry mouth, and urinary retention.

Drug Interactions

• Antihistamines can enhance the effect of other drugs that depress the CNS, such as barbiturates, tranquilizers, sleeping medications, and alcohol (present in many OTC preparations). If you are taking other depressant drugs, check with your doctor before you take Marezine. Avoid drinking alcohol if you are taking Marezine.

• Antihistamines can affect the results of skin and blood tests. Notify your health care professional before scheduling these tests if you are taking Marezine.

Food Interactions

None known.

Usual Dose

Each tablet of Marezine contains 50 mg of cyclizine hydrochloride.

Adult and Child (age 12 and over): 50 mg every 4–6 hours, not to exceed 200 mg in 24 hours.

Child (age 6–11): 25 mg every 6–8 hours, not to exceed 75 mg in 24 hours.

Child (under age 6): not recommended.

To prevent motion sickness, take Marezine 1 hour before departure for travel.

Overdosage

Symptoms of antihistamine overdose in children include dilated pupils, flushed face, dry mouth, fever, excitability, hallucinations, loss of muscle coordination, and seizures.

In adults, severe overdose can cause drowsiness or coma, which may be followed by excitability or seizures. Eventually fluid can build up in the brain; the kidneys may fail, and the heart and lungs may stop working, resulting in death.

Symptoms may develop within 30 minutes to 2 hours following an overdose of Marezine, and death may occur within 18 hours.

Even if the victim is not displaying any of the symptoms listed above, do the following in case of accidental overdose: If the victim is unconscious or having convulsions, call for an ambulance immediately. If you take the victim to an emergency room, be sure to bring the bottle or container with you. If the victim is conscious, call your local poison control center or a health care professional. The poison control center may suggest inducing vomiting with ipecac syrup (available without a prescription at any pharmacy). DO NOT induce vomiting unless specifically instructed to do so.

Special Populations

Pregnancy/Breast-feeding

Antihistamines are not recommended for use during pregnancy unless directed by your doctor. Antihistamines are known to pass into the breast milk of nursing mothers and may cause side effects in infants. Check with your doctor before taking Marezine if you are or might be pregnant, or if you are breast-feeding.

Infants/Children

Because most studies involving antiemetics are conducted with adults, the use of these products in children is controversial. Some clinicians question whether children suffering from a temporary, minor disorder such as motion sickness should be treated at all.

Children may be more susceptible to the side effects of Marezine. They are also more susceptible to accidental antihistamine overdose. Do not give Marezine to a child under 6 unless directed by your doctor.

Seniors

Older persons may be more sensitive to the side effects of Marezine and may experience nervousness, irritability, and restlessness. Dizziness, sedation, and low blood pressure may also occur. Most mild reactions may be handled by either lowering your dose or trying another antihistamine.

Chapter 13: Baby Care

Pain and Fever

A child's normal body temperature depends on several factors, such as activity level, age, and time of day. An infant's temperature tends to be higher than an older child's, and all body temperatures rise in the afternoon and evening, and are lowest between midnight and the early morning. A normal temperature for a child under 3 can be as high as 100.4°F (taken rectally) or, for a child over 3, 100°F (taken rectally).

A fever by itself is not an illness. It is an indication that the body is battling an infection. Fever stimulates the production of white blood cells, which destroy bacteria. However, fever can make your child feel uncomfortable by increasing the pulse and breathing rate and the need for fluids.

Fever in children often accompanies ear infections, respiratory illnesses (e.g., pneumonia), flu, severe colds, sore throats, urinary tract infections, and viral illnesses.

Seek medical attention if any of the following applies to your child

- High fever
  - Over 100°F—taken rectally—for a child under 3 months old
  - Over 103°F—taken rectally—for a child over 3 months old
- Any fever accompanied by:
  - Changes in behavior (acts frightened, talks strangely)
  - Seeing things that are not there
- Fever lasts for more than 24 hours

Strategies for relieving fever

Sponge with tepid water
Shallow, tepid baths
Dress lightly
Drink extra fluids
Keep your child's room cool
Avoid fatty foods and foods that are hard to digest

Treatment for Pain and Fever

The main OTC product for relieving pain, aches, and fever in children is acetaminophen, available in products such as Tylenol, Panadol, and Tempra. Ibuprofen (Advil, Motrin) is suitable for children over 6 months. Read the label of all analgesic (pain-relieving) products carefully, and consult your physician about children under age 2 or those who weigh less than 24 pounds. Always check with your physician or pharmacist to find out the dosage that is right for your child. In determining the correct dose, a child's body weight is a more important factor than age.

Aspirin and Reye's Syndrome

Aspirin—even so-called children's aspirin—should not be taken by anyone under age 16 unless recommended by a doctor, because of the risk of a rare complication called Reye's syndrome. This disease, occurring mainly in children, causes damage to nerves, brain, and liver; in about 30% of cases, it is fatal.

OTC Products for Pain and Fever Relief

Acetaminophen
Ibuprofen

Coughs and Colds

The common cold is even more common among infants and children than adults. That's due in part to the fact that a child's immune system has not yet built up the resistance it needs to fight off ordinary infections. Another reason is that children spend much of their day in close contact with one another in schools or day-care centers, settings in which germs readily pass from one person to another. The problem is worse in the winter, when people spend more time indoors. (For more information about colds, see chapter 2.)

Viral infections such as colds and the flu can be spread by exposure to particles sneezed or coughed into the air, but more often, they are passed by contact with something that an infected person has touched. Babies, of course, are unable to prevent themselves from being exposed to such infections. Parents should do what they can to minimize risks, but it is impossible to prevent colds from occurring.

Treatment for Coughs and Colds

Most colds will get better over the course of a few days and vanish on their own. In the meanwhile, however, there are many steps you can take to relieve your baby's symptoms.

If the child's nose is congested, mucus can be loosened with the use of saline solution nose drops. OTC saline products are available in drugstores, or you can make your own (see box). The fluid can then be gently aspirated (sucked out) using a special bulb syringe, also available in drugstores.

Recipe for Saline Solution

- ¼ tsp salt
- ¾ cup (6 oz.) warm water
- Medicine dropper with suction end

Mix salt and water; stir. Apply as needed in nostrils, using medicine dropper. Suction each nostril gently with nasal bulb syringe.

Seek medical attention if any of the following applies to your child

- Changes in behavior
- Dehydration
- Difficulty breathing, wheezing, or rapid breathing not due to nasal congestion
- Difficulty swallowing
- Dry mouth (inside)
- Ear pain (child pulls at ears)
- Headache
- Unusual high-pitched crying
- Lethargy, marked irritability
- Persistent loss of appetite
- Seizures
- Skin rash
- Sore or swollen joints
- Sore throat
- Stiff neck
- Stomach pain
- Symptoms that get worse after 5 days of appropriate treatment
- Unresponsive or limp
- Vomiting or diarrhea

Humidifying the air in the child's bedroom can help keep nasal passages moist and break up thick mucus secretions. Ultrasonic humidifiers release cool, microscopic water particles into the air. There is some risk that standing water in a humidifier may allow bacteria to grow; this bacteria can then be spread by the humidifier and can cause infection. If you use a humidifier or vaporizer, be sure to clean it regularly according to the instructions that come with the product.

The time-honored advice for relief of colds—drink plenty of fluids—applies to infants as well. The child should be allowed to drink as much as possible. Fluid intake reduces the risk of dehydration and also helps keep mucus secretions thinner and easier to expel. Do not force or encourage a child to eat or drink if he or she is clearly not interested because this may provoke vomiting.

It may help to elevate one end of the crib or bed mattress by placing an object underneath it so that the child sleeps with the head higher than the feet. This promotes easier breathing and reduces coughing. Keeping the window open for coolness during sleep can relieve swollen tissues in the throat, thus making coughing less harsh and painful.

To relieve cough, children over the age of 2 years can be encouraged to sip 1/2 to 1 teaspoonful of a mixture of 2 parts honey to 1 part lemon juice.

No OTC medications will cure a cold or shorten its duration. As is true of adult colds, these products provide—at best—some short-term relief of symptoms. However, they must be used with extreme caution because children are more susceptible to the active ingredients and are more likely to experience side effects. No cold medications should be given to any child under 6 months old unless specifically prescribed by a physician. In older children, these products should be administered only in recommended doses. Treatment should stop if no improvement is seen or if side effects develop.

Cold products contain antihistamines, medications that work by counteracting histamine, a chemical released by the body's cells in response to exposure to an allergen (a substance that triggers an allergic reaction). (For more information, see chapters 2 and 7.) These products relieve congestion and runny nose. However, they can cause too much dryness, which can make such problems as sore throat or cough worse. Antihistamines also cause drowsiness and are used as sleep-inducing medications (see chapter 6). In most cases, if OTC antihistamines are given to children, they should be administered only at night. Even if the medication does not help relieve the symptoms of a cold, it may help the child get a good night's sleep—an important part of getting well. Dryness or other side effects may not be noticed during this time.

Many OTC cold relief products contain antitussives (cough suppressants). Generally, these work against the body's natural healing process. Coughing is necessary to loosen and expel mucus. Suppressing that natural reflex is counterproductive. However, you might consider giving an antitussive if the cough is so severe that it keeps the child awake at night.

Expectorants are drugs that break up mucus secretions and make them easier to expel through coughing. Generally these are not effective and are not needed for treatment of children's colds. Drinking fluids and keeping the air humidified are usually enough to achieve this goal. The pain and fever that often accompany coughs and colds can be treated with OTC analgesics. (See previous section in this chapter for more information on pain and fever relief.)

OTC Products for Coughs and Colds

Saline solutions and nasal bulb syringe
Analgesics (e.g., acetaminophen and ibuprofen)
Decongestants
Cough suppressants

Diaper Rash

Diaper rash is a skin irritation of the groin and buttocks that affects infants and children who wear diapers. The rash can develop from a combination of causes.

The main factor in diaper rash is prolonged exposure of the skin to fecal matter or urine. Children with diarrhea or frequent bowel movements are more likely to suffer from diaper rash. Feces is alkaline (the opposite of acidic), and apparently this quality contributes to its ability to cause skin irritation. A fungus called *Candida albicans* may also cause or contribute to the complications of diaper rash. This fungus, a form of yeast, is normally found in the mouth, the digestive tract, and the vagina. If the number of fungus cells becomes too great, an infection can develop such as thrush (mouth infection), a vaginal yeast infection, or diaper rash.

Contrary to common belief, the ammonia in urine does not appear to be a significant factor in diaper rash. Furthermore, urine is not likely to cause bacterial infection because urine (except in people with a urinary tract infection) is actually sterile. Instead, it is simply the presence of wetness in the diaper that causes rash. If the skin in the diaper area becomes waterlogged, the sweat glands are unable to release moisture. The pores of the skin can become plugged, which causes feelings of irritation (also known as prickly heat) and which can lead to the development of small fluid-filled blisters called vesicles.

The rash can also develop, or can be made worse, because of friction or chafing from tight-fitting diapers or from plastic pants with elastic bands. Certain soaps, detergents, or bleach used in laundry products can contribute to diaper rash.

Other microorganisms besides fungi can also trigger a diaper rash. Bacteria such as staphylococcal germs may be involved, causing enlarged, circular blistered lesions. In this case, prescription antibiotics may be needed.

Preventing Diaper Rash

- Check diapers frequently.
- Change diapers as soon as possible after they become soiled, especially after a bowel movement.
- If rash develops, try switching the type of diapers, soaps, wipes, or detergents you are using.
- Keep the diaper area clean, cool, and dry.
- Avoid using plastic pants; these increase heat and prevent moisture from evaporating.
- For cleaning, use clean soft cloths and plain warm (not hot) water.
- Use mild soap (or no soap at all).
- Do not use bubble bath or bath oil.
- Avoid using wipes that contain alcohol or scents.
- Allow skin to dry completely before putting on the new diaper. Some experts suggest the careful use of a hair blow-dryer, set to the lowest setting.
- If you use disposable diapers, try the extra-absorbent variety.
- If you use cloth diapers and do not subscribe to a diaper laundry service, boil the diapers for 15 minutes after laundering to remove traces of soap or detergents.

Dealing with Existing Rash

- If possible, leave the diaper area uncovered and exposed to air for several hours a day. For example, allow the child to nap while sleeping on an open diaper or thick, absorbent towel.
- Apply protective creams or ointments (such as petroleum jelly or zinc oxide) as barriers to the moisture.

Seek medical attention if any of the following applies to your child

- Rash involving pimples, blisters, raised patches, or small open sores
- Fever
- Poor appetite or weight loss
- Rash spreading to other parts of the body
- Rash worsening or failing to heal despite 3 to 7 days of appropriate treatment

Treatment for Diaper Rash

Mild cases of diaper rash usually improve if diapers are changed frequently (at least every couple of hours), if the diaper area is cleaned thoroughly using warm water and soft cloths or cotton balls, and if the use of plastic pants or other restrictive or impermeable garments is avoided.

Ointments are oil-based products that form a protective layer and prevent moisture from coming in contact with the skin. The main OTC ointments available for treatment and prevention of diaper rash are those containing zinc oxide (such as Desitin) and those with petrolatum (such as A and D Ointment). Zinc oxide products appear to work better for keeping skin dry and are less likely to cause irritation. Do not use OTC topical corticosteroids (e.g., hydrocortisone skin cream) for diaper rash unless advised by your pediatrician (see box).

A Word About Hydrocortisone: No

The topical corticosteroid hydrocortisone is widely used as a safe and effective OTC product for treating the redness and irritation of everyday skin problems. However, it is not appropriate for routine use in babies with diaper rash. The inflamed and raw skin, coupled with the use of a diaper that covers the area, means that the medication may be absorbed at higher levels than are safe for tiny bodies. Generally, hydrocortisone is of potential value only in serious cases where a zinc oxide cream has not been effective. Infants with moderate or severe rash should be under the care of a physician. Also, avoid using any skin care products that contain other ingredients that may irritate an infant's tender skin, such as

- benzoin tincture
- boric acid
- camphor
- methyl salicylate
- topical diphenhydramine

For decades, talcum powder has been applied to absorb moisture and reduce skin friction. However, there is some danger that the baby can inhale powders and develop respiratory problems such as pneumonia. There is also controversy over whether the use of cornstarch can contribute to the severity of an infection. Ask your doctor or pharmacist for advice. If you choose to use powders, do not allow the child to bring the container near to his or her face. Never use a powder if the diaper rash involves broken skin or open, oozing sores.

The FDA recently reviewed the scientific data and concluded that medications intended for use in fighting bacterial or fungal infections are not appropriate for treating diaper rash. (This assessment may change depending on the results of ongoing studies.) One reason for not allowing manufacturers to claim that their OTC products are effective in diaper rash is to encourage parents to receive an accurate diagnosis of the problem from a health care professional. Therefore, if the rash is moderate or severe, or if it persists for more than a few days despite treatment, have the child seen by a physician.

OTC Products for Diaper Rash

Skin protectants containing zinc oxide or petrolatum
Powders (talcum, cornstarch)

Teething Pain

When a baby's teeth begin to emerge from the gums, usually at about 4 to 6 months of age, it marks a significant landmark in the child's development. It can also mean a time of enormous pain and suffering—not just for the child but for the parents, who may search frantically for anything that will provide relief.

The teething process usually continues until the child is about 2 1/2 or 3 years old, when all 20 of the baby teeth are in place. Teething pain is not inevitable. Many infants survive the process without any signs of trouble. Others, however, experience redness, irritation, and sensitivity in the gums. Naturally, this can make them cranky and irritable. While teething, children tend to cry more frequently and to be clingy and fretful. Copious drooling is another sign of teething. The child may try to chew on anything in sight, since gentle pressure seems to ease the symptoms (see box).

Strategies for Easing Teething Pain

- Rub the gums with your finger; a wet gauze pad; a small, clean, cool spoon; or a cloth wrapped around ice chips.
- Cuddle, rock, or walk with your child.
- Give the child a fluid-filled teething ring or a wet washcloth to bite on. Coldness helps; chill these objects in the refrigerator. Do not freeze teething rings or other objects prior to use for relief of teething pain. Frozen objects can damage the skin if held in one place for too long.
- To prevent skin rash:

  Wipe up drool.

  Keep the child's clothing dry—use a bib and change shirts as needed.

  Apply an ointment containing petrolatum around the mouth and chin (not the lips).
- If the child is in serious pain or is unable to sleep, use an OTC pain reliever (such as acetaminophen) or an oral discomfort product as directed by your physician.

Seek medical attention if any of the following applies to your child

Contrary to popular belief, teething does not usually cause the following symptoms. If they occur during the teething stage, they are usually signs that some other medical problem is present and that the child should be seen by a physician.

- Fever
- Vomiting
- Diarrhea
- Loss of appetite
- Nasal congestion
- Earache
- Lack of energy, general sluggishness
- Convulsions
- Diaper rash

Treatment for Teething Pain

Topical local anesthetics work by numbing the nerve endings in gum tissue and blocking the transmission of pain signals to the brain. The main active ingredient in OTC products for local anesthesia is benzocaine, available in concentrations ranging from 5% to 20%. Benzocaine is considered safe for infants age 4 months or older and can be applied up to 4 times a day (every 6 hours). (For more information about mouth pain and OTC products, see chapter 8.)

Another ingredient that provides relief is phenol. Phenol is a counterirritant, which means it causes other sensations (such as cooling or stimulation) that help to mask the pain. In concentrations of up to 0.5%, phenol can be used up to 6 times a day (every 4 hours).

In some cases teething pain responds well to treatment with an oral analgesic such as acetaminophen in very small (pediatric) doses. Before giving these medications, ask your physician. Although ibuprofen is also available OTC, it should never be given to children except on the advice of a doctor.

OTC Products for Teething Pain

- Analgesics
  - Acetaminophen
  - Ibuprofen
- Oral discomfort products

Diaper Rash Products

BRAND NAME	ANTIMICROBIAL INGREDIENTS							
	8-hydroxy-quinoline	benzalko-nium chloride	benzetho-nium chloride	calcium undecy-lenate	cetylpyri-dinium chloride	chloroxy-lenol	methylben-zethonium chloride	methylparaben, polyparaben, imidazolidinyl urea
A and D Medicated Powder			X					
Ammens Medicated Original Fragrance	X							
Caldesene Medicated (powder)				10%				
Care-Creme Cream						0.8%		
Diapa-Kare							X	
Diaparene Diaper Rash								X
Diaper Guard		X						
Johnson's Baby Diaper Rash Ointment			X					
Lobana Peri-Guard						X		
Mexsana Medicated			X					
Spectro-Jel					0.1%			
Zeasorb						X		

Protectants

BRAND NAME	PROTECTANT INGREDIENTS									
	calamine	cod liver oil	dimethi-cone	lanolin	mineral oil	oatmeal	petro-latum	silicone	vitamin A & D	zinc oxide
A and D Medicated Ointment		x			x		x			x
A and D Medicated Powder										x
A and D Ointment		x			x		x		x	
ActiBath Soak Oatmeal Treatment						x				
Ammens Medicated Original Fragrance										9.1%
Ammens Medicated Shower Fresh Scent										9.1%
Aveeno Bath Treatment Soothing Formula					x	x				
Balmex										x
Calamine	8%									8%
Caldesene Medicated (ointment)							53.9%			15%
Care-Creme Cream		x		x			x		x	
Clocream									x	
Desitin		x		x			x			40%
Desitin Cornstarch Baby Powder										10%
Desitin Daily Care			x		x		x			10%
Diaparene Diaper Rash										15.8%
Diaper Guard			1%			x	66%			x
Diaper Rash Ointment		x								40%
DML Lotion							x			
Dyprotex		x	2.5%				31.1%			40%
First Aid Medicated Powder										x
Flanders Buttocks							x			x

Gold Bond Baby Powder									x
Gold Bond Medicated									x
Hydropel						x	30%		
Johnson's Baby Cream		2%	x	x					
Johnson's Baby Diaper Rash Ointment						x			x
Johnson's Baby, Medicated									x
Lantiseptic Skin Protectant			50%						
Little Bottoms		x		x		x			15%
Lobana Derm-ADE							x	x (plus vitamin E)	
Lobana Peri-Guard						x		x	
Mexsana Medicated									10.8%
Nutra Soothe Medicated					x				x
Plexolan Lanolin			15.5%	x		x			x
Resinol Diaper Rash	x								12%
Schamberg's Anti-Itch									x
Triple Paste						52%			x
Vaseline Pure Petroleum Jelly						100%			
ZBT Baby Powder				x					

Powder

BRAND NAME	POWDER				
	cornstarch	kaolin	sodium bicarbonate	talc	zinc stearate
A and D Medicated Powder	X	X			
ActiBath Soak Oatmeal Treatment			X		
Ammens Medicated Original Fragrance	X			X	
Ammens Medicated Shower Fresh Scent	X			X	
Caldesene Medicated (ointment)				X	
Desitin				X	
Desitin Cornstarch Baby Powder	88.2%				
Diapa-Kare	X		X		
Diaparene Cornstarch Baby Powder	88%				
Dyprotex					X
First Aid Medicated Powder	X				
Gold Bond Baby Powder			X		
Gold Bond Medicated				X	
Johnson's Baby Powder				X	
Johnson's Baby Powder Cornstarch	95%				
Johnson's Baby, Medicated	X				
Mexsana Medicated	X	X			
Nutra Soothe Medicated	X				
Velvet Fresh Powder	X				
ZBT Baby Powder	X				
Zeasorb	X				

Brand Name

A and D Medicated Diaper Rash Ointment

Generic Ingredients

Cholecalciferol
Cod liver oil
Mineral oil
White petrolatum
Zinc oxide

Type of Drug

Topical skin astringent and protectant; and antiseptic.

Used for

Treatment of diaper rash, abrasions, and minor burns; prevention of diaper rash; and protection of chafed skin due to diaper rash or other irritants.

General Information

Zinc oxide is used to shield the skin surface from irritants by providing a protective coating that does not dissolve in water or alcohol. It promotes healing by attracting protein to the affected area and thus encouraging new tissue growth. It also helps to dry the skin by hastening removal of skin-surface moisture, which further promotes healing.

Zinc oxide is also included in a number of skin care products to thicken lotions and creams and make them easier to apply.

Petrolatum (also known as mineral jelly or petroleum jelly), derived from petroleum, is commonly used in ointments and other skin care products. It soothes the skin surface, protects against outside irritants, and prevents the evaporation of moisture. It is more easily removed from the skin than substances such as zinc oxide and calamine. Petrolatum (sometimes called yellow petrolatum) has a yellowish tinge; "white" petrolatum is the same substance that has been processed to remove this coloring so it is clearer and more cosmetically pleasing. Products containing petrolatum have many uses, such as protecting an infant's genital area from the irritating effects of urine and fecal matter, thus relieving diaper rash discomfort; maintaining moisture in the skin and promoting its health by assisting the skin's natural defenses against infection.

Cod liver oil is a pale yellow, fatty oil extracted from the livers of cod fish and other related species. High in vitamins A and D, the oil is useful in preventing and treating diaper rash.

Cholecalciferol is the body's natural form of vitamin D. It is created in the skin from cholesterol during exposure to the ultraviolet radiation from the sun. It has properties of both a vitamin and a hormone. Cholecalciferol is used in skin ointments as a natural protectant and healing agent.

Mineral oil is used in skin preparations as an emollient, to protect the natural moisture content of damaged skin and promote healing. When added to products containing petrolatum, it allows the petrolatum to melt more easily at body temperature and makes the product easier to apply.

Cautions and Warnings

If the condition worsens or there is no improvement in the affected area within 7 days, or if an allergic reaction develops, discontinue using A and D and contact your doctor.

Do not exceed the recommended daily dosage of A and D.

Do not apply A and D to areas of broken skin, over deep or puncture wounds, or cuts. This enhances the internal absorption of the product, which might cause systemic complications.

Possible Side Effects

▼ Rare: local skin irritations.

Drug Interactions

None known.

Usual Dose

Diaper Rash

Remove soiled diaper promptly. Wash the genital and anal area thoroughly with water; pat dry. Apply A and D liberally with each diaper change and after baths, especially at night to prevent long exposure to moisture.

Minor Burns or Skin Conditions

Adult and Child (age 2 and over): Apply 3–4 times per day as needed, or as directed by your doctor.

Child (under age 2): not recommended unless directed by your doctor.

If possible, use bandages or other dressing to protect A and D from accidental removal before it has had a chance to work.

Overdosage

Do the following in case of accidental ingestion: If the victim is unconscious or having convulsions, call for an ambulance immediately. If you take the victim to an emergency room, be sure to bring the bottle or container with you. If the victim is conscious, call your local poison control center or a health care professional. The poison control center may suggest inducing vomiting with ipecac syrup (available without a prescription at any pharmacy). DO NOT induce vomiting unless specifically instructed to do so.

Special Populations

Pregnancy/Breast-feeding

It is not generally recommended that pregnant women take any drugs, particularly during the first 3 months after conception. Check with your doctor before using A and D if you are or might be pregnant, or if you are breast-feeding.

Infants/Children

Do not use A and D on children under age 6 for conditions other than diaper rash without first consulting your doctor.

Seniors

Seniors should exercise the same caution as younger adults when using A and D.

Brand Name

Desitin Ointment (DESS-i-tin)

Generic Ingredients

Cod liver oil
Lanolin
Petrolatum
Talc
Zinc oxide

Type of Drug

Topical skin astringent and protectant; and antiseptic.

Used for

Treatment and prevention of diaper rash; and treatment of chafed skin, superficial wounds and burns, and minor skin irritations.

General Information

Zinc oxide is used to shield the skin surface from chemical irritants and harmful sun overexposure. It provides a protective coating that does not dissolve in water or alcohol.

It promotes healing by attracting protein to the affected area and thus encouraging new tissue growth. It also helps to dry the skin by hastening removal of skin-surface moisture, which further promotes healing. Zinc oxide is also used in a number of skin care products to thicken lotions and creams and make them easier to apply.

Petrolatum (also known as mineral jelly or petroleum jelly) is a substance derived from petroleum that is commonly used in ointments and other skin care products. It soothes the skin surface, protects it against outside irritants, and prevents the evaporation of moisture. It is more easily removed from the skin than substances such as zinc oxide and calamine. Petrolatum (sometimes called yellow petrolatum) has a yellowish tinge. Products containing petrolatum are used to protect an infant's genital area from the irritating effects of urine and fecal matter, thus relieving diaper rash discomfort, and to maintain moisture in the skin and promote health by assisting the skin's natural defenses against infection.

Cod liver oil is a pale yellow, fatty oil extracted from the livers of cod fish and other related species. High in vitamins A and D, the oil is useful in preventing and treating diaper rash.

Lanolin is a fatty substance obtained from sheep's wool. Lanolin is used as a skin protectant in Desitin Ointment. People who are allergic to lanolin may be better able to tolerate products formulated with refined lanolin.

Cautions and Warnings

If there is no improvement in the affected area within 7 days or an allergic reaction develops, discontinue using Desitin and contact your doctor.

Do not exceed the recommended daily dosage of Desitin.

Desitin is for external use only.

Some individuals may become sensitized to the lanolin in Desitin and develop a rash. Should this occur, discontinue using Desitin and contact your doctor.

Do not apply Desitin to areas of broken skin, over deep or puncture wounds, or cuts. This would enhance the internal absorption of the product, and might cause systemic (whole-body) complications.

Products containing petrolatum have been shown to impair the natural healing process of superficial burns, which need exposure to oxygen. Consult your doctor before using petrolatum products on burns.

Possible Side Effects

▼ Rare: local skin irritation.

Drug Interactions

None known

Usual Dose

Diaper Rash

Remove soiled diaper promptly. Wash the genital and anal area thoroughly with water; pat dry. Apply Desitin liberally with each diaper change and after baths, especially at night to prevent long exposure to moisture. The ointment tends to be most easily removed with the use of mineral oil.

Skin Conditions

Adult and Child (age 6 and over): Apply 3–4 times a day as needed, or as directed by a doctor.

Child (under age 6): Consult your physician.

If possible, protect Desitin from accidental removal before it has had a chance to work by using bandages or other dressing.

Overdosage

Do the following in case of accidental ingestion: If the victim is unconscious or having convulsions, call for an ambulance immediately. If you take the victim to an emergency room, be sure to bring the bottle or container with you. If the victim is conscious, call your local poison control center or a health care professional. The poison control center may suggest inducing vomiting with ipecac syrup (available without a prescription at any pharmacy). DO NOT induce vomiting unless specifically instructed to do so.

Special Populations

Pregnancy/Breast-feeding

Since zinc oxide is not absorbed into the skin, there is little risk to either pregnant women or nursing mothers and their babies. However, if you are using Desitin to soothe and heal nipples that are cracked and irritated from nursing, be certain to remove all traces of the product from the skin prior to breast-feeding to prevent accidental ingestion by your infant.

Infants/Children

Zinc oxide products are generally safe when used as directed for diaper rash (see "Cautions and Warnings"). However, Desitin should not be used in children under age 6 to treat skin conditions without first consulting your doctor.

Seniors

Seniors should exercise the same caution as younger adults when using Desitin.

Orajel Baby Teething Pain Medication (OR-uh-jel)

see **Benzocaine,** page 686

Tylenol Infant's Suspension Drops (TYE-leh-nol)

see **Acetaminophen,** page 659

Chapter 14: Future OTC Medications

Sales of over-the-counter (OTC) drugs in the United States are expected to exceed 20 billion dollars in 1997 and expected to increase to around 30 billion dollars by the year 2000.

United States citizens depend on OTC drugs to treat many common, less serious ailments. Of approximately 3.5 billion health-care problems suffered by U.S. residents each year, about 2 billion, or 57%, are treated with an OTC drug; and more than 50% of all medications taken in the United States are OTC drugs.

This increase in the use and importance of OTC drugs has been recognized by the U.S. Food and Drug Administration. In 1993 the FDA established an Office of OTC Drug Evaluation to address the increasing volume of OTC matters. Recently the FDA has proposed improvements in the labels of OTC drugs. These improvements include greater uniformity in label design as well as standardized headings, subheadings, and order of information. Simplified language is being adopted to make it easier for consumers to understand the benefits and risks of OTC medications. A minimum type size has also been proposed to make it easier for individuals with vision problems to read OTC labels.

One of the pivotal trends in health care in the 1990s has been the increased involvement of people in their own care. This trend is evident in the large number of OTC drugs available to the consumer. There are more than 300,000 OTC drug formulations on the market, giving people more choices—and more opportunities to assume responsibility for their health care—than ever before. The need for quality information about OTC drugs has never been greater.

The number and range of OTC products is due in part to another trend: the reclassification of many drugs from prescription to OTC status, known in the industry as *switching.* More than 600 products previously available only by prescription have become available as OTC drugs in the last 30 years. At any given time there are at least 20 prescription drugs under consideration for reclassification by the FDA.

There are many advantages to the increased availability of therapeutic drugs which has resulted from the greater number of OTC products on the market. The average American reportedly experiences a health problem suitable for self-medication (i.e., a condition not serious enough to require medical supervision) every 3 to 4 days. More than 400 medical conditions are treatable with OTC drugs (see box for some of the most common). This is good news for time—and money—conscious people who don't want to run to the doctor every time they get the sniffles.

Health Problems Most Likely to Be Treated with an OTC Drug

- Headache
- Common cold
- Muscle aches and pains (including sprains and strains)
- Skin conditions
  - Acne
  - Athlete's foot
  - Cold sores
  - Dandruff
  - Dry skin
  - Jock itch
- Cuts, scrapes, and other minor wounds
- Premenstrual and menstrual symptoms
- Upset stomach
- Sleeping problems

The increased availability of powerful, formerly prescription-only drugs means that consumer awareness also needs to be increased. That is the concern of industry analysts, and consumer watchdog groups such as the National Consumer League, who fear that the public's knowledge of drugs—and awareness of potential dangers if drugs are misused—is not keeping up with the OTC switches.

Making the Switch

The FDA does not casually reclassify a drug from prescription to OTC status. Switching is a lengthy, involved process in which many factors are considered, including the drug's toxicity, its potential for misuse and abuse, and whether the condition is suited to self-diagnosis and self-treatment. As with a new prescription drug awaiting approval, the benefits of switching to OTC status must be weighed against potential risks; specifically, the benefits of *availability* must outweigh possible risks.

Before even being considered for OTC status, a prescription drug must have a history of safety and effectiveness, and the manufacturers seeking the switch must show that people can both diagnose their condition and use the product correctly without a doctor's supervision.

There are two methods manufacturers can use to apply for OTC status for a product: They can conduct new clinical studies of a lower strength of the medication for a specific OTC use; or they can submit a supplement to a prescription drug's original approved application, often at the prescription strength. In either case, the FDA determines whether the medication has been shown to be safe for use without physician supervision, whether it is safe at high doses, if there is potential for abuse, and whether there are serious drug interactions to consider.

Helping the Consumer

Americans today are more health-conscious and knowledgeable than Americans 20 years ago; they want more control over their health and they are increasingly capable of responsibly exercising that control. Industry-conducted surveys indicate that people—85% according to one poll—support access to OTC drugs to treat minor medical conditions or problems.

There are many benefits to OTC drugs when they are used appropriately. They can spare a person with a minor ailment a time-consuming visit to the doctor's office. That same doctor visit can also be expensive; even with health insurance there is often a co-payment or a deductible to be met. In addition, the doctor may prescribe a drug, which can mean another co-payment. So, in the final analysis, OTC drugs can save consumers money. (Although it should be noted that health insurance rarely reimburses for OTC products, and that generic drugs obtained by prescription are often less expensive than a similar brand-name OTC product, particularly when they are used for lengthy periods of time.)

OTC drugs may be cost-effective for the nation's health care system as well. According to one research firm, OTC drugs saved $10.5 billion in 1987 and will save $34.1 billion annually by the year 2000, all this while accounting for less than 2 cents of every dollar spent on health care.

Drug therapy has long been a successful mainstay of health care. With the switching of new and improved prescription drugs, OTC drugs have moved beyond relieving minor, transient aches and pains. Drugs formerly available only by prescription can be used to actually cure some conditions (e.g., athlete's foot) and help manage chronic and recurring illnesses, which account for 80% of illnesses in the U.S. Given all these factors, it is clear that OTC drugs are poised to play a major therapeutic role.

Helping the Manufacturers

Manufacturers rightfully promote the increased control and savings that OTC drugs offer consumers; however, industry watchdogs realize that manufacturers may not be disinterested parties in the debate.

When a prescription-strength drug is about to go off patent (meaning that generic drug companies can manufacture the product and sell it at a lower cost), a switch to OTC status can sometimes help the initial manufacturer keep the patent. Particularly when a manufacturer conducts a new clinical study—for instance, a study of a drug for specific OTC use at a strength lower than the prescription strength—the original manufacturer can retain market exclusivity because of the new study. (This strategy doesn't always pan out for the manufacturer. Minoxidil [Rogaine] was switched to OTC status in February 1996, just before its patent was to expire. The manufacturer requested 3 more years of marketing exclusivity on the grounds that it had done additional research to prove minoxidil was safe for OTC use, but the FDA denied them the right. Minoxidil is currently available OTC by brand and generic name.)

There are other business-savvy reasons for switching a prescription drug to OTC status. Former prescription-only drugs have recognizable names that help the product to outsell other OTC products used to treat the same condition. For example, the cold and allergy product Benadryl had sales of $20 million in 1985, the year before it was switched. Within 10 years of its availability as an OTC drug, its sales had risen to $140 million annually. This kind of increase in sales is due in part to a dramatic increase in distribution. When a prescription drug is switched to an OTC drug, its outlets can leap from 55,000 pharmacies to more than 750,000 retail locations (e.g., supermarkets and convenience stores).

The abundance of OTC switches has consumer groups, pharmacists, and doctors worried that an uneducated public will misuse OTC drugs, with potentially dangerous side effects. But as drug manufacturers are quick to point out, adverse effects are less likely to occur if label directions are followed carefully.

The Responsible Consumer

OTC drugs that have been switched are usually made in lower dosages than their prescription counterparts, but when used improperly they can still cause serious adverse effects. Whatever the dosage, these are potent chemicals at work. The same factors taken into consideration with prescription drugs—contraindications, drug interactions, side effects, recommendations for different populations—must also be taken into consideration when the drugs are purchased over the counter.

Approximately 30% to 50% of *prescribed* drugs are taken incorrectly; the resulting drug-induced problems cost billions of dollars in hospital and doctor visits annually. If drugs whose dosages are prescribed by a doctor are so commonly misused, what hope is there for OTC drugs, which can be bought in a convenience store as casually as a bar of soap?

The Label

Without a doctor's supervision, it's up to the individual to use OTC drugs in an informed, appropriate, and responsible manner. Cautions are outlined on the package labels—which is why so much attention is being focused on OTC labels. The consumer should read the label thoroughly *and* follow the directions carefully.

A common misuse of an OTC drug is taking it for a longer period of time or in larger doses than recommended on the label, or neglecting to see a doctor when advised to do so on the label. Adverse effects may result.

Overuse of laxatives, for example, can lead to laxative dependence. People who regularly take a nonsteroidal anti-inflammatory drug (NSAID), such as aspirin, to ease chronic pain (e.g., from arthritis) run the risk of serious gastrointestinal (GI) disorders, such as bleeding ulcers. Approximately 10,000 to 20,000 deaths occur each year from severe GI bleeding caused by NSAIDs.

Prolonged use of some products can continue to relieve symptoms and make an individual feel better, but all consumers should realize that by taking an OTC medication they could be masking a serious illness which might be causing the symptoms. Cimetidine, which in its prescription strength is used to treat ulcers, is now available in lowered dosages as an OTC heartburn remedy. However, the stomach pains that it relieves could indicate a serious GI disorder, such as cancer or, ironically, an ulcer. If the individual continues to take cimetidine to relieve the presumed heartburn longer than the 2 weeks recommended on the label, he or she runs the risk of delaying diagnosis of the more serious underlying disorder.

There are other dangers associated with self-medicating without reading the packaging label: The label of an OTC vaginal yeast infection medication, for instance, tells the consumer that the infection should not be self-treated unless previously diagnosed by a doctor. Vaginal infections can be caused by any of several different pathogens and a drug indicated for fungal yeast infections cannot and should not be used to treat a vaginal infection caused by a bacteria.

Labels also inform consumers of particularly serious drug and food interactions—which can be present where they are least expected. The popular analgesic acetaminophen is regarded as a very safe drug, but when taken regularly by people who also consume alcohol regularly (even in moderate amounts), it can cause serious liver damage. The brand Tylenol, currently used by more than 55 million people a year, now carries a warning to that effect written by the FDA.

The Pharmacist

Communication is perhaps the best way to disseminate information about OTC products. As the health care professional who is best educated on the use of drugs, a pharmacist can give sound advice based on the information a consumer provides. From the start, he or she can help determine whether a consumer should seek medical attention rather than self-medicate, and whether an OTC drug might potentially mask a serious underlying condition.

Once the decision has been made to self-medicate, the pharmacist can help the consumer make an informed choice from among the many products used to treat a particular condition, and answer any questions about the chosen product. Of course, interaction with the pharmacist is only possible if the consumer chooses to go to a pharmacy rather than a supermarket—and chooses to speak up.

Improving the Lot

There are steps to take—some already in progress—to ensure that OTC drugs will continue to give people the choices and savings they enjoy without posing undue risks.

Better Labels

The FDA and manufacturers are both working to improve the readability of labels. Among the measures under consideration are *standardization,* by which all OTC labels will provide essential information in the same order and in the same place, and *uniformity* of print size, type face, paragraph spacing, and other design elements. Special consideration for people who cannot see well (e.g., seniors) may lead to larger type size for certain crucial information.

One continuing obstacle is the size of labels: Small packages are convenient for consumers, but leave little room for label text. Even if the packages were larger, however, and the text more comprehensive and easier to read, a label can never address every possible issue for every consumer. One solution that has been suggested is enclosing inserts in OTC products, as with prescription drugs.

A Third Class

A long-standing suggestion that has never been adopted is the introduction of a third class of drugs: one that could be sold without a prescription, but only by a pharmacy (i.e., not by a supermarket or convenience store). A drug's classification in this third category would be based on its side-effect profile, its potential for drug interactions, and the potential for its misuse or abuse. The American Pharmaceutical Association has been in favor of a three-class system since 1964, and since 1987 it has proposed that all drugs under consideration for an OTC switch be placed in a third category for a trial period of at least 2 years. Several countries—England, Denmark, France, the Netherlands, Canada—have a third and even fourth category of drugs.

In 1995, after completing a 3-year study of 10 countries, the General Accounting Office of the U.S. Congress concluded that a third class of drugs would not result in significant benefits. The FDA also rejects the idea, arguing that if they have determined that a drug is safe for OTC use, then it is indeed safe.

Consumer and pharmaceutical groups will probably continue to lobby for additional safety measures, as well as the third-category idea. Their object is not to curb self-medication, but to make it more intelligent, and thus safer and more effective.

Looking to the Future

In 1995, 6 drugs were switched from prescription to OTC status; 6 more were switched in 1996. There are at least 20 prescription drugs currently awaiting OTC clearance from the FDA. While there is no telling exactly how many drugs will be switched in 1997, industry experts believe that the following 7 drugs are likely to be granted OTC status in the near future.

NSAIDs

There are 5 NSAIDs that may soon be approved for OTC use: etodolac (prescription name, Lodine), diflunisal (prescription name, Dolobid), nabumetone (prescription name, Relafen), sulindac (prescription name, Clinoril), and piroxicam (prescription name, Feldene). In prescription strength, these drugs are used to treat various kinds of pain, such as that resulting from rheumatoid arthritis, osteoarthritis, and tendinitis. These drugs also have antipyretic (fever-reducing) properties. In the past when the FDA has allowed what was formerly a prescription NSAID to be sold OTC the dose has generally been cut in half. The indications have generally been restricted to fever reduction and relief of pain associated with headache, colds, toothache, muscle ache, minor arthritis, and menstrual cramps.

While the five prescription drugs mentioned above are all NSAIDs, they differ in their indications and warnings. Some are used primarily for arthritic conditions such as rheumatoid arthritis or osteoarthritis, while diflunisal is used for other kinds of pain relief. Some of these drugs are less irritating to the stomach than OTC NSAIDs. For example, nabumetone is a "pro-drug," which means that it must be converted by the body's metabolism in order to become an active NSAID. Pro-drugs are considered to have less adverse effects on the stomach.

Triazole Antifungal Drugs

Several of the azole or triazole class of drugs are already available OTC for the treatment of *vaginal candidiasis* (yeast infection). When used for yeast infection, these drugs are very effective and can achieve cure rates in excess of 90% for most women. Fluconazole (prescription name, Diflucan), is a triazole antifungal agent currently available only by prescription. Oral fluconazole has been effective in preventing and curing a wide variety of fungal infections, including some that are life-threatening. In clinical yeast infection studies, a single dose of oral fluconazole has been shown to be just as effective as a multi-day treatment of topical vaginal cream or ointment. Most women in these studies reported that they preferred fluconazole because it was more convenient to use and relieved their symptoms (e.g., itching) faster. It should be noted that none of these studies compared a single dose of oral fluconazole to a single-dose vaginal cream such as Vagistat-1, which is available OTC. In general, oral drugs such as fluconazole that have a systemic (whole-body) effect present a greater risk of side effects (in this case, nausea, vomiting, diarrhea, abdominal pain, and headache) than do topical creams or ointments, although it should be noted that fluconazole has proven to be safe when used to treat yeast infection.

Topical Antimicrobial Ointment

Mupirocin (prescription name, Bactroban) is an antibacterial agent available by prescription as a 2% topical ointment for the treatment of impetigo (common skin infection) due to common bacteria such as *Staphaureus, Streptococcus pyogenes,* and other *streptococci* bacteria. It is also available by prescription as mupirocin calcium 2% (prescription name, Bactroban Nasal) and is used for the eradication of methicillin-resistant *Staphaureus* (MRSA) from nasal passages. It is reasonable to expect that the topical ointment of mupirocin will be approved for the OTC treatment of minor skin infections. One major concern the FDA may have before giving approval for OTC mupirocin is that increased use of mupirocin may hasten the development of mupirocin resistance in MRSA. Should this be the case, the ability of mupirocin to eradicate MRSA from nasal passages could be impaired.

Part II

Generic Name

Acetaminophen (uh-SEAT-uh-MIN-uh-fen)

Brand Names

Acephen
Aceta [C]
†Actamin
*Actifed
*†Alka-Seltzer
*Allerest
Aminofen [C] [S]
Anacin Aspirin Free
Arthriten [S]
Arthritis Foundation Aspirin Free
Aspirin Free [C]
Backaid [C] [S]
*†Bayer Select Aspirin-Free
*†Benadryl
†Bromo-Seltzer
Buffets II
Chlor-Trimeton Allergy, Sinus, Headache
Clear Cough Night Time [A] [S]
*†Codimal
Coldonyl
†Comtrex
*Contac
*Coricidin
DayGel
Dent's Double-Action Kit
*†Dimetapp
*†Diurex
*Dristan
*Drixoral
Duadacin
*Dynafed
Dyspel [C]
Ed-APAP [A] [C]
Emagrin Forte
Excedrin
Fem-1
Fendol
Feverall [C]
Flu-Relief
Goody's
*Kolephrin
Legatrin PM
Liquiprin [A] [C]
Lurline PMS [C] [S]
†Midol
ND-Gesic
Neopap
NiteGel
Oranyl
Ornex
Pamprin [C]
†Panadol
PediApap [A] [C] [S]
Percogesic [C]
Premsyn PMS [C]
Pyrroxate
Rid-a-Pain
*†Robitussin
Sinapils
Sinarest
*Sine-Aid
Sine-Off
Singlet
Sinulin [S]
*Sinutab
Sinutol Maximum Strength
Sominex Pain Relief Formula
Stanback AF [C]
†Sudafed

Supac [S]
Tapanol
Tempra
Tetrahist
TheraFlu
Tranquil Plus
Triaminic Sore Throat, Throat Pain & Cough [A]
Triaminicin
Tycolene [C]
†Tylenol
Unisom Pain Relief
†Valorin
Vanquish
*†Vicks

**Not all products in this brand-name group contain acetaminophen.*

†Consult the OTC ingredient charts to determine whether different formulations in this brand-name group are alcohol-, caffeine-, or sugar-free.

Type of Drug

Analgesic (pain reliever) and antipyretic (fever reducer).

Used for

Symptomatic relief of pain and reduction of fever.

General Information

Acetaminophen is used to relieve pain and fever associated with the common cold, flu, viral infections, or other disorders (neuritis, neuralgia, bursitis, arthritis, rheumatism, simple headache, menstrual cramps, tooth and periodontic pain, sprains, and minor muscular aches). In many studies, acetaminophen and aspirin have been proven equally effective in reducing most types of pain, and their antipyretic effects are the same. However, there are important differences between these 2 common pain relievers that should be considered when choosing which one to take. Acetaminophen is associated with less gastrointestinal (GI) irritation, erosion, and bleeding than aspirin or the other salicylates (magnesium salicylate, sodium salicylate, sodium thiosalicylate, choline salicylate, and magnesium salicylate), and is usually well tolerated by people who are allergic to aspirin; it can also be taken by those who cannot use aspirin because of potential interactions with other drugs such as oral anticoagulants (blood-thinning agents). However, unlike aspirin or the other nonsteroidal anti-inflammatory drugs

(NSAIDs), acetaminophen does not reduce inflammation.

Acetaminophen is also available in nonprescription combination products, where it is combined with aspirin, caffeine, or another agent. It has not been clearly established that these combinations are any more effective in reducing pain than acetaminophen alone.

Cautions and Warnings

Do not take acetaminophen for more than 10 consecutive days (5 days for children) or, in the presence of fever, for more than 3 days, unless directed by your doctor.

Do not exceed the recommended daily dosage of acetaminophen.

In doses of more than 4 grams per day, acetaminophen is potentially toxic to the liver. Use acetaminophen with caution if you have kidney or liver disease or viral infections of the liver. Studies have shown that the risk of liver damage with acetaminophen is associated with fasting and alcohol use. People with pre-existing liver disease who are taking other drugs that are potentially damaging to the liver, who do not eat regularly, or who drink alcohol (even moderately) are especially at risk. If you take acetaminophen regularly, avoid drinking alcoholic beverages and/or fasting.

People who cannot digest phenylalanine (phenylketonurics) should be aware that some chewable tablet forms of acetaminophen contain aspartame (Nutrasweet), which breaks down in the GI tract to phenylalanine after the tablet is taken.

Extra-strength formulations of acetaminophen are not for use in children under age 12.

The effectiveness of acetaminophen may be decreased if you smoke, and you may need a higher dose to achieve the desired effect.

Possible Side Effects

- ▼ Most common: lightheadedness.
- ▼ Less common: trembling and pain in lower back or side.
- ▼ Rare: extreme fatigue, rash, itching, or hives; sore throat or fever; unexplained bleeding or bruising; anemia; yellowing of the skin or eyes; blood in urine; painful or frequent urination; and decreased output of urine volume.

Drug Interactions

• Acetaminophen's effects may be reduced by long-term use or large doses of barbiturate drugs; the anticonvulsants carbamazepine and phenytoin (and other similar drugs); rifampin, used to treat tuberculosis (TB) and sulfinpyrazone, used to treat gout. These drugs may also increase the chances of liver toxicity if taken with acetaminophen.

• Taking chronic, large doses of acetaminophen with isoniazid (used to treat TB) may increase the risk of liver damage.

• If acetaminophen is taken with an anticoagulant such as warfarin, it may increase the blood-thinning effect of the anticoagulant agent. This does not occur with occasional use.

• Alcohol increases the liver toxicity caused by large doses of acetaminophen (see "Cautions and Warnings"). If you take acetaminophen regularly, avoid alcohol.

• It has been reported that patients with AIDS and AIDS-related complex taking zidovudine (AZT) with acetaminophen have an increased incidence of bone marrow suppression. However, studies performed to try to determine if a harmful interaction exists have not shown that short-term use of acetaminophen (less than 7 days) increases the risk of bone marrow suppression or causes a decrease in white blood cells in AIDS patients taking AZT. Acetaminophen, when taken on a short-term basis or only as needed, is the recommended OTC pain-relieving drug for these patients.

Food Interactions

None known.

Usual Dose

Adult and Child (age 12 and over): 325–650 mg every 4–6 hours as necessary. Do not take more than 4 grams in 24 hours.

Child (age 6–11): 150– 300 mg 3–4 times a day.

Child (under age 6): Consult your doctor.

Acetaminophen is also available as rectal suppositories for those who cannot tolerate oral medication. The same dosage used for oral acetaminophen can be used for the suppositories, but you may need a higher dose to get the same effect.

For those who have difficulty swallowing acetaminophen capsules, they can be opened and the contents mixed with a spoonful of liquid or soft food. The liquid should not be hot, because this may result in a bitter taste. Do not try to stir the capsule contents into a glass of liquid; they may stick to the sides of the glass.

If you are taking the extended-release form of acetaminophen tablets, they should not be crushed, chewed, or dissolved in a liquid.

Overdosage

The first signs of acetaminophen overdose, which can include nausea, vomiting, drowsiness, confusion, and abdominal pain, usually occur within 2 to 3 hours but may not be seen for as long as 2 days after the overdose is taken. Other effects of overdose include low blood pressure, yellowing of the skin and eyes, and liver damage.

Even if the victim is not displaying any of the symptoms listed above, do the following in case of accidental overdose: If the victim is unconscious or having convulsions, call for an ambulance immediately. If you take the victim to an emergency room, be sure to bring the bottle or container with you. If the victim is conscious, call your local poison control center or a health care professional. The poison control center may suggest inducing vomiting with ipecac syrup (available without a prescription at any pharmacy). DO NOT induce vomiting unless specifically instructed to do so.

Special Populations

Allergies

Some OTC forms of acetaminophen contain sulfites as a preservative, which may cause allergic-type reactions in people who are sensitive to these ingredients; these reactions include anaphylactic shock (respiratory symptoms, fainting, itching, and rash) and severe asthmatic episodes. People with asthma may be more likely to have sulfite sensitivity.

Pregnancy/Breast-feeding

It is not generally recommended that pregnant women take any drugs, particularly during the first 3 months after con-

ception. Although taking normal dosages of acetaminophen is considered relatively safe for the expectant mother and her baby, taking continual high doses may cause birth defects or interfere with the baby's development.

Acetaminophen is considered acceptable for use during breast-feeding by the American Academy of Pediatrics. Although acetaminophen does pass into breast milk when taken by nursing mothers, the only side effect reported in infants is a rash that goes away when the mother stops taking the drug.

Check with your doctor before taking acetaminophen if you are or might be pregnant, or if you are breast-feeding.

Infants/Children

Acetaminophen is available in liquid or chewable tablets for young children.

Acetaminophen is not recommended for children under 6 unless directed by a doctor. Extra-strength formulations of acetaminophen are not for use in children under age 12.

Because these formulations come in different strengths, do not use the dropper from one bottle to measure the dose from another. Also, the correct dose for your child may need to be recalculated as he or she grows and gains weight.

Seniors

Because acetaminophen may clear the body more slowly in older adults, the drug's side effects may be more noticeable.

Generic Name

Acetone (ASS-eh-tone)

Definition

A solvent (a fluid that dissolves other chemicals) used in OTC foot-care products for treatment of corns, calluses, and warts. Acetone dissolves the active ingredient (e.g., salicylic acid) and helps it spread across and adhere to the affected area so the medication can produce the desired effects. Acetone is also used in some acne treatment pads for cleaning and disinfecting the skin.

Generic Name

Alcohol (AL-kuh-hall)

Definition

A clear, colorless liquid used in OTC products as an antiseptic, a solvent (a fluid that dissolves other chemicals), and a preservative. The FDA has classified alcohol as safe and effective for first-aid use in the home. In various forms (e.g., cetearyl alcohol and cetyl alcohol), alcohol is found in preparations designed to alleviate the pain and itching of fever blisters and cold sores. It is also included in formulations that aid in treating corns, calluses, and warts. *(see **Isopropyl Alcohol,** page 858.)*

The drinkable form of alcohol found in alcoholic beverages is called ethyl alcohol, or ethanol. This form is used in mouthwashes to add bite and freshness, enhance flavor, make other ingredients more soluble, destroy bacteria, and cleanse tissues. Not all mouthwashes contain alcohol; in those that do, the alcohol content is 27% or less. These products are not meant to be swallowed, but children might be tempted to drink them because of their flavors and bright colors. Because the amounts of alcohol present in mouthwashes can cause serious injury, such products should be stored out of reach of children.

Generic Name

Aluminum (ah-LUE-mih-num)

Definition

A metallic element that is found in small amounts in the body but whose biological function is unknown. Different forms of aluminum are used in various OTC products (see below).

Generic Name

Aluminum Acetate (ah-LUE-mih-num ASS-eh-tate)

Definition

Also known as Burow's solution, aluminum acetate is a mild astringent (drying agent) used to relieve minor skin irritations such as poison ivy and insect bites. It is also effective in relieving itching and inflammation caused by external ear infections. Aluminum acetate is available in tablets or powders with 5% active ingredient; in either of these forms, it must be diluted in water in a ratio of 1:10 to 1:40 prior to use. Treatment of skin irritations involves applying a wet compress soaked with aluminum acetate. When used to treat ear infections, a dosage of 4 to 6 drops every 4 to 6 hours is used until itching or burning subsides. The acid level of aluminum acetate restores the normal pH level in the infected ear, which helps to kill bacteria. The treatment can be used on adults and children over age 2. Adverse reactions are rare.

Generic Name

Aluminum Chloride

(ah-LUE-mih-num KLOR-ide)

Definition

A common ingredient in antiperspirants. Some people develop an allergic reaction and dermatitis (skin inflammation) when aluminum chloride comes in contact with their skin.

Generic Name

Aluminum Hydroxide

(ah-LUE-mih-num hye-DROKS-ide)

Brand Names

ALternaGEL [S]
Aluminum Hydroxide Concentrate
Amphojel
Basaljel
Dialume
*Di-Gel
†Gaviscon
Gelusil
Kudrox
*Maalox
Magnesia and Alumina
Magnalox
*Mylanta
Nephrox
Simaal
Tempo Drops

**Not all products in this brand-name group contain aluminum hydroxide.*

†Consult the OTC ingredient charts to determine whether different formulations in this brand-name group are alcohol-, caffeine-, or sugar-free.

Type of Drug

Antacid.

Used for

Relief of heartburn, sour stomach, acid indigestion, upset stomach, and flatulence associated with these symptoms.

General Information

All antacids work in the same way, by neutralizing gastric acid. However, they differ in potency: Aluminum antacids such as aluminum hydroxide are the least potent of these products, after calcium carbonate, sodium bicarbonate, and magnesium antacids. The higher the potency of an antacid, the less of it you will need to take to achieve the desired effect.

Antacids also vary according to adverse effects and drug interactions, as well as onset and duration of action. Aluminum antacids dissolve more slowly in stomach acid than do sodium bicarbonate and magnesium hydroxide, and thus may take longer to begin working. It can take up to 30 minutes for the acid-neutralizing effect of an aluminum acid to take place.

How long an antacid product works depends on how long it remains in the stomach. Possibly because they delay gastric emptying, aluminum antacids have a longer duration of action than magnesium antacids or sodium bicarbonate. In general, an antacid taken on an empty stomach leaves the stomach rapidly and works for only 20 to 40 minutes. However, when taken after a meal, it leaves the stomach more slowly. When taken 1 hour after a meal, an antacid can work for up to 3 hours.

Aluminum hydroxide is one of 4 types of aluminum antacid; the others are carbonate, phosphate, and aminoacetate. Aluminum hydroxide is the most potent of the group.

Generic aluminum hydroxide is available in liquid (suspension) form only; brand name products are available in suspension and tablet form. While the suspension is more potent than the tablet, some people do not like the taste of the liquid and also prefer the convenience of the pill form when taking multiple doses throughout the day. Aluminum hydroxide is also available in combination products containing one of 3 other antacids: magnesium hydroxide, magnesium trisilicate, or magnesium carbonate.

Cautions and Warnings

Do not take the maximum daily dosage of aluminum hydroxide for more than 2 weeks continuously except under a doctor's supervision. Antacids may relieve symptoms of a serious condition such as peptic ulcer disease. If you take an antacid for a prolonged period, you run the risk of unknowingly masking the symptoms of a serious gastrointestinal (GI) disease and delaying diagnosis.

Do not exceed the recommended daily dosage of aluminum hydroxide.

Call your doctor if you do not get relief from aluminum hydroxide, or if your stool is black or tarry or looks like coffee grounds, which indicates bleeding in the intestines or stomach. These may be signs of a serious GI disorder that cannot and should not be treated unsupervised with an OTC product.

Because some of the aluminum in aluminum hydroxide is absorbed into the bloodstream and then eliminated through the kidneys, people with impaired kidney function should not take this product for prolonged periods. Excretion of aluminum is decreased during chronic use by these people, and the aluminum may accumulate in bones, lungs, and nerve tissue.

Excessive amounts of an aluminum antacid taken for a prolonged period can lead to low blood phosphate levels, which are characterized by loss of appetite, malaise, and muscle weakness.

Possible Side Effect

▼ Most common: constipation.

Drug Interactions

• Aluminum hydroxide decreases the absorption of the following drugs, reducing their effect: allopurinol, an antigout medication; nitrofurantoin, an antibiotic; tetracycline antibiotics; quinolone antibiotics, such as ciprofloxacin; cimetidine and ranitidine, used to treat peptic ulcers, heartburn, and acid indigestion; indomethacin, a nonsteroidal anti-inflammatory drug (NSAID); digoxin, used to treat congestive heart failure; iron; and ketoconazole, an antifungal agent. It may also decrease the bioavailability of the beta blocker atenolol, used to treat high blood pressure. If you are taking aluminum hydroxide at the same time as any of these drugs, separate your dose of each drug by at least 2 hours; with quinolone antibiotics, 4 to 6 hours is preferable.

• Aluminum hydroxide increases the absorption of the anticonvulsant valproic acid, creating the potential for valproic acid toxicity, and of the benzodiazepine tranquilizer diazepam, increasing its sedative effect. If you are taking valproic acid or diazepam, consult your doctor before taking aluminum hydroxide.

• Aluminum hydroxide increases the body's elimination of aspirin and other salicylates, reducing their effect. Conversely, it increases the absorption of enteric-coated aspirin.

Food Interactions

Aluminum hydroxide is best taken after meals (see "General Information").

Usual Dose

Adult and Child (age 12 and over): 15–60 ml, 1–3 hours after meals and at bedtime, as needed.

Child (age 6–11): 5–15 ml, 1–3 hours after meals and at bedtime, as needed.

Child (under 6): not recommended.

Take aluminum hydroxide as symptoms occur, but do not exceed the recommended daily dosage specified on the package. If you are taking the chewable tablet, be sure to chew it completely and drink a full glass of water afterward to ensure maximum benefit.

Overdosage

Do the following in case of accidental overdose: If the victim is unconscious or having convulsions, call for an ambulance immediately. If you take the victim to an emergency room, be sure to bring the bottle or container with you. If the victim is conscious, call your local poison control center or a health care professional. The poison control center may suggest inducing vomiting with ipecac syrup (available without a prescription at any pharmacy). DO NOT induce vomiting unless specifically instructed to do so.

Special Information

Patients with a history of diarrhea may choose aluminum hydroxide over other antacids because it can cause constipation.

Because magnesium antacids may cause diarrhea, they are often taken concurrently with aluminum hydroxide to regulate bowel function.

Storage Instructions

The suspension form of aluminum hydroxide may be stored at room temperature, but to improve its taste, refrigerate it. Do not freeze it.

Special Populations

Pregnancy/Breast-feeding

It is not generally recommended that pregnant women take any drugs, particularly during the first 3 months after conception. However, antacids can be safely taken in small doses for short periods of time during pregnancy and while breast-feeding. Check with your doctor before self-medicating with aluminum hydroxide if you are or might be pregnant, or if you are breast-feeding.

Infants/Children

The safety of antacid use in infants and children has not been established. Children under age 6 should not be given aluminum hydroxide unless directed by a doctor.

Seniors

Seniors may safely take antacids. Be advised that many older patients are at high risk for complications from ulcers, yet often do not show classic ulcer symptoms. Discuss the possible causes of your gastric discomfort with your pharmacist before self-medicating with an antacid and possibly delaying diagnosis of an ulcer. Be aware of possible interactions with other medications you may be taking.

Because constipation is a common complaint in seniors, aluminum hydroxide is not the preferred antacid for this age group.

Generic Name

Aluminum Silicate

(ah-LUE-mih-num SILL-ih-kate).

Definition

A tooth and denture cleanser.

Generic Name

Aluminum Sulfate

(ah-LUE-mih-num SULL-fate)

Definition

An astringent (drying agent) in OTC products used for treatment of dermatitis.

Generic Name

Ammonia (ah-MOE-nyah)

Definition

A colorless, strong-smelling gas consisting of nitrogen and hydrogen, used in smelling salts, detergents, and analgesic (pain-relieving) solutions. Stronger ammonia water (also known as stronger ammonium hydroxide solution, and Spirit of Hartshorn) is a solution containing 27% to 30% by weight of ammonia in a water base. It should be used with extreme caution. If the caustic vapors are inhaled they can irritate and damage the lungs. For safe use, stronger ammonia water must be diluted to a solution of 1.0% to 2.5% ammonia and must not be inhaled more than 3 or 4 times a day.

Aromatic ammonia spirit—also known as smelling salts—contains 1.9 g of total ammonia and other ingredients such as lavender oil, lemon oil, nutmeg oil, and alcohol. It is inhaled as a mild stimulant to treat or prevent fainting. It should be stored at room temperature and protected from light. In oral form, aromatic ammonia spirit can also relieve gas and act as an antacid. The oral dose is 2 to 4 ml diluted with at least 30 ml of water.

Generic Name

Ammonium Chloride

(ah-MOE-nee-um KLOR-ide)

Definition

A salt used as a diuretic and expectorant. In combination with a xanthine diuretic such as caffeine or pamabrom, ammonium chloride is used for the short-term relief of water weight gain or bloating associated with menstrual periods.

Generic Name

Aspirin (ASS-prin)

Brand Names

Adprin B [C]
*†Alka-Seltzer
*Anacin
Anodynos
*Arthritis Foundation
Arthritis Pain Formula [C]
Ascriptin [C]
Aspercin [C]
Aspergum [C]
Aspermin [C]
Aspirtab [C]
Back-Quell [C]
*Bayer [C]
BC
Buffaprin [C]
Buffasal [C]
Bufferin [C]
Buffetts II
Buffinol [C]
Cope
Ecotrin
Emagrin
Empirin [C]
*Excedrin
Goody's
Halfprin
Heartline
Norwich Aspirin [C]
P-A-C
Regiprin
Rid-a-Pain with Codeine
St. Joseph Low Dose Adult Aspirin
Stanback
Supac [C]
Vanquish

** Not all products in this brand-name group contain aspirin.*

† Consult the OTC ingredient charts to determine whether different formulations in this brand-name group are alcohol-, caffeine-, or sugar-free.

Type of Drug

Nonsteroidal anti-inflammatory drug (NSAID), analgesic (pain reliever), and antipyretic (fever reducer).

Used for

Temporary relief of mild to moderate pain and fever associated with the common cold, flu, and viral infections. It is also useful in treating mild to moderate pain associated with a variety of disorders including neuritis, neuralgia, bursitis, arthritis, rheumatism, simple headache, menstrual cramps, tooth and periodontic pain, sprains, and minor muscular aches. It may also be taken to relieve arthritis or inflammation of bones, joints, or other body tissues. There are certain populations that may benefit from aspirin taken under their doctor's supervision. Check with your doctor if you think the following may apply to you: Men (and possibly women) who have had a stroke or transient ischemic attack (TIA)—(oxygen shortage to the brain) because of a problem with blood coagulation may use aspirin to reduce the risk of having another attack. Aspirin may also be used as an anticoagulant (blood-thinning) drug in people with unstable angina, to protect against heart attack. The long-term effect of aspirin in preventing cataracts and colon cancer is now being studied.

General Information

NSAID is the general term used for a group of drugs that is effective in reducing inflammation and pain. Other OTC drugs in this group are ibuprofen, ketoprofen, and naproxen sodium. NSAIDS are generally quickly absorbed into the bloodstream. Pain and fever relief usually occurs within 1 hour of taking the first dose and lasts for 4 to 6 hours. Aspirin is also a member of the group of drugs called salicylates. Other OTC members of this group include sodium salicylate, choline salicylate, and magnesium salicylate. These drugs are no more effective than regular aspirin, although choline salicylate, sodium salicylate, and magnesium salicylate may be a little less irritating to the stomach. The other salicylates are also more expensive than aspirin.

Aspirin reduces fever by acting on the heat-regulating center in the brain. This causes the blood vessels in the skin to dilate, allowing heat to leave the body more rapidly. Aspirin's effects on pain and inflammation are thought to be related to its ability to prevent the manufacture of complex body hormones called prostaglandins, which sensitize pain receptors and stimulate the inflammatory response. Of all the salicylates, aspirin has the greatest effect on prostaglandin production.

Aspirin and acetaminophen have been proven equally effective in reducing most types of pain, and their fever-reducing effects are the same. However, unlike acetaminophen, aspirin presents risks to certain populations: Aspirin is associated with gastrointestinal (GI) irritation, erosion, and bleeding, and should not be used by individuals with a GI bleeding disorder or a history of peptic ulcers. Because it has been shown to be harmful to the developing fetus, aspirin should not be taken by pregnant women. Finally, aspirin should not be used by children under age 16 because of the risk of Reye's syndrome (see "Cautions and Warnings").

Aspirin is available by generic and brand name in the following forms. Generic name: tablets—buffered, chewable, and enteric; and rectal suppositories. Brand name: caplets—both regular and extended release; tablets—buffered, chewable, delayed-release, effervescent, and extended-release; chewing gum; powder; and rectal suppositories.

Cautions and Warnings

Do not take aspirin for more than 10 consecutive days or, in the presence of fever, for more than 3 days, unless directed by your doctor. Notify your doctor if this product does not relieve your symptoms in that time. Aspirin chewing gum should not be used for longer than 2 days because they may cause erosions in the mouth with long-term use.

Do not exceed the recommended daily dosage of aspirin.

Many OTC combination products contain aspirin. The following cautions and warnings also apply to those products.

People with liver damage or severe kidney failure should avoid aspirin.

Aspirin should not be used by patients with a history of bleeding disorders or by patients taking drugs for anticoagulation (blood thinning) without checking with a physician or pharmacist.

Aspirin should be avoided prior to surgery to reduce the risk of bleeding. Check with your physician regarding the duration of time to avoid aspirin use prior to a surgical procedure.

Alcohol can aggravate the stomach irritation caused by aspirin. The risk of aspirin-related ulcers is increased by alcohol.

Aspirin should not be used by patients with a history of ulcer disease.

If any of the following conditions develop, aspirin use should be stopped immediately and physician notified: continuous stomach pain, dizziness, hearing loss, and ringing or buzzing in the ears.

Patients with a history of asthma should not use aspirin without checking with a physician.

Children with the flu or chicken pox who are given aspirin or other salicylates may develop Reye's syndrome, a life-threatening condition characterized by vomiting, progressive damage to the central nervous system, liver injury, and abnormally low blood sugar. Up to 30% of those who develop Reye's syndrome die and permanent brain damage is possible in those who survive. Because of the risk of Reye's syndrome, do not give aspirin or other salicylates to children under age 16. Acetaminophen can usually be substituted.

Patients with AIDS and AIDS-related complex who take zidovudine (AZT) should avoid using aspirin because it may increase their risk of bleeding. For these patients, acetaminophen (taken as needed or for no longer than 7 consecutive days, unless recommended by a physician) is the recommended alternative for relief of pain.

Effervescent aspirin (e.g., some Alka-Seltzer products) is very high in sodium, which can lead to fluid retention. If you must restrict your sodium intake because of high blood pressure, heart failure, or kidney failure, choose another form of aspirin.

Possible Side Effects

▼ Common: nausea, upset stomach, heartburn, loss of appetite, and appearance of small amounts of blood in the stool.

Possible Side Effects *(continued)*

▼ Rare: hives, rashes, liver damage, fever, thirst, and difficulties with vision. Aspirin may contribute to the formation of stomach ulcers and bleeding. People who are allergic to aspirin and those with a history of nasal polyps, asthma, or rhinitis may experience breathing difficulty and a stuffy nose.

Drug Interactions

• Aspirin should not be taken by individuals currently taking methotrexate, which is used to treat cancer, severe psoriasis, severe rheumatoid arthritis, and to induce abortion, or valproic acid, an anticonvulsant. It can increase the toxicity of these drugs.

• Aspirin should also not be taken with anticoagulant (blood-thinning) drugs, such as warfarin and dicumarol. It will exaggerate the effects of these drugs and increase the risk of abnormal bleeding.

• The possibility of a stomach ulcer is increased if aspirin is taken together with an adrenal corticosteroid, such as hydocortisone; phenylbutazone, another NSAID; or alcoholic beverages. Taking aspirin with another NSAID has no benefit and carries a greatly increased risk of side effects.

• Aspirin will counteract the effects of the antigout medications probenecid and sulfinpyrazone and may counteract the effects of angiotensin-converting enzyme (ACE) inhibitors and beta blockers, which work to lower blood pressure. Aspirin may also counteract the effects of some diuretics in people with severe liver disease.

• Combining nitroglycerin tablets and aspirin may lead to an unexpected drop in blood pressure.

Food Interactions

Take aspirin with food, milk, or water to reduce the chance of upset stomach or bleeding.

Usual Dose

Caplet, Tablet, Powder, or Suppositories

Adult (age 16 and over): 325–650 mg every 4 hours, as needed; the total dose should not exceed 4000 mg in 24 hours.

Child (under age 16): not recommended because of the risk of Reye's syndrome (see "Cautions and Warnings").

Chewing Gum

Adult (age 16 and over): The usual dose is 454 mg, repeated as needed; the total dose should not exceed 3630 mg in 24 hours.

Child (under age 16): not recommended because of the risk of Reye's syndrome (see "Cautions and Warnings").

Highly Buffered Effervescent Solution

Adult (age 16 and over): The usual dose is 648 mg every 4–6 hours, as needed; the total dose should not exceed 2590 mg in 24 hours.

Child (under age 16): not recommended because of the risk of Reye's syndrome (see "Cautions and Warnings").

Extended-release Tablets

Adult (age 16 and over): The usual dose is 650–1300 mg every 8 hours, as needed; the total dose should not exceed 3900 mg in 24 hours. If you find it difficult to swallow these tablets, you may gently break them up or crumble them, either while they are in your mouth or just before you are ready to take them. However, they must not be ground up if they are to work properly.

Child (under age 16): not recommended because of the risk of Reye's syndrome (see "Cautions and Warnings").

If your doctor recommends aspirin for the prevention of stroke, TIA, or heart attack, he or she will design a dosage schedule to meet your needs.

Overdosage

Symptoms of mild overdosage include rapid or deep breathing, nausea, vomiting, dizziness, ringing or buzzing in the ears, flushing, sweating, thirst, headache, drowsiness, diarrhea, and rapid heartbeat. Severe overdose may cause fever, excitement, low blood sugar, confusion, convulsions, liver or kidney failure, coma, and bleeding.

Even if the victim is not displaying any of the symptoms listed above, do the following in case of accidental overdose: If the victim is unconscious or having convulsions, call for an ambulance immediately. If you take the victim to an emergency room, be sure to bring the bottle or container with you. If the victim is conscious, call your local poison control center or a health care professional. The poison control center may suggest inducing vomiting with ipecac syrup (available without a prescription at any pharmacy). DO NOT induce vomiting unless specifically instructed to do so.

Special Information

A strong vinegary smell means that the aspirin has started to break down in the bottle and should be discarded.

Special Populations

Allergies

If you are allergic to indomethacin, sulindac, ibuprofen, ketoprofen, fenoprofen, naproxen, tolmetin, or meclofenamate sodium, or to products containing tartrazine (a commonly used orange food coloring), you may also be allergic to aspirin.

People with asthma and/or nasal polyps are more likely to be allergic to aspirin.

Pregnancy/Breast-feeding

Aspirin can cause bleeding problems in the developing fetus and can lead to a low-birth-weight infant; it can also cause bleeding problems in the mother before, during, or after pregnancy. Do not take aspirin if you are pregnant.

Aspirin passes into breast milk. If you are nursing, call your doctor before self-medicating with aspirin. Acetaminophen may be a better choice.

Infants/Children

Aspirin should not be taken by children younger than age 16 unless directed by a doctor, due to the risk of Reye's syndrome (see "Cautions and Warnings").

Seniors

Seniors may find aspirin irritating to the stomach, especially in larger doses. Older adults with liver disease or severe kidney impairment should not use aspirin.

Generic Name
Attapulgite (ATT-uh-PULL-gite)

Brand Names

Diasorb
Donnagel
Kaopectate
Parepectolin
Rheaban

Type of Drug

Antidiarrheal.

Used for

Control and symptomatic relief of acute diarrhea.

General Information

The average, healthy individual defecates anywhere from 3 times a day to 3 times a week. Diarrhea is characterized by abnormal frequency or consistency of stool, and can be caused by any one of several conditions, either gastrointestinal (GI) or non-GI. These include bacterial and viral infections, food intolerance, gastroenteritis, and side effects of prescription and OTC drugs. The cause of the diarrhea determines which drug therapy is best.

It should be emphasized that diarrhea is a symptom. Antidiarrheal medications provide symptomatic relief, which generally is sufficient for the treatment of temporary, uncomplicated diarrhea, such as that caused by an allergic reaction to dairy products. Persistent or recurrent diarrhea, however, can be a sign of a more serious condition requiring the attention of a health care professional and treatment geared toward the underlying condition. Persistent diarrhea can also lead to dehydration. Self-medication with attapulgite or another antidiarrheal does not preclude the fluid, electrolyte, and nutritional therapies necessary for the treatment of more serious, chronic diarrhea.

Attapulgite is one of several GI adsorbents, which work by adsorbing, or binding, toxins, bacteria, and various noxious materials in the GI tract—although their action is not limited to undesirable substances (see "Cautions and Warnings").

Adsorbents are the OTC antidiarrheal products prescribed most often. However, attapulgite, along with other adsorbents, is currently being evaluated for safety and efficacy by the FDA's OTC Center for Drug Evaluations and Research. Consult your pharmacist regarding possible reclassification and labeling changes before self-medicating with attapulgite.

Generic attapulgite is available in liquid form; brand name products are available in tablet, chewable tablet, caplet, and liquid form. Because large doses are generally used, attapulgite products are most commonly available in flavored liquid form to improve palatability.

Cautions and Warnings

Do not use attapulgite for more than 2 days, unless directed by your doctor. Uncomplicated, acute diarrhea usually improves within 24 to 48 hours. Persistent diarrhea can lead to dehydration, which may require the administration of appropriate fluid and electrolyte therapy.

Do not exceed the recommended daily dosage of attapulgite.

Do not take attapulgite if your diarrhea is accompanied by high fever (higher than 101°F), vomiting, or blood in the stool. Call your doctor if fever develops during self-medication with attapulgite.

Because attapulgite's action is not selective, this product may adsorb desirable substances such as nutrients along with toxins. It may also adsorb oral medications being taken at the same time (see "Drug Interactions").

Possible Side Effects

▼ Most common: constipation, bloating, fullness.

Drug Interactions

• Because attapulgite's GI adsorption is not selective, it may adsorb any other oral medication being taken at the same time, thus decreasing the absorption of the other medication. It is generally advised to take other oral medications 2 hours before or 3–4 hours after taking attapulgite. You may have to change the dosing interval of your other medication. Talk to your physician or pharmacist.

Food Interactions

None known.

Usual Dose

Adult and Child (age 12 and over): 1200–3000 mg up to 7 doses, or 9000 mg a day.

Child (age 6–11): 600–1500 mg up to 7 doses, or 4500 mg a day.

Child (age 3–5): 300–750 mg up to 7 doses, or 2250 mg a day.

Child (under age 3): not recommended unless directed by your doctor.

Take attapulgite after the first loose bowel movement. You may take additional doses after subsequent loose bowel movements, but do not exceed the recommended daily dosage.

Be sure to shake the liquid well before using.

Do not take attapulgite for more than 2 days.

Be sure to drink plenty of clear liquids to help prevent dehydration, which may accompany diarrhea.

Overdosage

Do the following in case of accidental overdose: If the victim is unconscious or having convulsions, call for an ambulance immediately. If you take the victim to an emergency room, be sure to bring the bottle or container with you. If the victim is conscious, call your local poison control center or a health care professional. The poison control center may suggest inducing vomiting with ipecac syrup (available without a prescription at any pharmacy). DO NOT induce vomiting unless specifically instructed to do so.

Special Populations

Pregnancy/Breast-feeding

It is not generally recommended that pregnant women take any drugs, particularly during the first 3 months after conception. Check with your doctor before self-medicating with attapulgite if you are or might be pregnant, or if you are breastfeeding. Also talk to your physician regarding fluid and electrolyte management if you are suffering from diarrhea.

Infants/Children

Infants and children with acute or chronic diarrhea are at particular risk for severe and possibly dangerous dehydration and electrolyte imbalance. Over-reliance on antidiarrheal drugs may lead to the loss of essential nutritional factors and dehydration. Antidiarrheal medications in general have not been shown to be especially effective in children.

Attapulgite should not be used for self-medication in children under age 3 unless directed by a doctor.

Seniors

Attapulgite should not be used for self-medication by individuals older than age 60. If, in addition to diarrhea, you are suffering from other ailments that make you weak, it is beneficial to consult your physician regarding fluid and electrolyte management.

Generic Name

Bacitracin Zinc (BASS-uh-TRAY-sin zink)

Brand Names

Bacigvent
Betadine First Aid
  Antibiotic Plus Moisturizer
Campho-phenique
  Triple Antibiotic
Clomycin
Lanabiotic
Medi-Quik Triple
  Antibiotic
Mycitracin
Neomixin
*Neosporin
Polysporin
Tribiotic Plus

**Not all products in this brand-name group contain bacitracin zinc.*

Type of Drug

Topical antibiotic.

Used for

Treatment of skin infection in minor cuts, scrapes, and burns.

General Information

Topical antibiotics are used to prevent or treat infections caused by bacteria that grow in wounds and cause inflammation, itching, and oozing. If left untreated, such infections can progress to more serious infections involving the deeper tissue of the skin.

There are many types of antibiotics available, each effective against different forms of bacteria. Many OTC products combine different antibiotics so that they have a broad spectrum of effectiveness against a range of disease-causing bacteria.

Bacitracin is used to treat or prevent wound infections caused by various bacteria, including staphylococcus and streptococcus germs. It is usually available in combination with other antibiotics, such as polymyxin B sulfate and neomycin. Bacitracin is available by generic and brand name in cream, ointment, powder, and spray form.

Applied within 4 hours after an injury, antibiotics may reduce the risk of infection by killing any bacteria that have contaminated the wound. If infection is prevented or a minor infection contained, then the wound can heal more quickly.

Cautions and Warnings

If there is no improvement in the infected area within 5 days of continuous use or if an allergic reaction develops, discontinue using bacitracin and contact your doctor.

Do not exceed the recommended daily dosage of bacitracin products.

This drug is for external use on minor wounds only.

Do not use bacitracin products over large areas of injured skin, on open wounds, or in large quantities.

OTC formulations of bacitracin are not meant for treatment of eye infections. Topical ointment containing antibiotics should never be used on the eyes. Be sure to read labels carefully.

In the case of deep puncture wounds or animal bites, contact your doctor immediately.

Bacitracin rarely causes any allergic reaction on its own, but the drug is often combined with drugs such as neomycin, which can cause a secondary rash or inflammation.

Use of bacitracin may allow certain fungal infections to develop, especially involving the fungus *Candida*. These infections may require treatment with products that work against fungi. Consult your doctor.

Possible Side Effects

- ▼ Most common: general itching, burning, swelling of the lips and face, sweating, and chest tightness.
- ▼ Rare: low blood pressure, fainting, difficulty breathing, and cardiac arrest.

Drug Interactions

None known.

Usual Dose

Adult and Child (age 2 and over): Cleanse the wound before applying. Apply a fingertip-sized amount of the product 1–3 times a day, as needed. The affected area may be covered with a sterile bandage.

Child (under age 2): Consult a doctor.

Overdosage

Most of this medication is absorbed by the skin tissues. Very little is absorbed by the rest of the body. Consequently there is a low risk of overdose.

Do the following in case of accidental ingestion: If the victim is unconscious or having convulsions, call for an ambulance immediately. If you take the victim to an emergency room, be sure to bring the bottle or container with you. If the victim is conscious, call your local poison control center or a health care professional. The poison control center may suggest inducing vomiting with ipecac syrup (available without a prescription at any pharmacy). DO NOT induce vomiting unless specifically instructed to do so.

Special Populations

Allergies

People who are sensitive to neomycin may also be sensitive to bacitracin.

Pregnancy/Breast-feeding

It is not generally recommended that pregnant women take any drugs, particularly during the first 3 months after con-

ception. However, there is no indication that bacitracin has any abnormal effects on pregnant women and their fetuses or on nursing mothers and their infants.

Infants/Children

Combination medications containing bacitracin may also contain neomycin. These products should never be used on diaper rash in infants unless recommended by your doctor. There is a possibility of allergic reaction to the neomycin. In addition, these products should not be used over large areas of the body. These factors can lead to serious internal complications in a child.

Do not use bacitracin in children younger than age 2 without first consulting your doctor.

Seniors

Products containing bacitracin should never be used on large areas of the body in older individuals.

Generic Name

Benzalkonium Chloride

(BEN-zal-KOE-nee-um KLOR-ide)

Definition

An anti-infective used in OTC solutions and sprays for the treatment of minor injuries and infected wounds. The area being treated must be thoroughly free of soap residue, since soap renders benzalkonium chloride ineffective. Benzalkonium chloride is also used in ophthalmic (eye) solutions to preserve sterility.

Generic Name

Benzethonium Chloride

(BEN-zeh-THOE-nee-um KLOR-ide)

Definition

An anti-infective ingredient found in a wide range of OTC products. As an antibacterial agent in first-aid skin care products, it prevents secondary infection that can result when people scratch insect bites and bee stings. Because it acts as a detergent, benzethonium chloride is used in shampoos for control of mild cases of dandruff. In eye care products, it serves to kill microorganisms, but these products should be used with caution because benzethonium chloride can weaken the ability of tears to keep the eye moist. It is the active ingredient in products for maintaining sterility in stomas (surgical openings in the skin) and for deodorizing ostomy bags.

In douche products, benzethonium chloride acts as a preservative but is present in amounts that are too low to provide the antimicrobial action that some manufacturers claim. Although benzethonium chloride does not usually cause skin irritation, some women who use douches may be highly sensitive to the chemical. If irritation develops, stop using the product. Although some hemorrhoid preparations might contain benzethonium chloride, the FDA has not yet determined whether it is safe and effective for this use.

A similar ingredient, methylbenzethonium chloride, is used as a topical anti-infective in diaper rash treatments and other skin care products.

Generic Name

Benzocaine (BEN-zoe-kane)

Brand Names

Aerocaine
Aerotherm
Americaine
†Anbesol
Babee Teething
Benzodent Denture Analgesic
Bicozene External Analgesic Creme
Boil Ease
Burntame
*Cepacol
Cetacaine
Chigger-Tox
Chiggerex
Chloraseptic
*Dent's
Dent-Zel-Ite Oval Mucosal Analgesic
Dermacoat
Dermoplast
Dr. Scholl's
Foille
HDA Toothache Gel
†Hurricaine
Kank-A Professional Strength
Lagol

Lanacane
Little Teethers Oral Pain Relief [A] [S]
Medadyne
Medicated First Aid Burn
Mycinettes Lozenge
Numzident Adult Strength
Numzit
*†Orajel
Outgro Pain Relieving
*Ovabase
Ovasol
†Protac
Red Cross Canker Sore Medication
*Rhuli Spray
Rid-a-Pain Dental Drops
SensoGARD [A]
Solarcaine
Spec-T Sore Throat
Sting-Eze
*Tanac
Vicks Chloraseptic Sore Throat [A]
Zilactin B

**Not all products in this brand-name group contain benzocaine.*

†Consult the OTC ingredient charts to determine whether different formulations in this brand-name group are alcohol-, caffeine-, or sugar-free.

Type of Drug

Local anesthetic.

Used for

Temporary relief of sore throat pain, pain associated with various dental conditions (toothache, sore gums, denture irritation, teething), or pain and itching from minor burns, sunburns, minor cuts or scrapes, insect bites, minor skin irritations, or hemorrhoids.

General Information

Topical anesthetics work by blocking pain signals in the skin and keeping them from traveling along the nerves to the brain. The duration of relief from pain from OTC anesthetics for skin conditions is often short, lasting only 15 to 45 minutes. However, these medications should be applied only 3 or 4 times a day. Consequently, they will not always provide around-the-clock relief.

When applied to the skin or gums or taken as a lozenge, benzocaine temporarily numbs pain by blocking the pain impulses to that area. Because the sensation of itching is produced by the nerve fibers that carry pain impulses, benzocaine also relieves itching at the same time as it reduces pain.

Benzocaine was included in OTC weight control products for nearly 40 years, but has been removed from most of these products following the FDA's advisory letter to manufacturers stating that the agency intends to classify the drug as ineffective for weight loss.

Benzocaine is available by generic and brand name in a variety of forms (aerosols, lozenges, gels, pastes, lotions, solutions), depending on the condition for which it is intended to be used. Although benzocaine is included in products to temporarily relieve ear pain, it has not been proven to be effective for this indication.

Cautions and Warnings

If your condition worsens or symptoms persist for more than 7 days, or clear up and recur within a few days, or if you develop an infection or irritation, stop using benzocaine immediately and call your doctor.

Do not exceed the recommended daily dosage of benzocaine.

Topical benzocaine is for external use only. Avoid getting it into your eyes.

Don't use topical benzocaine for deep or puncture wounds or for serious burns.

If you develop sensitivity to benzocaine, the second time you use it, you will notice an itchy, possibly oozing, rash that can appear minutes to hours after exposure. If this occurs, stop using benzocaine immediately. Wash the area gently to remove any traces of benzocaine and apply compresses of cool tap water if the area is oozing. Calamine lotion, colloidal oatmeal baths, and hydrocortisone cream may help relieve the itching and inflammation. Call your doctor if you have a severe reaction, if the reaction covers a large area of your body, or if the rash does not begin to improve in a few days or worsens.

Phenylketonurics (people who cannot digest the amino acid phenylalanine) should be aware that some oral formulations of benzocaine contain aspartame (Nutrasweet), which breaks down in the gastrointestinal tract to phenylalanine after the drug is taken.

Benzocaine should not be used by individuals with known or suspected hypersensitivity to it or to other ester-type local anesthetics (such as proparacaine hydrochloride or tetracaine).

Individuals with methemoglobinemia (a rare blood disorder) should not use benzocaine.

Benzocaine lozenges or spray aerosols for sore throat pain should be used only at intervals between eating or drinking. The benzocaine numbs your throat and can make it hard to swallow, increasing the risk of choking.

Possible Side Effects

In about 1% of people, benzocaine can cause a hypersensitivity reaction leading to allergic contact dermatitis (rash). This reaction will not be apparent the first time you use benzocaine; an initial sensitizing exposure is necessary.

Drug Interactions

- Benzocaine can react with the chemicals in hair dyes and with sunscreens containing para-aminobenzoic acid (PABA); this may result in allergic contact dermatitis.

Food Interactions

None known.

Usual Dose

Oral Preparations

Adult and Child (age 3 and over): Dissolve 1 lozenge in the mouth; repeat as needed (e.g., every hour).

Child (under age 3): not recommended.

Topical Preparations

Adult and Child (age 2 and over): Apply to the affected area as needed, usually 3–4 times daily, or as directed by your doctor.

Child (under age 2): not recommended unless directed by a doctor.

Overdosage

Do the following in case of accidental ingestion or overdose: If the victim is unconscious or having convulsions, call for an ambulance immediately. If you take the victim to an emergency room, be sure to bring the bottle or container with you. If the victim is conscious, call your local poison control center or a health care professional. The poison control center may suggest inducing vomiting with ipecac syrup (available without a prescription at any pharmacy). DO NOT induce vomiting unless specifically instructed to do so.

Special Populations

Allergies

Some oral benzocaine preparations also contain the dye tartrazine, which may cause allergic reactions (including bronchial asthma) in some people. Those who are allergic to aspirin are more likely to react to tartrazine.

Pregnancy/Breast-feeding

It is not generally recommended that pregnant women take any drugs, particularly during the first 3 months after conception. Check with your doctor if you are or might be pregnant, or if you are breast-feeding.

Infants/Children

Oral benzocaine preparations should not be used by children under 3 years of age, and topical benzocaine should not be used by children under 2 years of age, unless directed by a doctor.

Seniors

Seniors should exercise the same caution as younger adults when using benzocaine.

Generic Name

Benzoic Acid (ben-ZOE-ik ASS-id)

Brand Names

Antinea Cream
Blis-To-Sol Powder
Rid-Itch
Whitfield's Ointment

Type of Drug

Antimicrobial and antifungal agent.

Used for

Treatment of fungal infections on the skin.

General Information

Benzoic acid works against fungal infections by damaging the cell walls of the fungus, thus killing the cell and stopping the fungus from spreading. Besides deterring fungal growth, benzoic acid acts as a mild antiseptic.

Benzoic acid is usually combined with salicylic acid in OTC products used to treat a number of common fungal conditions of the skin: Athlete's foot, jock itch, and ringworm are infections caused by various kinds of fungus that develop on the feet, crotch, and scalp, respectively. These infections cause itching, burning, and inflammation. In severe cases the infected area can ooze, and the skin can break and peel.

Thrush is a form of infection caused by the *Candida* fungus. It appears on mucous membranes or moist skin, such as in the crotch or under the breasts. Men are at risk of developing thrush on the penis which can be passed on to sexual partners. Thrush can also develop in association with diaper rash. Symptoms on the skin include inflammation and itchy red rash with flaky white patches.

Benzoic acid is a weak antifungal agent. Due to the availability of other highly effective topical antifungal agents, such as clotrimazole, miconazole, and tolnaftate, benzoic acid is considered a second-line agent.

Benzoic acid is available by brand name as a cream and by brand and generic name as an ointment.

Cautions and Warnings

Antifungal drugs are for use on the skin. If there is no improvement in the infected area within 7 days or if an allergic reaction develops, discontinue using the drug and contact your doctor.

Do not exceed the recommended daily dosage of benzoic acid products.

Do not use benzoic acid products on or near the eyes unless directed by your doctor. Do not use over large areas of inflamed skin or in large doses.

Possible Side Effects

▼ Rare: increased skin irritation, stinging, or inflammation. These are actually signs that the medication is working, because they are due in part to benzoic acid's destructive action on the fungus. The discomfort or stinging in the affected area should stop after the first few applications. If it does not, discontinue using the product and contact your doctor.

Drug Interactions

None known.

Usual Dose

For use in the treatment of fungal infections of the skin, drugs containing benzoic acid should be applied once or twice daily to the affected area after the area is washed and thoroughly patted dry. To avoid the accumulation of moisture, after application the skin should be allowed to air-dry before replacing clothing or footware.

Overdosage

Do the following in case of accidental ingestion: If the victim is unconscious or having convulsions, call for an ambulance immediately. If you take the victim to an emergency room, be sure to bring the bottle or container with you. If the victim is conscious, call your local poison control center or a health care professional. The poison control center may suggest inducing vomiting with ipecac syrup (available without a prescription at any pharmacy). DO NOT induce vomiting unless specifically instructed to do so.

Special Information

After bathing or showering the affected area should be dried last to avoid spread of the infection from the towel to other parts of the body. Wash towels in hot water after each use. The area should then be kept as dry as possible. Cotton balls or cotton gauze can be wedged between toes or under the breasts to aid in keeping the affected sites aired.

Wash your hands after applying the medication to avoid the possibility of accidentally getting these products in your mouth or eyes.

Special Populations

Pregnancy/Breast-feeding

It is not generally recommended that pregnant women take any drugs, particularly during the first 3 months after conception.

However, there is no indication that benzoic acid poses a risk to pregnant women, nursing mothers or their infants. If you are or might be pregnant, or you are breast-feeding, check with your doctor prior to using benzoic acid.

Infants/Children

When using this product on children, care should be taken to prevent the child from putting the treated area in their mouth, risking accidental ingestion.

Seniors

Seniors should exercise the same caution as younger adults when using these products.

Generic Name

Benzoyl Peroxide (BEN-zoil per-OKS-ide)

Brand Names

AMBI 10 Acne Medication
Benoxyl
*Clean & Clear
*Clearasil
Clear By Design
*ExACT
*Fostex 10%
Loroxide
Neutrogena Acne
On-The-Spot
*Oxy
Pan Oxyl
Vanoxide

**Not all products in this brand-name group contain benzoyl peroxide.*

Type of Drug

Topical acne medication.

Used for

Treatment and prevention of mild to moderate acne vulgaris.

General Information

Acne is a common skin disorder, usually arising during puberty. Acne blemishes (pimples and blackheads) are formed when a pore in the skin becomes blocked, trapping sebum (an oily skin secretion). Bacteria can grow in this closed area, causing infection. The body sends white blood cells and other cells of the immune system to the site to destroy the bacteria. The debris from this process builds up, causing the area to become swollen and irritated, creating a pimple.

Acne occurs in areas of the body that have a high number of oil glands, such as the face, chest, upper back, and shoulders.

Benzoyl peroxide fights acne infection in several ways. It stimulates skin, which causes it to shed cells more quickly and thus prevents the pore from closing around the oil plug. This in turn makes the oil and debris easier to remove through gentle scrubbing. It also mildly irritates the tissue surfaces within the pore itself. By doing so, it promotes the rapid turnover of cells inside the pore, which helps flush out any excess skin oils and debris.

This drug also destroys or prevents the growth of the acne-causing bacteria inside infected pores. It reduces the formation of fatty substances that contribute to blemishes. Finally, benzoyl peroxide has a drying effect on the skin, which aids in keeping the excess oils under control and encourages the skin to heal by producing new cells more rapidly.

Benzoyl peroxide only works so long as it is in contact with the skin. Merely washing the area does not produce long-lasting effects. Products should be chosen that remain on the skin for a period of time so the medication has a chance to work.

Lotions are recommended for dry or sensitive skin and are appropriate for use during dry winter weather. However, gels are the most effective formulations, because they have strong drying properties and remain active on the skin surface for longer periods of time.

The FDA recently stated that there is insufficient evidence to conclude whether benzoyl peroxide is indeed safe and effective. Studies to resolve the question are under way, but results will take a few years.

Cautions and Warnings

If benzoyl peroxide is not effective after 3 months you may need to try a different product.

Do not exceed the recommended daily dosage of benzoyl peroxide.

Products containing benzoyl peroxide are for external use only. Do not use these products if you have very sensitive skin or have had an adverse reaction to this chemical.

Keep these products away from your eyes, lips, and mouth. Do not let them come into contact with cuts, scrapes, or other abrasions, since benzoyl peroxide can irritate these areas and cause pain.

Individuals with sensitive skin may first want to try products with lower concentrations (5% or less) of benzoyl peroxide to test for sensitivity to the chemical. Apply only to a small area and see if your skin develops a reaction over the next 24 hours. Do not reapply until you are sure there is no adverse reaction.

Benzoyl peroxide achieves its results in part by causing mild skin irritation. However, if excessive stinging or burning occurs, wash the affected area with a mild soap and water. Do not reapply the product for 24 hours.

Avoid exposure to sunlamps and sunlight while using benzoyl peroxide, unless recommended by your doctor. Ultraviolet light can aggravate acne conditions.

Benzoyl peroxide can act as a bleaching agent on clothes and hair. Take appropriate precautions while applying benzoyl peroxide to avoid contact with clothes and thus reduce risk of discoloration.

In recent years scientists have become concerned that use of benzoyl peroxide may be a factor in certain kinds of skin cancer. The drug does not appear to cause tumors to develop; the cause of most skin cancers is ultraviolet radiation. However, benzoyl peroxide may contribute to the growth of tumors once they start to form.

Possible Side Effects

▼ Most common: redness, burning, itching, peeling, or possible swelling. If these side effects develop, you may need to use the product less frequently or in a lower strength. If the irritation becomes severe or continues even after you stop using benzoyl peroxide, contact your doctor.

Drug Interactions

• Do not use products containing benzoyl peroxide at the same time as other acne medications. This can result in excessive drying or irritation of the skin, which can increase the risk of infection.

Usual Dose

Adult and Child (age 12 and over): The affected area should be gently cleansed with a nonmedicated soap and water, then patted dry. Apply a thin layer of the product and massage it into the affected area. Apply once or twice per day, as needed or as directed.

Child (under age 12): not recommended unless directed by a doctor.

Overdosage

Accidental ingestion of large amounts of these products is not likely. In theory, however, these products may cause nausea, vomiting, abdominal discomfort, and diarrhea.

Even if the victim is not displaying any of the symptoms listed above, do the following in case of accidental ingestion: If the victim is unconscious or having convulsions, call for an ambulance immediately. If you take the victim to an emergency room, be sure to bring the bottle or container with you. If the victim is conscious, call your local poison control center or a health care professional. The poison control center may suggest inducing vomiting with ipecac syrup (available without a prescription at any pharmacy). DO NOT induce vomiting unless specifically instructed to do so.

Special Populations

Pregnancy/Breast-feeding

It is not generally recommended that pregnant women take any drugs, particularly during the first 3 months after conception. Check with your doctor before using benzoyl peroxide if you are or might be pregnant, or if you are breast-feeding.

Infants/Children

Benzoyl peroxide is not recommended for children under 12 unless directed by a doctor.

Seniors

Seniors should exercise the same caution as younger adults when using benzoyl peroxide.

Generic Name

Benzyl Alcohol (BEN-zil AL-kuh-hall)

Definition

A clear, colorless, oily liquid used as a topical anesthetic. In low concentrations (0.05% to 0.1%), benzyl alcohol is used to treat the pain of canker sores. It is available in concentrations of 5% to 25% for relief of pain caused by hemorrhoids. At higher concentrations (10% to 33%), it is an effective remedy for pain from external skin problems, including fever blisters, cold sores, and minor burns or sunburn.

Generic Name

BHT

Definition

Abbreviation for butylated hydroxytoluene (BYU-til-ATE-ed hye-DROK-see-TOL-yew-een), a chemical preservative used in OTC products (e.g., vaginal lubricants).

Generic Name

Bisacodyl (bis-uh-KOE-dill)

Brand Names

Bisco-Lax
*Correctol
Deficol
Dulcolax
Evac-Q-Kwik
Feen-A-Mint
*†Fleet
Gentle Laxative

**Not all products in this brand-name group contain bisacodyl.*

†*Consult the OTC ingredient charts to determine whether different formulations in this brand-name group are alcohol-, caffeine-, or sugar-free.*

Type of Drug

Laxative.

Used for

Relief of occasional constipation (irregularity).

General Information

The average, healthy individual defecates anywhere from 3 times a day to 3 times a week. Constipation is determined, not necessarily by the frequency of bowel movements, but by the consistency of the stool, how difficult it is to eliminate, and symptoms such as dull headache, low back pain, and abdominal distention (swelling). Evaluate your condition carefully and discuss your symptoms and their possible causes with your pharmacist before self-medicating with a laxative. Laxatives are not always necessary, and when used improperly can either prevent the desired effect or result in laxative dependency. If you are indeed constipated, your condition may be best managed through proper diet, adequate fluid intake, and exercise. If you must use a laxative, choose the mildest effective product.

Laxatives may be classified by their mechanism of action: bulk-forming, emollient (stool softeners), lubricant, saline, hyperosmotic, and stimulant. Bisacodyl is a stimulant laxative. According to different studies, stimulant laxatives work by either increasing the propulsive activity of the intestine or stimulating the secretion of water and electrolytes in the intestine, thus leading to evacuation of the colon. Bisacodyl is specifically a diphenylmethane laxative, which produces a more intense effect than other stimulant laxatives, such as the anthraquinone stimulant senna.

Bisacodyl generally produces a bowel movement in 6 to 12 hours if taken orally and in 15 to 60 minutes if taken rectally.

Generic bisacodyl is available in tablet form; brand name products are available in tablet, caplet, suppository, and enema form. Bisacodyl is also available in several combination products containing other laxatives/ingredients.

Cautions and Warnings

Do not use bisacodyl for more than 7 days, unless directed by your doctor. Long-term use of laxatives has been linked with laxative dependence, chronic constipation, and loss of normal bowel function. Using laxatives too frequently can result in persistent diarrhea, hypokalemia (abnormally low potassium in the blood), loss of essential nutrients, and dehydration.

Do not exceed the recommended daily dosage of bisacodyl.

Of all the types of laxatives, stimulant laxatives such as bisacodyl are particularly habit-forming, and are the most likely to cause adverse effects such as diarrhea, gastrointestinal (GI) irritation, and fluid and electrolyte depletion with long-term use. The higher the dose of bisacodyl, the more likely you are to experience adverse effects.

Do not take bisacodyl if you have abdominal pain, nausea, vomiting, or kidney disease, unless directed by your doctor.

If you notice a marked change in bowel habits lasting for more than 2 weeks, do not take bisacodyl until you have spoken to your doctor. Also contact your doctor if there is blood in your stool, so that colon cancer or other significant disease can be ruled out before you begin self-medication with bisacodyl.

If you have had a disease or surgery affecting the GI tract, using a laxative may affect your condition adversely.

If you have rectal bleeding after using bisacodyl, or if you do not have a bowel movement after 7 days of using this medication, you may have a serious condition. Stop using the product and call your doctor.

Laxatives may decrease the absorption of other drugs that pass through the GI tract (see "Drug Interactions").

Bisacodyl tablets are coated to prevent stomach irritation. Do not chew them, or the medication will possibly irritate your stomach and cause you to vomit. People who cannot swallow pills without chewing or crushing them should not take bisacodyl unless directed by a doctor.

If you are using a bisacodyl enema product, be sure to follow the directions on the package carefully. An enema that is incorrectly administered can have adverse effects.

Possible Side Effects

- ▼ Most common: abdominal discomfort, faintness, nausea, cramps, pinching and spasmodic pain in the bowels, colic, increased mucus secretion.
- ▼ Less common (chronic use of product only): metabolic acidosis or alkalosis (imbalances of acid and base in body fluids), hypocalcemia (too little calcium in the blood), tetany (characterized by foot spasms, muscular twitching, and cramps), loss of protein in the small intestine, electrolyte and fluid deficiencies (characterized by vomiting and muscle weakness), impaired intestinal absorption of nutrients, burning sensation in the rectum (suppository only), cathartic colon (weak or dilated colon).

Drug Interactions

• All laxatives potentially decrease the absorption of any oral drug taken at the same time. If you are currently taking an oral medication, talk to your pharmacist before self-medicating with bisacodyl.

• To avoid stomach irritation and possible vomiting, do not take bisacodyl within 1 hour of taking an antacid.

• Bisacodyl should not be taken with drugs that increase gastric pH, such as cimetidine and ranitidine (used to treat peptic ulcers, heartburn, and acid indigestion) and omeprazole, a proton pump inhibitor (used to treat ulcers).

Food Interactions

To avoid stomach irritation and possible vomiting, do not take bisacodyl within 1 hour of drinking milk.

Usual Dose

Doses should be adjusted to individual usage. Take bisacodyl as needed, but do not exceed the recommended daily dosage. Take on an empty stomach for rapid effect.

Tablet

Adult and Child (age 12 and over): 10–30 mg once a day. Do not chew or crush. Oral bisacodyl is best taken at night if a morning bowel movement is desired.

Child (age 6–11): 5–10 mg once a day.

Child (under age 6): not recommended unless directed by a doctor.

Suppository

Adult and Child (age 6 and over): 10 mg once a day. Administer the suppository at the time a bowel movement is desired. Remove the wrapper from the suppository. Lie on your side and, with pointed end up, push the suppository high into the rectum. Retain it for 15–20 minutes. If you feel the suppository slipping out, push it higher into the rectum. If you suffer from hemorrhoids or anal fissures, coat the tip of the suppository with petroleum jelly.

Child (under age 6): not recommended unless directed by a doctor.

Enema

Adult and Child (age 6 and over): Follow the directions on the package carefully. To administer an enema, lie on your side with your knees bent. Allow the solution to flow into the rectum *slowly*. Retain the solution until you feel stomach cramps.

Child (under age 6): not recommended unless directed by a doctor.

Overdosage

Symptoms of overdosage include persistent diarrhea and dehydration.

Even if the victim is not displaying any of the symptoms listed above, do the following in case of accidental overdose: If the victim is unconscious or having convulsions, call for an ambulance immediately. If you take the victim to an emergency room, be sure to bring the bottle or container with you. If the victim is conscious, call your local poison

control center or a health care professional. The poison control center may suggest inducing vomiting with ipecac syrup (available without a prescription at any pharmacy). DO NOT induce vomiting unless specifically instructed to do so.

Special Information

If your bisacodyl suppository feels too soft to insert, hold it under cold water, still in the wrapper, for a couple of minutes.

Special Populations

Pregnancy/Breast-feeding

Stimulant laxatives such as bisacodyl should be avoided during pregnancy. Only bulk-forming or emollient laxatives are recommended for pregnant women. Also consider talking to your doctor about diet and mild exercise in the management of constipation.

Bisacodyl passes into breast milk in very small amounts. Check with your doctor before taking bisacodyl if you are breast-feeding.

Infants/Children

Observe your child carefully for patterns of bowel movements and the pain or difficulty with which the bowel movements are made before deciding whether the child is actually constipated. As with adults, "normal" bowel habits vary in children. If your child is indeed constipated, increasing fluid intake and adding fiber to his or her diet may be ways to manage the condition. In general, the use of laxatives should be avoided in children.

Do not give bisacodyl to children under age 6 unless directed by a doctor.

Seniors

Seniors commonly experience constipation, and consequently may become laxative-dependent. Be cautious of chronically turning to laxatives to ease constipation, and instead look to diet and increased fluid intake as therapeutic measures (see "Cautions and Warnings").

Stimulant laxatives such as bisacodyl may not be the best choice for this group because they alter fluid and electrolyte balance, placing some seniors at risk for side effects. Bulk-forming laxatives are usually preferred for seniors.

Generic Name

Bismuth Formic Iodide

(BIZ-muth FOR-mick EYE-oe-dide)

Definition

An antiseptic found in OTC first-aid antibiotic products.

Generic Name

Bismuth Subsalicylate

(BIZ-muth sub-SAL-ih-SILL-ate)

Brand Name

†Pepto-Bismol

†*Consult the OTC ingredient charts to determine whether different formulations in this brand-name group are alcohol-, caffeine-, or sugar-free.*

Type of Drug

Antidiarrheal; general stomach remedy.

Used for

Control and symptomatic relief of acute diarrhea, including traveler's diarrhea; relief of heartburn, indigestion, and upset stomach; relief of nausea associated with dyspepsia, heartburn, and fullness (gas) caused by overindulgence in food and drink.

General Information

The average, healthy individual defecates anywhere from 3 times a day to 3 times a week. Diarrhea is characterized by abnormal frequency or consistency of stool, and can be caused by any one of several conditions, either gastrointestinal (GI) or non-GI. These include bacterial and viral infections, food intolerance, gastroenteritis, and side effects of prescription and OTC drugs. The cause of the diarrhea determines which drug therapy is best.

It should be emphasized that diarrhea is a symptom. Antidiarrheal medications provide symptomatic relief, which is generally sufficient for the treatment of temporary, uncomplicated diarrhea, such as that caused by an allergic reaction to dairy products. Persistent or recurrent diarrhea, however, can be a sign of a more serious condition requiring the attention of a health professional and treatment geared toward the underlying condition. Persistent diarrhea can also lead to dehydration. Self-medication with bismuth subsalicylate or another antidiarrheal does not preclude the fluid, electrolyte, and nutritional therapies necessary for the treatment of more serious, chronic diarrhea.

Bismuth subsalicylate has been used for more than 200 years to treat ailments of the stomach. It has been clinically proven in double-blind, placebo-controlled trials for relief of upset stomach symptoms and diarrhea.

For diarrhea, bismuth subsalicylate is believed to work by several mechanisms in the GI tract, including normalizing fluid movement, binding bacterial toxins, and inhibiting antimicrobial activity. Besides controlling diarrhea, bismuth subsalicylate relieves the cramps associated with it. It has also proven effective in preventing traveler's diarrhea. Bismuth subsalicylate should control diarrhea within 24 hours.

For upset stomach symptoms, bismuth subsalicylate is believed to work by coating the stomach lining.

Bismuth subsalicylate is thought to have some value in treating peptic ulcers because of its perceived ability to suppress *Helicobacter pylori* (the bacteria that causes most ulcers), but it is not indicated for this use. However, it is a component of several oral antibiotic–based regimens for treating *H. pylori.*

Generic bismuth subsalicylate is available in chewable tablet and liquid form; brand name products are available in caplet, chewable tablet, and liquid form.

Cautions and Warnings

Do not use bismuth subsalicylate for more than 2 days, unless directed by your doctor. Uncomplicated, acute diarrhea usually improves within 24 to 48 hours. Persistent diarrhea can lead to dehydration, which may require the administration of appropriate fluid and electrolyte therapy.

Do not exceed the recommended daily dosage of bismuth subsalicylate.

Do not take bismuth subsalicylate if your diarrhea is accompanied by high fever (higher than 101°F). Call your doctor if fever develops during self-medication with bismuth subsalicylate.

There is a slight potential for systemic bismuth subsalicylate absorption and toxicity, which can cause neurotoxicity (destruction to nerve tissue), but this is more of a concern with the other bismuth subsalicylate salts, such as the subnitrate and the subgallate. Only a few cases of bismuth subsalicylate neurotoxicity have been reported.

Bismuth subsalicylate, as the name implies, contains salicylate. Although it does not contain aspirin, which is a salicylate, you should exercise some of the same caution you would if taking aspirin (see "Drug Interactions" and "Special Populations").

If you have ringing in your ears after taking bismuth subsalicylate at the same time as aspirin, stop taking the bismuth subsalicylate.

Possible Side Effects

▼ Rare: Mild tinnitus (ringing in the ears) may be associated with moderate to severe salicylate toxicity.

Drug Interactions

• Do not take bismuth subsalicylate if you are currently taking aspirin or another salicylate-containing medication. Toxic levels of salicylate may be reached even if you follow the dosage directions of each product.

• Bismuth subsalicylate may interact adversely with oral anticoagulants (blood-thinning) drugs, such as warfarin; methotrexate, which is used to treat cancer, severe psoriasis, severe rheumatic arthritis, and to induce abortion; probenicid, an antigout medication; toblutamide, an oral sulfonylurea antidiabetes drug; and any other drug that potentially interacts with aspirin. Talk to your doctor or pharmacist before taking bismuth subsalicylate if you are taking any of these medications.

Food Interactions

None known.

Usual Dose

Liquid

Adult and Child (over age 16): 2 tbs.

Child (under 16): not recommended due to the risk of Reye's syndrome (see "Special Populations").

Caplet or Chewable Tablet

Adult and Child (age 16 and over): 2 tablets.

Child (under 16): not recommended due to the risk of Reye's syndrome (see "Special Populations").

For either the liquid or the tablet, repeat dosage every 30–60 minutes as needed, to a maximum of 8 doses in 24 hours.

To prevent traveler's diarrhea, the adult dose is 2 tbs. or 2 tablets taken 4 times a day with meals and at bedtime during the first 2 weeks of travel.

Be sure to drink plenty of clear liquids to help prevent dehydration, which may accompany diarrhea.

Shake the liquid well before using.

Chewable tablets may be dissolved in the mouth.

Overdosage

Do the following in case of accidental overdose: If the victim is unconscious or having convulsions, call for an ambulance immediately. If you take the victim to an emergency room, be sure to bring the bottle or container with you. If the victim is conscious, call your local poison control center or a health care professional. The poison control center may suggest inducing vomiting with ipecac syrup (available without a prescription at any pharmacy). DO NOT induce vomiting unless specifically instructed to do so.

Special Information

Bismuth subsalicylate may cause a temporary and harmless darkening of the tongue and/or stool. This should not be confused with melena (black and tarry stools due to GI bleeding).

Special Populations

Allergies

Although bismuth subsalicylate does not contain aspirin, you should not take it if you are allergic to aspirin or any nonaspirin salicylate.

Pregnancy/Breast-feeding

It is not generally recommended that pregnant women take any drugs, particularly during the first 3 months after conception.

Do not take bismuth subsalicylate if you are pregnant or nursing without consulting your physician. If you are suffering from diarrhea, talk to your doctor regarding fluid and electrolyte management.

If you must take bismuth subsalicylate, bottle-feed your baby with formula.

Infants/Children

Infants and children with acute or chronic diarrhea are at particular risk for severe and possibly dangerous dehydration and electrolyte imbalance. Over-reliance on antidiarrheal drugs may lead to the loss of essential nutritional factors and dehydration. Antidiarrheal medications in general have not been shown to be especially effective in children.

Children with the flu or chicken pox who are given aspirin or other salicylates may develop Reye's syndrome, a life-threatening condition characterized by vomiting, progressive damage to the central nervous system, liver injury, and abnormally low blood sugar. Up to 30% of those who develop Reye's syndrome can die, and permanent brain damage is possible in those who survive. Because of the risk of Reye's syndrome and the lack of documented benefits of bismuth, OTC products containing bismuth should not be given to children under 16 without first consulting your doctor.

Seniors

Seniors should generally exercise the same caution as younger adults when using bismuth subsalicylate. If, in addition to diarrhea, you are suffering from other ailments that make you weak, it may be beneficial to consult your physician regarding fluid and electrolyte management.

Generic Name

Boric Acid (BOR-ik ASS-id)

Brand Names

20/20 Drops
AK-NaCl
Allerest Eye Drops
Clear Eyes
Collyrium
Dri-Ear Drops
Ear-Dry
Eye-Sed
EyeSine
GenTeal Lubricant
Moisture Drops
Murocel Lubricant
OcuHist
Opcon-A
Sensitive Eyes
Soothe
Star-Otic Ear Solution
Swim-Ear
Tearisol
Visine

Type of Drug

Topical antiseptic.

Used for

Relieving tired or irritated eyes.

General Information

Boric acid is a common ingredient in OTC products for eye care. In a liquid solution, it helps soothe irritated eyes; as an ointment, it relieves irritated or swollen eyelids. It is used as an antiseptic in some artificial tear products, and in irrigants for the removal of foreign bodies from the eye. Some ear care products include boric acid for its anti-infective property. In some products boric acid acts as a buffer to maintain the proper acid level.

Soft contact lens cleaning solutions include boric acid because it helps remove oil and protein deposits that can build up on the surface of the lens, obscuring vision and inviting infection.

Boric acid is listed as an ingredient in some vaginal douches. However, the concentration of the drug in these products is so weak that it is probably ineffective as a bacteria fighter.

Cautions and Warnings

Do not use these products for more than 3 to 4 days unless under the direction of your doctor.

Do not exceed the recommended daily dosage of boric acid products.

If you experience pain or visual disturbances while using an eye product containing boric acid, discontinue use and contact your doctor.

Do not apply to damaged skin or open wounds. The risk of toxicity is also increased when high concentrations of boric acid are applied repeatedly or in large amounts to damaged skin.

If your condition persists or recurs, discontinue use of the product and contact your doctor.

To prevent spread of infection, only 1 person should use a bottle of a product such as eyedrops or eardrops.

To avoid contamination, do not touch the tip of the container to any surface.

Possible Side Effects

Side effects from the use of boric acid in OTC products are rare. Other ingredients in these products may cause an adverse reaction.

Drug Interactions

- Eye washes containing boric acid (e.g., Collyrium for Fresh Eyes) should not be used with a wetting solution for contact lenses or any other ophthalmic products containing polyvinyl alcohol.

Usual Dose

Eyedrops

Adult and Child (age 12 and over): 1 to 2 drops up to 4 times daily. Replace cap after using.

Child (under age 12): Consult your doctor for the appropriate dose.

Eyewash

Adult and Child (age 12 and over): Fill an eyecup halfway with the product, then lean forward and place the eyecup firmly over your eye. Tilt or lean your head back and open your eye, rotating your eye in a circular motion to ensure proper irrigation. To prevent eye infection, it is important to thoroughly clean and dry the eyecup after each use.

Child (under age 12): Consult your doctor for the appropriate dose.

Eye Ointment

Adult and Child (age 12 and over): Apply a small amount of the ointment to the inner surface of the lower eyelid once or twice daily.

Child (under age 12): not recommended.

Overdosage

Do the following in case of accidental ingestion: If the victim is unconscious or having convulsions, call for an ambulance immediately. If you take the victim to an emergency room, be sure to bring the bottle or container with you. If the victim is conscious, call your local poison control center or a health care professional. The poison control center may suggest inducing vomiting with ipecac syrup (available without a prescription at any pharmacy). DO NOT induce vomiting unless specifically instructed to do so.

Special Populations

Pregnancy/Breast-feeding

It is not generally recommended that pregnant women use any drugs, particularly during the first 3 months after conception. If you are or might be pregnant, or you are breast-feeding, check with your doctor before using a product containing boric acid.

Infants/Children

Eyedrops and ear drops with boric acid should not be used in children under age 12 unless the dosage is determined by a doctor.

Seniors

Seniors should exercise the same caution as younger adults when using a product containing boric acid.

Generic Name

Brompheniramine Maleate

(BROM-fen-EER-ah-meen MAL-ee-ate)

Brand Names

*Alka-Seltzer Plus
Bromatapp
†Bromfed [A]
Bromotap
Dimetane Allergy
*†Dimetapp
*Dristan Cold Multi-Symptom Maximum Strength
Vicks DayQuil Allergy Relief 12-Hour

**Not all products in this brand-name group contain brompheniramine maleate.*

†*Consult the OTC ingredient charts to determine whether different formulations in this brand-name group are alcohol-, caffeine-, or sugar-free.*

Type of Drug

Antihistamine.

Used for

Temporary relief of runny nose, sneezing, itchy eyes, scratchy throat, and other symptoms associated with cold and allergy.

General Information

Histamine is one of the substances released by the body tissues during an allergic reaction. When it is released, the body reacts with a variety of symptoms, including itching and sneezing. Antihistamines work by competitively inhibiting the pharmacological action of histamine, which makes them very effective for relieving the symptoms of allergic reactions. Antihistamines may also help relieve a runny nose. However, because antihistamines do not work against the other substances released by the body during an allergic reaction, they can reduce only about 40% to 60% of allergic symptoms. They are also not effective in clearing up a stuffy nose.

If you have seasonal allergies, antihistamines work best if you take them before your allergy season begins. Those who suffer from allergies regardless of the season may need to take antihistamines all year.

Antihistamines will not cure or prevent allergies, viral infections (colds), or bacterial infections. The best you can hope for is symptomatic relief.

Brompheniramine is classified as an alkylamine antihistamine. Others in this group include chlorpheniramine and pheniramine. Of the antihistamines available without a prescription, these are the least likely to make you sleepy. However, drowsiness is still a significant side effect of brompheniramine. Newer antihistamines such as terfenadine, astemizole, cetirizine, and loratadine do not have the common antihistamine side effect of drowsiness, but they are currently available only by prescription.

Relief of symptoms usually begins within 15 to 30 minutes after taking brompheniramine and lasts for 3 to 6 hours.

In cold and allergy products, brompheniramine is often combined with a nasal decongestant such as phenylpropanolamine or pseudoephedrine. In these combination products, brompheniramine may also be used in a related form called dexbrompheniramine.

Brompheniramine is available by generic and brand name in tablets, softgel, and liquid forms, both alone and in combination products.

Cautions and Warnings

Do not exceed the recommended daily dosage of brompheniramine.

Unless prescribed by a doctor, brompheniramine and other antihistamines should not be used by people who have a breathing problem such as emphysema or chronic bronchitis or by individuals with asthma.

Brompheniramine should be used with caution by people with glaucoma, hyperthyroidism, heart disease, high blood pressure, or an enlarged prostate. If you have any of these conditions, consult your doctor before taking brompheniramine.

Brompheniramine's effects on the central nervous system (CNS) can make you feel sleepy or reduce your concentration. Your ability to perform activities that require your full alertness and coordination, such as driving a motor vehicle or operating machinery, may be affected. Drinking alcohol while you are taking brompheniramine can add to these effects.

Phenylketonurics (people who cannot digest the amino acid phenylalanine) should be aware that some formulations of brompheniramine contain aspartame (Nutrasweet), which breaks down in the gastrointestinal tract to phenylalanine after the drug is taken.

Possible Side Effects

▼ Most common: restlessness, nervousness, sleeplessness or drowsiness, excitability, dizziness, poor coordination, and upset stomach.

▼ Less common: dry eyes, nose, and mouth; blurred vision; difficulty urinating; irritability (at high doses); increased or irregular heart rate; and heart palpitations.

Drug Interactions

• Brompheniramine's effects can combine with those of other drugs that depress the CNS, including barbiturates, tranquilizers, sleeping medications, and alcohol (present in many OTC preparations). If you are taking other depressant drugs, check with your doctor before you take brompheniramine or any other antihistamine. Avoid drinking alcohol if you are taking brompheniramine or any other antihistamine.

• Brompheniramine should not be used at the same time as a monoamine oxidase inhibitor (MAOI) or within 2 weeks of stopping treatment with an MAOI. MAOIs are used to treat depression, other psychiatric or emotional conditions, and Parkinson's disease. If you are not sure whether you are or have been taking an MAOI, check with your doctor or pharmacist before you use brompheniramine or any other antihistamine.

• Antihistamines can affect the results of skin and blood tests. Notify your health care professional before scheduling these tests if you are taking brompheniramine.

Food Interactions

None known.

Usual Dose

Because histamine is released nearly continuously, it is best to take antihistamines on a schedule rather than as needed.

Adult and Child (age 12 and over): 4 mg every 4–6 hours. Do not take more than 24 mg in 24 hours. For extended-release tablets containing 8 or 12 mg of brompheniramine, take 1 tablet every 8–12 hours (8-mg tablet) or every 12 hours (12-mg tablet).

Child (age 6–11): 2 mg every 4–6 hours. Do not give more than 12 mg in 24 hours.

Child (under age 6): not recommended unless directed by a doctor.

The inconvenience of the sedating effects of brompheniramine may be minimized by either taking a full dose at bedtime or using the smallest recommended doses, combined with a decongestant, during the day. Another alternative is to start with the lowest dose when you begin taking the drug and gradually increase the dosage over several days. When normal doses of brompheniramine cause significant sedation (i.e., 4 mg), try breaking the tablet in half and try a 2 mg dose. Many people find this still offers relief of symptoms and not as much sedation. This does not apply to sustained release products.

If you forget to take a dose of brompheniramine, do so as soon as you remember. If it is almost time for your next dose, skip the one you forgot and continue with your regular schedule. Do not take a double dose.

Overdosage

Symptoms of antihistamine overdose in children include dilated pupils, flushed face, dry mouth, fever, excitability, hallucinations, loss of muscle coordination, and seizures.

In adults, severe overdose can cause drowsiness or coma, which may be followed by excitability or seizures. Eventually fluid can build up in the brain; the kidneys may fail, and the heart and lungs may stop working, resulting in death. Symptoms may develop within 30 minutes to 2 hours following an overdose, and death may occur within 18 hours.

Even if the victim is not displaying any of the symptoms listed above, do the following in case of accidental overdose: If the victim is unconscious or having convulsions, call for an ambulance immediately. If you take the victim to an emergency room, be sure to bring the bottle or container with you. If the victim is conscious, call your local poison control center or a health care professional. The poison control center may suggest inducing vomiting with ipecac syrup (available without a prescription at any pharmacy). DO NOT induce vomiting unless specifically instructed to do so.

Special Populations

Pregnancy/Breast-feeding

Antihistamines are not recommended for use during pregnancy unless directed by your doctor. Antihistamines are known to pass into the breast milk of nursing mothers and may cause side effects in infants. Check with your doctor before taking brompheniramine if you are or might be pregnant, or if you are breast-feeding.

Infants/Children
Children may be more susceptible to the side effects of brompheniramine. They are also more susceptible to accidental antihistamine overdose. Do not give brompheniramine to a child under 6 unless directed by your doctor.

Seniors
Older persons may be more sensitive to the side effects of brompheniramine and other antihistamines and may experience nervousness, irritability, and restlessness. Dizziness, sedation, and low blood presssure may also occur. Older men may experience difficulty in urinating. Most mild reactions may be handled by either lowering your dose or trying another antihistamine.

Generic Name

Butamben Picrate

(bew-TAM-ben PYE-krate)

Definition

A local anesthetic found in first-aid products used for relief of pain from minor burns and sunburn. Such products generally are short-acting; relief lasts up to 45 minutes. They should not be applied more than 3 or 4 times per day.

Generic Name

Caffeine (kaff-EEN)

Brand Names

20/20
357 Magnum II
Caffedrine
Dexitac
*†Diurex
King of Hearts
*†Midol
No Doz
Overtime
Pep-Back
Quick-Pep
Vivarin

**Not all products in this brand-name group contain caffeine.*

†Consult the OTC ingredient charts to determine whether different formulations in this brand-name group are alcohol-, caffeine-, or sugar-free.

Type of Drug

Central nervous system (CNS) stimulant; diuretic.

Used for

As a stimulant, to fight against drowsiness and produce mental alertness; decreasing water retention.

General Information

Caffeine is a common ingredient in tea, coffee, colas, and chocolate, consumed by well over half the adults in the U.S. every day and by many children as well. As a mild CNS stimulant, caffeine is used in medications to help fight off sleep and increase mental alertness, and can improve coordination. It is also combined with analgesics such as acetaminophen and aspirin to treat headache or the fluid retention, tension, and fatigue that can accompany menstruation.

With some exceptions (see "Special Populations"), moderate consumption of caffeine is generally considered to be safe.

Cautions and Warnings

If you are taking caffeine to help you stay awake, see your doctor if your sleep problems last longer than 7 to 10 days.

Do not exceed the recommended daily dosage of caffeine stimulant products.

Caffeine should be used with caution by individuals with a history of peptic ulcer.

Caffeine may have the potential to cause cardiac arrhythmia (irregular heartbeats), although this effect is still under investigation. As a precaution, it is recommended that caffeine be avoided by individuals with symptomatic cardiac arrhythmias and/or palpitations and during the first several days to weeks after a heart attack.

Potential effects of caffeine on mood include a decrease in aggressive behavior, worsened symptoms in people with anxiety or panic disorder, and worsened symptoms in women with moderate to severe premenstrual syndrome.

Over the long term, high caffeine intake can lead to tolerance of and psychological dependence on the drug. If caffeine is stopped abruptly, physical signs of withdrawal may occur. The most common symptoms of caffeine withdrawal are fatigue and a throbbing headache, followed by vomiting, impaired physical coordination, irritability, restlessness, drowsiness, and sometimes yawning and a runny nose. These symptoms usually begin 12 to 24 hours after caffeine is stopped and reach their maximum in 20 to 48 hours; they may last for as long as a week.

Caffeine may have adverse effects on the quality of your sleep. You may wake up more frequently during the night or may be awakened more easily by noises or other disturbances.

Contrary to popular belief, caffeine will not help a person who has had too much to drink to become sober more quickly and can lead to adverse gastrointestinal (GI) effects if taken with alcohol (see "Drug Interactions").

Possible Side Effects

At usual therapeutic doses (100 to 200 mg), caffeine can have adverse effects on both the CNS and the GI system. CNS effects include insomnia, restlessness, nervousness, light-headedness, tremors, headache, and irritability; GI effects include nausea, vomiting, and upset stomach. These effects are usually more severe in children than in adults.

Large doses of caffeine (up to 500 mg) can produce headache, excitement, agitation, shakiness, irritability, anxiety, scintillating scotoma (a sensation of light before the eyes), hyperesthesia (unusual sensitivity of the skin or of a particular sense), ringing in the ears, muscle tremors or twitches, increased urination, and rapid or premature heartbeat or other cardiac arrhythmias.

Drug Interactions

• The body's metabolism of caffeine is inhibited by the following drugs: mexiletine, an antiarrhythmic; cimetidine, used to treat peptic ulcers, heartburn, and acid indigestion; the fluoroquinolone anti-infectives norfloxacin, enoxacin, and ciprofloxacin; and oral contraceptives containing estrogen. This effect is also seen when caffeine is ingested with alcohol or the drug disulfiram, which is used in the treatment of chronic alcoholism. Alcohol, nonsteroidal anti-inflammatory drugs (NSAIDs), and corticosteroids can also increase the adverse GI effects of caffeine.

• Because caffeine may decrease the body's absorption of iron, iron supplements should be taken 1 hour before or 2 hours after caffeine is taken.

• Coadministration of caffeine and phenylpropanolamine, a decongestant, may increase blood pressure.

• Dangerous heart problems may occur if monoamine oxidase inhibitors (MAOIs) are taken with caffeine. MAOIs are used to treat depression, other psychiatric or emotional conditions, and Parkinson's disease. If you are not sure whether you are taking an MAOI, contact your doctor before taking caffeine.

• Caffeine may interfere with the therapeutic benefit of drugs given to regulate heart rhythm, such as quinidine and propranolol.

• Caffeine may increase the breakdown of phenobarbital or aspirin, thus decreasing the efficacy of these drugs.

• The effects of both the benzodiazepine tranquilizer diazepam and caffeine may either be increased or decreased (depending on dose and specific behavioral tests used) when these drugs are taken together.

• Caffeine may cause false-positive results in tests performed to diagnose pheochromocytoma (tumor of the adrenal gland) or neuroblastoma (tumor of the nervous system), and may also affect readings of uric acid concentrations.

Food Interactions

To avoid the potential danger of caffeine overdose, be aware of your consumption of coffee, tea, cola drinks, chocolate, and other caffeine-containing foods if you are taking caffeine as an OTC drug. Check with your doctor or other health care professional about a safe level of caffeine intake for you.

Usual Dose

Adult and Child (age 12 and over): 100–200 mg no more than every 3–4 hours. For timed-release formulations, 200–250 mg once daily. Do not take the timed-release formulation less than 6 hours before bedtime.

Child (under age 12): not recommended unless directed by a doctor.

Overdosage

Caffeine toxicity can occur when doses greater than 250 mg are ingested. Symptoms of overdose include stomach pain, nervousness, restlessness, excitement, increased heart rate, sleeplessness, frequent urination, flushing, muscle twitching, and disordered thoughts and speech. More serious symptoms include irregular heartbeat and seizures.

Even if the victim is not displaying any of the symptoms listed above, do the following in case of accidental overdose: If the victim is unconscious or having convulsions, call for an ambulance immediately. If you take the victim to an emergency room, be sure to bring the bottle or container with you. If the victim is conscious, call your local poison control center or a health care professional. The poison control center may suggest inducing vomiting with ipecac syrup (available without a prescription at any pharmacy). DO NOT induce vomiting unless specifically instructed to do so.

Special Populations

Pregnancy/Breast-feeding

It is not generally recommended that pregnant women take any drugs, particularly during the first 3 months after conception. Caffeine has been shown to cross the placenta in pregnant women, which means that it passes from the mother to the fetus. In rat studies, caffeine has been shown to have harmful effects on the developing fetus. Although these effects have not been seen in humans, the FDA recommends that women limit their caffeine intake or avoid caffeine during pregnancy. Studies in humans suggest that the adverse effect of caffeine during pregnancy is related to the amount ingested; doses of more than 300 mg per day have been linked to slowed growth and low birth weight of the infant.

Caffeine passes into breast milk and may cause wakefulness and irritability in nursing infants of mothers taking high doses (600 mg per day). Because the highest concentrations of caffeine in breast milk occur within 1 hour of caffeine intake, you may want to take caffeine immediately *after* you nurse. Keep your caffeine intake at moderate levels, especially if your child is under 4 months old. Another alternative is simply to avoid caffeine entirely until your child is weaned.

Check with your doctor before self-medicating with a caffeine-containing medication if you are or might be pregnant or if you are breast-feeding.

Infants/Children

The adverse CNS effects of caffeine (see "Possible Side Effects") are usually more severe in children than in adults. Because the liver metabolic pathways are still immature in newborns, their metabolism of caffeine is very slow, and dangerous plasma concentrations of caffeine can build up. Do not give caffeine to children under age 12 unless directed by your doctor.

Seniors

Seniors may be more sensitive to caffeine's stimulant effects and may be more likely to have nervousness, anxiety, sleeplessness, and irritability. Be especially cautious about your caffeine intake if you are taking other CNS stimulants, such as theophylline (used as a bronchodilator), amantadine (used to treat Parkinson's disease), tricyclic antidepressants, or appetite suppressants.

Generic Name

Calamine (KAL-uh-mine)

Brand Names

Aveeno Anti-Itch
Caladryl
Ivarest 8-Hour Medicated
Resinol Medicated
Rhuli Spray

Type of Drug

Topical astringent (drying agent), antiseptic, antibacterial, antipruritic (anti-itch agent), skin protectant.

Used for

Protecting skin from irritants; temporary relief from itching caused by poison ivy and insect bites; and healing of skin inflammation.

General Information

Calamine is a combination of zinc oxide, the active ingredient; and ferrous oxide, which has no medicinal value, but is added to give a pink coloration to the product and make it cosmetically more pleasing.

Calamine shields the skin surface from chemical irritants and harmful sun overexposure. It also provides a protective coating that does not dissolve or wash away with water.

The product also promotes healing by attracting protein to the affected area, which encourages new tissue growth. As an astringent, calamine absorbs moisture from oozing rashes, such as poison ivy, which promotes further healing.

Calamine is used in combination products containing such ingredients as topical anesthetics, corticosteroids, or antihistamines to reduce pain and inflammation. Certain bandages contain calamine as a means of protecting against leg ulcers.

Calamine-containing products are safe and effective remedies for a range of skin conditions, such as:

- diaper rash
- poison ivy, oak, and sumac exposure
- dermatitis (skin inflammation)
- chicken pox
- insect bites

Calamine is available by brand and generic name in the form of ointment, lotion, and dusting powder.

Cautions and Warnings

If there is no improvement in the infected area within 7 days or if an allergic reaction develops, discontinue using calamine and contact your doctor.

Do not exceed the recommended daily dosage of calamine.

This drug is for external use only.

Calamine is sometimes used in combination products containing lanolin. While calamine itself has no tendency to cause allergic reactions, some individuals may become sensitized to the lanolin and develop a rash. Should this occur, discontinue using the product and contact your doctor.

People who are sensitive to any ingredient in a calamine preparation should avoid using the product. Be sure to read the ingredients on the label.

Do not apply calamine ointments to areas of broken skin, over deep or puncture wounds, or to cuts.

When using baby powders containing calamine, keep the powder away from the child's face to prevent accidental inhalation.

Do not use calamine by itself as a protectant for treatment of external hemorrhoids. Products designed for hemorrhoid relief that contain calamine should also contain from 1 to 3 other protectant ingredients.

Possible Side Effects

The thickness and consistency of calamine prevents it from being absorbed into the skin. Consequently topical and systemic (whole-body) side effects or allergic reactions, even with long-term use, are rare.

▼ Hemorrhoid ointments containing calamine (or its main active ingredient, zinc oxide) may cause a burning sensation in some people, especially if the skin in the affected area is not intact.

Drug Interactions

None known.

Usual Dose

Calamine has a great many uses, and the doses and applications are varied.

Diaper Rash

Clean the affected area and dry it as much as possible. Apply a thin layer of calamine product to the area. Extend the application a small distance past the affected area. Allow it to dry before putting on a fresh diaper. If you apply calamine a subsequent time, be sure to remove the remainder of the previous application by gentle use of mineral oil.

Chicken Pox

Adult and Child (age 6 and over): Apply a small dot of the product to skin eruptions as often as needed. Children should be instructed not to pick at the medication as it dries, since this can cause additional irritation and make the symptoms of chicken pox worse.

Child (under age 6): not recommended unless directed by a doctor.

Insect Bites, Dermatitis, or Itchy Skin Rashes Caused by Poison Ivy, Oak, or Sumac

Adult and Child (age 6 and over): Apply as needed to affected areas. Allow to dry.

Child (under age 6): not recommended unless directed by a doctor.

Hemorrhoids

Adult and Child (age 12 and over): If using an ointment or cream, apply up to 4 times a day, particularly at night, in the morning, or after bowel movements.

Child (under age 12): Consult your doctor.

Overdosage

Calamine, due to its density of substance, is not readily absorbed through the pores of the skin and presents minimal risk of overdose.

Do the following in case of accidental ingestion: If the victim is unconscious or having convulsions, call for an ambulance immediately. If you take the victim to an emergency room, be sure to bring the bottle or container with you. If the victim is conscious, call your local poison control center or a health care professional. The poison control center may suggest inducing vomiting with ipecac syrup (available without a prescription at any pharmacy). DO NOT induce vomiting unless specifically instructed to do so.

Special Populations

Pregnancy/Breast-feeding

It is not recommended that pregnant women take any drugs, particularly during the first 3 months after conception.

However, since calamine is not absorbed into the skin, there is little risk to either pregnant women and their fetuses or nursing mothers and their infants.

Infants/Children

Calamine products are generally safe when used as directed for diaper rash. However, consult a physician before using hemorrhoid products on children under age 12, and before using skin products on children under age 6.

Due to the possibility of accidental ingestion, these products should not be used on children under age 2 without close adult supervision.

Seniors

Seniors using calamine should exercise the same caution as younger adults.

Generic Name

Calcium Acetate (KAL-see-um ASS-eh-tate)

Definition

An astringent (drying agent) used in OTC skin care products for treatment of dermatitis (skin inflammation).

Generic Name

Calcium Carbonate

(KAL-see-um KAR-buh-nate)

Brand Names

Acid-X
Alka-Mints
*†Alka-Seltzer
Alkets
Amitone
Chooz
Dicarbosil
Di-Gel
Equilet
Gas-X Chewable Tablet
Maalox Caplet $
Marblen
Mylanta
Rolaids
Tempo Drops
Titralac
Tums
Tylenol Headache Plus Extra Strength

**Not all products in this brand-name group contain calcium carbonate.*

†Consult the OTC ingredient charts to determine whether different formulations in this brand-name group are alcohol-, caffeine-, or sugar-free.

Type of Drug

Antacid.

Used for

Relief of heartburn, sour stomach, acid indigestion, upset stomach, and flatulence (gas) associated with these symptoms. Calcium carbonate has also been recommended as a source of extra calcium to prevent osteoporosis.

General Information

All antacids work in the same way, by neutralizing gastric acid. However, they differ in potency: Calcium carbonate is the most potent of these products, followed by sodium bicarbonate, magnesium antacids, and aluminum antacids. The higher the potency of an antacid, the less of it you will need to take to achieve the desired effect.

Antacids also vary according to adverse effects and drug interactions, as well as onset and duration of action. Calcium carbonate dissolves more slowly in stomach acid than do sodium bicarbonate and magnesium hydroxide, and thus may take longer to begin working. It can take up to 30 minutes for the acid-neutralizing effect of calcium carbonate to begin working.

How long an antacid product works depends on how long it remains in the stomach. Calcium carbonate has a longer duration of action than magnesium antacids or sodium bicarbonate. In general, an antacid taken on an empty stomach leaves the stomach rapidly and works for only 20 to 40 minutes. However, when taken after a meal, it leaves the stomach more slowly. When taken 1 hour after a meal, an antacid can work for up to 3 hours.

Generic calcium carbonate is available in chewable tablet and suspension (liquid) form; brand name products are available in chewable tablet and gum form. Calcium carbonate is also available in combination products containing either magnesium hydroxide or magnesium carbonate.

Cautions and Warnings

Do not take the maximum daily dosage of calcium carbonate for more than 2 weeks continuously except under a doctor's supervision. Antacids may relieve symptoms of a serious condition such as peptic ulcer disease. If you take an antacid for a prolonged period, you run the risk of unknowingly masking the symptoms of a serious gastrointestinal (GI) disease and delaying diagnosis.

Do not exceed the recommended daily dosage of calcium carbonate.

Call your doctor if you do not get relief from calcium carbonate, or if your stool is black or tarry or looks like coffee grounds, which indicates bleeding in the intestines or stomach. These may be signs of a serious GI disorder that cannot and should not be treated with an OTC product without your doctor's supervision.

Calcium carbonate, unlike other antacids, can have a rebound effect; that is, more gastric acid is secreted after the drug has been emptied by the stomach. This limits long-term use.

Large doses of calcium carbonate may lead to hypercalcemia (an excess of calcium in the blood), which can cause nausea, vomiting, loss of appetite, weakness, headache, dizziness, and change in mental state.

Calcium carbonate has also caused milk-alkali syndrome, which occurs when there is a high intake of calcium combined with anything producing alkalosis (imbalance of acid and base in body fluids). Symptoms include headache, nausea, irritability, dizziness, and vomiting. Left unchecked, the syndrome can cause irreversible kidney damage. Hypercalcemic and milk-alkali syndrome are more likely to occur in people with impaired kidney function.

Possible Side Effects

▼ Most common: constipation, diarrhea.

▼ Less common: belching, flatulence.

Drug Interactions

• Because antacids interact with a number of orally administered drugs, it is best to separate doses of other medications by 1 to 2 hours (or check with your pharmacist about possible interactions).

• Calcium carbonate decreases the absorption of the following drugs, reducing their effect: tetracycline antibiotics; quinolone antibiotics, such as ciprofloxacin; and iron. It may also decrease the bioavailability of the beta blocker atenolol, used to treat high blood pressure. If you are taking calcium carbonate at the same time as any of these drugs, separate your dose of each drug by at least 2 hours; with quinolone antibiotics, 4 to 6 hours is preferable.

• Calcium carbonate increases the body's elimination of aspirin and other salicylates, reducing their effect.

• Calcium carbonate decreases the elimination of the antiarrhythmic quinidine, raising the serum concentration of quinidine to potentially dangerous levels. If you are taking quinidine, consult your doctor before taking calcium carbonate.

• Concurrent use of calcium carbonate with sodium polystyrene sulfonate, a potassium remover, may be dangerous. Separate your dose of each drug by at least 2 hours.

Food Interactions

Calcium carbonate is best taken after meals (see "General Information").

Usual Dose

Antacid

Adult and Child (age 6 and over): Take calcium carbonate as symptoms occur, but do not exceed the recommended daily dosage specified on the package. Be sure to chew the tablet completely and drink a full glass of water afterward to ensure maximum benefit.

Child (under age 6): Consult your doctor.

Calcium Supplement

Adult and Child (age 6 and over): Chew 2 tablets after meals, or as directed by your physician.

Child (under age 6): Consult your doctor.

Overdosage

Do the following in case of accidental overdose: If the victim is unconscious or having convulsions, call for an ambulance immediately. If you take the victim to an emergency room, be sure to bring the bottle or container with you. If the victim is conscious, call your local poison control center or a health care professional. The poison control center may suggest inducing vomiting with ipecac syrup (available without a prescription at any pharmacy). DO NOT induce vomiting unless specifically instructed to do so.

Special Populations

Pregnancy/Breast-feeding

It is not generally recommended that pregnant women take any drugs, particularly during the first 3 months after conception. However, antacids can be safely taken in small doses for short periods of time during pregnancy and while breast-feeding. Since pregnant women often increase their milk or calcium intake, they should be especially aware of the risk of milk-alkali syndrome (see "Cautions and Warnings") before choosing calcium carbonate as an antacid.

Check with your doctor before taking calcium carbonate if you are or might be pregnant, or if you are breast-feeding.

Infants/Children

The safety of antacid use in infants and children has not been established. Children under age 6 should not be given calcium carbonate unless directed by a doctor.

Seniors

Seniors may safely take antacids. However, be advised that many older patients are at high risk for complications from ulcers, yet often do not show classic ulcer symptoms. Discuss with your pharmacist the possible causes of your gastric discomfort before using an antacid and possibly delaying diagnosis of an ulcer. Be aware of possible interactions with other medications you may be taking.

Seniors may be more likely than younger adults to have diarrhea caused by calcium carbonate.

Generic Name

Calcium Polycarbophil

(KAL-see-um pol-ee-KAR-buh-fill)

Brand Names

Equalactrin
Fiberall
FiberCon $
Fiber-Lax
Konsyl Fiber
Mitrolan

Type of Drug

Laxative.

Used for

Relief of occasional constipation (irregularity).

General Information

The average, healthy individual defecates anywhere from 3 times a day to 3 times a week. Constipation is determined not necessarily by the frequency of bowel movements, but by the consistency of the stool, how difficult it is to eliminate, and other symptoms associated with constipation, such as dull headache, low back pain, and abdominal distention (swelling). Evaluate your condition carefully and discuss your symptoms and their possible causes with your pharmacist before taking a laxative. Laxatives are not always necessary, and when used improperly can either prevent the desired effect or result in laxative dependency. If you are indeed constipated, it may be best managed through proper diet, adequate fluid intake (6 to 8 classes of water daily), and exercise. If you must use a laxative, choose the mildest effective product.

Laxatives may be classified by their mechanism of action: bulk-forming, emollient (stool softeners), lubricant, saline, hyperosmotic, and stimulant. Calcium polycarbophil is a bulk-forming laxative. Bulk-forming laxatives work by dissolving or swelling in water to form an emollient gel. The increased bulk of the fecal material helps the intestine to contract in waves, forcing the feces out. Of all laxatives, bulk-forming products most closely approximate the natural, physiologic mechanism of defecation. Consequently, they are considered by most doctors to be the best initial therapy for simple constipation, which is generally caused by a low-fiber or low-fluid diet.

Bulk-forming laxatives are recommended for people with colostomies and irritable bowel syndrome, and for people who should avoid straining during defecation (e.g., individuals with hernias). However, they are not recommended for treating constipation associated with hard, dry stools. They are also not the best choice when a prompt or complete emptying of the bowel is desired.

Bulk-forming laxatives generally begin to work within 12 to 24 hours, but the full effect may not be achieved for 2 to 3 days.

Generic calcium polycarbophil is available in tablet form; brand-name products are available in tablet and chewable tablet form.

Cautions and Warnings

Do not use for more than 7 days, unless directed by your doctor. Long-term use of laxatives has been linked with laxative dependence, chronic constipation, and loss of normal bowel function. Using laxatives too frequently can result in persistent diarrhea, hypokalemia (abnormally low potassium in blood), loss of essential nutrients, and dehydration.

Do not exceed the maximum daily dosage of calcium polycarbophil. The higher the dose, the more likely you are to experience adverse effects.

Do not take calcium polycarbophil if you have abdominal pain, nausea, vomiting, or kidney disease, unless directed by your doctor.

If you notice a marked change in bowel habits lasting for more than 2 weeks, do not take calcium polycarbophil until you have spoken to your doctor. Also contact your doctor if there is blood in your stool, so that colon cancer or other significant disease can be ruled out before you begin taking calcium polycarbophil.

If you have had a disease or surgery affecting the gastrointestinal (GI) tract, using a laxative may affect your condition adversely.

If you have rectal bleeding after using calcium polycarbophil, or if you do not have a bowel movement after 7 days of using this medication, you may have a serious condition. Stop using the product and call your doctor.

Calcium polycarbophil should not be used by people with partial bowel obstruction.

People at risk for hypercalcemia should exercise caution when using calcium polycarbophil.

People with diabetes or with carbohydrate-restricted diets should be aware that calcium polycarbophil preparations may contain large amounts of sugar. Be sure to read the label carefully.

Each dose of calcium polycarbophil must be taken with at least 8 oz. of water or other fluid. If you do not drink enough fluid with your bulk-laxative dose, a semisolid mass can form, resulting in bowel and/or esophageal obstruction, swelling or blockage of the throat, choking, or asphyxiation. Calcium polycarbophil should not be used by people with throat problems or those who have difficulty swallowing or strictures of the esophagus. Call your doctor if, after taking this product, you have chest pain or pressure, you regurgitate or vomit, or you have difficulty swallowing or breathing.

Possible Side Effects

Calcium polycarbophil, when used properly, rarely causes adverse effects. However, a dose of calcium polycarbophil taken without enough fluid (8 oz.) can result in bowel and/or esophageal obstruction, swelling or blockage of the throat, choking, or asphyxiation (see "Cautions and Warnings").

▼ Less common: diarrhea, abdominal discomfort, flatulence (gas), excessive loss of fluid.

Drug Interactions

• All laxatives have the potential to decrease the absorption of any oral drug taken at the same time. If you are taking the heart medication digitalis, oral anticoagulants (e.g., warfarin), the urinary anti-infective nitrofurantoin, or a salicylate such as aspirin, consult your doctor or pharmacist before beginning to take calcium polycarbophil. Some physicians recommend separating doses by at least 3 hours if you take calcium polycarbophil at the same time as any of the above drugs.

• If you are taking any form of tetracycline, take your dose of tetracycline at least 1 hour before or 2 to 3 hours after you have taken the calcium polycarbophil.

Food Interactions

None known.

Usual Dose

Doses should be adjusted to individual usage. Do not exceed the maximum daily dosage.

Each dose of calcium polycarbophil must be taken with at least 8 oz. water or other fluid (see "Cautions and Warnings").

Adult and Child (age 12 and over): 1g 4 times a day up to 6g a day.

Child (age 6–11): 500mg 1–3 times a day up to 3g a day.

Child (under age 6): not recommended unless directed by a doctor.

If you are taking the maximum daily dosage of calcium polycarbophil, take it in divided doses.

Overdosage

Do the following in case of accidental overdose: If the victim is unconscious or having convulsions, call for an ambulance immediately. If you take the victim to an emergency room, be sure to bring the bottle or container with you. If the victim is conscious, call your local poison control center or a health care professional. The poison control center may suggest inducing vomiting with ipecac syrup (available without a prescription at any pharmacy). DO NOT induce vomiting unless specifically instructed to do so.

Special Populations

Pregnancy/Breast-feeding

It is not generally recommended that pregnant women take any drugs, particularly during the first 3 months after conception. However, stool softeners and bulk-forming laxatives such as calcium polycarbophil are the only laxatives recommended for use by pregnant women.

Check with your doctor before using calcium polycarbophil if you are, or might be, pregnant, or if you are breast-feeding. Also consider talking to your doctor about diet and mild exercise in the management of constipation.

Infants/Children

Observe your child carefully for patterns of bowel movements and the pain or difficulty with which the bowel movements are made before deciding whether the child is actually constipated. As with adults, "normal" bowel habits vary in children. If your child is indeed constipated, increasing fluid intake and adding fiber to his or her diet may help to manage the condition. In general, the use of laxatives should be avoided in children.

Consult your doctor before giving calcium polycarbophil to a child under 6.

Seniors

Seniors commonly experience constipation, and consequently may become laxative-dependent. Be cautious of chronically turning to laxatives to ease constipation, and instead look to diet and increased fluid intake as therapeutic measures.

Although esophageal obstruction has occurred in seniors taking bulk-forming laxatives, these products are usually the preferred choice for older individuals.

Generic Name

Calcium Undecylenate

(KAL-see-um UN-des-UHL-en-ate)

Definition

An antifungal used to treat and/or prevent diaper rash, intertrigo (rashes on skin in contact with other skin surfaces, such as between the toes or under the breasts), prickly heat, athlete's foot, and jock itch, and to soothe itchy or "burning" skin resulting from minor fungal infections. When combined with neomycin and hydrocortisone acetate, calcium undecylenate is used to treat fungal infections that affect existing skin conditions. If the area being treated is cut or scraped, calcium undecylenate may cause a mild stinging sensation.

Generic Name

Camphor (KAM-for)

Brand Names

Arthricare Double Ice Pain Relieving Rub
Aveeno Anti-Itch
Banalg
*Benadryl Itch Stopping
Ben-Gay Ultra Strength Pain Relieving
Betuline
Blue Star
Campho-phenique Pain Relieving Antiseptic
Carmex
Deep-Down
Dencorub Cream
Heet
Mentholatum Ointment
Minit-Rub
Noxzema
Numol
Ostiderm
Rhuli
Sarna
Soltice Quick Rub
Sports Spray Extra Strength
TheraPatch
Vaporizer in a Bottle Air Wick Inhaler
*Vicks

**Not all products in this brand-name group contain camphor.*

Type of Drug

Topical analgesic (pain reliever); antitussive (cough suppressant).

Used for

Relief of soreness, stiffness, and pain in muscles, joints, and tendons; suppression of a dry, hacking, nonproductive cough (a cough that does not bring up any mucus).

General Information

Camphor is a common OTC drug ingredient with a variety of uses. In concentrations of 3% to 11%, camphor is used as a counterirritant topical analgesic. Counterirritation is the production of a less severe pain to distract from a more intense pain. When a counterirritant medication is applied to the skin, it produces a feeling of warmth or cold that reduces the perception of more deep-seated pain in a muscle or joint. The smell or the feelings of warmth or coolness that counterirritant analgesics produce may also contribute to a placebo effect; that is, if you believe they will work to relieve your pain, they probably will.

Camphor's aromatic vapors work as an antitussive when this product is rubbed as an ointment on the throat or chest (in strengths of 4.7% to 5.3%). Camphor is also commonly found in solutions for steam inhalation.

Camphor is available by brand name in cream and liniment, ointment as well as in liquid products to be used in a vaporizer. Depending on the intended use of the product, camphor is usually combined with other topical analgesics such as methyl salicylate or with menthol, which also has both analgesic and antitussive properties.

Cautions and Warnings

If your cough lasts longer than 7 days, is recurrent, or is accompanied by fever, rash, or persistent headache, call your doctor. A persistent cough may be a sign of a serious condition.

Do not exceed the recommended daily dosage of camphor.

Topical preparations containing high strengths (over 11%) of camphor can be dangerous to children; 5 ml of a 20% camphor liniment can cause slowed breathing, resulting in death or seizure. You may want to consider choosing another analgesic or antitussive for children. Accidental ingestion of camphor can also lead to seizures in both children and adults..

If your skin becomes irritated or red, or your pain gets worse or is constant and felt in any position, stop using this product and call your doctor.

Camphor preparations should be used only on the skin. Don't apply them near your eyes or to mucous membranes (i.e., inside the mouth, nose, rectum, or vagina).

Camphor preparations should not be used with a heating pad, hot water bottle, or any other heating device. You should also avoid sunlight and sunlamps after using these products.

Don't use camphor (or any other topical analgesic) after intense exercise, especially during hot and humid weather, when you will probably be flushed and warm. If you have a sore muscle from working out and want to use a topical analgesic to relieve the pain, wait until you cool down. You should also avoid applying this product before using a sauna or getting a professional massage.

To avoid the risk of irritation, redness, or blistering, don't use a tight bandage or dressing over the skin where you apply camphor or any other counterirritant analgesic.

Don't use camphor on broken, irritated, or sunburned skin, or on an open wound.

If you wear contact lenses, don't take them out or put them in your eyes after you use a camphor preparation without first washing your hands.

If you are using camphor in a steam inhalation to treat a child's cough, to avoid the risk of serious burns, never leave the child unsupervised.

Never expose camphor steam inhalation solution to a flame or try to microwave it.

Possible Side Effects

▼ Most common: temporary burning and stinging, sneezing.

Some people may overreact to the skin irritation caused by counterirritant medications such as camphor and may develop rashes and blisters. This may be more likely to occur in sensitive areas of the skin, such as behind your knees. Counterirritants may also cause the skin to become over sensitive. If you develop any skin irritation while using camphor, stop using it immediately.

Drug Interactions

None known.

Usual Dose

Topical Analgesic

Adult and Child (age 12 and over): Gently massage a small amount of a 3%–11% concentration of camphor over the area on the skin where pain is felt. Make sure to wash your hands thoroughly afterward. If you are treating your hands, wait 30 minutes before washing. Reapply as needed, no more than 3 or 4 times a day.

Child (under age 12): not recommended unless directed by a doctor.

Topical Antitussive

Adult and Child (age 2 and over): As a 4.7%–5.3% camphor ointment, rub on the throat and chest as a thick layer. Repeat up to 3 times daily, or as directed by your doctor. For steam inhalation, add 1 tbs. of a 6.2% camphor solution per quart of water directly to the water in a hot steam vaporizer. Breathe in the vapors. Repeat up to 3 times daily, or as directed by your doctor.

Child (under age 2): not recommended unless directed by a doctor.

Overdosage

Do the following in case of accidental ingestion: If the victim is unconscious or having convulsions, call for an ambulance immediately. If you take the victim to an emergency room, be sure to bring the bottle or container with you. If the victim is conscious, call your local poison control center or a health care professional. The poison control center may suggest inducing vomiting with ipecac syrup (available without a prescription at any pharmacy). DO NOT induce vomiting unless specifically instructed to do so.

Special Information

Besides using a topical preparation, there are also physical methods of producing counterirritation, such as by gently massaging the injured area. In fact, some of the benefit gained from using counterirritants may simply be due to the fact that they are applied by being rubbed and massaged into the skin. Another way to produce counterirritation is to apply heat to the skin with a hot water bottle or heating pad; in addition to reducing pain, heat helps the collagen in your skin regain its elasticity and lose its stiffness after a stretching injury. However, you should never use a counterirritant such as camphor with a heating device (see "Cautions and Warnings").

Special Populations

Pregnancy/Breast-feeding

It is not generally recommended that pregnant women use any drugs, especially during the first 3 months after conception. If you are pregnant or breast-feeding, check with a doctor before using camphor.

Infants/Children
It is not recommended that high strengths (over 11%) of camphor be used in children (see "Cautions and Warnings").

Keep external preparations containing camphor away from children. When camphor is taken internally, it is highly toxic and difficult to treat.

Seniors
Seniors should exercise the same caution as younger adults when using a product containing camphor.

Generic Name

Capsaicin (kap-SAY-eh-sin)

Brand Names

Capzasin-P
Dencorub Liquid
Heet
Menthacin
Pain Doctor
Rid-a-Pain Cream
Sloan's
Zostrix

Type of Drug

Topical analgesic (pain reliever).

Used for

Temporary relief of minor aches and pains of muscles and joints related to arthritis or neuralgias (including the pain following shingles or associated with diabetic neuropathy), simple backache, strains, and sprains.

General Information

Topical analgesics are one of the most popular types of OTC drugs, and the number of these drugs sold continues to increase year after year. Many of the people using these products are over age 50; in fact, 40% of individuals in this age group use topical analgesics on a regular basis, and 75% have arthritis. Younger people may use topical analgesics to relieve pain and soreness brought on by exercising or playing sports.

Capsaicin is derived from the fruit of plants in the nightshade family. Other medications in this family are capsicum and capsicum oleoresin. Capsaicin works by depleting the chemical substance P, which is thought to mediate pain sensation. Capsaicin is the same ingredient that makes chili peppers hot. When it is applied to the skin, capsaicin produces a feeling of warmth without causing blistering or reddening; in high concentrations, it can cause a sensation of burning pain.

You should feel pain relief within 2 weeks after you start using capsaicin; however, sometimes it may take up to 4 to 6 weeks to notice an effect. Capsaicin remains effective for 4 to 6 hours after it is applied.

Capsaicin is available by brand name in liquid, liniment, and cream form. It is often found in combination products with other topical analgesics such as menthol and methyl salicylate.

Cautions and Warnings

Do not exceed the recommended daily dosage of a capsaicin preparation.

Capsaicin preparations should be used only on the skin. Don't apply them near your eyes or to mucous membranes (i.e., inside the mouth, nose, rectum, or vagina).

If your pain gets worse or is constant and felt in any position, call your doctor.

Some people may overreact to the skin irritation caused by capsaicin and develop rashes and blisters. This may be more likely to occur in sensitive areas of the skin, such as behind your knees. If you develop any skin irritation or redness while using capsaicin, stop using it immediately and call your doctor.

Capsaicin should not be used with a heating pad, hot water bottle, or any other heating device. You should also avoid sunlight and sunlamps after using this product.

Don't use capsaicin (or any other topical analgesic) after intense exercise, especially during hot and humid weather, when you will probably be flushed and warm. If you have a sore muscle from working out and want to use capsaicin to relieve the pain, wait until you cool down. You should also avoid applying this product before using a sauna or getting a professional massage.

To avoid the risk of irritation, redness, or blistering, don't use a tight bandage or dressing over the skin where you apply capsaicin.

Don't use capsaicin on broken, irritated, or sunburned skin, or on an open wound.

If you wear contact lenses, don't take them out or put them in your eyes after you use a capsaicin preparation without first washing your hands.

Possible Side Effects

You may notice a temporary burning sensation when you apply capsaicin to your skin. This reaction should go away in a few days.

Some people may overreact to the skin irritation caused by capsaicin (see "Cautions and Warnings").

Drug Interactions

None known.

Usual Dose

Adult and Child (age 2 and over): Capsaicin is available in topical preparations in concentrations ranging from 0.025% –0.25%. Gently massage a small amount over the area on the skin where pain is felt. Make sure to wash your hands thoroughly afterward. (If you are treating pain in your hands, wait 30 minutes before washing.) Reapply as needed, no more than 3 or 4 times a day.

Child (under age 2): not recommended.

Overdosage

Do the following in case of accidental ingestion: If the victim is unconscious or having convulsions, call for an ambulance immediately. If you take the victim to an emergency room, be sure to bring the bottle or container with you. If the victim is conscious, call your local poison control center or a health care professional. The poison control center may suggest inducing vomiting with ipecac syrup (available without a prescription at any pharmacy). DO NOT induce vomiting unless specifically instructed to do so.

Special Information

Besides using a topical preparation, there are also physical methods of easing the pain of an overworked muscle, such as gently massaging the injured area. In fact, some of the benefit gained from using topical medications may simply be due to the fact that they are applied by being rubbed and massaged into the skin. Another way to ease pain is to apply heat to the skin with a hot water bottle or heating pad; in addition to reducing pain, heat helps the collagen in your skin regain its elasticity and lose its stiffness after a stretching injury. However, you should never use a heating pad or other heating device after applying capsaicin (see "Cautions and Warnings").

Special Populations

Pregnancy/Breast-feeding

If you are or might be pregnant, or you are breast-feeding, check with a doctor or other health care professional before using capsaicin.

It is not generally recommended that pregnant women take any drugs, particularly during the first 3 months after conception.

Infants/Children

Capsaicin should not be used by children younger than age 2.

Seniors

Seniors should exercise the same caution as younger adults when using capsaicin.

Generic Name

Capsicum Oleoresin

(KAP-sih-kum OE-lee-oe-REZ-in)

Definition

A concentrated liquid derived from the fruit of plants in the nightshade family. Used as an ingredient in topical analgesics (pain relievers), it produces a warm sensation when rubbed on the skin.

Generic Name

Carbamide Peroxide

(KAR-buh-mide per-OKS-ide)

Brand Names

Auro
Aurocaine
Cankaid
Debrox
Dent's Ear Wax Drops
E.R.O.
Gly-Oxide
Mollifene
Murine Ear Wax Removal System
Orajel Perioseptic

Type of Drug

Topical antiseptic.

Used for

Prevention of bacterial infection in canker sores and mouth irritations; ear wax removal.

General Information

Carbamide peroxide is an antibacterial agent used as a disinfectant for minor mouth irritations. It has a deodorant effect as well due to its ability to inhibit bacteria that cause odor.

It is also used in products that remove cerumen (ear wax) from the ear canal. The FDA has approved products containing 6.5% carbamide peroxide for the removal of ear wax.

When carbamide peroxide comes into contact with bacteria, a chemical reaction occurs in which oxygen and hydrogen peroxide are released in the form of bubbles. The activity of these bubbles, or fizzing, acts to loosen and scrub away dead tissue or ear wax, carrying it up and away from the wound or ear canal. This creates a clearer path for antibiotic and antibacterial medications to reach the affected area and to treat infection.

Carbamide peroxide is only effective as long as it is producing bubbles. Once the fizzing stops, the product no longer has any therapeutic benefit.

Carbamide peroxide is available by brand name as a solution or gel.

Cautions and Warnings

For treatment of canker sores, carbamide peroxide products should not be used for more than 7 days continuously, unless under the supervision of a doctor.

Ear wax removal products containing carbamide peroxide should not be used for longer than 4 days continuously, unless under the supervision of a doctor.

Do not exceed the recommended dose of carbamide peroxide.

Carbamide peroxide is for external use only. It should not be used in the eyes. If used in a gargle or mouthwash preparation, care should be taken to avoid swallowing. Ingestion of significant amounts of carbamide peroxide can cause ulcers (open wounds) in internal organs.

Do not use carbamide peroxide for ear wax removal if you are experiencing dizziness, rash, ear pain, ear drainage or discharge, or if you have had ear surgery within the past 6 weeks. If you suspect that you have an infection or that your eardrum is perforated (which causes symptoms such as hearing loss or pain), contact your doctor immediately.

Carbamide peroxide is also used as a bleach (e.g., in hair products). If used as a tooth whitening agent, it can seriously damage the enamel surface of the teeth.

Possible Side Effects

In some instances, the skin at the edges of a mouth sore will become white and remain so after the removal of the carbamide peroxide. This is not harmful; instead, it is an indication that dead tissue surrounding the wound has absorbed the chemical. The dead tissue will dry up and be sloughed off (shed) as the sore continues healing.

Drug Interactions

- When a carbamide peroxide gargle or toothpaste product is used, there is a chance that other chemicals in the mouth might exert more powerful activity. For example, residues from smoking or tobacco chew might become even more likely to cause cancer than they normally are.

Food Interactions

After applying this product to the affected area of the mouth, do not drink or rinse your mouth for at least 5 minutes.

Usual Dose

Ear Wax Removal

Adult and Child (age 12 and over): Tilt your head sideways and place 5–10 drops in your ear. The tip of the applicator should not enter the ear canal. Keep the drops in your ear for several minutes by keeping your head tilted or placing cotton in your ear. Any wax remaining after treatment may be removed by gently flushing the ear with *warm* (not hot) water, using a soft-bulb ear syringe.

Child (under age 12): Consult your doctor.

Oral Solution or Gel

Adult and Child (age 2 and over): Dry the affected area as much as possible. This allows the gel to adhere to the skin surface. Apply several drops of liquid or a small amount of gel to the sore or irritation and allow it to remain undisturbed for at least 1 minute. Wipe the affected area gently to remove the gel and dead tissue. Use up to 4 times per day—after meals and at bedtime, or as directed by a doctor.

Child (under age 2): Consult your doctor.

Overdosage

The swallowing of this chemical can result in serious internal organ damage. In case of accidental ingestion, DO NOT MAKE THE VICTIM VOMIT.

Do the following in case of accidental ingestion: If the victim is unconscious or having convulsions, call for an ambulance immediately. If you take the victim to an emergency room, be sure to bring the bottle or container with you. If the victim is conscious, call your local poison control center or a health care professional.

Special Information

The fizzing of the chemical reaction produced by carbamide peroxide can be frightening to small children and some adults. Before treating these individuals, it is a good idea to explain what is about to happen and offer assurance that the product is not an acid and will not cause pain.

Storage Instructions

The strength of carbamide peroxide deteriorates when exposed to light, repeated shaking, and heat.

Special Populations

Pregnancy/Breast-feeding

It is not generally recommended that pregnant woman take any drugs, particularly during the first 3 months after conception. Check with your doctor if you are or might be pregnant, or if you are breast-feeding.

Infants/Children

Since carbamide peroxide can be irritating to skin tissue, consult your doctor before using ear wax removal products on children under age 12, and before using oral products containing carbamide peroxide on children under age 2.

Children under 12 should be supervised by an adult when using carbamide peroxide gel.

Seniors

Seniors should exercise the same caution as younger adults when using carbamide peroxide.

Generic Name

Carboxymethylcellulose Sodium

(kar-BOK-see-METH-il-SELL-yue-loes SOE-dee-um)

Definition

A synthetic form of cellulose. Because it helps tissues retain moisture, it is used in artificial tears for relief of dry eyes and in artificial salivas for relief of dry mouth. Similar substances found in artificial tears include hydroxyethylcellulose, hydroxypropyl methylcellulose, and methylcellulose. Cellulose is also used as a moistening and bulking ingredient in laxative products.

Generic Name

Cascara Sagrada

(kass-KAR-ah sah-GRAH-dah)

Brand Names

Caroid
Milk of Magnesia Cascara
Nature's Remedy

Type of Drug

Laxative.

Used for

Relief of occasional constipation (irregularity).

General Information

The average, healthy individual defecates anywhere from 3 times a day to 3 times a week. Constipation is determined not necessarily by the frequency of bowel movements, but by the consistency of the stool, how difficult it is to eliminate, and symptoms such as dull headache, low back pain, and abdominal distention (swelling). Evaluate your condition carefully and discuss your symptoms and their possible causes with your pharmacist before self-medicating with a laxative. Laxatives are not always necessary and, when used improperly, can either prevent the desired effect or result in laxative dependency. If you are indeed constipated, your condition may be best managed through proper diet, adequate fluid intake (6 to 8 glasses a day), and exercise. If you must use a laxative, choose the mildest effective product.

Laxatives may be classified by their mechanism of action: bulk-forming, emollient (stool softeners), lubricant, saline, hyperosmotic, and stimulant. Cascara sagrada is a stimulant laxative. According to different studies, stimulant laxatives work by either increasing the propulsive activity of the intestine or stimulating the secretion of water and electrolytes in the intestine, thus leading to evacuation of the colon.

Cascara, made from the dried bark of the buckthorn tree, is specifically an anthraquinone laxative. It is milder than other stimulant laxatives, such as the diphenylmethane stimulant phenolphthalien. Cascara is also milder and less likely to cause abdominal cramps than another commonly used anthraquinone, senna.

The intensity of action of stimulant laxatives is dose-proportional. Cascara generally produces a bowel movement in 6 to 12 hours, but may take as long as 24 hours.

Casanthranol, a mixture of glycosides extracted from cascara, is found in several combination products containing the stool softener docusate sodium.

Cascara is available by generic name in tablet and fluidextract forms. The fluidextract tastes very bitter but appears to be more effective than the tablet. An aromatic fluidextract form improves on the taste but is not as effective. Cascara is also available by brand name in tablet and suspension form.

Cautions and Warnings

Do not use cascara for more than 7 days unless directed by your doctor.

Do not exceed the recommended daily dosage of cascara. The higher the dose, the more likely you are to experience adverse effects.

Long-term use of laxatives has been linked with laxative dependence, chronic constipation, loss of normal bowel function, and, in severe cases, nerve, muscle, and tissue damage to the intestines. Using laxatives too frequently can result in persistent diarrhea, hypokalemia (abnormally low potassium in the blood), loss of essential nutritional factors, and dehydration.

Of all the types of laxatives, stimulant laxatives such as cascara are particularly habit-forming and with long-term use are the most likely to cause adverse effects such as diarrhea, gastrointestinal (GI) irritation, and fluid and electrolyte depletion.

Do not take cascara if you have abdominal pain, nausea, vomiting, or kidney disease unless directed by your doctor.

If you notice a marked change in bowel habits lasting for more than 2 weeks, do not take cascara until you have spoken to your doctor. Also contact your doctor if there is blood in your stool so that colon cancer or other significant disease can be ruled out before you begin self-medication with cascara.

If you have had a disease or surgery affecting the GI tract, using a laxative may affect your condition adversely.

If you have rectal bleeding after using cascara or if you do not have a bowel movement after 7 days of using this medication, you may have a serious condition. Stop using cascara and call your doctor.

Laxatives may decrease the absorption of other drugs that pass through the GI tract (see "Drug Interactions").

Possible Side Effects

Stimulant laxatives like cascara are more likely to cause abdominal cramping than other types.

▼ Most common: abdominal discomfort, faintness, nausea, cramps, pinching and spasmodic pain in the bowels, colic, and increased mucus secretion.

▼ Less common (associated with chronic use of cascara): metabolic acidosis or alkalosis (imbalances of acid and base in body fluids), hypocalcemia (too little calcium in the blood), tetany (foot spasms and muscular twitching/cramps), electrolyte and fluid deficiencies (vomiting and muscle weakness), impaired intestinal absorption of nutrients, cathartic colon (weak or dilated colon).

Drug Interactions

• All laxatives potentially decrease the absorption of any oral drug taken at the same time. If you are currently taking an oral medication, talk to your doctor or pharmacist before self-medicating with cascara.

Food Interactions

None known.

Usual Dose

Doses should be adjusted to individual usage. Take cascara as needed, but do not exceed the recommended daily dosage. Take cascara tablets with a full glass (8 oz.) of water.

Fluidextract

Adult and Child (age 12 and over): 2–6 ml a day.

Child (age 6–11): 1–3 ml a day.

Child (under age 6): not recommended unless directed your doctor.

Tablets
Adult and Child (age 12 and over): 300–1000mg a day.

Child (age 6–11): 150–500mg a day.

Child (under age 6): not recommended unless directed by your doctor.

Overdosage

Symptoms of overdosage include persistent diarrhea and dehydration.

Even if the victim is not displaying any of the symptoms listed above, do the following in case of accidental overdose: If the victim is unconscious or having convulsions, call for an ambulance immediately. If you take the victim to an emergency room, be sure to bring the bottle or container with you. If the victim is conscious, call your local poison control center or a health care professional. The poison control center may suggest inducing vomiting with ipecac syrup (available without a prescription at any pharmacy). DO NOT induce vomiting unless specifically instructed to do so.

Special Information

Cascara may cause your urine to appear pink, red, brown, or black. This is not a cause for alarm.

Storage Instructions

Store liquid cascara at room temperature in a light-resistant container. Do not expose it to direct sunlight.

Special Populations

Pregnancy/Breast-feeding
Cascara should be avoided during pregnancy. Only bulk-forming or emollient laxatives are recommended for pregnant women.

Cascara passes into breast milk, but has not been reported to cause problems in nursing infants. Check with your doctor if you are breast-feeding before using cascara.

Also, consider talking to your doctor about diet and mild exercise in the management of constipation.

Infants/Children

In general, the use of laxatives should be avoided in children.

Do not give cascara to children under age 6 unless directed by a doctor.

Observe your child carefully for patterns of bowel movements and the pain or difficulty with which the bowel movements are made before deciding whether the child is actually constipated. As with adults, "normal" bowel habits vary in children. If your child is indeed constipated, increasing fluid intake and adding fiber to his or her diet may help to manage the condition.

Seniors

Seniors commonly experience constipation, and may become laxative-dependent. Avoid chronically using laxatives to ease constipation, and instead look to diet and increased fluid intake as therapeutic measures.

Stimulant laxatives such as cascara may not be the best choice for this age group because they alter fluid and electrolyte balance, placing some seniors at risk for side effects. Bulk-forming laxatives are usually preferred for seniors.

Generic Name

Castor Oil (KASS-tor)

Brand Names

Emulsoil
Kellogg's [A]
Neoloid
Purge [S]

Type of Drug

Laxative.

Used for

Preparation of the bowel for X-ray, surgery, and proctological procedures; and constipation.

General Information

The average, healthy individual defecates anywhere from 3 times a day to 3 times a week. Constipation is determined not necessarily by the frequency of bowel movements, but by the consistency of the stool, how difficult it is to eliminate, and other symptoms associated with constipation, such as dull headache, low back pain, and abdominal distention (swelling). Evaluate your condition carefully and discuss your symptoms and their possible causes with your pharmacist before self-medicating with a laxative. Laxatives are not always necessary, and when used improperly can either prevent the desired effect or result in laxative dependency. If you are indeed constipated, your condition may be best managed through proper diet, adequate fluid intake (6 to 8 glasses of water daily), and exercise. If you must use a laxative, choose the mildest effective product.

Laxatives may be classified by their mechanism of action: bulk-forming, emollient (stool softeners), lubricant, saline, hyperosmotic, and stimulant. Castor oil is a stimulant laxative, specifically a glyceride. According to different studies, stimulant laxatives work by either increasing the propulsive activity of the intestine or stimulating the secretion of water and electrolytes in the intestine, thus leading to evacuation of the colon. Castor oil also increases activity of the small intestine.

Castor oil has a very pronounced, sometimes violent laxative effect. This medication is mainly used when a complete evacuation of the gastrointestinal (GI) tract is desired (see "Used for") and is rarely used for routine constipation.

Castor oil generally produces a loose bowel movement in 2 to 3 hours.

Castor oil is available by brand name in oil or liquid form. The liquid and aromatic preparations of the oil taste somewhat better than the plain oil.

Cautions and Warnings

Do not use castor oil for more than 7 days unless directed by your doctor. Long-term use of laxatives has been linked with laxative dependence, chronic constipation, and loss of normal bowel function. Using laxatives too frequently can result in persistent diarrhea, hypokalemia (abnormally low potassium in the blood), loss of essential nutritional factors, and dehydration. The higher the dose of castor oil, the more likely you are to experience adverse effects.

Do not exceed the recommended daily dosage of castor oil.

Of all the types of laxatives, stimulant laxatives, such as

castor oil, are particularly habit-forming and are the most likely to cause adverse effects, such as diarrhea, GI irritation, and fluid and electrolyte depletion, with long-term use. Because it acts mainly on the small intestine, using castor oil for extended periods may result in excessive loss of fluids, electrolytes, and nutrients.

Do not take castor oil if you have abdominal pain, nausea, vomiting, or kidney disease, unless directed by your doctor.

If you notice a marked change in bowel habits lasting for more than 2 weeks, do not take castor oil until you have spoken to your doctor. Also contact your doctor if there is blood in your stool so that colon cancer or other significant disease can be ruled out before you begin self-medication with castor oil.

If you have had a disease or surgery affecting the GI tract, using a laxative may affect your condition adversely.

If you have rectal bleeding after using castor oil or if you do not have a bowel movement after 1 week of using this medication, you may have a serious condition. Stop using the product and call your doctor.

Castor oil should not be used by menstruating women.

Laxatives may decrease the absorption of other drugs that pass through the GI tract (see "Drug Interactions").

Possible Side Effects

- ▼ Most common: abdominal discomfort, faintness, nausea, cramps, pinching and spasmodic pain in the bowels, colic, increased mucus secretion, excessive irritation of the colon.
- ▼ Less common (chronic use of product only): metabolic acidosis or alkalosis (imbalances of acid and base in body fluids), hypocalcemia (too little calcium in the blood), tetany (characterized by foot spasms, muscular twitching, and cramps), loss of protein in the small intestine, electrolyte and fluid deficiencies (characterized by vomiting and muscle weakness), impaired intestinal absorption of nutrients, cathartic colon (weak or dilated colon).
- ▼ Rare: pelvic congestion.

Drug Interactions

• All laxatives potentially decrease the absorption of any oral drug taken at the same time. If you are currently taking an oral medication, talk to your pharmacist before taking castor oil.

Food Interactions

Castor oil is most effective when taken on an empty stomach.

Usual Dose

Doses should be adjusted to individual usage. Castor oil is not generally recommended for treating routine constipation.

If you are using plain castor oil, take it with fruit juice or a carbonated drink to mask the unpleasant taste, or refrigerate (at least 1 hour).

Adult and Child (age 12 and over): 2–4 tbs.
Child (age 6–11): 1 tbs.
Child (under age 6): Consult your doctor.

Overdosage

Symptoms of overdosage include persistent diarrhea and dehydration.

Do the following in case of accidental overdose: If the victim is unconscious or having convulsions, call for an ambulance immediately. If you take the victim to an emergency room, be sure to bring the bottle or container with you. If the victim is conscious, call your local poison control center or a health care professional. The poison control center may suggest inducing vomiting with ipecac syrup (available without a prescription at any pharmacy). DO NOT induce vomiting unless specifically instructed to do so.

Special Information

Do not take castor oil right before going to bed; it works quickly and will interrupt your sleep.

Storage Instructions

Do not store above room temperature to avoid rancidity.

Special Populations

Pregnancy/Breast-feeding

Do not use castor oil if you are or might be pregnant. This medication has been associated with premature labor. Only bulk-forming or emollient laxatives are recommended for pregnant women. Also consider talking to your doctor about diet and mild exercise in the management of constipation during pregnancy.

It is not known if castor oil passes into breast milk. Check with your doctor before using castor oil if you are breast-feeding.

Infants/Children

Observe your child carefully for patterns of bowel movements and the pain or difficulty with which the bowel movements are made before deciding whether the child is actually constipated. As with adults, "normal" bowel habits vary in children. If your child is indeed constipated, increasing fluid intake and adding fiber to his or her diet may help to manage the condition. In general, the use of laxatives should be avoided in children.

Castor oil is not generally recommended for treating constipation in adults; it should be used with particular caution in constipated children and only after consulting a doctor.

Seniors

Seniors commonly experience constipation and consequently may become laxative-dependent. Be cautious of chronically turning to laxatives to ease constipation, and instead look to diet and increased fluid intake as therapeutic measures.

Stimulant laxatives, such as castor oil, may not be the best choice for this group because they alter fluid and electrolyte balance, placing some seniors at risk for side effects. Bulk-forming laxatives are usually preferred for seniors.

Generic Name

Cetearyl Alcohol (SEE-tah-reel AL-kuh-hall)

Definition

*see **Alcohol,** page 665*

Generic Name

Cetyl Alcohol (SEE-til AL-kuh-hall)

Definition

*see **Alcohol,** page 665*

Generic Name

Cetylpyridinium Chloride

(SEE-til-pye-rih-DIN-ee-uhm KLOR-ide)

Definition

An anti-infective ingredient found in a wide range of OTC products, including douches, diaper rash treatments and lozenges. As an antibacterial ingredient in first aid skin care products, it prevents secondary infection that can result when people scratch insect bites and bee stings. Cetylpyridinium chloride is included in some mouthwashes designed to fight plaque, although this ingredient does not penetrate plaque well.

Generic Name

Charcoal, Activated

(CHAR-kole)

Brand Names

Actidose
CharcoAid [S]
Charcoal Plus DS
†CharcoCaps
Liqui Char

†*Consult the OTC ingredient charts to determine whether different formulations in this brand-name group are alcohol-, caffeine-, or sugar-free.*

Type of Drug

Adsorbent.

Used for

Emergency treatment of acute poisoning by ingestion. Activated charcoal may also be used for symptomatic relief of intestinal gas, although its value in this capacity has not been conclusively established.

General Information

Activated charcoal works as a poison antidote by adsorbing, or binding, toxic substances and preventing them from being absorbed from the gastrointestinal (GI) tract into the bloodstream. The charcoal itself is not absorbed from the GI tract or metabolized.

Activated charcoal is recommended for treating acute poisoning caused by the following substances: acetaminophen, aspirin, atropine, barbiturates, dextropropoxyphene, digoxin, poisonous mushrooms, oxalic acid, phenol, phenylpropanolamine, phenytoin, propantheline, strychnine, and tricyclic antidepressants. Multiple doses of activated charcoal are recommended to increase the elimination of phenobarbital from the body.

Activated charcoal is best used immediately (within 30 minutes) after the poison has been ingested, although it may still be beneficial even after several hours have passed.

In the past 10 years, the use of activated charcoal in the treatment of acute poisoning has surpassed the use of ipecac syrup. However, the effectiveness of activated charcoal may be enhanced by using it after a dose of ipecac (see "Cautions and Warnings").

Activated charcoal is available by brand name in suspension (liquid) and caplet forms. The suspension form is more effective in the treatment of acute poisoning.

Cautions and Warnings

When used as an antiflatulent, do not take the maximum daily dosage of activated charcoal for more than 24 hours except under a doctor's supervision.

Do not exceed the recommended daily dosage of activated charcoal.

In an acute poisoning emergency, first try to contact an emergency room, local poison control center, or doctor. If outside help cannot be obtained quickly enough, take or administer the activated charcoal, carefully following the directions on the label. Some health care professionals recommend using ipecac syrup first to induce vomiting. Again, read the label carefully before taking or administering ipecac. Because activated charcoal adsorbs ipecac, it is crucial to take the ipecac first and vomit before taking the charcoal. After taking or administering the ipecac and/or charcoal, try again to contact a health care professional.

Activated charcoal should not be used for oral poisonings involving corrosive agents, cyanide, iron, mineral acids, or organic solvents (e.g., alcohol, acetone, paint thinner, etc.).

Activated charcoal adsorbs enzymes, vitamins, amino acids, minerals, and other nutrients. This is not a cause for concern when the product is being used only to treat acute poisoning, but should be taken into consideration if the product is being taken regularly to treat flatulence. Activated charcoal may also decrease the absorption, and thus the effectiveness, of other orally administered drugs.

The so-called universal antidote of 2 parts activated charcoal, 1 part magnesium oxide, and 1 part tannic acid does not work as well as activated charcoal alone, and the tannic acid is, in fact, potentially toxic.

Possible Side Effects

Activated charcoal, taken regularly for flatulence, adsorbs enzymes, vitamins, amino acids, minerals, and other nutrients.

Drug Interactions

Antiflatulent

- Activated charcoal may decrease the absorption and reduce the effectiveness of other orally administered medications. Space doses by at least 1 hour.

Food Interactions

Do not use milk, ice cream, or sherbet as a flavoring agent if you are using charcoal in powder form; they substantially decrease the effectiveness of the activated charcoal.

Usual Dose

Poison Antidote

Adult and Child (age 12 and over): Use only in case of emergency. If you are using a commercially prepared suspension, shake the bottle vigorously for at least 15 seconds and drink the entire contents. If you are using a powder, mix it with enough water to form a slurry (usually about 60–100 g of activated charcoal). To improve the taste of the slurry, add a small amount of concentrated fruit juice or chocolate powder.

Child (under age 12): as directed by your doctor.

Antiflatulent

Adult and Child (age 12 and over): Take activated charcoal after eating or as symptoms occur, but do not exceed the maximum daily dosage specified on the package.

Child (under age 12): not recommended.

Overdosage

When used as a poison antidote, there is no maximum dose limit with activated charcoal. There are no reports of overdosage with activated charcoal used for flatulence.

Special Information

Contrary to popular belief, burnt toast is not a form of activated charcoal and may not be used as a substitute for it in treating acute poisoning.

Storage Instructions

Store in a tightly sealed glass or metal container.

Special Populations

Pregnancy/Breast-feeding

When treating acute poisoning, use activated charcoal as directed by a health care professional.

It is not generally recommended that pregnant women take any drugs, particularly during the first 3 months after conception. Check with your doctor before treating flatulence with activated charcoal if you are or might be pregnant or if you are breast-feeding.

Infants/Children

When treating an infant or child for acute poisoning, use activated charcoal as directed by a health care professional. Children should receive about a third of the dose that an adult would take. Some health care professionals recommend ipecac syrup over activated charcoal for home use in children because the ipecac is easier to administer.

Activated charcoal is not recommended for use as an antiflatulent in children under 12.

Seniors

Seniors should exercise the same caution as younger adults when using activated charcoal.

Generic Name

Chlorhexidine Gluconate

(klor-HEKS-ih-deen GLUE-kon-ate)

Definition

A chemical used as an antiseptic in first-aid skin care products and as a preservative in vaginal lubricant products and contact lens cleaning solutions. People who wear contact lenses made of silicone or styrene should avoid lens care products with chlorhexidine gluconate, which can make the lens surface more difficult to wet and can cause clouding on the lens surface.

Generic Name

Chlorobutanol (KLOR-oe-BEW-tah-nol)

Definition

White crystals primarily used as a preservative in solutions of epinephrine and other OTC drugs. It has local anesthetic properties and is sometimes used topically, as a 25% solution in clove oil, to relieve dental pain. It has also been administered orally as a sedative and to allay vomiting due to gastritis.

Generic Name

Chloroxylenol (KLOR-oe-ZYE-leh-nol)

Brand Names

Care-Creme Cream
Dermacoat
*Foille Medicated First Aid Burn
*Undelenic
Vaseline Medicated Antibacterial Petroleum Jelly
Zeasorb

**Not all products in this brand-name group contain chloroxylenol.*

Type of Drug

Antifungal agent.

Used for

Cure of tinea pedis (athlete's foot), tinea cruris (jock itch), and tinea corporis (ringworm), and relief of the itching, cracking, burning, and discomfort accompanying these conditions; prevention of the recurrence of athlete's foot.

General Information

A fungus is an organism that obtains nutrients from other living organisms or from dead organic matter in order to survive. Fungi can cause both systemic and cutaneous (skin) infection. Chloroxylenol is an OTC antifungal drug used only for fungal infection of the skin. It is important to understand that fungi are different from bacteria and that drugs (antibiotics) that cure bacterial infection have no effect on, and cannot relieve the symptoms of, a fungal infection. Similarly, antifungal drugs have no effect on, and cannot relieve the symptoms of a bacterial infection. Generally, cutaneous fungal infections occur in warm, moist areas of the body, such as the vagina, the groin area, and between the toes. Chloroxylenol is not recommended or approved by the FDA as a treatment for vaginal yeast infections.

Chloroxylenol is not considered safe and effective by the FDA for use as an antimicrobial or skin disinfectant.

Chloroxylenol is available by brand name in creams, ointments, and solutions.

Cautions and Warnings

Do not use chloroxylenol products to treat athlete's foot, jock itch, or ringworm for more than 12 weeks unless directed by your doctor.

Do not exceed the recommended daily dosage of chloroxylenol products.

Chloroxylenol products are for external use only. Avoid contact with your eyes. After applying one of these products, wash your hands with soap and water.

If irritation, itching, or swelling occurs, stop using chloroxylenol and call your doctor.

Chloroxylenol is not effective in treating fungal infections of the scalp or nails.

Although some antifungal agents have been shown to be effective in treating diaper rash when the rash is caused by the *Candida* fungus, the OTC products available are not approved for this use by the FDA.

Possible Side Effects

▼ Rare: mild skin irritation, burning, and stinging.

Drug Interactions

None known.

Usual Dose

Adult and Child (age 2 and over): Clean the affected area with soap and water, and dry thoroughly. Apply a thin layer of the product over the affected area twice daily (morning and night) or as directed by a doctor.

If you are treating athlete's foot, be sure to thoroughly dry the feet and in-between the toes and apply the cream, ointment, or solution to the spaces between or under the toes.

Athlete's foot almost always affects both feet. Be sure to treat all areas of both feet that itch, hurt, or appear red.

For best results, use chloroxylenol for the length of time indicated on the package directions. Treatment of athlete's foot and ringworm should be complete within 4 weeks; treatment of jock itch, 2 weeks. Call your doctor if any of these conditions persists despite treatment.

Child (under age 2): not recommended.

Overdosage

Do the following in case of accidental ingestion: If the victim is unconscious or having convulsions, call for an ambulance immediately. If you take the victim to an emergency room, be sure to bring the bottle or container with you. If the victim is conscious, call your local poison control center or a health care professional. The poison control center may suggest inducing vomiting with ipecac syrup (available without a prescription at any pharmacy). DO NOT induce vomiting unless specifically instructed to do so.

Special Information

When treating athlete's foot, certain measures can be taken, in addition to using an antifungal agent, to assist in curing the infection:

- Wash your feet with soap and water every day, and thoroughly dry them (but be careful not to scrub too hard between the toes and irritate the skin).
- Wear well-fitting, ventilated shoes and light socks.
- Change your shoes and socks at least once daily, and wash the socks thoroughly.
- Try not to wear canvas, leather, or rubber-soled shoes for too long.
- Keep your feet dry.
- Air your feet out as often as possible.

Special Populations

Pregnancy/Breast-feeding

It is not generally recommended that pregnant women take any drugs, particularly during the first 3 months after conception. Check with your doctor if you are or might be pregnant, or if you are breast-feeding.

Infants/Children

Do not use chloroxylenol on children under 2 years of age unless directed by a doctor. Supervise older children under the age of 12 in the use of these products.

Seniors

Seniors should exercise the same caution as younger adults when using chloroxylenol products.

Generic Name

Chlorpheniramine Maleate

(KLOR-fen-EER-ah-meen MAL-ee-ate)

Brand Names

A.R.M.
*Alka-Seltzer
*Allerest
Allergy Relief
BC Allergy-Sinus-Cold
Cerose-DM
Cheracol Plus
*Chlor-Trimeton

*†Codimal
*Comtrex
*Contac
Coricidin
*†Creomulsion
Dallergy-D [A]
†Demazin
Diabetic Tussin [A] [S] Allergy Relief
Dristan Cold Multi-Symptom
Duadacin
Efidac 24 Chlorpheniramine
Fedahist
Hayfebrol [A] [S]
Histatab Plus
*†Kolephrin
Kophane [A]
Napril
*Novahistine
*†PediaCare
Prominicol
Protac SF [A]
Pyrroxate
Quelidrine Cough
Robitussin Pediatric Night Relief [A]
Scot-Tussin DM [A] [S]
Sinapils
*Sinarest
Sine-Off Sinus
Singlet
Sinulin [S]
Sinus Relief Extra Strength
Sinutab Sinus Allergy Medication Maximum Strength
Teldrin
Tetrahist
*TheraFlu
Tri-Nefrin
*†Triaminic
Triaminicin
Triaminicol [A]
†Tricodene
Tussar-DM [A]
*†Tylenol
*†Vicks

**Not all products in this brand-name group contain chlorpheniramine maleate.*

†Consult the OTC ingredient charts to determine whether different formulations in this brand-name group are alcohol-, caffeine-, or sugar-free.

Type of Drug

Antihistamine.

Used for

Temporary relief of runny nose, sneezing, itchy eyes, scratchy throat, and other symptoms (skin rash, itching, or hives) associated with seasonal allergy.

General Information

Histamine is one of the substances released by the body tissues during an allergic reaction. When it is released, the body reacts with a variety of symptoms, including itching and sneezing. Antihistamines work by competitively inhibiting the pharmacological actions of histamine, which makes them very effective for relieving the symptoms of allergic reactions. Antihistamines may also help relieve a runny nose. However, because antihistamines do not work against the other substances released by the body during an allergic reaction, they can reduce only about 40% to 60% of allergic symptoms. They are also not effective in clearing up a stuffy nose.

If you have seasonal allergies, antihistamines work best if you take them before your allergy season begins. Those who suffer from allergies regardless of the season may need to take antihistamines all year.

Antihistamines will not cure or prevent allergies, viral infections (colds), or bacterial infections. The best you can hope for is symptomatic relief.

Chlorpheniramine is classified as an alkylamine antihistamine. Others in this group include brompheniramine and pheniramine. Of the antihistamines available without a prescription, these are the least likely to make you sleepy. However, drowsiness is still a significant side effect of chlorpheniramine. Newer antihistamines do not have the common antihistamine side effect of drowsiness, but they are currently available only by prescription.

In cold and allergy products, chlorpheniramine is often combined with a nasal decongestant, such as phenylpropanolamine or pseudoephedrine. In these combination products, chlorpheniramine may also be used in a related form, called dexchlorpheniramine. Chlorpheniramine is available by brand and generic name in capsule and syrup form.

Cautions and Warnings

Do not take the maximum daily dosage of chlorpheniramine for more than 7 days continuously except under a doctor's supervision.

Do not exceed the recommended daily dosage of chlorpheniramine.

Unless prescribed by a doctor, chlorpheniramine and other antihistamines should not be used by people who have a breathing problem, such as emphysema or chronic bronchitis, or by individuals with asthma.

Chlorpheniramine should be used with caution by people with glaucoma, hyperthyroidism, heart disease, high blood pressure, or enlargement of the prostate gland. If you have any of these conditions, consult your doctor before taking chlorpheniramine.

Chlorpheniramine's effects on the central nervous system (CNS) can make you feel sleepy or reduce your concentration. Your ability to perform activities that require your full alertness and coordination, such as driving a motor vehicle or operating machinery, may be affected. Drinking alcohol or taking other sedative drugs while you are taking chlorpheniramine can add to these effects.

Phenylketonurics (people who cannot digest the amino acid phenylalanine) should be aware that some formulations of chlorpheniramine contain aspartame (Nutrasweet), which breaks down in the gastrointestinal tract to phenylalanine after the drug is taken.

Possible Side Effects

▼ Most common: restlessness, nervousness, sleeplessness or drowsiness, sedation, excitability, dizziness, poor coordination, and upset stomach.

▼ Less common: dry eyes, nose, and mouth; blurred vision; difficulty urinating; irritability (at high doses); increased or irregular heart rate; and heart palpitations.

Drug Interactions

• Chlorpheniramine's effects can combine with those of other CNS depressants, including barbiturates, tranquilizers, sleeping medications, and alcohol (present in many OTC preparations). If you are taking other depressant drugs, check with your doctor before you take chlorpheniramine or any other antihistamine. Avoid drinking alcohol if you are taking chlorpheniramine or any other antihistamine.

• Chlorpheniramine should not be used at the same time as a monoamine oxidase inhibitor (MAOI) or within 2 weeks of stopping treatment with an MAOI. MAOIs are used to treat depression, other psychiatric or emotional conditions, and Parkinson's disease. If you are not sure whether you are or have been taking an MAOI, check with your doctor or pharmacist before you use chlorpheniramine or any other antihistamine.

• Antihistamines can affect the results of skin and blood tests. Notify your health care professional before scheduling these tests if you are taking chlorpheniramine.

Food Interactions

None known.

Usual Dose

Because histamine is released nearly continuously, it is best to take antihistamines on a schedule rather than as needed.

Chlorpheniramine

Adult and Child (age 12 and over): 4 mg every 4–6 hours. Do not take more than 24 mg in 24 hours. For extended-release formulations containing 8 or 12 mg of chlorpheniramine, take 1 tablet twice daily in the morning and evening. Do not take more than 24 mg in 24 hours. For extended-release tablets containing a 12-mg core and a 4-mg outer coating of chlorpheniramine (16 mg total), take 1 tablet once a day. This tablet should be swallowed whole with fluid and should not be crushed, chewed, or dissolved.

Child (age 6–11): 2 mg every 4–6 hours. Do not give more than 12 mg in 24 hours.

Child (under age 6): Consult your doctor.

Child (under age 2): not recommended.

The sedating effects of chlorpheniramine may be minimized by either taking a full dose at bedtime or using the smallest recommended doses, combined with a decongestant, during the day. Another alternative is to start with the lowest dose when you begin taking the drug and gradually increase the dosage over several days.

If you forget to take a dose of chlorpheniramine, do so as soon you remember. If it is almost time for your next dose, skip the one you forgot and continue with your regular schedule. Do not take a double dose.

Overdosage

Symptoms of antihistamine overdose in children include dilated pupils, flushed face, dry mouth, fever, excitability, hallucinations, loss of muscle coordination, and seizures.

In adults, overdose can cause drowsiness or coma, which may be followed by excitability or seizures. Eventually fluid can build up in the brain; the kidneys may fail, and the heart and lungs may stop working, resulting in death. Symptoms may develop within 30 minutes to 2 hours following an overdose, and death may occur within 18 hours.

Even if the victim is not displaying any of the symptoms listed above, do the following in case of accidental overdose: If the victim is unconscious or having convulsions, call for an ambulance immediately. If you take the victim to an emergency room, be sure to bring the bottle or container with you. If the victim is conscious, call your local poison control center or a health care professional. The poison control center may suggest inducing vomiting with ipecac syrup (available without a prescription at any pharmacy). DO NOT induce vomiting unless specifically instructed to do so.

Special Populations

Allergies

Some chlorpheniramine preparations also contain the dye tartrazine, which may cause allergic reactions (including bronchial asthma) in some people. Individuals who are allergic to aspirin are likely to react to tartrazine.

Pregnancy/Breast-feeding

Chlorpheniramine and other antihistamines are not recommended for use during pregnancy unless prescribed by your doctor. Antihistamines are known to pass into the breast milk of nursing mothers and may cause side effects in infants. Check with your doctor before taking chlorpheniramine if you are or might be pregnant, or if you are breast-feeding.

Infants/Children

Extended release preparations of chlorpheniramine should not be used by children under 12 unless directed by a doctor.

Children may be more susceptible to the CNS-stimulant effects of chlorpheniramine. Chlorpheniramine is not recommended for children under 2.

Seniors

Seniors may be more sensitive to the side effects of chlorpheniramine and other antihistamines and may experience nervousness, irritability, and restlessness. Dizziness, sedation, and low blood pressure may also occur. Older men may experience difficulty in urinating. Most mild reactions may be handled by either lowering your dose or trying another antihistamine.

Generic Name

Chlorothymol (KLOR-oe-THYE-mol)

Definition

A white, granular powder used as an antiseptic in OTC products for the treatment of minor skin irritation and infection.

Generic Name

Cholecalciferol (KOE-lah-kal-SIH-far-ol)

Definition

White, odorless crystals known as vitamin D3 and having the same function as vitamin D.

Cholecalciferol, which is obtained from natural sources or is prepared synthetically, is available as a clear solution in an edible vegetable oil. Like vitamin D, cholecalciferol is used to prevent or treat rickets or osteomalacia (softening of the bones). It is also used to treat hypocalcemia (reduction of calcium in the blood). Because of the risk of toxicity, cholecalciferol's use should be closely monitored; consult your doctor. Cholecalciferol should not be used in people with kidney failure.

Generic Name

Citric Acid Solution (SIH-trik ASS-id)

Definition

When used in combination with sodium citrate, it serves as a systemic (affecting the entire body) and urinary alkalizer (acid neutralizer). Citric acid is also used as a component in anticoagulant (blood-thinning) solutions.

Generic Name

Clotrimazole (kloe-TRIM-ah-zole)

Brand Names

Desenex AF
Femizole-7
Gyne-Lotrimin
*Lotrimin AF
Mycelex-7

**Not all products in this brand-name group contain clotrimazole.*

Type of Drug

Antifungal agent.

Used for

Topical Products
Curing tinea pedis (athlete's foot), tinea cruris (jock itch), and tinea corporis (ringworm) and relieving the itching, cracking, burning, and discomfort accompanying these conditions.

Vaginal Products
Treating vaginal yeast infection.

General Information

A fungus is an organism that obtains nutrients from other living organisms or from dead organic matter in order to survive. Fungi can cause both systemic and cutaneous (skin) infection. Over-the-counter antifungal drugs are used only for fungal infection of the skin and vagina. It is important to understand that fungi are different from bacteria and that drugs (antibiotics) that cure bacterial infection have no effect on, and cannot relieve the symptoms of, a fungal infection. In a similar fashion, antifungal drugs have no effect on, or cannot relieve the symptoms of, a bacterial infection. Generally, cutaneous fungal infections occur in warm, moist areas of the body, such as the vagina, the groin area, and between the toes.

Clotrimazole is one of 4 antifungal agents known as imidazoles; 3 others in the group, butoconazole, tioconazde, and miconazole, are also available without a prescription. The imidazoles inhibit the growth of and kill fungi and also relieve the symptoms of the infection caused by the fungi.

Studies have shown that the 4 OTC imidazoles are equally effective in inhibiting the growth of and killing the fungus known as *Candida,* which causes vaginal yeast infections. They have an effectiveness rate of about 85% to 90%. One advantage of butoconazole is that it is taken for only 3 days; clotrimazole and miconazole must be taken for 7 days to cure a vaginal yeast infection.

Clotrimazole is equal in efficacy to miconazole in treating athlete's foot, and both are as effective as tolnaftate (Tinactin), the standard topical antifungal medication.

All 4 OTC imidazoles are well tolerated.

Clotrimazole topical products are available by brand name in cream, solution, and lotion forms. Be aware that products of the same brand name do not necessarily contain the same active ingredient. For example, the active ingredient in Lotrimin AF cream is clotrimazole, but the active ingredient in Lotrimin AF spray powder is miconazole.

Clotrimazole vaginal products are available by brand name in cream and vaginal tablet forms. The cream may be preferable if your vulva (outer genital tissue) has been significantly affected by the infection; it can be applied externally, to relieve itching, as well as internally. The brand Mycelex-7 is available in a combination pack of vaginal tablets and cream. The vaginal tablets, used internally, treat the fungus; and the cream, used externally, relieves the itching in the vulva.

Cautions and Warnings

Do not exceed the recommended daily dosage of clotrimazole products.

Clotrimazole topical and vaginal products are for external use only. Avoid contact with your eyes. After applying, wash your hands with soap and water.

Topical Products

If there is no improvement in your athlete's foot or ringworm within 4 weeks or in your jock itch within 2 weeks, stop using the product and call your doctor.

If irritation, itching, or swelling occurs, stop using the product and call your doctor.

Clotrimazole is not effective on the scalp or nails.

Although some antifungal agents have been shown to be effective in treating diaper rash caused by the *Candida* fungus, the OTC products available are not approved for this use by the FDA.

Vaginal Products

If you do not improve after 3 days of treatment with clotrimazole or if you do not get well in 7 days, you may have a condition other than a yeast infection. Call your doctor.

Self-medicate with a clotrimazole vaginal product only if you have had a doctor diagnose a vaginal yeast infection previously and you recognize the same symptoms now. If this is the first time you have had vaginal itch and discomfort, DO NOT SELF-MEDICATE WITH CLOTRIMAZOLE. Call your doctor, and have him or her determine whether what you have is truly a yeast infection and not another type of vaginal infection, such as one caused by bacteria, which can't be effectively treated with clotrimazole.

Do not use a clotrimazole vaginal product if you have abdominal pain, fever, or foul-smelling discharge. Call your doctor immediately.

Stop using the product and call your doctor if you develop abdominal cramping, headache, hives, or skin rash.

If your symptoms return within 2 months or if you have infections that do not clear up easily with treatment, call your physician. You could be pregnant, or there could be a serious underlying medical reason for your infections, such as diabetes or an impaired immune system (such as that associated with HIV infection).

If you are using the combination pack of vaginal tablets and external vulvar cream, do not use the cream to relieve vulvar itching due to causes other than a yeast infection.

You must use these products for 7 consecutive days in order for them to cure your fungal infection. Do not stop therapy before then even if your symptoms disappear right away, as often happens.

You may use clotrimazole vaginal products during your period, but do not use tampons. If your period begins after you have started your 7-day treatment, do not stop treatment.

It is recommended that you avoid sexual intercourse during your 7-day treatment. Be aware that clotrimazole can damage condoms, diaphragms, and cervical caps, thus increasing your risk of pregnancy.

Possible Side Effects

Topical Products

▼ Rare: mild skin irritation, burning, and stinging.

Vaginal Products

▼ Rare: abdominal cramps, headache, itching, irritation, and allergic reactions.

Drug Interactions

None known.

Usual Dose

Topical Products

Adult and Child (age 2 and over): Clean the affected area with soap and water, and dry thoroughly. Apply a thin layer of the product over the affected area twice daily (morning and night) or as directed by a doctor.

If you are treating athlete's foot, be sure to apply the cream, lotion, or solution to the spaces between the toes.

Athlete's foot almost always affects both feet. Be sure to treat both feet with equal thoroughness even if one foot looks worse than the other.

For best results, use clotrimazole for the length of time indicated on the package directions. Treatment of athlete's foot and ringworm should be complete within 4 weeks; treatment of jock itch, 2 weeks. Call your doctor if any of these conditions persists despite treatment.

Child (under 2): not recommended.

Vaginal Products

Wash your entire vaginal area with mild soap and water and dry thoroughly before applying the cream or insert.

Adult and Child (age 12 and over): Read the package carefully before using a clotrimazole vaginal product.

Child (under age 12): not recommended.

Vaginal Cream

Adult and Child (age 12 and over): 1 full application into the vagina at bedtime. Attach the applicator to the tube and squeeze the tube from the bottom to force the cream into the applicator. Once the applicator is full, remove it from the tube and insert it as high up into the vagina as possible.

Child (under age 12): not recommended.

Vaginal Tablets

Adult and Child (age 12 and over): Unwrap 1 tablet, place it in the barrel of the applicator, and insert the applicator into your vagina. Press the plunger on the applicator until it deposits the tablet in your vagina.

Repeat the procedure daily for 7 consecutive days.

Be sure to wash the applicator in soap and water and air-dry so that it is clean for use the next day. (The brand Mycelex-7 is available in disposable applicator form.)

If you are using the combination pack of vaginal tablets and external cream, squeeze a small amount of cream onto your finger and gently spread it onto the irritated area of the vulva. Use it once or twice daily, as needed, for up to 7 days.

It is best to use these products at bedtime to avoid the dripping or leaking that occurs when you are upright. Since there may still be some leakage, you may want to wear a sanitary pad. Do not use a tampon to prevent leakage.

Child (under age 12): not recommended.

Overdosage

Do the following in case of accidental ingestion: If the victim is unconscious or having convulsions, call for an ambulance immediately. If you take the victim to an emergency room, be sure to bring the bottle or container with you. If the victim is conscious, call your local poison control center or a health care professional. The poison control center may suggest inducing vomiting with ipecac syrup (available without a prescription at any pharmacy). DO NOT induce vomiting unless specifically instructed to do so.

Special Information

Topical Products

When treating athlete's foot, certain measures can be taken, in addition to using an antifungal agent, to assist in curing the infection:

- Wash your feet with soap and water every day, and thoroughly dry them (but be careful not to scrub too hard between the toes and irritate the skin).
- Wear well-fitting, ventilated shoes and light socks.
- Change your shoes and socks at least once daily, and wash the socks thoroughly.
- Try not to wear canvas, leather, or rubber-soled shoes for too long.
- Keep your feet dry.
- Air your feet out as often as possible.

Special Populations

Pregnancy/Breast-feeding

It is not generally recommended that pregnant women take any drugs, particularly during the first 3 months after conception. Check with your doctor if you are or might be pregnant, or if you are breast-feeding.

Infants/Children

Topical Products

Do not use clotrimazole topical cream, lotion, or solution on children under 2 years of age unless directed by a doctor. Supervise older children under the age of 12 in the use of these products.

Vaginal Products

Children under 12 years of age should not use clotrimazole vaginal cream or inserts.

Seniors

Seniors should exercise the same caution as younger adults when using clotrimazole products.

Generic Name

Coal Tar

Brand Names

Aquatar
Balnetar
Cutar
Denorex
*DHS
Doctar
Duplex-T
Estar
Fototar
Glover's Medicated
*Ionil T
*MG217
*Neutrogena T/Gel
Oxipor VHC
Pentrax
Polytar
Psoriasin
Psoriasis Tar
Psorigel
Sebex-T
Sebutone
SLT Lotion
Tar Scalp Solution
Tar Shampoo Maximum Strength
Taraphilic
Tarsum Shampoo/Gel
Tegrin
Vanseb T
*X-Seb
Zetar

** Not all products in this brand-name group contain coal tar.*

Type of Drug

Keratolytic agent (topical skin cell remover); and skin irritant.

Used for

Treatment and control of skin and scalp disorders, such as dandruff, seborrhea, and psoriasis.

General Information

Coal tar is a byproduct of coal production. In medicinal applications, it works as a mild irritant. By robbing skin cells of oxygen, coal tar slows their rate of reproduction. It also helps produce smaller cells. These effects thus reduce the severity of common skin conditions that involve overproduction of skin cells, such as dandruff and seborrhea. Coal tar relieves the itching, irritation, and flaking of seborrheic dermatitis and the itching, redness, and scaling of psoriasis.

Coal tar is available in a variety of forms, each formulated to mask the unpleasant odor, color, and staining properties of this chemical. Most OTC products containing coal tar are used as shampoos. Coal tar is also available in some OTC and prescription formulations for use elsewhere on the body.

Tar gels are the most cosmetically pleasing form of coal tar, and are nongreasy, nonstaining and almost colorless. Their only drawback is that they are drying to the skin, and may require the addition of a moisturizing product to your skin-care routine to counteract this problem.

Cautions and Warnings

Do not take the maximum daily dosage of coal tar for more than 7 days unless under the supervision of a doctor.

Do not exceed the recommended daily dosage of coal tar.

Coal tar products are for external use only. Care should be taken to avoid contact with the eyes. If this occurs, flush the eyes well with water.

Coal tar can increase the skin's sensitivity to sunlight for up to 24 hours after use.

You should avoid exposure to sunlight and sunlamps while using any of these products. If this cannot be avoided, remove all traces of the product before exposure.

If your condition persists or worsens with regular use as directed, stop using the product and consult your doctor.

Products containing coal tar should not be used over large areas of the body or on broken or already inflamed skin. If you are experiencing an intense inflammation of psoriasis, do not use coal tar products, because this can cause a shedding of healthy skin cells over the entire body. After the condition has subsided and the usual scales appear, a coal tar product may then be used to help remove the scaly skin.

Many physicians advise switching from dandruff shampoo to regular shampoo on alternate days or using dandruff shampoos no more than twice a week.

Using these products more frequently than directed can cause excessive dryness of skin or scalp. Scalp and skin irritation is possible, with the development of inflamed hair follicles.

Coal tar applied to the skin poses a risk of skin cancer if used over large areas of the body other than the scalp for long periods of time.

Possible Side Effects

There is a risk that coal tar can cause excessive dryness of the skin, scalp, or hair. Also, products containing this chemical might cause irritation and dermatitis, resulting in a hardening of the skin surface or mild scabbing. Allergic reactions are rare.

Certain products containing coal tar tend to stain. This can particularly affect people with blond, bleached, dyed, or gray hair.

These products may cause folliculitis (inflammation of the pores containing the hair follicle). Pustules or pimplelike eruptions may occur.

Drug Interactions

- Coal tar products should not be used at the same time as other photosensitizing drugs, such as tetracyclines, phenolthiazines, thiazides, and sulfanomides.

Usual Dose

Dandruff or Seborrheic Dermatitis

Adult and Child (age 2 and over): Use a lotion shampoo product with a 0.5%–5.0% coal tar concentration. Apply to the scalp, massage in thoroughly, rinse, and repeat the application. Use at least twice a week or as directed by a doctor.

Child (under age 2): Consult a doctor.

Psoriasis

Adult and Child (age 2 and over): Use a product with a 0.5%–5.0% coal tar concentration for mild to moderately severe cases. Apply a thin layer to the affected skin surface. Follow the package directions for frequency of application. For more severe, thicker-scaled outbreaks, a concentration of 5% salicylic acid in combination with 20% juniper tar and 10% sulfur may be more efficient.

Child (under age 2): Consult a doctor.

Overdosage

Do the following in case of accidental ingestion: If the victim is unconscious or having convulsions, call for an ambulance immediately. If you take the victim to an emergency room, be sure to bring the bottle or container with you. If the victim is conscious, call your local poison control center or a health care professional. The poison control center may suggest inducing vomiting with ipecac syrup (available without a prescription at any pharmacy). DO NOT induce vomiting unless specifically instructed to do so.

Special Information

Coal tar and ultraviolet radiation have been used by doctors since 1925 in a procedure called the Goeckerman treatment and induced remissions from psoriasis for up to 12 months. This procedure is complicated and should be performed only by your doctor. You should not attempt to use coal tar preparations and sunlight or sunlamps to mimic this treatment, since serious complications may occur from unsupervised self-treatment.

Special Populations

Pregnancy/Breast-feeding

It is not generally recommended that pregnant women use any drugs, especially during the first 3 months of pregnancy. Check with your doctor if you are or might be pregnant, or if you are breast-feeding.

Infants/Children

Coal tar products should not be used in children under age 2 unless directed by a doctor.

Seniors

People with gray hair should be aware of the possibility that coal tar may discolor their hair.

Generic Name

Cocoa Butter (KOE-koe)

Definition

The fat obtained from the roasted seeds of *Theobroma*

cacao. It is used as a skin protectant and softener, and as a base for suppositories. It is also used in cosmetics, for its emollient (skin-softening/soothing) properties.

Generic Name

Cod Liver Oil

Definition

A pale yellow, fatty oil from the livers of fresh codfish and other related species. High in vitamins A and D, the oil is given to infants as a nutritional supplement to ensure the healthy development of bones and skin. It is also available in capsule form and in a malt extract. Cod liver oil is also used as a skin protectant in hemorrhoid products and diaper rash treatments.

Generic Name

Codeine (KOE-deen)

Brand Names

Codimal PH
*Novahistine
Tricodene No. 1 [A]
*†Tussar

** Not all products in this brand-name group contain codeine.*

† Consult the OTC ingredient charts to determine whether different formulations in this brand-name group are alcohol-, caffeine-, or sugar-free.

Type of Drug

Antitussive (cough suppressant).

Used for

Suppression of a dry, hacking, nonproductive cough.

General Information

Codeine belongs to a class of drugs known as opiate agonists, which stimulate the opiate receptors in the brain to relieve pain and produce a number of other effects on the central nervous system. Among these effects is suppression of the cough reflex. In addition to this suppression, codeine appears to dry up respiratory tract mucous membranes and make bronchial secretions more fluid. Although products containing codeine are available without a prescription in some states, they are considered controlled substances under the Federal Controlled Substances Act.

Codeine is used specifically to suppress nonproductive coughs: dry coughs in which there is no mucus to be expelled. However, some cough syrups may contain both an antitussive such as codeine and an expectorant (which loosens and clears secretions from the respiratory tract) such as guaifenesin. The combination of these ingredients is counterproductive because the action of the antitussive may make it harder for you to cough up the secretions loosened by the expectorant.

In limited studies, neither codeine nor dextromethorphan, another antitussive, has been shown to be more effective than a placebo in controlling coughs associated specifically with the common cold. However, these medications may be useful to suppress dry coughs that interfere with sleep.

Codeine is also used as an analgesic (pain reliever) and has mild sedative effects.

When used as an antitussive, codeine starts to work within 1 to 2 hours and its effects last for up to 4 hours.

Codeine is combined with other ingredients in many cough and cold preparations available by brand name in liquid form.

Cautions and Warnings

Do not exceed the recommended dosage of your codeine preparation.

If you have asthma, pulmonary emphysema, or shortness of breath, do not use codeine unless it is prescribed by your doctor. Unmonitored use may lead to thicker lung secretions and suppressed coughing, to such an extent that breathing becomes difficult.

Long-term use of codeine can lead to tolerance (decreased efficacy) of and physical dependence on the drug.

Codeine's effects on the central nervous system can make you feel sleepy or light-headed. Your ability to perform activities that require your full alertness and coordination, such as driving a motor vehicle or operating machinery, may be affected. Drinking alcohol while you are taking codeine can add to these effects.

If your cough lasts longer than 7 days, is recurrent, or is accompanied by fever, rash, or persistent headache, call your doctor. A persistent cough may be a sign of a more serious condition.

Possible Side Effects

- ▼ Most common: nausea, vomiting, constipation (with repeated doses), light-headedness, and sedation.
- ▼ Less common: itching and allergic reactions.
- ▼ Rare: excessive sweating and agitation.

Drug Interactions

• The sedating effects of codeine are enhanced when it is used with other drugs that depress the central nervous system (cause drowsiness). These drugs include other narcotic analgesics (pain relievers), muscle relaxants, tranquilizers, sedatives and hypnotics, antidepressants, monoamine oxidase inhibitors (MAOIs) (used to treat depression, other psychiatric or emotional conditions, and Parkinson's disease), and antipsychotics. If you are taking any of these other medications, do not use a codeine preparation unless it is prescribed by your doctor.

Food Interactions

None known.

Usual Dose

To minimize the risk of tolerance and physical dependence with codeine, preparations containing this drug should be given in the smallest effective dose and as infrequently as possible.

Adult and Child (age 12 and over): 10–20 mg every 4–6 hours. Do not take more than 120 mg in 24 hours.

Child (age 6–11): 5–10 mg every 4–6 hours. Do not give

more than 60 mg in 24 hours.

Child (age 2–5): Use only as directed by a physician.

Child (under age 2): not recommended unless prescribed by a doctor (see "Special Populations").

If you are buying a preparation with codeine to give to a child age 2–6 years, you should receive a dispensing device, such as a dropper, calibrated for age or weight. Make sure you use this device to measure your child's dose, and be extremely careful to measure the right amount. Do not give more than the recommended daily dosage because serious side effects could occur.

Overdosage

Do the following in case of accidental overdose: If the victim is unconscious or having convulsions, call for an ambulance immediately. If you take the victim to an emergency room, be sure to bring the bottle or container with you. If the victim is conscious, call your local poison control center or a health care professional. The poison control center may suggest inducing vomiting with ipecac syrup (available without a prescription at any pharmacy). DO NOT induce vomiting unless specifically instructed to do so.

Special Populations

Pregnancy/Breast-feeding

If large amounts of codeine are taken for a long time during pregnancy and/or breast-feeding, the baby may become dependent on the drug and may show withdrawal symptoms.

It is not generally recommended that pregnant women take any drugs, particularly during the first 3 months after conception. If you are or might be pregnant, check with your doctor before you take a preparation containing codeine.

Codeine has been shown to pass into breast milk. If you must take codeine, bottle-feed your baby with formula.

Infants/Children

It is especially important not to give any product containing codeine to a child under age 2 unless you are specifically told to do so by your doctor. Children in this age group are more susceptible to codeine's respiratory depressant effects, which include respiratory arrest, coma, and death.

Seniors
Seniors may be more susceptible to codeine's effects and should take reduced doses. Check with your doctor about the appropriate dose.

Generic Name
Cornstarch

Definition

A powdery substance made from corn, used to treat diaper rash because of its ability to absorb moisture. Cornstarch and other powders should not be used on a severe, oozing rash because they may cause secondary crusting and infection. Parents should apply the powder carefully: Avoid sprinkling powder too close to the infant's head, since inhaling the dust can cause chemical pneumonia and breathing problems. Cornstarch is also used as a vehicle (carrier) for antifungal drugs for the treatment of athlete's foot.

Generic Name
Dexbrompheniramine Maleate
(DEKS-brom-fen-EER-ah-meen MAL-ee-ate)

Definition

*see **Brompheniramine Maleate,** page 711*

Generic Name
Dextran **(DEKS-tran)**

Definition

An ingredient in artificial tear products used to enhance the ability of the product to remain on the eye tissue and thus provide moisture.

Generic Name

Dextromethorphan

(DEKS-troe-meth-OR-fan)

Brand Names

*Alka-Seltzer Plus
Anti-Tuss DM
Babee Cof
†Benylin
Cerose-DM
Cheracol
Clear Cough [A] [S]
ClearTussin 30 [A]
Codimal DM [A] [S]
*Comtrex
Contac Severe Cold & Flu Maximum Strength
Coricidin Cough & Cold
Cough-X
Creomulsion [A]
Daygel
Delsym Extended Release [A]
Diabe-tuss DM [A] [S]
*†Diabetic Tussin
Dimacol
*†Dimetapp
Dorcol Children's Cough [A]
Dristan Cold & Cough Liqui-Gels
*Drixoral
GuiaCough CF
Hold
Ipsatol [A]
*†Kolephrin
Kophane Cough Cold Medication [A]
*†Naldecon
NiteGel
Novahistine DMX
*†PediaCare
*†Pediacon
Pertussin
Pinex
Prominicol Cough
†Protac
Quelidrine Cough
REM [A]
*†Robitussin
Safe Tussin 30 [A] [S]
*†Scot-Tussin
Spec-T Sore Throat Cough Suppressant
St. Joseph Cough Suppressant for Children [A]
Sucrets 4-Hour Cough Suppressant
*†Sudafed
Tetrahist
*TheraFlu
Tolu-Sed DM
*†Triaminic
Triaminicol Multi-Sympton Relief [A]
*†Tricodene
Tuss-DM
*†Tussar
*†Tylenol
*†Vicks

**Not all products in this brand-name group contain dextromethorphan.*

†Consult the OTC ingredient charts to determine whether different formulations in this brand-name group are alcohol-, caffeine-, or sugar-free.

Type of Drug

Antitussive (cough suppressant).

Used for

Suppressing a dry, hacking cough.

General Information

Dextromethorphan is a very common antitussive used in OTC cough preparations. Like codeine, dextromethorphan suppresses the cough reflex by acting directly on the cough center in the brain. However, unlike codeine, dextromethorphan does not have pain-relieving effects, does not depress breathing, and has a low potential for addiction.

Antitussives are used to suppress nonproductive coughs (a cough that does not bring up any mucus). Some cough syrups may contain both an antitussive such as dextromethorphan and an expectorant such as guaifenesin. However, the combination of these ingredients is counterproductive, because the action of the antitussive may make it harder for you to cough up the secretions loosened by the expectorant.

In limited studies, neither dextromethorphan nor codeine has been shown to be more effective than a placebo in controlling coughs associated specifically with the common cold. However, these medications may be useful to suppress dry coughs that interfere with sleep. Dextromethorphan and codeine are generally thought to be equally effective.

Cautions and Warnings

If your cough lasts longer than 7 days, is recurrent, or is accompanied by fever, rash, or persistent headache, call your doctor. A persistent cough may be a sign of a serious condition.

Do not exceed the recommended daily dosage of dextromethorphan.

If you experience fever, rash, or persistent headache while taking dextromethorphan, stop taking it immediately and call your doctor.

Dextromethorphan should not be used for persistent or chronic cough, such as that associated with smoking, asthma, chronic bronchitis, or emphesema, or for coughs associated with excessive mucus, unless prescribed by your doctor.

Do not take dextromethorphan if you are confined to bedrest or are under sedation.

Do not use dextromethorphan to treat a productive cough.

Dextromethorphan should be used with caution by individuals with asthma or liver disease.

Possible Side Effects

▼ Rare: nausea or other gastrointestinal (GI) upset, slight drowsiness, and dizziness.

Drug Interactions

• Dextromethorphan should not be used at the same time as a monoamine oxidase inhibitor (MAOI) or within 2 weeks of stopping treatment with an MAOI. MAOIs are used to treat depression, other psychiatric or emotional conditions, and Parkinson's disease. If you are not sure whether you are or have been taking an MAOI, check with your doctor or pharmacist before you use dextromethorphan.

Food Interactions

None known.

Usual Dose

Adult and Child (age 12 and over): 10–20 mg every 4–8 hours, or 30 mg every 8 hours. Do not take more than 120 mg in 24 hours.

Child (age 6–12): 5–10 mg every 4 hours, or 15 mg every 6–8 hours. Do not give more than 60 mg in 24 hours.

Child (age 2–6): 2.5 mg every 4 hours, or 7.5 mg every 8 hours. Do not give more than 30 mg in 24 hours.

Child (under age 2): not recommended unless directed by a doctor.

Dextromethorphan is also available as dextromethorphan polistrex in an extended-release oral suspension. Usual doses are as follows:

Adult and Child (age 12 and over): 60 mg twice daily.

Child (age 6–12): 30 mg twice daily.

Child (age 2–6): 15 mg twice daily.

Child (under age 2): not recommended unless directed by a doctor.

Overdosage

Signs of dextromethorphan overdose include nausea, vomiting, drowsiness, dizziness, blurred vision, rapid rolling of the eyeballs, uncoordinated muscular movements, shallow breathing, urinary retention, stupor, toxic psychosis, and coma.

Even if the victim is not displaying any of the symptoms listed above, do the following in case of accidental overdose: If the victim is unconscious or having convulsions, call for an ambulance immediately. If you take the victim to an emergency room, be sure to bring the bottle or container with you. If the victim is conscious, call your local poison control center or a health care professional. The poison control center may suggest inducing vomiting with ipecac syrup (available without a prescription at any pharmacy). DO NOT induce vomiting unless specifically instructed to do so.

Special Populations

Allergies

Some preparations with dextromethorphan also contain the dye tartrazine, which may cause allergic reactions (including bronchial asthma) in some people. Individuals who are allergic to aspirin are more likely to react to tartrazine.

Phenylketonurics (people who cannot digest phenylalanine) should be aware that some dextromethorphan preparations contain the artificial sweetener aspartame (Nutrasweet), which breaks down in the GI tract to phenylalanine.

Pregnancy/Breast-feeding

It is not generally recommended that pregnant women take any drugs, particularly during the first 3 months after conception. Check with your doctor before taking dextromethorphan if you are or might be pregnant, or if you are breast-feeding.

Infants/Children

Lozenges containing dextromethorphan should not be given to children under age 6.

Dextromethorphan should not be given to children under age 2 unless directed by a doctor.

Seniors

Seniors should exercise the same caution as younger adults when using dextromethorphan.

Generic Name

Dibucaine (DYE-bew-kane)

Brand Name

Nupercainal

Type of Drug

Topical anesthetic.

Used for

Temporary relief of pain and itching from minor cuts and burns, insect bites, hemorrhoids, minor skin irritations, fever blisters, and cold sores.

General Information

Topical anesthetics work by blocking pain signals in the skin and keeping them from traveling along the nerves to the brain.

Dibucaine starts to work within 15 minutes but the duration of relief from pain is short, lasting only 2 to 4 hours. However, since these medications should be applied only 3 or 4 times a day, they will not always provide around-the-clock relief.

Dibucaine belongs to the same drug class as benzocaine.

Dibucaine is available by generic and brand name in cream and ointment form.

Cautions and Warnings

Do not use dibucaine for more than 2 consecutive weeks. If your symptoms persist or worsen within 7 days, stop using the drug and contact your doctor.

Do not exceed the recommended daily dosage of dibucaine. Using the product more often or in higher amounts than recommended increases the risk of developing an allergic reaction or internal side effects.

Topical anesthetics should not be used for serious burns or puncture wounds, which need more appropriate medical attention.

Do not apply dibucaine to large areas of your body or use it near the eyes or nose.

Unless otherwise directed, the hemorrhoid product is for external use only and should not be inserted into the rectum.

Do not apply if you are allergic or have a reaction to other amide topical anesthetics (e.g., benzocaine, lidocaine).

Do not apply to raw or blistered areas.

If pain, bleeding, redness, irritation, rash, or swelling occurs, discontinue use of the product and contact your doctor.

Possible Side Effects

Topical application of anesthetics can cause temporary burning or stinging in sensitive individuals, due to the skin inflammation.

Drug Interactions

None known.

Usual Dose

Pain-relief Product

Adult and Child (age 12 and over): Clean the affected area with mild soap and warm water. Rinse thoroughly. *Gently* dry the area with a soft cloth or tissue; do not rub or irritate the area. Take a liberal amount of the medication on your fingertip, apply it to the affected area, and rub it in thoroughly. Repeat as needed, but do not use more than 1 oz. in 24 hours. When used for treatment of skin pain, the area may be covered with a light dressing.

Hemorrhoid Product

Adult and Child (age 12 and over): Apply up to 3–4 times a day after each bowel movement.

Pain-relief or Hemorrhoid Product

Child (age 2–11): Do not use except with a doctor's recommendation. If the pain relief medication is used, do not apply more than 7.5 g in 24 hours.

Child (under age 2): Do not use.

Overdosage

Do the following in case of accidental ingestion: If the victim is unconscious or having convulsions, call for an ambulance immediately. If you take the victim to an emergency room, be sure to bring the bottle or container with you. If the victim is conscious, call your local poison control center or a health care professional. The poison control center may suggest inducing vomiting with ipecac syrup (available without a prescription at any pharmacy). DO NOT induce vomiting unless specifically instructed to do so.

Special Information

This drug darkens with exposure to light, but this does not affect the efficacy of the product.

Special Populations

Allergies

Dibucaine is not very likely to cause allergic reactions. However, formulations of dibucaine that include sulfites (such as Nupercainal pain relief cream) may cause allergic reactions in sensitive individuals.

Pregnancy/Breast-feeding

It is not generally recommended that pregnant women take any drugs, particularly during the first 3 months after conception. Ask your doctor before using this or any medication.

If you experience dry, sore, or cracked nipple tissues while breast-feeding, do not use an OTC anesthetic except on advice from a physician. There is a chance the infant could accidentally ingest the medication during feeding.

Infants/Children

Children under age 2 should not use OTC topical anesthetics except under a doctor's supervision.

The hemorrhoid medication should not be used in children younger than 12 except on advice from a physician. No more than 7.5 g (1/6 of a 1.5-ounce tube) per day of the pain relief product should be used in treating children.

Children treated with dibucaine should be instructed not to put the affected area in the mouth, to avoid accidental ingestion of the anesthetic.

Seniors
Seniors should exercise the same caution as younger adults when using dibucaine.

Generic Name

Dimenhydrinate (DYE-muhn-HYE-drin-ate)

Brand Names

Calm-X
†Dramamine
Triptone

†*Consult the OTC ingredient charts to determine whether different formulations in this brand-name group are alcohol-, caffeine-, or sugar-free.*

Type of Drug

Antihistamine; antiemetic.

Used for

The prevention and treatment of nausea, vomiting, and dizziness associated with motion sickness.

General Information

Nausea and vomiting (emesis) may be caused by various disorders: some minor, some serious. Various antiemetics are used to treat nausea and vomiting caused by motion sickness; pregnancy; mild infectious disease; radiation therapy; cancer chemotherapy; and metabolic, central nervous system (CNS), gastrointestinal (GI), and endocrine disorders.

Dimenhydrinate is only approved for the prevention and treatment of nausea and vomiting associated with traveling (motion sickness).

Dimenhydrinate is one of a group of drugs called antihistamines. Besides having many other uses, including the relief of allergy symptoms, antihistamines are the primary OTC products used as antiemetics. While it is not known precisely how dimenhydrinate works, certain antihistamines have a depressant effect on overstimulated labyrinth (inner ear) function, which causes motion sickness. Dimenhydrinate is equal in effectiveness to the antihistamine/antiemetic meclizine, but causes drowsiness (a common side effect of antihistamines) more frequently.

Dimenhydrinate is indicated for the prevention as well as the treatment of motion sickness. Motion sickness is much easier to prevent than to treat once it has begun.

Dimenhydrinate begins working within 15 to 30 minutes and continues to work for 3 to 6 hours.

Dimenhydrinate is available by generic name in tablet form and by brand name in tablet, chewable tablet, and children's syrup forms.

Cautions and Warnings

Do not use dimenhydrinate too frequently or for a prolonged period unless directed by a health care professional. A decrease in this product's effectiveness has been noted after prolonged use.

Do not exceed the recommended daily dosage of dimenhydrinate.

Dimenhydrinate, like all antihistamines, may cause extreme drowsiness, which may be exacerbated by the concurrent use of alcoholic beverages, sedatives, hypnotics, or tranquilizers (see "Drug Interactions"). If you are taking dimenhydrinate, use caution when performing activities that require mental alertness or physical coordination, such as driving a motor vehicle or operating machinery.

People with the following conditions should not take dimenhydrinate without first consulting a health care professional: emphysema, chronic bronchitis, or other breathing problems; glaucoma; difficulty urinating because of enlargement of the prostate gland; or obstructive disease of the GI tract. Dimenhydrinate should be used with caution by individuals with seizure disorders.

Nausea and vomiting associated with radiation therapy; cancer chemotherapy; and metabolic, CNS, GI, and endocrine disorders are serious conditions that should not be self-medicated with dimenhydrinate. Consult your doctor. This product should also not be used for treating nausea and vomiting caused by pregnancy (see "Special Populations").

Phenylketonurics (people who cannot digest phenylalanine) should note the inactive ingredients in the chewable dimenhydrinate product. Phenylketonurics should avoid sugar-free chewable products containing aspartame (NutraSweet). Be sure to read the label.

Possible Side Effects

▼ Most common: drowsiness, excitability (characterized by restlessness, insomnia, tremors, nervousness, rapid heartbeat, headache, blurred vision, tinnitus (ringing or buzzing in the ears), dry mouth, lack of coordination, dizziness, and hypotension (abnormally low blood pressure).

▼ Less common: loss of appetite, constipation or diarrhea, and difficult or painful urination.

Drug Interactions

• Antihistamines can enhance the effect of other drugs that depress the CNS, such as barbiturates, tranquilizers, sleeping medications, and alcohol (present in many OTC preparations). If you are taking other depressant drugs, check with your doctor before you take dimenhydrinate. Avoid drinking alcohol if you are taking dimenhydrinate.

• People taking drugs with anticholinergic effects (e.g., tricyclic antidepressants, antihistamines) are more likely to experience side effects such as blurred vision, dry mouth, constipation, or difficulty urinating with concurrent use of dimenhydrinate.

• Dimenhydrinate may mask symptoms of ototoxicity (a condition affecting the organs of hearing and balance). Use with caution if you are taking an ototoxic drug, such as an aminoglycoside antibiotic or high doses of aspirin.

Food Interactions

None known.

Usual Dose

Adult and Child (age 12 and over): 50–100 mg every 4–6 hours. Do not exceed 400 mg in 24 hours.

Child (age 6–11): 25–50 mg every 6–8 hours. Do not exceed 150 mg in 24 hours.

Child (age 2–5): 12.5–25 mg every 6–8 hours. Do not exceed 75 mg in 24 hours.

Child (under age 2): Consult your doctor.

To prevent motion sickness, take dimenhydrinate 1/2–1 hour before departure for travel. Continue to take the product during travel.

Overdosage

Symptoms of antihistamine overdose in children include dilated pupils, flushed face, dry mouth, fever, excitability, hallucinations, loss of muscle coordination, and seizures.

Overdose in adults (individuals taking 500 mg or more of dimenhydrinate) may be characterized by extreme difficulty in speech and swallowing, confusion, and hallucinations. In adults, severe overdose can cause drowsiness or coma, which may be followed by excitability or seizures. Eventually fluid can build up in the brain; the kidneys may fail, and the heart and lungs may stop working, resulting in death. Symptoms may develop within 30 minutes to 2 hours following an overdose of dimenhydrinate, and death may occur within 18 hours.

Even if the victim is not displaying any of the symptoms listed above, do the following in case of accidental overdose: If the victim is unconscious or having convulsions, call for an ambulance immediately. If you take the victim to an emergency room, be sure to bring the bottle or container with you. If the victim is conscious, call your local poison control center or a health care professional. The poison control center may suggest inducing vomiting with ipecac syrup (available without a prescription at any pharmacy). DO NOT induce vomiting unless specifically instructed to do so.

Special Populations

Allergies

Some people are allergic to tartrazine, a dye found in Dramamine chewable tablets. Be sure to read the label if you are taking a generic chewable product, in case it contains tartrazine.

Pregnancy/Breast-feeding

Antihistamines are not recommended for use during pregnancy unless directed by your doctor. Antihistamines are known to pass into the breast milk of nursing mothers and may cause side effects in infants. Check with your doctor before taking dimenhydrinate if you are or might be pregnant, or if you are breast-feeding.

Infants/Children

Because most studies involving antiemetics are conducted with adults, the use of antiemetics in children is controversial. Some clinicians question whether children suffering from a temporary, minor disorder such as motion sickness should be treated with dimenhydrinate.

Children may be more susceptible to the side effects of dimenhydrinate. They are also more susceptible to accidental antihistamine overdose.

Children may become excited rather than drowsy after taking dimenhydrinate (see "Possible Side Effects").

Consult your doctor before giving dimenhydrinate to a child under 2 years of age. In young children, one alternative to drug therapy in treating motion sickness caused by automobile travel is to place the child in a car seat positioned so that he or she can see out the front window.

Seniors

Older persons may be more sensitive to the side effects of dimenhydrinate and may experience nervousness, irritability, and restlessness. Dizziness, sedation, and low blood pressure may also occur. Most mild reactions may be handled by either lowering your dose or trying another antihistamine.

Generic Name

Dimethicone (dye-METH-ih-kone)

Definition

An ingredient in skin care products that helps prevent dry skin. It is also used as a skin protectant ingredient in diaper rash products.

Generic Name

Diphenhydramine

(DYE-fen-HYE-druh-meen)

Brand Names

Aller-med
Anacin P.M. Asprin Free
Arthriten PM
Arthritis Foundation Nightime
Backaid PM Pills
Bayer PM Extra Strength
Benadryl Itch Stopping Extra Strength
Cala-gel Clearly Calamine
Compoz
Contac Day & Night Allergy/Sinus
Dermamycin
Dermapax
Dermarest Plus
Di-Delamine
Diphenadryl
Diphenylin
Doan's P.M. Extra Strength
Dormarex
Dormin
Excedrin PM
Excedrin PM LiquiGels
Genahist
HC-DermaPax
Hydramine Cough
Hydrosal
Ivarest
Legatrin PM
Midol PM Night Time Formula
Nauzene [S]
Nervine Nighttime Sleep-Aid
Nytol
Sleep-eze 3
Sleepinal
Snooze Fast
Sominex Maximum Strength
Sominex Original
Tranquil
Twilite
Tylenol PM Extra Strength
Unisom Pain Relief

Type of Drug

Antihistamine, also used as an antitussive (cough suppressant), sleep aid, and antiemetic (motion sickness aid).

Used for

Temporary relief of runny nose, sneezing, itchy eyes, scratchy throat, and other symptoms (skin rash, itching, or hives) associated with cold and allergy; temporary relief of cough caused by minor throat and bronchial irritation; short-term management of insomnia; and prevention and treatment of motion sickness.

General Information

Histamine is one of the substances released by the body tissues during an allergic reaction. When it is released, the body reacts with a variety of symptoms, including itching and sneezing. Antihistamines work by competitively inhibiting the pharmacological action of histamine, which makes them very effective for relieving the symptoms of allergic reactions. Antihistamines may also help relieve a runny nose. However, because antihistamines do not work against the other substances released by the body during an allergic reaction, they can reduce only about 40% to 60% of allergic symptoms. They are also not effective in clearing up a stuffy nose.

If you have seasonal allergies, antihistamines work best if you take them before your allergy season begins. Those who suffer from allergies regardless of the season may need to take antihistamines all year.

Antihistamines will not cure or prevent allergies, viral infections (colds), or bacterial infections. The best you can hope for is symptomatic relief.

Diphenhydramine is classified as an ethanolamine antihistamine. Others in this group include doxylamine and phenyltoloxamine. Of the antihistamines available without a prescription, these are the most likely to make you sleepy. Newer antihistamines do not have the common antihistamine side effect of drowsiness, but for now they are available only by prescription.

Besides relieving allergy and cold symptoms, diphenhydramine has a number of other indications. Diphenhydramine's sleep-inducing effects are used in OTC sleep aids. Creams, lotions, and solutions containing diphenhydramine are used to temporarily relieve itching. Diphenhydramine is also used to prevent and treat nausea, vomiting, and dizziness associated with motion sickness.

In combination products, diphenhydramine may be used in the related forms bromodiphenhydramine or diphenhydramine citrate.

Diphenhydramine is available by generic and brand name in tablet, caplet, softgel, liquid, powder, gel, cream, and ointment form, both alone and in combination products.

Cautions and Warnings

If you are taking diphenhydramine for cough and the cough lasts longer than 7 days, is recurrent, or is accompanied by fever, rash, or persistent headache, call your doctor. A persistent cough may be a sign of a serious condition.

If you are using topical diphenhydramine for a skin condition that worsens or lasts longer than 7 days, or your symptoms go away but come back within a few days, stop using the topical preparation and call your doctor.

If you are taking diphenhydramine as a sleep aid, call your doctor if your insomnia lasts longer than 2 weeks. Insomnia may be a sign of a serious underlying physical, emotional, or psychological condition that needs medical attention.

Do not exceed the recommended daily dosage of a diphenhydramine product.

Unless prescribed by a doctor, diphenhydramine and other antihistamines should not be used by people who have a breathing problem such as emphysema or chronic bronchitis or by individuals with asthma.

Diphenhydramine should be used with caution by people with glaucoma, hyperthyroidism, heart disease, high blood pressure, or enlargement of the prostate gland. If you have any of these conditions, consult your doctor before taking diphenhydramine.

Even if you are not taking diphenhydramine specifically to help you sleep, its effects on the central nervous system (CNS) can make you feel sleepy or reduce your concentration. Your ability to perform activities that require your full alertness and coordination, such as driving a motor vehicle or operating machinery, may be affected. Drinking alcohol or taking other sedative drugs while you are taking diphenhydramine can add to these effects.

Phenylketonurics (people who cannot digest the amino acid phenylalanine) should be aware that some formulations of diphenhydramine contain aspartame (Nutrasweet), which breaks down in the gastrointestinal tract to phenylalanine after the drug is taken.

Some formulations of diphenhydramine may contain sodium bisulfite, which may cause allergic-type reactions, in some people, including anaphylaxis and life-threatening or less severe asthmatic episodes. Individuals with asthma are more likely to be sensitive to sodium bisulfite.

Topical diphenhydramine solutions that contain high concentrations of ethanol (alcohol) are flammable and should not be exposed to an open flame, lighted cigarettes, or other ignited materials.

One study of diphenhydramine's effects on different ethnic groups has indicated that Asians may need as much as 1.7 times the amount of diphenhydramine as Caucasians to experience the same level of sedation. If diphenhydramine is used as a sleep aid by Asians, a larger nightly dose may be needed if there is no response to smaller doses.

Possible Side Effects

▼ Most common: restlessness, nervousness, sleeplessness or drowsiness, sedation, excitability, dizziness, poor coordination, and upset stomach.

▼ Less common: dry eyes, nose, and mouth, blurred vision, difficulty urinating, irritability (at high doses), increased or irregular heat rate; and heart palpitations.

Drug Interactions

• Diphenhydramine's effects can combine with those of other CNS depressants, including barbiturates, tranquilizers, sleeping medications and alcohol (present in many OTC preparations.). If you are taking other depressant drugs, check with your doctor before you take diphenhydramine or any other antihistamine. Avoid drinking alcohol if you are taking diphenhydramine or any other antihistamine.

• Diphenhydramine should not be used at the same time as a monoamine oxidase inhibitor (MAOI) or within 2 weeks of stopping treatment with an MAOI. MAOIs are used to treat depression, other psychiatric or emotional conditions, and Parkinson's disease. If you are not sure whether you are or have been taking an MAOI, check with your doctor or pharmacist before you use diphenhydramine or any other antihistamine.

• Antihistamines can affect the results of skin and blood tests. Notify your health care professional before scheduling these tests if you are taking diphenhydramine.

Food Interactions

None known.

Usual Dose

Because histamine is released nearly continuously, it is best to take antihistamines on a schedule rather than as needed.

Cold and Allergy or Motion Sickness

Adult and Child (age 12 and over): 25–50 mg every 4–6 hours. Do not take more than 300 mg in 24 hours.

Child (age 6–11): 12.5–25 mg every 4–6 hours. Do not give more than 150 mg in 24 hours.

Cough

Adult and Child (age 12 and over): 25 mg (or 38 mg of diphenhydramine citrate) every 4 hours. Do not take more than 150 mg (228 mg of diphenhydramine citrate) in 24 hours.

Child (age 6–11): 12.5 mg (19 mg of diphenhydramine citrate) every 4 hours. Do not give more than 75 mg (114 mg of diphenhydramine citrate) in 24 hours.

Sleep Aid

Adult and Child (age 12 and over): 50 mg (76 mg of diphenhydramine citrate), as needed.

Child (age 6–11): not recommended unless directed by your physician.

Itching

Adult and Child (age 6 and over): Apply creams, lotions, or solutions containing 1%–2% diphenhydramine 3–4 times daily.

Child (under age 6): not recommended unless directed by your doctor.

You may minimize the inconvenience of the sedative effects of diphenhydramine by either taking a full dose at bedtime or using the smallest recommended doses, combined with a decongestant, during the day. Another alternative is to start with the lowest dose when you begin taking the drug and gradually increase the dosage as needed over several days.

If you forget to take a dose of diphenhydramine, do so as soon as you remember. If it is almost time for your next dose, skip the one you forgot and continue with your regular schedule. Do not take a double dose.

Overdosage

Symptoms of antihistamine overdose in children include dilated pupils, flushed face, dry mouth, fever, excitability, hallucinations, loss of muscle coordination, and seizures.

In adults, severe overdose can cause drowsiness or coma, which may be followed by excitability or seizures. Eventually fluid can build up in the brain; the kidneys may fail, and the heart and lungs may stop working, resulting in death. Symptoms may develop within 30 minutes to 2 hours following an overdose, and death may occur within 18 hours.

Even if the victim is not displaying any of the symptoms listed above, do the following in case of accidental ingestion or overdose: If the victim is unconscious or having convulsions, call for an ambulance immediately. If you take the victim to an emergency room, be sure to bring the bottle or container with you. If the victim is conscious, call your local poison control center or a health care professional. The poison control center may suggest inducing vomiting with ipecac syrup (available without a prescription at any pharmacy). DO NOT induce vomiting unless specifically instructed to do so.

Special Populations

Pregnancy/Breast-feeding

Antihistamines are not recommended during pregnancy unless directed by your doctor. Antihistamines are known to pass into the breast milk of nursing mothers and may cause side effects in infants. Check with your doctor before taking diphenhydramine if you are or might be pregnant, or if you are breast-feeding.

Infants/Children

Children may be more susceptible to the side effects of diphenhydramine. They are also more susceptible to accidental antihistamine overdose. Diphenhydramine used for cold, cough, allergy, motion sickness, and for itching should not be given to a child under 6 unless directed by your doctor. Diphenhydramine used as a sleep aid should not be given to a child under 12.

Seniors

Seniors may be more sensitive to the side effects of diphenhydramine and other antihistamines and may experience nervousness, irritability, and restlessness. Dizziness, sedation, and low blood pressure may also occur. Most mild reactions may be handled by either lowering the dose or trying another antihistamine. However, persons over age 80 and those with acute physical disorders or dementia may be at risk of developing delirium from even small doses of diphenhydramine. Older men may experience difficulty urinating.

Generic Name
Docusate (DOK-yew-sate)

Brand Names

Colace
Correctol Extra Gentle
Dialose
Dialose Plus
Dioctolose
Docu-K Plus
Doxidan
Dulcolax
Ex-Lax Extra Gentle
Femixal
Gentlax S
Kasof
Modane Plus
Modane Soft
Peri-Colace
Phillip's
Pro-Cal-Sof
Pro-Sof
Pro-Sof-Plus
Regulace
Regulax
Senokot-S
Sof-Lax
Surfak
Therevac [A]
Unilax [S]

Type of Drug

Laxative.

Used for

Relief of occasional constipation (irregularity) and prevention of constipation.

General Information

The average, healthy individual defecates anywhere from 3 times a day to 3 times a week. Constipation is determined not necessarily by the frequency of bowel movements, but by the consistency of the stool, how difficult it is to eliminate, and symptoms such as dull headache, low back pain, and abdominal distention (swelling). Evaluate your condition carefully and discuss your symptoms and their possible causes with your pharmacist before taking a laxative. Laxatives are not always necessary, and when used improperly can either prevent the desired effect or result in laxative dependency. If you are indeed constipated, it may be best managed through proper diet, adequate fluid intake (6 to 8 glasses of water daily), and exercise. If you must use a laxative, choose the mildest effective product.

Laxatives may be classified by their mechanism of action: bulk-forming, emollient (stool softeners), lubricant, saline, hyperosmotic, and stimulant. Docusate is an emollient laxative, or stool softener. Stool softeners, as the name implies, work by drawing water into fecal material, thus softening it and easing defecation. They do not stimulate bowel movements. There are 3 different docusate salts; docusate calcium, docusate potassium, and docusate sodium.

Docusate laxatives are recommended for people who have hard, dry stools, or for people who should avoid straining during defecation (e.g., people with hernias). While mineral oil is recommended for the same purpose, docusate laxatives are regarded as the safer and more effective choice.

Docusate laxatives, taken orally, generally produce softening of the feces within 1 to 3 days.

Docusate is available by brand name in capsule form. This medication is also commonly used in combination form with a stimulant laxative, casanthranol; this combination is available by both generic and brand name.

Cautions and Warnings

Do not use docusate for more than 7 days, unless directed by your doctor. Long-term use of laxatives has been linked with laxative dependence, chronic constipation, and loss of normal bowel function. Using laxatives too frequently can result in persistent diarrhea, hypokalemia (abnormally low potassium in blood), loss of essential nutrients, and dehydration.

Do not exceed the maximum daily dosage of docusate. The higher the dose, the more likely you are to experience adverse effects.

Do not take docusate if you have abdominal pain, nausea, vomiting, or kidney disease, unless directed by your doctor.

If you notice a marked change in bowel habits lasting for more than 2 weeks, do not take docusate until you have spoken to your doctor. Also contact your doctor if there is blood in your stool, so that colon cancer or other significant disease can be ruled out before you begin self-medication with docusate.

If you have had a disease or surgery affecting the gastrointestinal tract, using a laxative may affect your condition adversely.

If you have rectal bleeding after using docusate, or if you do not have a bowel movement after 7 days of using this medication, you may have a serious condition. Stop using the product and call your doctor.

Docusate laxatives may enhance the absorption of many orally administered drugs (see "Drug Interactions").

Possible Side Effects

▼ Rare: mild, temporary stomach cramps; and rash.

Drug Interactions

• In theory, docusate laxatives may enhance the absorption of many orally administered drugs. Consult your doctor or pharmacist before taking docusate if you are currently taking any other medication, including OTC products.

• Docusate should not be taken at the same time as oral mineral oil.

• Taking docusate with aspirin has reportedly caused greater intestinal mucosal damage than taking aspirin alone.

• Some clinicians recommend that docusate laxatives not be taken at the same time as oral drugs having low therapeutic indices (i.e., drugs for which the median lethal dose is very close to the median effective dose). Docusate laxatives may increase the toxicity of these drugs.

Food Interactions

None known.

Usual Dose

Adult and Child (age 12 and over): 100–300 mg daily.

Child (age 6–11): 100 mg at bedtime.

Child (under age 6): not recommended unless directed by a doctor.

Doses should be adjusted to individual usage, but should be taken in doses only large enough to produce softening of the stool. Do not exceed the maximum daily dosage.

Docusate may be taken in divided doses, but 1 dose taken at bedtime is usually sufficient.

Be sure to drink lots of fluids when taking docusate, to facilitate the softening of your stool.

Overdosage

Do the following in case of accidental overdose: If the victim is unconscious or having convulsions, call for an ambulance immediately. If you take the victim to an emergency room, be sure to bring the bottle or container with you. If the victim is conscious, call your local poison control center or a health care professional. The poison control center may suggest inducing vomiting with ipecac syrup (available without a prescription at any pharmacy). DO NOT induce vomiting unless specifically instructed to do so.

Special Populations

Pregnancy/Breast-feeding

It is not generally recommended that pregnant women take any drugs, particularly during the first three months after conception. However, bulk-forming laxatives and stool softeners such as docusate potassium are the only laxatives recommended for use by pregnant women.

Check with your doctor before taking docusate potassium if you are or might be pregnant, or if you are breast-feeding. Also consider talking to your doctor about diet and mild exercise in the management of constipation.

Infants/Children

Observe your child carefully for patterns of bowel movements and the pain or difficulty with which the bowel movements are made before deciding whether the child is actually constipated. As with adults, "normal" bowel habits vary in children. If your child is indeed constipated, increasing fluid intake and adding fiber to his or her diet may help to manage the condition. In general, the use of laxatives should be avoided in children.

Docusate laxatives are recommended for children with constipation associated with hard, dry stools, but consult your physician before giving this product to a child under 6 years of age.

Seniors

Seniors commonly experience constipation, and consequently may become laxative-dependent. Be cautious of chronically turning to laxatives to ease constipation, and instead look to diet and increased fluid intake as therapeutic measures.

There are no restrictions regarding use of stool softeners by older people, although you should exercise caution if you are currently taking other oral medications (see "Drug Interactions"). Bulk-forming laxatives are usually preferred for seniors.

Generic Name

Doxylamine Succinate

(doks-ILL-uh-meen SUK-sih-nate)

Brand Names

Alka-Seltzer Plus Night-Time Cold Medicine Liqui-Gels
Clear Cough Night Time
NiteGel
Nytol Maximum Strength
Robitussin Night-Time Cold Formula
Unisom Nighttime Sleep Aid
†*Vicks NyQuil

**Not all products in this brand-name group contain doxylamine succinate.*

†Consult the OTC ingredient charts to determine whether different formulations in this brand-name group are alcohol-, caffeine-, or sugar-free.

Type of Drug

Antihistamine and sleep aid.

Used for

Temporary relief of runny nose, sneezing, itchy eyes, scratchy throat, and other symptoms associated with cold and allergy; short-term management of insomnia.

General Information

Histamine is one of the substances released by the body tissues during an allergic reaction. When it is released, the body reacts with a variety of symptoms, including itching and sneezing. Antihistamines work by competitively inhibiting the pharmocological action of histamines, which makes them very effective for relieving the symptoms of allergic reactions. Antihistamines may also help relieve a runny nose. However, because antihistamines do not work against the other substances released by the body during an allergic reaction, they can reduce only about 40% to 60% of allergic symptoms. They are also not effective in clearing up a stuffy nose.

If you have seasonal allergies, antihistamines work best if you take them before your allergy season begins. Those who suffer from allergies regardless of the season may need to take antihistamines all year.

Antihistamines will not cure or prevent allergies, viral infections (colds), or bacterial infections. The best you can hope for is symptomatic relief.

Doxylamine succinate is classified as an ethanolamine antihistamine. Others in this group include diphenhydramine and phenyltoloxamine. Of the antihistamines available without a prescription, these are the most likely to make you sleepy. Newer antihistamines such as astemizole, cetirizine, and loratadine do not have the common antihistamine side effect of drowsiness, but for now they are available only by prescription.

Doxylamine is often combined with decongestants, antitussives (cough suppressants), and expectorants in combination products intended to treat cough and cold symptoms.

Like diphenhydramine, doxylamine is also used as an OTC sleep aid; however, doxylamine has *not* been proven to be safe and effective when used in this way. The FDA has nevertheless permitted doxylamine to remain on the market for this indication.

Doxylamine is available by generic and brand name in tablet, caplet, softgel, liqui-cap, and liquid forms, both alone and in combination products.

Cautions and Warnings

If you are taking doxylamine as a sleep aid, call your doctor if your insomnia lasts longer than 2 weeks. Insomnia may be a sign of a serious underlying physical, emotional, or psychological condition that needs medical attention.

Do not exceed the recommended daily dosage of doxylamine.

Unless prescribed by a doctor, doxylamine and other antihistamines should not be used by people who have a breathing problem such as emphysema or chronic bronchitis or by individuals with asthma.

Doxylamine should be used with caution by people with glaucoma, hyperthyroidism, heart disease, high blood pressure, or enlargement of the prostate gland. If you have any of these conditions, consult your doctor before taking doxylamine.

Even if you are not taking doxylamine specifically to help you sleep, its effects on the central nervous system (CNS) can make you feel sleepy or reduce your concentration. Your ability to perform activities that require your full alertness and coordination, such as driving a motor vehicle or operating machinery, may be affected. Drinking alcohol while you are taking doxylamine can add to these effects.

Possible Side Effects

- ▼ Most common: restlessness, nervousness, sleeplessness or drowsiness, sedation, excitability, dizziness, poor coordination, and upset stomach.
- ▼ Less common: blurred vision; difficulty urinating; irritability (at high doses); dry eyes, nose, and mouth; increased or irregular heart rate; and heart palpitations.

Drug Interactions

• Doxylamine's effects can combine with those of other CNS depressants, including barbiturates, tranquilizers, sleeping medications, and alcohol (present in many OTC preparations). If you are taking other depressant drugs, check with your doctor before you take doxylamine or any other antihistamine. Avoid drinking alcohol if you are taking doxylamine or any other antihistamine.

• Doxylamine should not be used at the same time as a monoamine oxidase inhibitor (MAOI) or within 2 weeks of stopping treatment with an MAOI. MAOIs are used to treat depression, other psychiatric or emotional conditions, and Parkinson's disease. If you are not sure whether you are or have been taking an MAOI, check with your doctor or pharmacist before you use doxylamine or any other antihistamine.

• Antihistamines can affect the results of skin and blood tests. Notify your health care professional before scheduling these tests if you are taking doxylamine.

Food Interactions

None known.

Usual Dose

If you are taking doxylamine for allergies, it is best to take it on a schedule rather than as needed, because histamine is released nearly continuously.

Cold and Allergy Relief

Adult and Child (age 12 and over): 7.5–12.5 mg every 4–6 hours. Do not take more than 75 mg in 24 hours.

Child (age 6–12): 3.75–6.25 mg every 4–6 hours. Do not give more than 37.5 mg in 24 hours.

Child (under age 6): not recommended unless directed by your doctor.

Sleep Aid

Adult and Child (age 12 and over): 25 mg taken 30 minutes before going to bed.

Child (under age 12): not recommended.

If you forget to take a dose of doxylamine, do so as soon as you remember. If it is almost time for your next dose, skip the one you forgot and continue with your regular schedule. Do not take a double dose.

Overdosage

Symptoms of antihistamine overdose in children include dilated pupils, flushed face, dry mouth, fever, excitation, hallucinations, loss of muscle coordination, and seizures.

In adults, overdose can cause drowsiness or coma, which may be followed by excitability or seizures. Eventually fluid can build up in the brain; the kidneys may fail, and the heart and lungs may stop working, resulting in death. Symptoms may develop within 30 minutes to 2 hours following an overdose, and death may occur within 18 hours.

Even if the victim is not displaying any of the symptoms listed above, do the following in case of accidental overdose: If the victim is unconscious or having convulsions, call for an ambulance immediately. If you take the victim to an emergency room, be sure to bring the bottle or container with you. If the victim is conscious, call your local poison control center or a health care professional. The poison control center may suggest inducing vomiting with ipecac syrup (available without a prescription at any pharmacy). DO NOT induce vomiting unless specifically instructed to do so.

Special Populations

Pregnancy/Breast-feeding

Doxylamine was formerly marketed (in combination with other drugs) to relieve nausea and vomiting associated with pregnancy, but was voluntarily taken off the market by the manufacturer because it was alleged to have harmful effects on the developing fetus.

Antihistamines are not recommended during pregnancy unless directed by your doctor. Antihistamines are known to pass into the breast milk of nursing mothers and may cause side effects in infants. Check with your doctor before taking doxylamine if you are or might be pregnant, or if you are breast-feeding.

Infants/Children

Children may be more susceptible to the side effects of doxylamine. They are also more susceptible to accidental antihistamine overdose. Doxylamine used for cold and allergy relief should not be given to a child under 6 unless directed by your doctor. Doxylamine used as a sleep aid should not be given to a child under 12.

Seniors

Seniors may be more sensitive to the side effects of doxylamine and other antihistamines and may experience nervousness, irritability, and restlessness. Dizziness, sedation, and low blood pressure may also occur. Most mild reactions may be handled by either lowering the dose or trying another antihistamine. Older men may experience difficulty in urinating.

Generic Name

Dyclonine Hydrochloride

(DYE-kloe-neen HYE-droe-KLOR-ide)

Brand Names

*Orajel Cover Med, Tinted
*Sucrets
Tanac Medicated

* *Not all products in this brand-name group contain dyclonine HCl.*

Type of Drug

Local anesthetic.

Used for

Relief of sore-throat pain; pain associated with various dental conditions (e.g., toothache, sore gums, denture irritation, teething); and pain and itching from minor burns, sunburns, minor cuts or scrapes, insect bites, minor skin irritations, and hemorrhoids.

General Information

When applied to the skin or taken in a tablet or lozenge, dyclonine temporarily relieves pain by blocking the pain impulses to that area. Dyclonine also relieves itching at the same time that it reduces pain, since the sensation of itching is produced by the same nerve fibers that carry pain impulses. The drug is available by brand name in a variety of forms (aerosols, lozenges, gels) depending on the condition it is intended to be used for. In an aerosol spray form, dyclonine starts to work within 2 to 10 minutes after you take it and its effects last for about 30 minutes.

Cautions and Warnings

You should not use dyclonine for longer than 2 days. If you do not feel better by that time, stop using it and consult your pharmacist or call your doctor.

Do not exceed the recommended daily dosage of dyclonine.

You should also stop using dyclonine and consult a doctor if the pain and irritation persists or worsens, if a rash develops, or if your symptoms clear up but reoccur within a few days.

Dyclonine lozenges or spray aerosols for sore-throat pain should be used only at intervals between eating or drinking. The drug numbs your throat and can make it hard to swallow, increasing the risk of choking.

Topical dyclonine is for external use only. Avoid getting it in your eyes.

Possible Side Effects

▼ Rare: skin bumps, itching, and swelling.

Drug Interactions

None known.

Food Interactions

None known.

Usual Dose

Oral Preparations

Adult and Child (age 12 and over): Slowly dissolve 1 lozenge in the mouth. An additional lozenge can be taken every 2 hours if necessary.

Child (under age 12): not recommended unless prescribed by a doctor.

Topical Preparations—Spray

Adult and Child (age 3 and over): Apply 0.1% solution 3–4 times a day, as needed.

Child (under age 3): not recommended unless prescribed by a doctor.

Topical Preparations—Gel

Adult and Child (age 2 and over): Apply 1% gel to the affected area up to 3–4 times daily.

Child (under age 2): not recommended unless prescribed by a doctor.

Overdosage

If high doses of dyclonine are taken, or if the drug is quickly absorbed, adverse central nervous system effects that can occur include excitability and/or depression, nervousness, dizziness, blurred vision, and tremors, followed by seizures, unconsciousness, drowsiness, or stopped breathing; effects on the cardiovascular system include depression of heart muscle, low blood pressure, slowed heartbeat, and stopped heartbeat.

Even if the victim is not displaying any of the symptoms listed above, do the following in case of accidental ingestion or overdose: If the victim is unconscious or having convulsions, call for an ambulance immediately. If you take the victim to an emergency room, be sure to bring the bottle or container with you. If the victim is conscious, call your local poison control center or a health care professional. The poison control center may suggest inducing vomiting with ipecac syrup (available without a prescription at any pharmacy). DO NOT induce vomiting unless specifically instructed to do so.

Special Populations

Pregnancy/Breast-feeding

It is not generally recommended that pregnant women take any drugs, especially during the first 3 months after conception.

If you are or might be pregnant, or you are breast-feeding, check with your doctor or other health care professional before using dyclonine.

Infants/Children

Oral preparations of dyclonine should not be used by children under age 12. The spray and gel formulations of dyclonine should not be used by children under age 3 and age 2, respectively.

Seniors

Seniors should exercise the same caution as younger adults when using these products.

Generic Name

8-Hydroxyquinoline

(hye-DROKS-ee-KWIN-oe-leen)

Brand Names

Ammens Medicated Original Fragrance
Burntame
*Lagol
New Skin Liquid Bandage
Vaginex Medicated

** Not all products in this brand-name group contain 8-Hydroxyquinoline.*

Type of Drug

Topical anti-infective.

Used for

Prevention of infection in minor scrapes, cuts, and burns; relief of symptoms of minor vaginal itching and irritation; and treatment of fungal skin infections.

General Information

8-Hydroxyquinoline is a germicide effective against both bacteria and fungi. It has many different uses, according to formulation.

Lagol, which is available in oil form, is marketed as antifungal medication. However, 8-Hydroxyquinoline is not one of the 7 OTC antifungal drug products regarded as safe and effective by the FDA.

New Skin Liquid Bandage, available as a liquid or spray, is applied to broken skin, where it quickly dries, forming a thin adhesive layer that protects the affected skin from bacteria.

Vaginex Medicated powder, which consists of 8-Hydroxyquinoline plus 8-Hydroxyquinoline sulfate, relieves vaginal itching and irritation.

8-Hydroxyquinoline is also combined with the anesthetic benzocaine in Burntame spray, used to treat minor burns and sunburns.

In the past, 8-Hydroxyquinoline has been used to treat athlete's foot. However, it is no longer regarded as safe and effective for this purpose.

Cautions and Warnings

Do not exceed the recommended daily dosage of 8-hydroxyquinolone.

These products are for external use only. Avoid contact with your eyes.

8-Hydroxyquinoline and 8-Hydroxyquinoline sulfate are combined with the protectant zinc oxide in Ammens Medicated powder, used to treat complicated diaper rash. However, the FDA does not regard any OTC topical antimicrobial product as safe and effective for the treatment and/or prevention of diaper rash. The agency maintains that diaper rash associated with bacterial infection must be diagnosed and treated by a physician, and not self-medicated.

Lagol

If you do not see substantial improvement of your fungal skin infection in 7 days, call your doctor. Recurring skin infections may be a sign of an underlying serious disease, such as diabetes or an immunodeficiency.

New Skin Liquid Bandage

In case of deep cuts, puncture wounds, or serious burns, consult your physician.

If redness, irritation, swelling, or pain persists or increases, or if infection occurs, stop using this product and call your doctor.

Avoid contact with floors, countertops, and other finished surfaces.

New Skin spray is flammable. Do not use or store it near heat or open flame, incinerate it, or puncture the container.

Possible Side Effects

None known.

Drug Interactions

None known.

Usual Dose

Use these products as needed.

New Skin

Clean and dry the broken skin area before applying New Skin. Spray the affected area from 6" away until the area is lightly coated, then let it dry. For added protection, apply a second coating. Keep knees, elbows, or knuckles bent when applying and while drying.

To remove New Skin, spray the area with a fresh coat and rub off quickly with a disposable wipe.

Overdosage

Do the following in case of accidental ingestion: If the victim is unconscious or having convulsions, call for an ambulance immediately. If you take the victim to an emergency room, be sure to bring the bottle or container with you. If the victim is conscious, call your local poison control center or a health care professional. The poison control center may suggest inducing vomiting with ipecac syrup (available without a prescription at any pharmacy). DO NOT induce vomiting unless specifically instructed to do so.

Storage Instructions

Exposing New Skin spray to temperatures above 120°F may cause it to burst. New skin is flammable and must be stored away from heat and open flame.

Special Populations

Pregnancy/Breast-feeding

It is not generally recommended that pregnant women take any drugs, particularly during the first 3 months after conception. Check with your doctor if you are or might be pregnant, or if you are breast-feeding.

Infants/Children

When treating children with 8-Hydroxquinoline, extra care should be taken to prevent accidental ingestion.

Seniors

Seniors should exercise the same caution as younger adults when using these products.

Generic Name

Ephedrine (eh-FED-rin)

Brand Names

Bronkaid
Dynafed Two-Way
Mini Thin Two-Way
Pretz-D
Primatene
Quelidrine Cough
Tedrigen

Type of Drug

Bronchodilator.

Used for

Treatment of mild forms of seasonal or chronic asthma.

General Information

During an asthma attack, the muscles in the bronchial tubes in the lungs contract spasmodically and make it difficult to breathe air into the lungs. Bronchodilator drugs such as ephedrine relax the bronchial muscles and expand their air passages, thus easing breathing.

Ephedrine has been used to illegally produce methamphetamine and methcathione, which are potent central nervous system (CNS) stimulators with the potential for abuse and dependence. By itself, ephedrine has been abused for its stimulant effects, often by adolescents and young adults. For these reasons, since November 1994 ephedrine has been regulated by the Chemical Diversion and Trafficking Act. Purchase of an ephedrine product now requires the buyer's signature and 2 forms of identification. The FDA is considering whether it should accept several recommendations that ephedrine no longer be available for sale without a prescription.

Ephedrine is combined with various ingredients in many OTC brand-name formulations used to treat respiratory symptoms. It is available generically in capsule form.

Cautions and Warnings

If your symptoms are not relieved within 1 hour of taking ephedrine, or become worse, stop using the drug and call your doctor immediately.

Do not exceed the recommended daily dosage of ephedrine.

You should use ephedrine only if you have been diagnosed with asthma by a doctor, you have never been hospitalized for asthma, and you are not taking any other asthma medications (unless prescribed by your doctor).

Discontinue ephedrine use if you experience persistent or worsening nervousness, tremors, sleeplessness, nausea, or loss of appetite.

Persons with heart disease, high blood pressure, thyroid disease, angle-closure glaucoma, diabetes, or difficulty urinating because of an enlarged prostate should take ephedrine only under the supervision of a doctor.

If you are taking a prescription drug for hypertension (high blood pressure) or are taking an antidepressant, check with your doctor before taking ephedrine (see "Drug Interactions").

Possible Side Effects

▼ Most common: CNS stimulation, nervousness, anxiety, apprehension, fear, tension, agitation, excitability, restlessness, weakness, irritability, talkativeness, insomnia, nausea, loss of appetite, tremors, rapid heartbeat, and difficulty urinating.

Drug Interactions

• Ephedrine should not be used at the same time as a monoamine oxidase inhibitor (MAOI) or within 2 weeks of stopping treatment with an MAOI. MAOIs are used to treat depression, other psychiatric or emotional conditions, and Parkinson's disease. If you are not sure whether you are or have been taking an MAOI, check with your doctor or pharmacist before you use ephedrine.

• Blood pressure may increase if ephedrine is taken with clonidine, used to treat high blood pressure; procarbazine, used to treat Hodgkin's disease; furazolidone, an anti-infective; or selegiline, used to treat Parkinson's disease.

• Ephedrine may increase the effect of ergotamine (used to treat migraines) on the heart and blood vessels and decrease the blood-pressure-lowering ability of guanethidine (an antihypertensive).

• Ephedrine's effects may be weakened if the drug is taken with methyldopa or reserpine, both antihypertensives. Tricyclic antidepressants may also have this effect on ephedrine.

• Concentrations of ephedrine may be increased if it is taken with acetazolamide or dichlorphenamide, both used to treat glaucoma, or sodium bicarbonate, an antacid—when it is taken in a large dose.

Food Interactions

None known.

Usual Dose

Adult and Child (age 12 and over): 12.5–25 mg every 4 hours. Do not take more than 150 mg in 24 hours.

Child (under age 12): Consult a doctor.

Overdosage

Do the following in case of accidental overdose: If the victim is unconscious or having convulsions, call for an ambulance immediately. If you take the victim to an emergency room, be sure to bring the bottle or container with you. If the victim is conscious, call your local poison control center or a health care professional. The poison control center may suggest inducing vomiting with ipecac syrup (available without a prescription at any pharmacy). DO NOT induce vomiting unless specifically instructed to do so.

Special Populations

Pregnancy/Breast-feeding

It is not generally recommended that pregnant women take any drugs, particularly during the first 3 months after conception. While it is unknown whether ephedrine can cause harm to the fetus if taken during pregnancy, this drug should be taken by pregnant women only if prescribed by a doctor.

Although no specific studies have been done, it is presumed that ephedrine passes into breast-milk. If you must take ephedrine, bottle-feed your baby with formula.

Infants/Children

Do not give ephedrine to children under 12 without consulting your doctor.

Seniors

Older men, especially those with an enlarged prostate, should be cautious about taking ephedrine.

Generic Name

Epinephrine (EP-ih-NEF-rin)

Brand Names

Asthma Haler [A]
Asthma Nefrin [A]
Breatheasy
Broncho Saline [A]
Bronkaid Mist and Refill
Bronkaid Mist Suspension
Dey-Vial Sodium [A] Chloride Solution
Epinephrine Mist
Micro NEFRIN
Primatene Mist

Type of Drug

Bronchodilator.

Used for

Treatment of mild forms of seasonal or chronic asthma.

General Information

During an asthma attack, the muscles in the bronchial tubes in the lungs contract spasmodically and make it difficult to bring air into the lungs. Inhaled bronchodilator drugs such as epinephrine relax the bronchial muscles and expand their air passages, thus easing breathing.

For many years, epinephrine was considered the gold standard for treatment of acute bronchospasm, but the availability of newer, prescription asthma medications has decreased its use. These drugs, known as beta$_2$ agonists, selectively stimulate the beta$_2$-adrenergic receptors, resulting in smooth muscle relaxation throughout the airway system of the lungs. Epinephrine also stimulates alpha and beta$_1$ receptors; this stimulation does not help to relieve bronchospasm and has some unwanted effects.

Epinephrine works for a relatively short time compared with newer bronchodilator drugs.

OTC epinephrine is available in inhalers.

Cautions and Warnings

If your symptoms are not relieved within 20 minutes of taking epinephrine, or become worse, stop using the drug and call your doctor immediately.

Do not exceed the recommended daily dosage of epinephrine.

Prolonged use of epinephrine may cause nervousness, rapid heartbeat, and adverse effects on the heart.

You should use epinephrine only if you have been diagnosed with asthma by a doctor, you have never been hospitalized for asthma, and you are not taking any other asthma medications (unless prescribed by your doctor).

Persons with heart disease, high blood pressure, thyroid disease, diabetes, or difficulty urinating because of an enlarged prostate should take epinephrine only under a doctor's supervision.

Epinephrine may increase certain symptoms of Parkinson's disease, such as tremors and rigidity.

If you are taking a prescription drug for hypertension (high blood pressure) or an antidepressant, check with your doctor before taking epinephrine (see "Drug Interactions").

Rinsing your mouth after using an epinephrine inhaler may prevent dry mouth and throat, as well as reduce the risk of oral *candidal* infections.

If you are using an epinephrine inhaler with a mouthpiece, wash the mouthpiece once daily with soap and hot water, rinse thoroughly, and dry with a clean, lint-free cloth.

Do not puncture the inhaler.

Do not use epinephrine solution if it is brown or cloudy.

Possible Side Effects

▼ Rare: central nervous system (CNS) stimulation (fear, anxiety, tenseness, restlessness, headache, tremors, dizziness, light-headedness, nervousness, sleeplessness, excitability, weakness, heart arrhythmia, and high blood pressure), nausea, vomiting, sweating, pale skin, difficulty breathing, and respiratory weakness or apnea.

Drug Interactions

• Epinephrine should not be used at the same time as a monoamine oxidase inhibitor (MAOI) or within 2 weeks of stopping treatment with an MAOI. MAOIs are used to treat depression, other psychiatric or emotional conditions, and Parkinson's disease. If you are not sure whether you are or have been taking an MAOI, check with your doctor or pharmacist before you use epinephrine.

• If epinephrine is taken with other drugs that stimulate the CNS, their effects could combine and lead to toxicity.

• If taken together with epinephrine, some drugs may increase epinephrine's effects on the body, particularly on heart rhythm and rate. These include tricyclic antidepressants (e.g., imipramine), some antihistamines (especially diphenhydramine, tripelennamine, and dexchlorpheniramine), and thyroid hormones.

• If you have diabetes and are using epinephrine, you may need increased dosages of insulin or oral hypoglycemic drugs, because epinephrine may cause hyperglycemia (abnormally increased blood sugar).

• Drugs used to treat high blood pressure, such as beta blockers (e.g., propranolol), and alpha blockers (e.g., phentolamine), may reduce epinephrine's effects. Ergot alkaloids (e.g., bromochitine) may also reduce epinephrine's effects.

Usual Dose

Adult and Child (age 4 and over): 1 inhalation from a metered-dose, aerosol inhaler, followed by a second inhalation if symptoms have not been relieved after 1 minute. Do not use again for at least 3 hours.

Epinephrine is also available in an aqueous solution at a concentration equivalent to 1% epinephrine base; the solution is used with a hand-held, rubber-bulb nebulizer (spraying device). The usual dose for adults and children age 4 and over is 1–3 inhalations no more than every 3 hours.

Children using epinephrine should always be supervised by an adult to ensure proper dosing.

Child (under age 4): Consult your doctor.

Overdosage

Symptoms of overdose include CNS stimulation (fear, anxiety, tenseness, restlessness, headache, tremors, dizziness, light-headedness, nervousness, sleeplessness, excitability, weakness, heart arrhythmia, and high blood pressure), nausea, vomiting, sweating, pale skin, difficulty breathing, and respiratory weakness or apnea.

Even if the victim is not displaying any of the symptoms listed above, do the following in case of accidental overdose or ingestion: If the victim is unconscious or having convulsions, call for an ambulance immediately. If you take the victim to an emergency room, be sure to bring the bottle or container with you. If the victim is conscious, call your local poison control center or a health care professional. The poison control center may suggest inducing vomiting with ipecac syrup (available without a prescription at any pharmacy). DO NOT induce vomiting unless specifically instructed to do so.

Storage Instructions

Keep epinephrine inhalers away from heat or open flames to avoid the risk of an explosion. Keep out of direct sunlight.

Special Populations

Pregnancy/Breast-feeding

It is not generally recommended that pregnant women take any drugs, particularly during the first 3 months after conception. While it is unknown whether epinephrine can cause harm to the fetus if taken during pregancy, this drug should be taken by pregnant women only if prescribed by a doctor.

Epinephrine passes into breast milk. If you must take epinephrine, bottle-feed your baby with formula.

Infants/Children

Epinephrine is not recommended in children under age 4 unless directed by your doctor.

Children using epinephrine should always be supervised by an adult to ensure proper dosing.

Seniors

Older men, especially those with an enlarged prostate, should be cautious about taking epinephrine.

Generic Name

Ether (EE-ther)

Definition

A solvent (a fluid that dissolves other chemicals) used in OTC foot care products for treatment of corns, calluses, and warts. By dissolving the active ingredient (e.g., salicylic acid) and then rapidly evaporating, ether helps the medication spread across and adhere to the affected area so it can produce the desired effects.

Generic Names

Eucalyptus Oil (YEW-kuh-LIP-tuss) Eucalyptol (YEW-kuh-LIP-tohl)

Brand Names

Cepacol, Menthol-Eucalyptus
Diabetic Tussin Cough Drops [S]
Eucalyptamint
First Aid Medicated Powder
*†Fisherman's Friend Lozenges
Halls
Herbal-Menthol [S]
Koldets Cough Drops
*†Luden's
Mentholatum Cherry Chest Rub for Kids
REM [A]
*†Robitussin Cough Drops
Vaporizer in a Bottle Air Wick Inhaler
*†Vicks

**Not all products in this brand-name group contain eucalyptus oil and eucalyptol.*

†Consult the OTC ingredient charts to determine whether different formulations in this brand-name group are alcohol-, caffeine-, or sugar-free.

Type of Drug

Topical analgesic (pain reliever) and antitussive (cough suppressant).

Used for

Relief of soreness, stiffness, and pain in muscles, joints, and tendons; suppression of a dry, hacking, nonproductive cough (i.e., a cough that does not bring up any phlegm or mucus); and as a flavoring agent in some OTCs.

General Information

Eucalyptus oil is a natural oil derived from eucalyptus leaves; eucalyptol is one of the main ingredients of the oil. When either is applied to the skin, it produces a feeling of warmth. Used in this way, eucalyptus oil and eucalyptol are counterirritant topical analgesics. Counterirritation is the production of a less severe pain to distract from a more intense pain. The smell or the feelings of warmth or coolness that counterirritant topical analgesics produce may also contribute to a placebo effect; that is, if you believe they will work to relieve your pain, they probably will. However, according to the FDA, eucalyptus oil has not been shown to be generally recognized as safe and effective when used as a counterirritant ingredient. Topical analgesic preparations of eucalyptus oil are available in ointment, gel, liquid, cream, and powder form.

As an antitussive ingredient, eucalyptus oil is also commonly found in ointments to be rubbed on the throat or chest, solutions for steam inhalation, and cough drops or lozenges, but its effectiveness in suppressing coughs is also not proven. In both topical analgesic and antitussive preparations, eucalyptus oil is usually combined with menthol, which has been confirmed by the FDA as effective for both of these indications.

Eucalyptol is also a common flavoring agent for mouthwashes.

Cautions and Warnings

Do not take the maximum dosage of eucalyptus oil for more than 7 days continuously except under a doctor's supervision.

Do not exceed the recommended daily dosage of a eucalyptus oil preparation.

Topical Analgesic

Topical preparations containing eucalyptus oil should be used only on the skin. Don't apply them near your eyes or to mucous membranes (i.e., inside the mouth, nose, rectum, or vagina).

If your skin becomes irritated or red, or your pain gets worse or is constant and felt in any position, call your doctor.

Eucalyptus oil preparations should not be used with a heating pad, hot water bottle, or any other heating device. You should also avoid sunlight and sunlamps after using one of these products.

Do not use eucalyptus oil (or any other topical analgesic) after intense exercise, especially during hot and humid weather, when you will probably be flushed and warm. If you have a sore muscle from working out and want to use eucalyptus oil to relieve the pain, wait until you cool down. You should also avoid applying this product before using a sauna or getting a professional massage.

To avoid the risk of irritation, redness, or blistering, don't use a tight bandage or dressing over the skin where you apply eucalyptus oil or any other counterirritant analgesic.

Don't use eucalyptus oil on broken, irritated, or sunburned skin, or on an open wound.

If you wear contact lenses, don't take them out or put them in your eyes after you use a eucalyptus oil preparation without first washing your hands.

Antitussive

If you are using eucalyptus oil in a steam inhalation to treat a child's cough, to avoid the risk of serious burns, never leave the child unsupervised.

Never expose eucalyptus oil steam inhalation solution to flame or try to microwave it.

If your cough lasts longer than 7 days, is recurrent, or is accompanied by fever, rash, or persistent headache, call your doctor. A persistent cough may be a sign of a serious condition.

Possible Side Effects

You may develop rashes and blisters if eucalyptus oil is applied to sensitive areas of the skin, such as behind your knees. If you develop any skin irritation while using eucalyptus oil, stop using it immediately.

Drug Interactions

None known.

Food Interactions

None known.

Usual Dose

Topical Analgesic

Adult and Child (age 2 and over): Gently massage a small amount over the area on the skin where pain is felt. Make sure to wash your hands thoroughly afterward. If you ae treating pain in your hands, wait 30 minutes before washing. Reapply as needed, no more than 3 or 4 times a day.

Child (under age 2): not recommended unless prescribed by a doctor.

Topical Antitussive

Adult and Child (age 2 and over): Rub on the throat and chest in a thick layer. Repeat up to 3 times daily or as directed by your doctor.

Child (under age 2): not recommended unless prescribed by a doctor.

Steam Inhalation

Adult and Child (age 6 and over): Add 1 tbs. of solution per quart of water directly to the water in a hot/warm steam vaporizer. Breathe in the vapors, but do not direct the steam at your face. Repeat up to 3 times daily or as directed by your doctor.

Child (under age 6): not recommended.

Overdosage

Do the following in case of accidental ingestion: If the victim is unconscious or having convulsions, call for an ambulance immediately. If you take the victim to an emergency room, be sure to bring the bottle or container with you. If the victim is conscious, call your local poison control center or a health care professional. The poison control center may suggest inducing vomiting with ipecac syrup (available without a prescription at any pharmacy). DO NOT induce vomiting unless specifically instructed to do so.

Special Information

Besides using a topical preparation, there are also physical methods of producing counterirritation, such as by gently massaging the injured area. In fact, some of the benefit gained from using counterirritants may simply be due to the fact that they are applied by being rubbed and massaged into the skin. Another way to produce counterirritation is to apply heat to the skin with a hot water bottle or heating pad; in addition to reducing pain, heat helps the collagen in your skin regain its elasticity and lose its stiffness after a stretching injury. However, you should never use a counterirritant such as eucalyptus oil with a heating device (see "Cautions and Warnings").

Special Populations

Pregnancy/Breast-feeding

It is not generally recommended that pregnant women take any drugs, particularly during the first 3 months after conception. Check with your doctor before using eucalyptus oil if you are or might be pregnant, or if you are breast-feeding.

Infants/Children

Eucalyptus oil is not recommended as a topical analgesic or a lozenge in children under 2 or as a steam inhalation in children under 6 unless prescribed by a doctor.

Mouthrinses containing eucalyptol should not be used by children under age 12 unless prescribed by a doctor.

Seniors

Seniors should exercise the same caution as younger adults when using products containing eucalyptus oil.

Generic Name

Eugenol (YEW-juhn-ol)

Definition

A counterirritant (an agent that causes superficial irritation or inflammation in one area of the body that relieves irritation or inflammation in another part) similar to menthol and phenol. It is sometimes used to alleviate the throbbing pain of a toothache. Although a few OTC products contain eugenol, the FDA has stated that this ingredient should be administered only by a dentist, because it can damage the teeth and soft tissue in the mouth. Eugenol is also found in some products for relief of canker sores, but these products should also be used under the supervision of a health care professional, because they pose a risk of tissue irritation and systemic toxicity.

Generic Name

Glycerin (GLISS-er-in)

Brand Name

Agoral
Docusate Sodium
Doxidan
Dulcolax
*Fiberall
*†Fleet
Fletcher's
Kasof
Kondremul
Modane Soft
Sani-Supp
Surfak
Therevac [A]

** Not all products in this brand-name group contain glycerin.*

† Consult the OTC ingredient charts to determine whether different formulations in this brand-name group are alcohol-, caffeine-, or sugar-free.

Type of Drug

Laxative.

Used for

Relief of occasional constipation (irregularity).

General Information

The average, healthy individual defecates anywhere from 3 times a day to 3 times a week. Constipation is determined not necessarily by the frequency of bowel movements, but by the consistency of the stool, how difficult it is to eliminate, and other symptoms associated with constipation, such as dull headache, low back pain, and abdominal distention (swelling). Evaluate your condition carefully and discuss your symptoms and their possible causes with your pharmacist before self-medicating with a laxative. Laxatives are not always necessary, and when used improperly can either prevent the desired effect or result in laxative dependency. If you are indeed constipated, your condition may be best managed through proper diet, adequate fluid intake (6 to 8 glasses of water daily), and exercise. If you must use a laxative, choose the mildest effective product.

Laxatives may be classified by their mechanism of action: bulk-forming, emollient (stool softeners), lubricant, saline, hyperosmotic, and stimulant. Glycerin is a hyperosmotic laxative. Hyperosmotic laxatives, which are generally taken rectally, work by drawing water from the tissues into the feces, thus stimulating evacuation of the bowels.

Glycerin, taken rectally, generally produces a bowel movement in 15 to 30 minutes.

Glycerin is available by generic and brand name in suppository and solution (for enema) forms. It is also available in several combination products containing other laxatives (e.g., Dulcolax, which combines glycerin, the stimulant laxative bisacodyl, and the stool softener docusate sodium).

Cautions and Warnings

Do not use glycerin for more than 7 days, unless directed by your doctor. Long-term use of laxatives has been linked with laxative dependence, chronic constipation, and loss of normal bowel function. Using laxatives too frequently can result in persistent diarrhea, hypokalemia (abnormally low potassium in the blood), loss of essential nutrients, and dehydration.

Do not exceed the recommended daily dosage of glycerin.

Do not use glycerin if you have abdominal pain, nausea, vomiting, or kidney disease, unless directed by your doctor.

If you notice a sudden change in bowel habits lasting for more than 2 weeks, do not use glycerin until you have spoken to your doctor. Also contact your doctor if there is blood in your stool, so that colon cancer or other significant disease can be ruled out before you begin self-medication with glycerin.

If you have had a disease or surgery affecting the gastrointestinal (GI) tract, using a laxative may affect your condition adversely.

If you have rectal bleeding after using glycerin, or if you do not have a bowel movement after 7 days of using this medication, you may have a serious condition. Stop using the product and call your doctor.

Laxatives may decrease the absorption of other drugs that pass through the GI tract (see "Drug Interactions").

If you are using a glycerin enema product, be sure to follow the directions on the package carefully. An enema that is incorrectly administered can have adverse effects.

Possible Side Effects

- ▼ Most common: rectal discomfort, irritation, burning, pinching, cramping pain, and straining.
- ▼ Less common: hemorrhaging (minimal) of the rectal mucosa, and mucus discharge.

Drug Interactions

• All laxatives have the potential to decrease the absorption of any oral drug taken at the same time. If you are currently taking an oral medication, talk to your pharmacist before self-medicating with glycerin.

Food Interactions

None known.

Usual Dose

Glycerin should be administered only at infrequent intervals, in single doses. Do not exceed the recommended daily dosage. Take a full glass of water (to provide enough liquid for the laxative to work properly).

Suppository

Adult and Child (age 6 and over): 3 g.

Child (age 2–5): 1–1.5 g.

Child (under age 2): 1–1.5 g.

Administer the suppository at the time a bowel movement is desired. Lie on your side and, with pointed end up, push the suppository high into the rectum. Retain it for as long as possible. If you feel the suppository slipping out, push it higher into the rectum.

Enema

Adult and Child (age 6 and over): 5–15 ml.

Child (age 2–5): 2–5 ml.

Child (under age 2): not recommended unless directed by a doctor.

Follow the directions on the package. To administer an enema, lie on your side with your knees bent. Allow the solution to flow into the rectum *slowly.* Retain the solution until you feel stomach cramps.

Overdosage

Symptoms of overdosage are probably exaggerated side effects.

Even if the victim is not displaying any of the symptoms listed above, do the following in case of accidental overdose: If the victim is unconscious or having convulsions, call for an ambulance immediately. If you take the victim to an emergency room, be sure to bring the bottle or container with you. If the victim is conscious, call your local poison control center or a health care professional. The poison control center may suggest inducing vomiting with ipecac syrup (available without a prescription at any pharmacy). DO NOT induce vomiting unless specifically instructed to do so.

Storage Instructions

Glycerin suppositories should be stored at cooler than room temperature.

Special Populations

Pregnancy/Breast-feeding

Osmotic agents such as glycerin should be avoided during pregnancy because they can possibly cause dangerous electrolyte imbalances. Only bulk-forming or emollient laxatives are recommended for pregnant women. Check with your doctor before you use glycerin if you are or might be pregnant. Also consider talking to your doctor about diet and mild exercise in the management of constipation.

It is not known if glycerin passes into breast milk. Check with your doctor before using glycerin if you are breast-feeding.

Infants/Children

Observe your child carefully for patterns of bowel movements and the pain or difficulty with which the bowel movements are made before deciding whether the child is actually constipated. As with adults, "normal" bowel habits vary in children. If your child is indeed constipated, increasing fluid intake and adding fiber to his or her diet may be ways to manage the condition.

In general, the use of laxatives should be avoided in children, but glycerin is one of the safer options among laxatives.

Enemas are not recommended for children under age 2.

Seniors

Seniors commonly experience constipation, and consequently may become laxative dependent. Be cautious of chronically turning to laxatives to ease constipation, and instead look to diet and increased fluid intake as therapeutic measures.

Glycerin suppositories are safe and effective in seniors. Seniors should exercise the same caution as younger adults when using glycerin.

Generic Name

Guaiacol (GWYE-uh-kol)

Definition

A counterirritant (an agent that causes superficial irritation or inflammation in one area of the body that relieves irritation or inflammation in another part) similar to menthol and phenol.

Generic Name

Guaifenesin (gwye-FEN-uh-sin)

Brand Names

Anti-Tuss
*†Benylin
Cheracol D
Clear Cough DM [A] [S]
Congestac
DayGel
*†Diabetic Tussin
Dimacol
Dorcol Children's Cough [A]
Dristan Cold & Cough
Dynafed Two-Way
Emagrin Forte
Fendol
GG-Cen
Guaifed [A]
GuiaCough
Hytuss
Ipsatol [A]
Kolephrin GG/DM [A]
Naldecon [A]
*Novahistine
Pediacon [A]
Protac DM
*†Robitussin
Safe Tussin 30 [A] [S]
*†Scot-Tussin

Sinutab Non-Drying [A]
*†Sudafed
Tolu-Sed DM
Triaminic Expectorant, Chest & Head Congestion [A]
Tuss-DM
*†Tussar
*†Vicks

**Not all products in this brand-name group contain guaifenesin.*

†*Consult the OTC ingredient charts to determine whether different formulations in this brand-name group are alcohol-, caffeine-, or sugar-free.*

Type of Drug

Expectorant.

Used for

Loosening and clearing secretions from the respiratory tract and management of coughs associated with colds, bronchitis, laryngitis, pharyngitis, and other conditions.

General Information

Guaifenesin is a very common ingredient in liquid cough preparations, but there is some controversy over whether it is effective in clearing mucus and other secretions from the respiratory tract. Even at high doses, guaifenesin has not been proven to thin sputum (respiratory discharge) or to increase the amount of sputum coughed up.

Some cough syrups may contain both guaifenesin and an antitussive (cough suppressant) such as codeine or dextromethorphan. However, the combination of these ingredients is counterproductive, because the suppressing action of the antitussive may make it harder to cough up the secretions loosened by the expectorant.

Guaifenesin is available by brand name. In addition to antitussives, guaifenesin is often combined with other ingredients, such as decongestants and analgesics (pain relievers), to ease cough and cold symptoms.

Cautions and Warnings

Do not exceed the recommended daily dosage of guaifenesin.

Guaifenesin should not be used for persistent or chronic cough, such as that associated with smoking, asthma, chronic bronchitis, or chronic emphysema, or for coughs associated with excessive mucus.

If your cough lasts longer than 1 week, is recurrent, or is accompanied by fever, rash, or persistent headache, call your doctor. A persistent cough may be a sign of a serious condition.

Possible Side Effects

▼ Rare: vomiting or other gastrointestinal side effects.

Drug Interactions

None known.

Food Interactions

None known.

Usual Dose

Adult and Child (age 12 and over): 200–400 mg every 4 hours. Do not take more than 2400 mg in 24 hours.

Child (age 6–11): 100–200 mg every 4 hours. Do not give more than 1200 mg in 24 hours.

Child (age 2–5): 50–100 mg every 4 hours. Do not give more than 600 mg in 24 hours.

Child (under age 2): not recommended.

Overdosage

Do the following in case of accidental overdose: If the victim is unconscious or having convulsions, call for an ambulance immediately. If you take the victim to an emergency room, be sure to bring the bottle or container with you. If the victim is conscious, call your local poison control center or a health care professional. The poison control center may suggest inducing vomiting with ipecac syrup (available without a prescription at any pharmacy). DO NOT induce vomiting unless specifically instructed to do so.

Special Information

If you have a cold, other ways to help get rid of respiratory tract secretions include drinking 6 to 8 8-oz. glasses of water or other fluids a day and using a humidifier.

Special Populations

Pregnancy/Breast-feeding

Animal studies with guaifenesin have shown it to have harmful effects on the fetus, but it is not known if the same effects occur in humans. It is not generally recommended that pregnant women take any drugs, particularly during the first 3 months after conception. If you are or might be pregnant, or you are breast-feeding, check with your doctor before taking guaifenesin.

Infants/Children

Unless prescribed by a doctor, guaifenesin should not be given to children under age 12 with persistent or chronic cough, such as that associated with asthma, or with cough accompanied by excessive mucus.

Seniors

Seniors should exercise the same caution as younger adults when using guaifenesin.

Generic Name

Hydrocortisone

(HYE-droe-KOR-tih-zone)

Brand Names

Aquanil HC
Bactine Hydrocortisone 1%
Caldecort
Cortaid
Corticaine
Cortizone
Dermarest DriCort
DermiCort
Dermtex HC
Earsol-HC
HC-DermaPax
Hytone
Kericort 10
Lanacort
Neutrogena T/Scalp Anti-Pruritic
No More Itchies
Preparation H Hydrocortisone 1% Anti-Itch
Procort
Scalp Relief Medicine
Scalpicin Anti-Itch
Scalpmycin

Type of Drug

Anti-inflammatory; antipruritic (anti-itch agent); and topical corticosteroid.

Used for

Reduction of pain, burning, swelling, and itching in skin tissues.

General Information

Hydrocortisone (also called cortisol) is a corticosteroid hormone produced naturally by the body's adrenal glands. If the body experiences an infection or an allergic response that causes inflammation, the glands release hydrocortisone, which then circulates to the affected area. Hydrocortisone can also be made synthetically.

Hydrocortisone has a number of effects in the body. Its primary use is as an anti-inflammatory agent. When skin is inflamed, nearby blood vessels swell, causing leakage of fluid into the tissue. This fluid causes the symptoms of inflammation: redness, pain, heat, swelling, and itch. By a variety of mechanisms, hydrocortisone relieves symptoms of inflammation.

(Note: Corticosteroids are different from anabolic steroids, which are derived from the major male hormone, testosterone. Anabolic steroids are prescribed to treat a number of conditions, including severe anemia, leukemia, and breast cancer. They are sometimes abused by athletes and body builders, because they can help increase muscle mass.)

How effective hydrocortisone is for skin inflammation depends on its concentration. At this time, most available OTC products containing hydrocortisone have concentrations of 0.5% or 1%. The FDA has stated that concentrations of 1% are probably needed to achieve therapeutic results. Anything less than that may not be very effective. Concentrations of more than 1% are available only with a prescription.

The ability of the skin to absorb hydrocortisone is affected by a number of factors. Skin wounds that are open (e.g., cuts) absorb more of the medication than skin wounds that do not break the surface (e.g., scrapes and burns).

The vehicle of the OTC product — the ingredient that carries the active medication — also determines how much hydrocortisone is absorbed. Hydrocortisone ointments, for example, are petrolatum-based and form a denser protective covering. The medication stays in place longer, permitting greater absorption. Creams and lotions are generally more pleasant to use, but the amount of medication absorbed may be somewhat lower.

Hydrocortisone creams and ointments are both absorbed quickly into the affected area. Ointments might be of more benefit than creams if your skin problem has a dry, rough appearance; ointments create a thin, moisturizing barrier to protect the skin surface from becoming too dried out as it attempts to heal.

Hydrocortisone is indicated for treating a number of skin conditions, such as:

- insect bites
- poison ivy, oak, and sumac
- contact dermatitis (rashes) caused by contact with soaps, cosmetics and jewelry
- psoriasis
- minor burns
- hemorrhoids

Hydrocortisone does not kill bacteria or fungi and thus is not used to fight infection. Wounds that are infected (marked by such symptoms as scaling, pus, and crusting) must be treated with the appropriate antibiotic or antifungal product. Use of hydrocortisone on infected skin can actually make the infection worse (see "Cautions and Warnings").

Cautions and Warnings

If your condition doesn't improve within 7 days, stop using the product and contact your doctor. You may need a different or stronger medication.

Do not exceed the recommended daily dosage of hydrocortisone products.

These products are for external use only.

Before you use hydrocortisone, you or a health care professional should determine that the area being treated is not infected. If the area is very hot to the touch, or oozing a milky pus or a clear yellowish fluid, it may be infected. Hydrocortisone can relieve the symptoms of infection, thus masking it. This would allow the infection to continue growing without your knowledge. If your condition doesn't improve within 7 days, stop using the product and contact your doctor. You may need a different or stronger medication.

The prolonged use of topical hydrocortisone can cause the skin to lose its elasticity. Hydrocortisone prevents the chemical collagen from getting to the tissues. Adequate amounts of collagen are necessary to keep the skin soft and supple.

Overuse of a hydrocortisone product can also cause it to lose its effectiveness. The body can become tolerant to hydrocortisone, which shortens the length of time the drug produces the desired effect. In some cases, stopping the medication can then cause a rebound effect, allowing the inflammation to return in a more severe form.

Using an occlusive dressing (a wound dressing that covers the skin and blocks out air and moisture) can increase absorption of hydrocortisone and thus increase the risk of side effects.

Do not use hydrocortisone in the genital area if you have vaginal discharge.

Do not use this drug for treatment of infant's diaper rash (see "Special Populations").

If you are using a product to treat itch in the anal area, be careful not to exceed the recommended daily dose. Do not use if bleeding is present, and do not insert hydrocortisone cream or ointment into the rectum.

Possible Side Effects

Because very little hydrocortisone is absorbed from the skin into the bloodstream, the risk of systemic side effects from use of hydrocortisone is very low. However, some people may experience local side effects (effects on the skin area where hydrocortisone is used), especially in such areas as the face or the folds of the skin (e.g., under the breast, between the legs).

Prolonged or excessive use of hydrocortisone may cause thinning of the skin, loss of collagen, and drying or cracking. The blood vessels near the surface of the skin may become fragile.

Some people might experience acnelike blemishes, itching, redness, burning, stinging, or loss of color. People who have poor blood circulation might develop open sores on the skin. In rare cases, contact dermatitis might develop as a reaction to hydrocortisone. Infection can set in, especially if occlusive dressings are used.

Most adverse reactions disappear after use of the medication is stopped.

Drug Interactions

None known.

Usual Dose

Adult and Child (age 2 and over): Hydrocortisone cream or ointment should be applied to the affected area no more than 3–4 times a day. Small amounts, gently massaged into the skin surface, are sufficient to treat the area.

Leave the skin area uncovered, to allow the outside air to circulate around the wound and assist in the healing process. If there are cosmetic reasons for covering the affected area, the bandage should be applied loosely, allowing air to pass through it.

Child (under age 2): not recommended unless prescribed by a doctor.

Overdosage

Do the following in case of accidental ingestion: If the victim is unconscious or having convulsions, call for an ambulance immediately. If you take the victim to an emergency room, be sure to bring the bottle or container with you. If the victim is conscious, call your local poison control center or a health care professional. The poison control center may suggest inducing vomiting with ipecac syrup (available without a prescription at any pharmacy). DO NOT induce vomiting unless specifically instructed to do so.

Special Populations

Pregnancy/Breast-feeding

It is not generally recommended that pregnant women take any drugs, particularly during the first 3 months after conception. Check with your doctor if you are or might be pregnant.

There is a potential risk that topical corticosteroids may be passed from mother to child during breast-feeding. If you must use hydrocortisone, bottle-feed your baby with formula.

Infants/Children

Children have a greater skin surface area in proportion to their size than adults. For this reason, they are at greater risk of complications from absorbing hydrocortisone. Use only the amount of hydrocortisone indicated for relief of symptoms.

Hydrocortisone is not recommended for children under age 2 unless prescribed by a doctor.

Hydrocortisone is not recommended for treatment of diaper rash, because the baby's delicate skin may absorb too much of the hormone. This risk is increased if tight fitting diapers or plastic pants are used, since these act the same way as occlusive dressings to increase absorption.

Seniors

Older individuals are at greater risk of skin thinning, loss of skin moisture, and dryness from use of hydrocortisone.

Generic Name

Hydrogen Peroxide

(HYE-droe-jen per-OKS-ide)

Brand Name

Peroxyl

Type of Drug

Topical antiseptic.

Used for

Prevention of bacterial infection in minor cuts, abrasions, mildly infected wounds, and irritations of the mouth.

General Information

Hydrogen peroxide is an antibacterial chemical used as a disinfectant for minor wounds and mouth irritations. It also has a deodorant effect. It works best on surface conditions rather than deep wounds. The FDA has approved this substance for use as a first-aid product.

When hydrogen peroxide comes into contact with bacteria, a chemical reaction occurs in which oxygen is released in the form of bubbles. The activity of these bubbles, or fizzing, acts to loosen and scrub away dead tissue, carrying it up and away from the wound or irritation. This creates a clearer path for antibiotic and antibacterial medications to reach the affected area and to treat infection.

Hydrogen peroxide is only effective as long as it is producing bubbles. Once the fizzing stops, the product no longer has any therapeutic benefit.

Hydrogen peroxide solution is available generically.

Cautions and Warnings

Do not use the maximum daily dosage of hydrogen peroxide for more than 5 days unless under the supervision of a doctor.

Do not exceed the recommended daily dosage of hydrogen peroxide.

This drug is for external use only. If used in a gargle or mouthwash preparation, care should be taken to avoid swallowing. Ingestion of significant amounts of hydrogen peroxide can cause ulcers (open wounds) in internal organs.

Solutions of more than 20% can be strongly irritating to skin and mucous tissues, and should be used infrequently and sparingly. Consult your doctor if any additional symptoms develop while using these stronger formulations.

Because it produces gas, hydrogen peroxide is not used to treat abscesses (closed wounds).

To prevent buildup of air at the wound site, bandages should not be applied until after the hydrogen peroxide has dried.

Hydrogen peroxide is also used as a bleach (e.g., in hair products). If used as a tooth whitening agent, it can seriously damage the enamel surface of the teeth.

Possible Side Effects

Special care should be taken when dealing with solutions of over 20% hydrogen peroxide. Overexposure of skin or mucous tissues to the harsh strength of this chemical could result in ulceration and secondary infections.

Drug Interactions

• When used in a gargle or mouthwash solution, there is a chance that other chemicals in the mouth might exert more powerful activity. For example, residues from smoking or tobacco chew might become even more likely to cause cancer than they normally are.

Food Interactions

None known.

Usual Dose

Solution

Adult and Child (age 2 and over): Saturate the wound with the solution using a cotton ball or cotton-tipped stick and allow the area to remain undisturbed until the chemical reaction has stopped. Wipe the surface of the affected area gently to remove the dead tissue, allow to dry, and proceed with whatever further medication or dressing is necessary.

Child (under age 2): not recommended unless prescribed by a doctor.

Oral Gel

Adult and Child (age 2 and over): Dry the affected area of the mouth or jaw tissues as much as possible. This allows the gel to adhere to the skin surface. Apply a small amount of gel to the wound, and allow it to remain undisturbed for at least 1 minute. Wipe the affected area gently to remove the gel and dead tissue. Wash hands prior to and after administration.

Child (under age 2): not recommended unless prescribed by a doctor.

Overdosage

The swallowing of this chemical can result in serious internal organ damage. In case of accidental ingestion, DO NOT MAKE THE VICTIM VOMIT.

Do the following in case of accidental ingestion: If the victim is unconscious or having convulsions, call for an ambulance immediately. If the victim is conscious, call your local poison control center or a health care professional. If you take the victim to an emergency room, be sure to bring the bottle or container with you.

Special Information

In some instances, the skin at the edges of the wound will become white and remain so after the removal of the hydrogen peroxide. This is not harmful; instead, it is an indication that dead tissue surrounding the wound has absorbed the chemical. The dead tissue will dry up and slough off as the wound continues healing.

The fizzing of the chemical reaction as hydrogen peroxide does its job can be frightening to small children and some adults. Before treating these individuals, it is a good idea to explain what is about to happen and offer assurance that the product is not an acid and will not cause pain.

Storage Instructions

The strength of hydrogen peroxide deteriorates when exposed to light, repeated shaking, and heat.

Special Populations

Pregnancy/Breast-feeding

It is not generally recommended that pregnant women take any drugs, particularly during the first 3 months after conception. Check with your doctor if you are or might be pregnant, or if you are breast-feeding.

Infants/Children

Since hydrogen peroxide can be irritating to skin tissue, consult your doctor before using this chemical on children under age 2.

Children under 12 should be supervised by an adult when using hydrogen peroxide gel.

Seniors

Seniors should exercise the same caution as younger adults when using a hydrogen peroxide product.

Generic Name

Hydrogenated Palm Oil Glyceride

(HYE-droe-jeh-NATE-ed PALM OIL GLISS-er-ide)

Definition

A lubricant used in OTC products for treatment of vaginal dryness.

Generic Name

Hydroxyethylcellulose

(hye-DROKS-ee-ETH-ill-SELL-yew-loes)

Definition

see ***Carboxymethylcellulose Sodium,*** *page 745*

Generic Name

Hydroxypropyl Methylcellulose

(hye-DROKS-ee-PROE-puhl METH-il-SELL-yew-loes)

Definition

see ***Carboxymethylcellulose Sodium,*** *page 745*

Generic Name

Ibuprofen (EYE-bew-PRO-fen)

Brand Names

Addaprin [C] [S]
†Advil
Arthritis Foundation Ibuprofen
Bayer Select Ibuprofen Pain Relief [C]
Dristan Sinus
Haltran
Midol IB Cramp Relief Formula [C]
†Motrin
Nuprin [C]
Sine-Aid
Ultraprin [C]
Valprin [C]
Vicks DayQuil Sinus Pressure & Pain Relief with Ibuprofen

†*Consult the OTC ingredient charts to determine whether different formulations in this brand-name group are alcohol-, caffeine-, or sugar-free.*

Type of Drug

Nonsteroidal anti-inflammatory drug (NSAID), analgesic (pain reliever), and antipyretic (fever reducer).

Used for

Temporary relief of mild to moderate pain associated with headache, colds, toothache, muscle ache, backache, arthritis, and menstrual cramps; and reduction of fever.

General Information

NSAID is the general term used for a group of drugs that are effective in reducing inflammation and pain. Other OTC drugs in this group are aspirin, ketoprofen, and naproxen sodium.

It is not known exactly how NSAIDs work. However, part of their action may be due to an ability to inhibit the body's production of a hormone called prostaglandin as well as other body chemicals (e.g., cyclooxygenase, lipoxygenase, leukotrienes, lysosomal enzymes) that sensitize pain receptors and stimulate the inflammatory response. NSAIDs are generally quickly absorbed into the bloodstream, and pain and fever relief usually occurs within 1 hour of taking the first dose and can last up to 6 hours. The anti-inflammatory effect of these agents generally takes longer to work (several days to 2 weeks) and may take a month or more to reach maximum effect.

Ibuprofen is especially effective in treating the cramps and headache associated with menstruation, which may be experienced by up to half of all women of childbearing age. In many clinical tests, ibuprofen has been shown to be better at relieving this type of pain than aspirin or other salicylates (choline salicylate, magnesium salicylate, sodium salicylate), and acetaminophen.

Ibuprofen is available by generic and brand name in tablet, caplet, and gelcap form, as well as in a suspension form for use in children to relieve aches and pains caused by colds, flu, sore throat, headache, and toothache. Ibuprofen is also an ingredient in combination drugs to relieve menstrual cramps or cold and flu symptoms.

Cautions and Warnings

Do not take ibuprofen for more than 10 consecutive days or, in the presence of fever, for more than 3 days, unless directed by your doctor. Notify your doctor if this product does not relieve your symptoms in that time.

Do not exceed the recommended daily dosage of ibuprofen.

Do not take acetaminophen or aspirin or any other NSAID, or any product containing them, while taking ibuprofen.

If you develop any severe gastrointestinal (GI) effects, blurred vision, or a rash while you are taking ibuprofen, call your doctor.

Because adverse effects of ibuprofen use occur most frequently in the GI tract, individuals who have active or previous ulcer disease of the stomach or duodenum (peptic ulcer disease) should be aware of the risk of using ibuprofen (or other NSAIDs).

Bronchospastic symptoms may worsen in people with asthma who take ibuprofen.

Ibuprofen use can have damaging effects on the kidneys. It may increase blood levels of urea nitrogen and serum creatinine and may also lead to sodium and water retention; these effects are especially dangerous in patients with existing kidney damage or congestive heart failure. However, with usual OTC doses, the risk of kidney damage is low unless you are a high-risk patient with pre-existing renal disease or you take the drug for prolonged periods of time. Kidney damage with ibuprofen use may also be more likely to occur in older people and in those with certain medical conditions. If any of the following applies to you do not take ibuprofen without first consulting with your doctor or pharmacist: high blood pressure, diuretic use, diabetes, and atherosclerotic heart disease.

In rare instances, severe effects on the liver, including jaundice and hepatitis, have been seen in people taking ibuprofen. If any signs or symptoms of liver damage occur (darkened urine, yellowed eyes) stop taking ibuprofen and contact your doctor.

Ibuprofen can slow down blood clotting and increase bleeding time by inhibiting platelet aggregation; however, this effect is reversible within 24 hours after ibuprofen use is stopped. People with a history of active GI bleeding should be cautious about taking ibuprofen or any NSAID.

Drinking alcoholic beverages has been shown to increase the prolongation of bleeding time associated with ibuprofen and should be avoided when you are taking this drug.

Ibuprofen can make you drowsy. Be careful when driving a motor vehicle or operating heavy machinery after taking ibuprofen.

Possible Side Effects

- ▼ Most common: GI problems (e.g., indigestion, heartburn, nausea, diarrhea, stomach irritation).
- ▼ Less common: stomach ulcers, GI bleeding, loss of appetite, hepatitis, gallbladder attacks, painful urination, poor kidney function, kidney inflammation, blood in the urine, dizziness, fainting, nervousness.
- ▼ Rare: severe allergic reactions, including closing of the throat, fever and chills, changes in liver function, jaundice, and kidney failure; ringing in the ears; blurred vision.

Drug Interactions

• If you are currently taking an anticoagulant (blood-thinning) drug, such as warfarin, you should not take ibuprofen without first consulting your doctor. Ibuprofen can increase the risk of bleeding if taken with an anticoagulant.

• In individuals taking ibuprofen and digoxin, a drug used to treat congestive heart failure, ibuprofen may increase the concentration of digoxin in the blood, although researchers are not sure of the implications of this effect. Ibuprofen may also increase the blood levels of phenytoin, a drug taken to control epilepsy. If you take either digoxin or phenytoin, consult your doctor before taking ibuprofen.

• Ibuprofen may work against the effects of drugs taken to lower blood pressure, including diuretics, angiotensin-converting enzyme (ACE) inhibitors, beta blockers, and others. If you are taking any of these drugs, acetaminophen may be a good alternative analgesic for you.

• If you are taking lithium, do not take ibuprofen without first consulting your doctor.

• Ibuprofen can increase the toxicity of methotrexate, which is used to treat cancer, severe psoriasis, severe rheumatic arthritis, and to induce abortion. If you are taking methotrexate, do not take ibuprofen or other NSAIDs without checking with your doctor.

Food Interactions

If ibuprofen upsets your stomach, take it with meals or with milk. You can also take an antacid containing aluminum hydroxide or magnesium hydroxide.

Usual Dose

Analgesic

Adult (age 12 and over): 200–400 mg every 4–6 hours (no more than 1200 mg in 24 hours). To prevent menstrual cramps as well as relieve the pain associated with menstruation, it is best to take ibuprofen on a schedule rather than only when you feel pain. A 200-mg dose can be taken every 4–6 hours for the first 48–72 hours after your period begins; if it is not effective, you may take a 400-mg dose every 6 hours.

Child (age 6 months–11 years): as directed by your doctor.

Antipyretic

Adult (age 12 and over): 200 mg every 4–6 hours. If your fever does not respond, the dosage can be increased to 400 mg every 4–6 hours, but it should not exceed 1200 mg a day unless prescribed by your doctor.

Child (age 6 months–11 years): as directed by your doctor.

Overdosage

Do the following in case of accidental overdose: If the victim is unconscious or having convulsions, call for an ambulance immediately. If you take the victim to an emergency room, be sure to bring the bottle or container with you. If the victim is conscious, call your local poison control center or a health care professional. The poison control center may suggest inducing vomiting with ipecac syrup (available without a prescription at any pharmacy). DO NOT induce vomiting unless specifically instructed to do so.

Special Populations

Allergies

People who are allergic to aspirin or to any other NSAID should not take ibuprofen.

Pregnancy/Breast-feeding

It is not generally recommended that pregnant women take any drugs, particularly during the first 3 months after conception.

Ibuprofen may cross into the circulation of a developing fetus, but it has not been proven that ibuprofen causes birth defects if taken during pregnancy. However, animal studies have shown that ibuprofen may have an effect on the developing heart, and its use may interfere with labor or delay birth. It is especially dangerous to take ibuprofen during the last 3 months of pregnancy. If you are or might be pregnant, do not take ibuprofen without your doctor's approval.

Ibuprofen has not been shown to pass into breast milk; however, it is not recommended that nursing mothers use this drug because of the risk of affecting the baby's heart or cardiovascular system. If you must take ibuprofen, bottle-feed your baby with formula.

Infants/Children

Ibuprofen has not been proven to be safe or effective in children younger than age 6 months. Ibuprofen should not be taken by children younger than age 12 unless directed by a physician.

Seniors

Seniors may be more likely to experience ibuprofen side effects, especially if they have poor kidney or liver function.

Generic Name

Imidazolidinyl Urea

(im-id-AZE-oe-LIH-din-il YEW-ree-uh)

Definition

An antimicrobial chemical used in some diaper rash products.

Generic Name

Iodine (EYE-oe-dine)

Brand Name

Efodine

Type of Drug

Topical antiseptic.

Used for

Prevention of infection in minor cuts and scrapes and as an ingredient in vaginal douche products.

General Information

Used externally, iodine is an efficient and fast-acting antimicrobial agent, applied to the skin to prevent infection in minor, superficial wounds. It is effective against bacteria, fungi, spores, protozoa, and yeast infections. Stronger solutions of iodine are also used to disinfect the skin before surgical procedures.

Iodine is often combined with a synthetic substance called povidone. Povidone is a vehicle (carrier of the active ingredient) that helps iodine stay in contact with the area being treated and releases the molecules of iodine over time. Povidone-iodine is an ingredient in some feminine hygiene products (such as douches) and in topical antifungals, used to combat common skin conditions such as athlete's foot and jock itch. Individuals whose skin cannot tolerate contact with iodine solutions may have better results with products containing a povidone-iodine mixture. This combination antiseptic is less irritating to skin and mucous membranes and encourages the natural immune responses that promote healing.

An iodine tincture contains 50% alcohol. This formulation also provides effective antisepsis, but is less preferable because it can be more irritating to the skin.

Iodine is available by brand name (in combination products) and generically in solution form as a combination of 2% iodine and 2.5% sodium iodine.

Cautions and Warnings

Do not use iodine skin preparations for more than 3 or 4 days continuously except under a doctor's supervision.

Do not exceed the recommended daily dosage of iodine.

These products are for external (or, in the case of douches, intravaginal) use only. While there is a small natural need for iodine in our daily diets, antiseptic iodine should never be ingested to meet that need. For this purpose, you should look for oral iodine supplements.

Iodine in high concentrations is an irritant, and can cause an "iodine burn" or a lasting stinging sensation after use, especially if a bandage is applied. You should leave the wound uncovered after treatment as much as possible to allow the iodine to evaporate.

Do not use iodine on severe burns or large wounds.

Iodine solutions may stain the skin. If this occurs, a compound called sodium thiosulfate solution may help remove the stain.

Possible Side Effects

Some people will develop an allergy, or sensitivity, to iodine during repeated contact with the substance. If you experience a rash, persistent burning sensation, or unusual warmth in the affected area, discontinue use and contact your doctor.

Drug Interactions

None known.

Usual Dose

Adult and child (age 6 and over): Apply iodine solution to the wound after cleansing with soap and water.

Child (age 2–5): Consult a doctor.

Child (under age 2): not recommended unless directed by a doctor.

In general, the wound should be left uncovered to avoid iodine irritation to the skin.

Overdosage

Iodine burns have occurred mainly with solutions that are 7% iodine or stronger. Strong iodine solutions should not be used as antiseptics.

Do the following in case of accidental ingestion: If the victim is unconscious or having convulsions, call for an ambulance immediately. If you take the victim to an emergency room, be sure to bring the bottle or container with you. If the victim is conscious, call your local poison control center or a health care professional. The poison control center may suggest inducing vomiting with ipecac syrup (available without a prescription at any pharmacy). DO NOT induce vomiting unless specifically instructed to do so.

Special Populations

Pregnancy/Breast-feeding

It is not generally recommended that pregnant women take any drugs, particularly during the first 3 months after conception. Check with your doctor if you are or might be pregnant, or if you are breast-feeding.

Infants/Children

Due to the skin-irritating qualities of iodine, it should not be used on children under 2 unless supervised by a doctor.

Seniors

Seniors may have skin that is especially sensitive to the irritating effects of iodine.

Generic Name

Ipecac Syrup (IP-uh-kak)

Type of Drug

Emetic.

Used for

Emergency treatment of acute poisoning by ingestion.

General Information

Emetics are substances that induce vomiting. They are used to evacuate potentially toxic substances from the stomach.

In an acute poisoning emergency, it is essential to contact a doctor, emergency room, or poison control center before taking or administering an emetic such as ipecac syrup in a home environment without medical supervision. The potential toxin ingested, the amount ingested, the time since ingestion, signs and symptoms, and the victim's age and weight all factor into whether the situation is potentially life-threatening or not. There are also many substances that should not be regurgitated (see "Cautions and Warnings"). If you do not have ipecac at home and are purchasing it specifically for immediate use, your pharmacist may be able to advise you whether to take the victim straight to the emergency room or treat the individual at home. Always follow up home treatment by contacting a health care professional.

Ipecac syrup is the emetic of choice in the treatment of acute poisoning, but in the past 10 years the use of ipecac has been surpassed by that of activated charcoal, an adsorbent. Some health care professionals believe that the effectiveness of ipecac may be enhanced by the consecutive use of activated charcoal. If you follow this procedure, you must be sure to induce vomiting with ipecac before administering the activated charcoal (see "Cautions and Warnings").

Ipecac generally induces vomiting in about 20 minutes. It is effective in 80% to 99% of the people who take it.

Ipecac is available by generic name only, in syrup form.

Cautions and Warnings

Do not take more than 2 consecutive doses of ipecac syrup.

Do not exceed the recommended daily dosage of ipecac.

In an acute poisoning emergency, first try to contact an emergency room, poison control center, or doctor. If outside help cannot be obtained quickly enough, take or administer the ipecac, carefully following the directions on the label.

Some health care professionals recommend using activated charcoal after you have induced vomiting with ipecac syrup. Because activated charcoal adsorbs (i.e., binds) ipecac, thus reducing its effectiveness, it is crucial that the poisoned individual take the ipecac first and vomit before taking the charcoal. Be sure the vomiting is completed before administration of the activated charcoal. After taking or administering the drug(s), try again to contact a health care professional.

Do not use ipecac if the poisoned individual is not fully conscious, is extremely inebriated, is in shock, is having seizures, or lacks the gag reflex. In such cases, the victim is at risk of breathing the vomit into his or her lungs.

If vomiting does not occur following administration of ipecac, the drug's emetine content may be absorbed and cause adverse systemic effects.

Unless you are advised to do so by a doctor, emergency room, or poison control center, do not give ipecac to individuals who have ingested any of the following substances: strychnine, kerosene, gasoline, paint thinner, fuel oil, cleaning fluid, an alkali such as lye, or a strong acid. Also contact a health care professional before giving ipecac to someone who has ingested a convulsant.

Ipecac may be used in poisonings with anti-emetic agents such as meclizine if it is given within 1 hour of ingestion, before toxic or anti-emetic effects appear.

Use ipecac with caution following overdosage of cardiac glycosides.

Ipecac is not recommended for use in individuals who have taken an overdose of an antidepressant, which may cause rapid unconsciousness, or of an amphetamine, which may rapidly produce seizures.

People with impaired cardiac function or hardening of the blood vessels should use ipecac with caution, because vomiting may cause an increase in blood pressure, leading to hemorrhage.

Vomiting may not eliminate all of the toxic material from the gastrointestinal tract. Be sure to have the victim carefully observed by a health care professional for signs of increasing intoxication.

ADMINISTRATION OF IPECAC SYRUP SHOULD NOT TAKE THE PLACE OF OTHER MEASURES USED IN THE EMERGENCY TREATMENT OF POISONING OR OVERDOSE. Always contact a physician, emergency room, or poison control center in cases of accidental overdose or poisoning.

Ipecac should be used in the management of poisoning and overdose only. Individuals who chronically abuse ipecac—such as individuals with anorexia nervosa, bulimia, or other eating disorders—have experienced serious, sometimes fatal adverse effects. These adverse effects can continue for months after discontinuance of the medication.

If you keep ipecac syrup in the house, periodically check the expiration date on the container. Ipecac used past its expiration may be ineffective. Since ipecac is used in emergency situations, it is best to be certain of its efficacy. However, if in an emergency the only ipecac available has passed its expiration date, use the product anyway; expired ipecac has been effective in some cases, although you should not depend on this as a general rule.

Ipecac syrup should not be confused with ipecac fluid extract, which is not currently commercially available in the U.S. The fluid extract is 14 times more potent than the syrup, and its administration has resulted in severe toxicity and death.

Possible Side Effects

▼ Rare: protracted vomiting, diarrhea, and drowsiness.

Drug Interaction

• The only potential drug interaction involves activated charcoal (see "Cautions and Warnings").

Food Interactions

None known.

Usual Dose

Adult and Child (age 12 and over): 30 ml.
Child (age 1–11): 15 ml.
Child (age 6–11 months): 5 ml, with professional guidance (see "Special Populations").
Child (under age 6 months): Consult a doctor.

If vomiting has not occurred within 20 minutes of ipecac administration, you may repeat the dose. If the second dose doesn't produce vomiting within another 30 minutes, contact a physician, emergency room, or poison control center. The victim should drink 12 to 16 oz. of water or another clear liquid immediately following administration of ipecac, to increase its effectiveness. He or she should also be kept moving or active after taking the drug.

Ipecac syrup is available over the counter in a container holding no more than 30 ml of the drug (i.e., 1 adult dose).

Overdosage

Most cases of ipecac overdosage have involved the fluid extract, which is not commercially available in the U.S. and should not be used. Symptoms of overdose with ipecac include nausea, bloody stools and vomit, cramping and abdominal pain, hypotension (abnormally low blood pressure), difficulty breathing, shock, seizures, coma, and congestive heart failure. The cause of death is usually heart failure.

Do the following in case of accidental overdose: If the victim is unconscious or having convulsions, call for an ambulance immediately. If the victim is conscious, call your local poison control center or a health care professional. If you take the victim to an emergency room, be sure to bring the bottle or container with you.

Special Populations

Pregnancy/Breast-feeding

It is not generally recommended that pregnant women take any drug, particularly during the first 3 months after conception.

It is not known whether ipecac syrup causes harm to fetuses or passes into breast milk. Pregnant women should use ipecac only if clearly needed. Be sure to contact your doctor before taking ipecac if you are or might be pregnant or if you are breast-feeding.

Infants/Children

When treating an infant or child for acute poisoning, use ipecac syrup as directed by a health care professional. Some health professionals recommend ipecac syrup over activated charcoal for home use in children because the ipecac is easier to administer.

In addition to being given smaller doses than adults, children treated with ipecac should drink less water (4 to 8 oz.). If the child refuses to drink water, some clinicians believe that a carbonated beverage, or even milk, will be more palatable to the child and will not significantly reduce the drug's effectiveness. You may also give the liquid to the child first, before the ipecac.

You may induce vomiting early by gently bouncing the child.

Before administering ipecac to a child age 6 months to 1 year, contact a health care professional regarding positioning, so the child doesn't breathe the vomit into his or her lungs.

Administer ipecac to an infant under age 6 months only under a doctor's supervision.

Seniors

Seniors should exercise the same caution as younger adults when using ipecac.

Generic Name

Isopropyl Alcohol

(EYE-soe-PROE-pill AL-kuh-hall)

Definition

A clear, colorless liquid that mixes well with water, ether, and ethyl alcohol; also called avantin, dimethyl carbinol, and isopropanol. Isopropyl alcohol is classified by the FDA as safe and effective for first-aid use in the home. It is used as a cleaner and disinfectant in contact lens products and is also found in topical products to prevent swimmer's ear and to dry water-clogged ears (although the FDA has not established that it is safe and effective for these uses). A solution of 70% isopropyl alcohol and water is used as a rubbing compound, known as isopropyl rubbing alcohol. In acne products, isopropyl alcohol helps the medication dry quickly to a filmlike consistency. It must never be taken internally! *(see also **Alcohol,** page 665)*

Generic Name

Kaolin and Pectin **(KAE-oe-lin and PEK-tin)**

Brand Names

Kaodene NN
Kaolin Pectin [S]
Kao-Spen
K-C

Type of Drug

Antidiarrheal.

Used for

Control and symptomatic relief of acute diarrhea.

General Information

The average, healthy individual defecates anywhere from 3 times a day to 3 times a week. Diarrhea is characterized by abnormal frequency or consistency of stool and can be caused by any one of several conditions, either gastrointestinal (GI) or non-GI. These include bacterial and viral infections, food intolerance, gastroenteritis, and drug adverse effects. The cause of the diarrhea should determine the choice of the best drug therapy.

It should be emphasized that diarrhea is a symptom. Antidiarrheal medications provide symptomatic relief, which is generally sufficient for the treatment of temporary, uncomplicated diarrhea, such as that caused by an allergic reaction to dairy products. Persistent or recurrent diarrhea, however, can be a sign of a more serious condition requiring the attention of a health care professional and treatment geared toward the underlying condition. Persistent diarrhea can also lead to dehydration. Self-medication with kaolin and pectin or another antidiarrheal does not preclude the fluid, electrolyte, and nutritional therapies necessary for the treatment of more serious, chronic diarrhea.

Kaolin and pectin, two substances that are used in combination, are GI adsorbents, which work by adsorbing, or binding, toxins, bacteria, and various noxious materials in the GI tract—although their action is not limited to undesirable substances (see "Cautions and Warnings").

Adsorbents are the OTC antidiarrheal products prescribed most often. However, the effectiveness of kaolin and pectin has not been demonstrated by controlled clinical studies. In one study, kaolin and pectin decreased the fluidity of stools in children with diarrhea, but did not decrease stool frequency or fecal weight and water content.

Kaolin and pectin, along with another adsorbent, attapulgite, are currently being evaluated for safety and efficacy by the FDA's OTC Center for Drug Evaluations and Research. The FDA may decide to remove pectin from the combination product because the evidence for kaolin alone is better than that for the kaolin and pectin combinations. The FDA is also considering including a warning not to take kaolin at the same time as other medications (see "Drug Interactions") and recommending that kaolin not be taken by children under age 12. Consult your pharmacist regarding possible reclassification and labeling changes before self-medicating with kaolin and pectin.

A kaolin and pectin combination is available in liquid form as a generic or brand-name product. Because large doses are generally used, kaolin and pectin products are most commonly available in flavored liquid form to improve palatability.

Cautions and Warnings

Do not use kaolin and pectin for more than 2 days unless directed by your doctor. Uncomplicated, acute diarrhea usually improves within 24 to 48 hours. Persistent diarrhea can lead to dehydration, which may require the administration of appropriate fluid and electrolyte therapy.

Do not exceed the recommended daily dosage of kaolin and pectin.

Do not take kaolin and pectin if your diarrhea is accompanied by high fever (higher than 101°F), vomiting, or blood in the stool.

Call your doctor if fever develops during self-medication with kaolin and pectin.

Because kaolin and pectin's action is not selective, this product may adsorb desirable substances, such as nutrients, along with toxins. It may also adsorb oral medications being taken at the same time (see "Drug Interactions").

Possible Side Effects

▼ Rare: mild and temporary constipation.

Drug Interactions

• Because kaolin and pectin's GI adsorption is not selective, it may adsorb any other oral medication being taken at the same time, thus decreasing the absorption of the other medication. It is generally advised to take oral medications 2 hours before or 3 to 4 hours after a dose of kaolin and pectin. You may have to change the dosing interval of your other medication. Talk to your doctor or pharmacist.

• Kaolin and pectin may also impair the absorption of digoxin, used to treat congestive heart failure. Take your kaolin and pectin dose several hours after your digoxin dose.

Food Interactions

None known.

Usual Dose

Adult and Child (age 12 and over): 60–120 ml after the first loose bowel movement. You may take additional doses after subsequent loose bowel movements, but do not exceed the recommended daily dosage.

Be sure to shake the liquid well before using.

Do not take kaolin and pectin for more than 2 days.

Be sure to drink plenty of clear liquids to help prevent dehydration, which may accompany diarrhea.

Child (age 3–11): Consult your doctor.

Child (under age 3): not recommended.

Overdosage

Do the following in case of accidental overdose: If the victim is unconscious or having convulsions, call for an ambulance immediately. If you take the victim to an emergency room, be sure to bring the bottle or container with you. If the victim is conscious, call your local poison control center or a health care professional. The poison control center may suggest inducing vomiting with ipecac syrup (available without a prescription at any pharmacy). DO NOT induce vomiting unless specifically instructed to do so.

Special Populations

Pregnancy/Breast-feeding

It is not generally recommended that pregnant women take any drugs, particularly during the first 3 months after conception. Check with your doctor before taking kaolin and pectin if you are or might be pregnant, or if you are breastfeeding. Also talk to your physician regarding fluid and electrolyte management if you are suffering from diarrhea.

Infants/Children

Infants and children with acute or chronic diarrhea are at particular risk for severe and possibly dangerous dehydration and electrolyte imbalance. Over-reliance on antidiarrheal drugs may lead to the neglect of crucial fluid and electrolyte management and nutritional therapy. Antidiarrheal medications in general have not been shown to be especially effective in children.

Presently, kaolin and pectin should not be given to children under age 3 unless directed by a doctor. However, the FDA is currently reviewing the safety and efficacy of kaolin (see "General Information") and may change this recommendation to apply to children under age 12.

Seniors
Kaolin and pectin should not be used by individuals over 60. If, in addition to diarrhea, you are suffering from other ailments that make you weak, consult your doctor regarding fluid and electrolyte management.

Generic Name

Ketoprofen (KEE-toe-PRO-fen)

Brand Names

Actron
Orudis KT [C]

Type of Drug

Nonsteroidal anti-inflammatory drug (NSAID), analgesic (pain reliever), and antipyretic (fever reducer).

Used for

Temporary relief of mild to moderate pain associated with headache, colds, toothache, muscle ache, backache, arthritis, and menstrual cramps; reduction of fever.

General Information

NSAID is the general term used for a group of drugs that are effective in reducing inflammation and pain. Other OTC drugs in this group are aspirin, ibuprofen, and naproxen sodium.

It is not known exactly how NSAIDs work. However, part of their action may be due to an ability to inhibit the body's production of a hormone called prostaglandin as well as other body chemicals (e.g., cyclooxygenase, lipoxygenase, leukotrienes, lysosomal enzymes) that sensitize pain receptors and stimulate the inflammatory response. NSAIDs are generally quickly absorbed into the bloodstream, and pain and fever relief usually occurs within 1 hour of taking the first dose. The anti-inflammatory effect of these agents generally takes longer to work (several days to 2 weeks) and may take a month or more to reach maximum effect.

Ketoprofen has a mechanism of action very similar to those of ibuprofen and naproxen sodium. It begins to work within 1 to 2 hours after it is taken and its pain-relieving effects last for approximately 3 to 4 hours.

Ketoprofen is available by brand name in caplet and tablet form.

Cautions and Warnings

Do not take ketoprofen for more than 10 consecutive days or, in the presence of fever, 3 days, unless directed by your doctor. Notify your doctor if this product does not relieve your symptoms in that time.

Do not exceed the recommended daily dosage of ketoprofen.

Ketoprofen can cause gastrointestinal (GI) bleeding, ulcers, and stomach perforation. This can occur at any time, with or without warning, in people who take this drug for a long period of time. People with a history of active GI bleedings should be cautious about taking any NSAID. Minor stomach upset, distress, or gas is common during the first few days of ketoprofen treatment. If you develop bleeding or ulcers, you should be aware of the risk of developing more serious drug toxicity.

Do not take acetaminophen or aspirin or any other NSAID, or any product containing them, while taking ketoprofen.

Ketoprofen can make you drowsy. Be careful when driving a motor vehicle or operating heavy machinery.

To avoid stomach irritation, don't lie down for 15 to 30 minutes after you take ketoprofen.

If you develop stomach pain, blurred vision, or any new, unusual, or unexpected symptoms while taking ketoprofen, call your doctor.

Consult your doctor if your pain or fever gets worse while you are taking ketoprofen or if the painful area becomes red or swollen.

People with a history of asthma attacks brought on by an NSAID, iodides, or aspirin should not take ketoprofen.

If you usually drink 3 or more alcoholic beverages a day, consult your doctor before taking ketoprofen.

Ketoprofen can have damaging effects on the kidneys. It may increase blood levels of urea nitrogen and serum creatinine and may also lead to sodium and water retention; these effects are especially dangerous in patients with existing kidney damage or congestive heart failure. However, the risk of kidney damage is low with usual OTC doses, unless you are a high-risk patient with pre-existing renal disease or you take the drug for prolonged periods of time. This may be more likely to occur in older people and in those with high blood pressure, diuretic use, diabetes, and/or atherosclerotic heart disease. If you have any of these conditions, you should not take ketoprofen without first consulting your doctor.

Ketoprofen can affect platelets and blood clotting at high doses, and should be avoided by people with clotting problems and by those taking warfarin, an anticoagulant (blood-thinning) drug.

Possible Side Effects

▼ Most common: stomach upset or irritation, diarrhea, nausea, vomiting, constipation, stomach gas, and loss of appetite.

▼ Less common: stomach ulcers, GI bleeding, hepatitis, gallbladder attacks, painful urination, poor kidney function, kidney inflammation, blood and protein in the urine, dizziness, fainting, nervousness, depression, hallucinations, confusion, disorientation, lightheadedness, tingling in the hands or feet, itching, increased sweating, dry nose and mouth, heart palpitations, chest pain, difficulty breathing, and muscle cramps.

▼ Rare: severe allergic reactions, including closing of the throat, fever and chills, headache, visual disturbances, swelling in the hands or feet, changes in liver function, jaundice, and kidney failure. If you experience any of these effects, or if you develop a severe skin reaction, see your doctor or go to a hospital emergency room immediately.

Drug Interactions

• If you are currently taking an anticoagulant (blood-thinning) drug, such as warfarin, you should not take ketoprofen without first consulting your doctor. Ketoprofen can increase the risk of bleeding if taken with an anticoagulant.

Ketoprofen may work against the effects of drugs taken to lower blood pressure, including diuretics, angiotensin-converting enzyme (ACE) inhibitors, beta blockers, and others. If you are taking any of these drugs along with ketoprofen, your dose of the blood-pressure-lowering drug may need to be reduced. Acetaminophen may be a good alternative analgesic for you.

When probenicid, an antigout medication, is taken with ketoprofen, concentrations of ketoprofen in the blood are increased. These drugs should not be taken together.

Do not take ketoprofen if you are taking lithium without checking with your doctor.

Ketoprofen can increase the toxicity of methotrexate, which is used to treat cancer, severe psoriasis, severe rheumatoid arthritis, and to induce abortion. Do not take ketoprofen or other NSAIDs if you are taking methotrexate without first checking with your doctor.

Food Interactions

If ketoprofen upsets your stomach, take it with meals or with milk. You can also take an antacid containing aluminum hydroxide or magnesium hydroxide.

Usual Dose

Adult (age 16 and over): 12.5 mg every 6–8 hours; a second 12.5-mg dose can be taken 1 hour after your initial dose. Some people may feel better with an initial 25-mg dose, but it is recommended that you take the smallest effective dose. Do not take more than 25 mg in any 4–6-hour period, or more than 75 mg in 24 hours.

To prevent menstrual cramps as well as relieve the pain associated with menstruation, it is best to take ketoprofen on a schedule rather than only when you feel pain. A 12.5- to 25-mg dose can be taken every 4–8 hours for the first 48–72 hours after your period begins. Do not take more than 25 mg in any 4–6 hour period, or more than 75 mg in 24 hours.

If you forget to take a dose of ketoprofen, do so as soon as you remember. If it is almost time for your next dose, skip the one you forgot and continue with your regular schedule. Do not take a double dose.

Child (under age 16): not recommended.

Overdosage

Do the following in case of accidental overdose: If the victim is unconscious or having convulsions, call for an ambulance immediately. If you take the victim to an emergency room, be sure to bring the bottle or container with you. If the victim is conscious, call your local poison control center or a health care professional. The poison control center may suggest inducing vomiting with ipecac syrup (available without a prescription at any pharmacy). DO NOT induce vomiting unless specifically instructed to do so.

Special Populations

Allergies

People who are allergic to aspirin or to any other NSAID should not take ketoprofen.

The tablet form of OTC ketoprofen contains the dye tartrazine, which may cause allergic reactions in some people, especially those who are allergic to aspirin. If you have any doubts, consult your doctor.

Pregnancy/Breast-feeding

There are no adequate or well-controlled studies of ketoprofen in pregnant women. Unless your doctor specifically directs you to do so, it is not recommended that ketoprofen be taken during pregnancy. This is especially important during the last 3 months of pregnancy; if ketoprofen is taken during this time, it may cause problems in the unborn child or complications during delivery.

Ketoprofen may pass into breast milk. Nursing mothers either should not take this drug, or should bottle-feed their babies with formula while taking it.

Infants/Children

Ketoprofen should not be taken by children younger than age 16 unless directed by a doctor.

Seniors

Because they usually have decreased kidney function, older adults may be more susceptible to the side effects of ketoprofen and may need to take a lower dose.

Generic Name

Lactulose (LACK-too-loes)

Definition

A white powder which is also available commercially as a sweet, viscous, yellow syrup. Lactulose is a disaccharide (complex sugar) made of the sugars fructose and galactose in equal parts. Lactulose is useful as a laxative in adult and geriatric patients because it reduces the ammonia in the colon, causing an increase of water in stools. Softer stools usually occur 24 to 48 hours after administration. In patients with chronic constipation, lactulose increases the number of bowel movements per day and the number of days bowel movements occur. While lactulose is an effective laxative, it is generally no more effective than milk of magnesia.

Generic Name

Lanolin (LAN-oe-lin)

Definition

A fatty substance obtained from sheep's wool, used as a skin protectant in OTC diaper rash ointments and hemorrhoid relief products. Lanolin protects the skin from coming in contact with fecal material and thus reduces itching, burning, and irritation. It is also an ingredient in many moisturizing products for dry skin. People who are allergic to lanolin may be able to tolerate products formulated with refined lanolin (check the product label).

Generic Name

Lidocaine Hydrochloride
(LYE-doe-kane HYE-droe-KLOR-ide)

Brand Names

Bactine First Aid
Banana Boat Sooth-A-Caine
Burn-O-Jel
Burnamycin
DermaFlex
Family Medic
Gold Bond Medicated Anti-Itch

Medi-Quik First Aid
Neosporin Plus Maximum Strength
No More
*Solarcaine Aloe Extra Burn Relief
Unguentine Plus
Xylocaine

Not all products in this brand-name group contain lidocaine HCl.

Type of Drug

Topical anesthetic.

Used for

Temporary relief of pain and itching from minor cuts and burns, insect bites, hemorrhoids, and minor skin irritations.

General Information

Topical anesthetics work by blocking pain signals in the skin and keeping them from traveling along the nerves to the brain. The duration of pain relief from OTC anesthetics for skin conditions is often short, lasting only 15 to 45 minutes. However, these medications should be applied only 3 or 4 times a day. Consequently, they will not always provide around-the-clock relief.

Lidocaine is one of 2 topical anesthetics most often used in OTC medicines; the other is benzocaine. Lidocaine is found in a variety of OTC products, including burn and sunburn treatments (liquids, gels, sprays, and creams), hemorrhoid treatments (creams, foams, and ointments), and products for treatment of insect bites and stings (sprays and creams).

Lidocaine is available in concentrations ranging from 0.5% to 4%. Higher concentrations of this drug are preferred for skin that is intact, and lower doses are better for skin that is broken or cut.

Cautions and Warnings

Do not use lidocaine for more than 4 consecutive weeks. If your symptoms persist or worsen within 7 days, discontinue using the drug and contact your doctor.

Do not exceed the recommended daily dosage of lidocaine.

Less than 1% of people using lidocaine products will experience an allergic reaction. However, using the product more often or in higher amounts than recommended increases the risk of developing an allergic reaction or internal side effects. The risk of systemic effects is higher with lidocaine than with benzocaine. Serious reactions are rare if the product is used properly (on small areas of intact skin for short periods of time).

These products are for external use only.

Topical anesthetics should not be used for serious burns or puncture wounds, which need more appropriate medical attention.

Lidocaine should not be used near the eyes or nose or applied to large areas of the body.

If the product is being used for relief of the discomfort of external hemorrhoids and increased pain or bleeding occurs, discontinue the use of the product and contact your doctor.

Topical anesthetics for hemorrhoid treatment should be used only in the anal area. Do not insert the product into the rectum, because there is a risk that too much of the drug can be absorbed, which can cause toxicity.

Do not use products containing lidocaine if you are allergic to any other ingredient the formulation contains.

Possible Side Effects

▼ Rare: rash, hives, and localized swelling. Should these symptoms develop, wash the area thoroughly with soap and water and discontinue use of the medication.

Topical application of anesthetics can cause temporary burning or stinging in sensitive individuals.

Drug Interactions

• The breakdown of lidocaine in the body can be affected by treatment with cimetidine, used for treating peptic ulcers, heartburn, and acid ingestion.

Usual Dose

Pain Relief

Adult and Child (age 2 and over): Apply 3–4 times a day or as directed by your doctor. The affected area should be cleansed and dried thoroughly before application of the medication. Apply a thin layer to extend to the edges of the inflammation. Pain relief should be felt within a few minutes.

Child (under age 2): Consult a doctor.

Hemorrhoid Product

Adult and Child (age 2 and over): Apply up to 6 times a day or after each bowel movement. Follow package directions for the specific product you are using.

Child (under age 2): not recommended unless directed by a doctor.

Overdosage

There is a possibility of an internal reaction with excessive use of lidocaine. Do not use these products in large quantities, especially on scraped or blistered skin. If a wound is sufficiently large or painful to require a high amount of the drug, the condition should be treated by a doctor.

Even if the victim is not displaying any of the symptoms listed above, do the following in case of accidental ingestion: If the victim is unconscious or having convulsions, call for an ambulance immediately. If you take the victim to an emergency room, be sure to bring the bottle or container with you. If the victim is conscious, call your local poison control center or a health care professional. The poison control center may suggest inducing vomiting with ipecac syrup (available without a prescription at any pharmacy). DO NOT induce vomiting unless specifically instructed to do so.

Special Populations

Pregnancy/Breast-feeding

It is not generally recommended that pregnant women take any drugs, particularly during the first 3 months after conception. Check with your doctor if you are or might be pregnant, or if you are breast-feeding.

If you experience dry, sore, or cracked nipple tissues while breast-feeding, do not use an OTC anesthetic except on advice from a physician. There is a chance the infant could accidentally ingest the medication during feeding.

Infants/Children

Children under age 2 should not use OTC topical anesthetics except under a doctor's supervision.

Children treated with lidocaine should be instructed not to put the affected area in the mouth to avoid accidental ingestion of the anesthetic.

Seniors
Seniors should exercise the same caution as younger adults when using lidocaine.

Generic Name

Loperamide Hydrochloride

(loe-PER-uh-mide HYE-droe-KLOR-ide)

Brand Names

Diar Aid
Imodium A-D
Kaodene A-D
Maalox Anti-Diarrheal
Pepto Diarrhea Control

Type of Drug

Antidiarrheal.

Used for

Control and symptomatic relief of acute diarrhea, including traveler's diarrhea.

General Information

The average, healthy individual defecates anywhere from 3 times a day to 3 times a week. Diarrhea is characterized by abnormal frequency or consistency of stool and can be caused by any one of several conditions, either gastrointestinal (GI) or non-GI. These include bacterial and viral infections, food intolerance, gastroenteritis, and drug adverse effects. The cause of the diarrhea determines which drug therapy is best.

It should be emphasized that diarrhea is a symptom. Antidiarrheal medications provide symptomatic relief, which is generally sufficient for the treatment of temporary, uncomplicated diarrhea, such as that caused by an allergic reaction to dairy products. Persistent or recurrent diarrhea, however, can be a sign of a more serious condition requiring the attention of a health care professional and treatment geared toward the underlying condition. Persistent diarrhea can also lead to dehydration. Using loperamide or another antidiarrheal does not preclude the fluid, electrolyte, and nutritional therapies necessary for the treatment of more serious, chronic diarrhea.

Loperamide works by slowing intestinal motility (the intestine's ability to move spontaneously), thus prolonging the transit time of intestinal contents. This action reduces the volume of fecal matter, increases the stool's viscosity (gummy consistency) and bulk, and reduces the loss of fluids and electrolytes. Loperamide also lessens the cramping caused by diarrhea. There is little scientific evidence proving that loperamide reduces the duration of diarrhea, except with regard to traveler's diarrhea. Loperamide generally provides relief, however, and is generally well tolerated. It is thus recommended by many health care professionals for the treatment of acute diarrhea.

Generic loperamide is available in caplet form; brand-name products are available in caplet and liquid forms.

Cautions and Warnings

Do not use loperamide for more than 2 days unless directed by your doctor.

Do not exceed the maximum daily dosage of loperamide.

Uncomplicated, acute diarrhea usually improves within 24 to 48 hours. Persistent diarrhea can lead to dehydration, which may require the administration of appropriate fluid and electrolyte therapy.

Do not take loperamide if your diarrhea is accompanied by high fever (higher than 101°F), if there is blood or mucus in your stool, or if you have had a rash or other allergic reaction to this medication. Call your doctor if fever develops while using loperamide.

Talk to your doctor before using this product if you are taking antibiotics or if you have a history of liver disease.

Do not use loperamide to treat diarrhea caused by certain infections (for example, infections caused by salmonella or shigella) or diarrhea associated with antibiotic-related colitis.

Use loperamide with caution if you have been diagnosed with acute ulcerative colitis.

Loperamide should not be used by individuals in whom constipation must be avoided.

Possible Side Effects

- ▼ Common: constipation, drowsiness, dizziness, fatigue, dry mouth, abdominal pain, distention (swelling), or discomfort, and nausea and vomiting. It should be noted that several of these effects are difficult to distinguish from characteristics normally associated with diarrhea.
- ▼ Children may be more sensitive than adults to adverse central nervous system (CNS) effects.

Drug Interactions

None known.

Food Interactions

None known.

Usual Dose

Adult and Child (age 12 and over): 4 mg after the first loose bowel movement, followed by 2 mg after each subsequent loose bowel movement. Do not exceed the maximum daily dosage of 8 mg.

Child (age 9–11): 2 mg after the first loose bowel movement, followed by 1 mg after each subsequent bowel movement. Do not exceed the maximum daily dosage of 6 mg.

Child (age 6–8): 2 mg after the first loose bowel movement, followed by 1 mg after each subsequent bowel movement. Do not exceed the maximum daily dosage of 4 mg.

Child (under age 6): not recommended unless directed by a doctor.

Do not take this product for more than 2 days.

Be sure to drink plenty of clear liquids to help prevent dehydration, which may accompany diarrhea.

Overdosage

Overdosage of loperamide may result in constipation, CNS depression, and nausea.

Even if the victim is not displaying any of the symptoms listed above, do the following in case of accidental overdose: If the victim is unconscious or having convulsions, call for an ambulance immediately. If you take the victim to an emergency room, be sure to bring the bottle or container with you. If the victim is conscious, call your local poison control center or a health care professional. The poison control center may suggest inducing vomiting with ipecac syrup (available without a prescription at any pharmacy). DO NOT induce vomiting unless specifically instructed to do so.

Special Populations

Allergies

Hypersensitivity reactions, including rash, have been reported after use of loperamide. Do not take this product if you have ever had an unusual or allergic reaction to it.

Pregnancy/Breast-feeding

It is not generally recommended that pregnant women take any drugs, particularly during the first 3 months after conception. Check with your doctor before taking loperamide if you are or might be pregnant, or if you are breast-feeding. Also consult your doctor regarding fluid and electrolyte management if you are suffering from diarrhea.

Infants/Children

Antidiarrheal drugs should not be used without the concurrent use of fluid and electrolyte management and nutritional therapy. Infants and children are at particular risk for severe and possibly dangerous dehydration and electrolyte imbalance when they are struck with diarrhea—acute as well as chronic. Antidiarrheal medications in general have not been shown to be especially effective in children.

Loperamide should be used with particular caution due to a variability of response to this medication among infants and young children. This product should not be used in children under 6 unless directed by a doctor.

Children may be more sensitive to the possible CNS adverse effects of loperamide than adults.

Seniors

Seniors should generally exercise the same caution as younger adults when using loperamide. If, in addition to diarrhea, you are suffering from other ailments that make you weak, it may be beneficial to consult your physician regarding fluid and electrolyte management.

Generic Name

Magaldrate (MAG-uhl-drate)

Brand Names

Losopan
Riopan

Type of Drug

Antacid.

Used for

Relief of heartburn, sour stomach, acid indigestion.

General Information

Magaldrate is a chemical mixture of the antacids magnesium hydroxide and aluminum hydroxide. Magnesium hydroxide and aluminum hydroxide are each used separately as single-ingredient products. They are also physically combined in several commercial products.

All antacids work in the same way, by neutralizing gastric acid. However, they differ in potency: Magnesium hydroxide and aluminum hydroxide, separately, are less potent than the antacids calcium carbonate and sodium bicarbonate. Magaldrate is less potent than a physical mixture of magnesium hydroxide and aluminum hydroxide (e.g., Maalox liquid). The higher the potency of an antacid, the less of it you will need to take to achieve the desired effect.

Antacids also vary according to adverse effects and drug interactions, as well as onset and duration of action. The main adverse effect associated with magnesium hydroxide is diarrhea; with aluminum hydroxide, constipation. Both of these side effects are dose-related. By combining magnesium hydroxide and aluminum hydroxide, high potency is achieved with low doses of each antacid, thus lessening the chances of side effects. It is also hoped that the diarrheal and constipating effects will cancel each other out. However, diarrhea is still reported in individuals taking combinations of magnesium hydroxide and aluminum hydroxide, but constipation is rarely reported.

How long an antacid product works depends on how long it remains in the stomach. In general, an antacid taken on an empty stomach leaves the stomach rapidly and works for only 20 to 40 minutes. However, when taken after a meal, it leaves the stomach more slowly. When taken 1 hour after a meal, an antacid can work for up to 3 hours.

Magaldrate is available by brand name in liquid form.

Cautions and Warnings

Do not take the maximum daily dosage of magaldrate for more than 2 weeks continuously except under a doctor's supervision. Antacids may relieve symptoms of a serious condition such as peptic ulcer disease. If you take an antacid for a prolonged period, you run the risk of unknowingly masking symptoms of a serious gastrointestinal (GI) disease and delaying diagnosis.

Do not exceed the recommended daily dosage of magaldrate.

Call your doctor if you do not get relief from magaldrate, or if your stool is black or tarry, which may indicate bleeding in the intestines or stomach. These may be signs of a serious GI disorder that cannot and should not be treated with an OTC product without your doctor's supervision.

Because some of the magnesium and aluminum in magnesium hydroxide and aluminum hydroxide, the components of magaldrate, is absorbed into the bloodstream and then eliminated through the kidneys, people with impaired kidney function should not use magaldrate. Such people are at high risk for magnesium toxicity, which can lead to nausea, vomiting, hypotension (abnormally low blood pressure), slowed heart rate, urinary retention, decreased muscle reflexes, central nervous system depression (sedation, coma), changes in breathing, or other life-threatening complications. In addition, excretion of aluminum is decreased during long-term use and the aluminum may accumulate in bones, lungs, and brain tissue.

Excessive amounts of aluminum taken for prolonged periods can lead to low blood phosphate levels, which are characterized by loss of appetite, malaise, and muscle weakness.

Avoid magaldrate if you have any conditions (e.g., decreased bowel mobility, dehydration, fluid restriction) or are taking any medications (e.g., narcotic analgesics) that may predispose you to bowel obstruction.

Possible Side Effects

Although in theory the constipating effect of aluminum hydroxide should balance the diarrheal effect of magnesium hydroxide, diarrhea has been reported in individuals taking magnesium-aluminum combination products. The same may be true for magaldrate.

Drug Interactions

• There is the potential for magaldrate to cause any of the drug interactions associated with its 2 components, magnesium hydroxide and aluminum hydroxide.

• Magnesium hydroxide and aluminum hydroxide both decrease the absorption of the following drugs, reducing their effect: tetracycline antibiotics; quinolone antibiotics, such as ciprofloxacin; indomethacin, a nonsteroidal anti-inflammatory drug (NSAID); digoxin, used to treat congestive heart failure; and iron. Magnesium hydroxide also decreases the absorption of phenytoin, an anticonvulsant, and dexamethasone, a corticosteroid. Aluminum hydroxide also decreases the absorption of allopurinol, an antigout medication; nitrofurantoin, an antibiotic; isoniazid, used to treat tuberculosis; cimetidine and ranitidine, used to treat peptic ulcers, heartburn, and acid indigestion; and ketoconazole, an antifungal agent; and it may decrease the bioavailability of the beta blocker atenolol, used to treat high blood pressure. If you are taking magaldrate at the same time as any of these drugs, separate your dose of each drug by at least 2 hours; with quinolone antibiotics, 4 to 6 hours is preferable.

• Magnesium hydroxide and aluminum hydroxide both increase the absorption of the anticonvulsant valproic acid, creating the potential for valproic acid toxicity. Aluminum hydroxide also increases the absorption of the benzodiazepine diazepam, increasing its sedative effect. If you are taking valproic acid or diazepam, consult you doctor before taking magaldrate.

• Magnesium hydroxide decreases the elimination of the antiarrhythmic quinidine, raising the serum concentration of quinidine. Toxicity has been reported. Do not take magaldrate if you are taking quinidine unless prescribed by your doctor.

• Concurrent use of magnesium hydroxide with sodium polystyrene sulfonate, a potassium remover, may be dangerous. Separate your dose of each drug by at least 2 hours.

• Aluminum hydroxide increases the body's elimination of aspirin and other salicylates, reducing their effect. Conversely, it increases the absorption of enteric-coated and buffered aspirin.

Food Interactions

Magaldrate is best taken after meals (see "General Information").

Usual Dose

Adult and Child (age 12 and over): 1–2 tsps. 1–3 hours after meals and at bedtime as needed. Do not exceed the recommended daily dosage specified on the package. Follow your dose with water. Shake magaldrate suspension well prior to use.

Child (under age 12): not recommended.

Overdosage

Do the following in case of accidental overdose: If the victim is unconscious or having convulsions, call for an ambulance immediately. If you take the victim to an emergency room, be sure to bring the bottle or container with you. If the victim is conscious, call your local poison control center or a health care professional. The poison control center may suggest inducing vomiting with ipecac syrup (available without a prescription at any pharmacy). DO NOT induce vomiting unless specifically instructed to do so.

Storage Instructions

Magaldrate may be stored at room temperature, but refrigeration improves its taste. Do not freeze magaldrate.

Special Populations

Pregnancy/Breast-feeding

Antacids can be safely taken in small doses for short periods of time during pregnancy and while breast-feeding.

However, it is not generally recommended that pregnant women take any drugs, particularly during the first 3 months after conception. Check with your doctor before self-medicating with magaldrate if you are or might be pregnant, or if you are breast-feeding.

Infants/Children

The safety of antacid use in infants and children has not been established. Children under age 12 should not be given magaldrate unless directed by a doctor.

Seniors

Seniors may safely take antacids. However, be advised that many older patients are at high risk for complications from ulcers, yet often do not show classic ulcer symptoms. You may want to discuss with your pharmacist the possible causes of your gastric discomfort before self-medicating with an antacid. Be aware of possible interactions with other medications you may be taking.

Seniors may be more likely than younger adults to have diarrhea caused by magnesium hydroxide, one of the components of magaldrate. Do not use magaldrate if you have decreased kidney function (see "Cautions and Warnings").

Generic Name

Magnesium Carbonate

(mag-NEE-zee-uhm KAR-bon-ate)

Brand Names

†Gaviscon
†Maalox
Marblen

†*Consult the OTC ingredient charts to determine whether different formulations in this brand-name group are alcohol-, caffeine-, or sugar-free.*

Type of Drug

Antacid.

Used for

Relief of heartburn, sour stomach, and acid indigestion.

General Information

All antacids work in the same way, by neutralizing gastric acid. However, they differ in potency: Magnesium antacids such as magnesium carbonate are more potent than aluminum antacids, but less potent than calcium carbonate and sodium bicarbonate. The higher the potency of an antacid, the less of it you will need to take to achieve the desired effect.

Antacids also vary according to adverse effects and drug interactions, as well as onset and duration of action. Magnesium antacids dissolve quickly in stomach acid and provide a rapid effect, unlike aluminum antacids, which dissolve more slowly in stomach acid and may take up to 30 minutes to begin working.

How long an antacid product works depends on how long it remains in the stomach. Magnesium antacids have a shorter duration of action than aluminum antacids and calcium carbonate. In general, an antacid taken on an empty stomach leaves the stomach rapidly and works for only 20 to 40 minutes. However, when taken after a meal, it leaves the stomach more slowly. When taken 1 hour after a meal, an antacid can work for up to 3 hours.

Magnesium carbonate is 1 of 4 types of magnesium antacid; the others are magnesium hydroxide, magnesium oxide, and magnesium trisilicate. Magnesium hydroxide is the most potent of the group.

Magnesium carbonate is commercially available in combination with either calcium carbonate or aluminum hydroxide.

Cautions and Warnings

Do not take the maximum daily dosage of magnesium carbonate for more than 2 weeks continuously except under a doctor's supervision. Antacids may relieve symptoms of a serious condition such as peptic ulcer disease. If you take an antacid for a prolonged period, you run the risk of unknowingly masking the symptoms of a serious gastrointestinal (GI) disease and delaying diagnosis.

Do not exceed the recommended daily dosage of magnesium carbonate.

Call your doctor if you do not get relief from magnesium carbonate, or if your stool is black or tarry or looks like coffee grounds, which indicates bleeding in the intestines or stomach. These may be signs of a serious GI disorder that cannot and should not be treated with an OTC product without your doctor's supervision .

Frequent use of magnesium carbonate alone (as opposed to in combination with an aluminum antacid) can cause diarrhea, which may lead to fluid and electrolyte imbalances.

Because some of the magnesium is absorbed into the bloodstream and eliminated through the kidneys, people with impaired kidney function should not use magnesium carbonate. Such people are at high risk for magnesium toxicity, which can lead to muscle paralysis, severe hypotension (abnormally low blood pressure), respiratory depression, and other life-threatening complications.

Possible Side Effect

▼ Most common: diarrhea.

Drug Interactions

• Magnesium carbonate decreases the absorption of the following drugs, reducing their effect: tetracycline antibiotics; quinolone antibiotics, such as ciprofloxacin; phenytoin, an anticonvulsant; dexamethasone, a corticosteroid; indomethacin, a nonsteroidal anti-inflammatory drug (NSAID); digoxin, used to treat congestive heart failure; and iron. If you are taking magnesium carbonate at the same time as any of these drugs, separate your dose of each drug by at least 2 hours; with quinolone antibiotics, 4 to 6 hours is preferable.

• Magnesium carbonate increases the absorption of the anticonvulsant valproic acid, creating the potential for valproic acid toxicity. If you are taking valproic acid, consult your doctor before taking magnesium carbonate.

• Magnesium carbonate decreases the elimination of the antiarrhythmic quinidine, raising the serum concentration of quinidine. Toxicity has been reported. If you are taking quinidine, consult your doctor before taking magnesium carbonate.

• Concurrent use of magnesium carbonate with sodium polystyrene sulfonate, a potassium remover, may be dangerous. Separate your dose of each drug by at least 2 hours.

Food Interactions

Magnesium carbonate is best taken after meals (see "General Information").

Usual Dose

Adult and Child (age 12 and over): Take magnesium carbonate as symptoms occur, but do not exceed the recommended daily dosage specified on the package.

Child (under age 12): not recommended.

Overdosage

Do the following in case of accidental overdose: If the victim is unconscious or having convulsions, call for an ambulance immediately. If you take the victim to an emergency room, be sure to bring the bottle or container with you. If the victim is conscious, call your local poison control center or a health care professional. The poison control center may suggest inducing vomiting with ipecac syrup (available without a prescription at any pharmacy). DO NOT induce vomiting unless specifically instructed to do so.

Special Information

Patients with a history of constipation or hemorrhoids may choose magnesium carbonate over other antacids because it can cause diarrhea. Diarrhea associated with magnesium carbonate, unlike diarrhea brought on by other causes, does not necessarily cause stomach cramps or nocturnal bowel movements.

Because aluminum antacids may cause constipation, they are often taken concurrently with magnesium carbonate to regulate bowel function.

Special Populations

Pregnancy/Breast-feeding

It is not generally recommended that pregnant women take any drugs, particularly during the first 3 months after conception. However, antacids can be safely taken in small doses for short periods of time during pregnancy and while breast-feeding. However, check with your doctor before using magnesium carbonate if you are or might be pregnant, or if you are breast-feeding.

Infants/Children

The safety of antacid use in infants and children has not been established. Children under age 12 should not be given magnesium carbonate unless directed by a doctor.

Seniors

Seniors may safely take antacids. However, be advised that many older patients are at high risk for complications from ulcers, yet often do not show classic ulcer symptoms. You may want to discuss with your pharmacist the possible causes of your gastric discomfort before self-medicating with an antacid and possibly delaying diagnosis of an ulcer. Be aware of possible interactions with other medications you may be taking.

Seniors may be more likely than younger adults to have diarrhea caused by magnesium carbonate. However, because constipation is a common complaint in this age group, magnesium carbonate may be a good choice, as long as the senior doesn't have severe kidney impairment.

Generic Name

Magnesium Citrate

(mag-NEE-zee-um SYE-trate)

Brand Name

Evac-Q-Kwik Liquid
*†Fleet

**Not all products in this brand-name group contain magnesium citrate.*

†*Consult the OTC ingredient charts to determine whether different formulations in this brand-name group are alcohol-, caffeine-, or sugar-free.*

Type of Drug

Laxative.

Used for

Relief of occasional constipation (irregularity).

General Information

The average, healthy individual defecates anywhere from 3 times a day to 3 times a week. Constipation is determined not necessarily by the frequency of bowel movements, but by the consistency of the stool, how difficult it is to eliminate, and other symptoms associated with constipation, such as dull headache, low back pain, and abdominal distention (swelling). Evaluate your condition carefully and discuss your symptoms and their possible causes with your pharmacist before taking a laxative. Laxatives are not always necessary, and when used improperly can either prevent the desired effect or result in laxative dependency. If you are indeed constipated, your condition may be best managed through proper diet, adequate fluid intake, and exercise. If you must use a laxative, choose the mildest effective product.

Laxatives may be classified by their mechanism of action: bulk forming, emollient (stool softeners), lubricant, saline, hyperosrnotic, and stimulant. Magnesium citrate is a saline laxative, which works by drawing water into the small intestine and increasing pressure and intestinal motility (ability to move spontaneously). Saline laxatives generally produce a bowel movement in 3 to 6 hours, or less. They are recommended for use when immediate and complete evacuation of the bowel is required; they are not recommended for the long-term management of constipation.

Magnesium citrate is available by generic and brand name in liquid form. It is also combined with bisacodyl, a stimulant laxative, in commercial enemas and suppositories.

Cautions and Warnings

Do not use magnesium citrate for more than 7 days, unless directed by your doctor. Long-term use of laxatives has been linked with laxative dependence, chronic constipation, and loss of normal bowel function. Using laxatives too frequently can result in persistent diarrhea, hypokalemia (abnormally low potassium in the blood), loss of essential nutritional factors, and dehydration.

Do not exceed the recommended daily dosage of magnesium citrate.

Do not take magnesium citrate if you have abdominal pain, nausea, vomiting, or kidney disease, unless directed by your doctor.

If you notice a sudden change in bowel habits lasting for more than 2 weeks, do not take magnesium citrate until you have spoken to your doctor. Also contact your doctor if there is blood in your stool, so that colon cancer or other significant disease can be ruled out before you begin self-medication with this product.

If you have had a disease or surgery affecting the gastrointestinal (GI) tract, using a laxative may affect your condition adversely.

If you have rectal bleeding after using magnesium citrate, or if you do not have a bowel movement after 7 days of using the product, you may have a serious condition. Stop using the product and call your doctor.

Laxatives may decrease the absorption of other drugs that pass through the GI tract (see "Drug Interactions").

Because some of the magnesium, when magnesium citrate is taken orally, is absorbed into the bloodstream and eliminated by the kidneys, people with impaired kidney function should not use magnesium citrate. Such people are at high risk for magnesium toxicity, which can lead to muscle paralysis, severe hypotension (abnormally low blood pressure), respiratory depression, and other life-threatening complications.

Possible Side Effects

▼ Most common: abdominal cramping, increased urination, nausea, vomiting, and dehydration.

Drug Interactions

• All laxatives potentially decrease the absorption of any oral drug taken at the same time. If you are currently taking an oral medication, talk to your pharmacist before taking magnesium citrate.

Food Interactions

None known.

Usual Dose

Doses should be adjusted to individual usage. In general, saline laxatives should be taken at infrequent intervals. Do not exceed the recommended daily dosage.

Be sure to follow your dose with a full glass (8 oz.) of liquid.

Adult and Child (age 12 and over): 240 ml once daily.

Child (age 6–11): 0.5 ml/kg once daily.

Child (under age 2): not recommended unless directed by a doctor.

Overdosage

Overdose with magnesium citrate can cause hypermagnesemia (an accumulation of magnesium in the blood), which may be characterized by muscle weakness, sedation, and confusion.

Even if the victim is not displaying any of the symptoms listed above, do the following in case of accidental overdose: If the victim is unconscious or having convulsions, call for an ambulance immediately. If you take the victim to an emergency room, be sure to bring the bottle or container with you. If the victim is conscious, call your local poison control center or a health care professional. The poison control center may suggest inducing vomiting with ipecac syrup (available without a prescription at any pharmacy). DO NOT induce vomiting unless specifically instructed to do so.

Storage Instructions

Magnesium citrate can be stored at room temperature, but may be refrigerated to improve the taste. Do not freeze it.

Special Populations

Pregnancy/Breast-feeding

Saline laxatives such as magnesium citrate can be absorbed into the mother's GI tract; both pregnant and nursing mothers should avoid using them. Toxicity with magnesium citrate could cause diarrhea, drowsiness, or respiratory difficulty. Only bulk-forming or emollient laxatives are recommended for pregnant women. Consider talking to your doctor about diet and mild exercise in the management of constipation.

Infants/Children

Observe your child carefully for patterns of bowel movements and the pain or difficulty with which the bowel movements are made before deciding whether the child is actually constipated. As with adults, "normal" bowel habits vary in children. If your child is indeed constipated, increasing fluid intake and adding fiber to his or her diet may be ways to manage the condition. In general, the use of laxatives should be avoided in children.

Children age 2 and over may be given magnesium citrate in smaller doses than those taken by adults. For children under age 2, consult a doctor.

Seniors

Seniors commonly experience constipation, and consequently may become laxative-dependent. Be cautious of chronically turning to laxatives to ease constipation, and instead look to diet and increased fluid intake as therapeutic measures.

Saline laxatives such as magnesium citrate may not be the best choice for this group because they alter fluid and electrolyte balance, placing some seniors at risk for side effects. They also should not be used by seniors with severe kidney impairment, which can affect the elimination of magnesium and lead to magnesium toxicity (see "Cautions and Warnings"). Bulk-forming laxatives are usually preferred for older individuals.

Generic Name

Magnesium Gluconate

(mag-NEE-zee-um GLUE-koe-nate)

Definition

A form of gluconic acid used as a magnesium replenisher.

Generic Name

Magnesium Hydroxide

(mag-NEE-zee-um hye-DROKS-ide)

Brand Name

Di-Gel
Gelusil
Haleys M-O [A]
Kudrox
*†Maalox
Magnalox
*Mylanta
†Phillips' Milk of Magnesia
*Rolaids
Simaal
Tempo Drops

**Not all products in this brand-name group contain magnesium hydroxide.*

†Consult the OTC ingredient charts to determine whether different formulations in this brand-name group are alcohol-, caffeine-, or sugar-free.

Type of Drug

Laxative/antacid.

Used for

Relief of occasional constipation (irregularity); and relief of heartburn, sour stomach, acid indigestion.

General Information

Laxative

Magnesium hydroxide is a mild saline laxative, which works by drawing water into the small intestine, increasing pressure and intestinal motility (ability to move spontaneously). It generally produces a bowel movement in 30 minutes to 6 hours. Saline laxatives are recommended for use when immediate and complete evacuation of the bowel is required; they are not recommended for the long-term management of constipation.

Antacid

All antacids work in the same way, by neutralizing gastric acid. However, they differ in potency: Magnesium antacids such as magnesium hydroxide are more potent than aluminum antacids, but less potent than calcium carbonate and sodium bicarbonate. The higher the potency of an antacid, the less of it you will need to take to achieve the desired effect.

Magnesium antacids dissolve quickly in stomach acid and provide a rapid effect, unlike aluminum antacids, which dissolve more slowly in stomach acid and may take up to 30 minutes to begin working. How long an antacid product works depends on how long it remains in the stomach. Magnesium antacids have a shorter duration of action than aluminum antacids and calcium carbonate. In general, an antacid taken on an empty stomach leaves the stomach rapidly and works for only 20 to 40 minutes. However, when taken after a meal, it leaves the stomach more slowly. When taken 1 hour after a meal, an antacid can work for up to 3 hours.

Magnesium hydroxide is one of 4 types of magnesium antacid; the others are magnesium carbonate, magnesium oxide, and magnesium trisilicate. Magnesium hydroxide is the most potent of the group.

Laxative or Antacid

Magnesium hydroxide is available by generic or brand name in suspension (liquid) and tablet form. While the suspension is more potent than the tablet, some people do not like the taste of the liquid and also prefer the convenience of the pill form when taking multiple doses throughout the day.

Magnesium hydroxide is also available in combination products containing another antacid, aluminum hydroxide.

Cautions and Warnings

Laxative

Do not use magnesium hydroxide for more than 7 days, unless directed by your doctor. Long-term use of laxatives has been linked with laxative dependence, chronic constipation, and loss of normal bowel function. Using laxatives too frequently can result in persistent diarrhea, hypokalemia (abnormally low potassium in the blood), loss of essential nutrients, and dehydration.

Do not take magnesium hydroxide if you have abdominal pain, nausea, vomiting, or kidney disease, unless directed by your doctor.

If you notice a marked change in bowel habits lasting for more than 2 weeks, do not take magnesium hydroxide until you have spoken to your doctor. Also contact your doctor if there is blood in your stool, so that colon cancer or other significant disease can be ruled out before you begin self-medication with magnesium hydroxide.

If you have had a disease or surgery affecting the gastrointestinal (GI) tract, using a laxative may adversely affect your condition.

If you have rectal bleeding after using magnesium hydroxide, or if you do not have a bowel movement after 7 days of using the product, you may have a serious condition. Stop using the product and call your doctor.

Laxatives may decrease the absorption of other drugs that pass through the GI tract (see "Drug Interactions").

Antacid

Do not take the maximum daily dosage for more than 2 weeks continuously except under a doctor's supervision. Antacids may relieve symptoms of a serious condition such as peptic ulcer disease. If you take an antacid for a prolonged period, you run the risk of unknowingly masking the symptoms of a serious GI disease and delaying diagnosis.

Call your doctor if you do not get relief from magnesium hydroxide, or if your stool is black or tarry, which indicates bleeding in the intestines or stomach. These may be signs of a serious GI disorder that cannot and should not be treated with an OTC product without your doctor's supervision.

Frequent use of magnesium hydroxide alone (as opposed to in combination with an aluminum antacid) can cause diarrhea, which may lead to fluid and electrolyte imbalances.

Laxative or Antacid

Do not exceed the recommended daily dosage of magnesium hydroxide.

Because some of the magnesium is absorbed into the bloodstream and eliminated through the kidneys, people with impaired kidney function should not use magnesium hydroxide. Such people are at high risk for magnesium toxicity, which can lead to muscle paralysis, severe hypotension (abnormally low blood pressure), respiratory depression, and other life-threatening complications.

Possible Side Effects

▼ Most common: diarrhea.

▼ Less common: abdominal cramping, increased urination, nausea, vomiting, and dehydration.

Drug Interactions

• Magnesium hydroxide, as a laxative, may decrease the absorption of any oral drug taken at the same time.

• Magnesium hydroxide decreases the absorption of the following drugs, reducing their effect: tetracycline antibiotics, quinolone antibiotics such as ciprofloxacin, isoniazid (INH), an antibiotic used to treat tuberculosis; phenytoin, an anticonvulsant; dexamethasone, a corticosteroid; indomethacin, a nonsteroidal anti-inflammatory drug (NSAID); digoxin, used to treat congestive heart failure; and iron. If you are taking magnesium hydroxide at the same time as any of these drugs, separate your dose of each drug by at least 2 hours; with quinolone antibiotics, 4 to 6 hours is preferable.

• Magnesium hydroxide increases the absorption of the anticonvulsant valproic acid, creating the potential for valproic acid toxicity. If you are taking valproic acid, consult your doctor before taking magnesium hydroxide.

• Magnesium hydroxide decreases the elimination of the antiarrhythmic quinidine, raising the serum concentration of quinidine to possibly dangerous levels. If you are taking quinidine, consult your doctor before taking magnesium hydroxide.

• Concurrent use of magnesium hydroxide with sodium polystyrene sulfonate, a potassium remover, may be dangerous. Separate your dose of each drug by at least 2 hours.

• Drugs with constipating side effects, such as tricyclic antidepressants and some calcium channel blockers (used to treat high blood pressure), may counteract the laxative effect of magnesium hydroxide when administered concurrently.

Food Interactions

When used as an antacid, magnesium hydroxide is best taken after meals (see "General Information").

Usual Dose

Laxative

Adult and Child (age 12 and over): 1–4 tbs. or 1866–2488 mg per day.

Child (age 6–11): 1–2 tbs. or 933–1244 mg per day.

Child (age 2–5): 1–3 tsp. or 311–622 mg per day.

Child (under age 2): Consult a doctor.

Be sure to follow your dose with 8 oz. of liquid.

Antacid

Adult and Child (age 12 and over): Take magnesium hydroxide as symptoms occur, but do not exceed the recommended daily dosage specified on the package. Follow your dose with water.

Child (under age 12): not recommended.

Overdosage

Do the following in case of accidental overdose: If the victim is unconscious or having convulsions, call for an ambulance immediately. If you take the victim to an emergency room, be sure to bring the bottle or container with you. If the victim is conscious, call your local poison control center or a health care professional. The poison control center may suggest inducing vomiting with ipecac syrup (available without a prescription at any pharmacy). DO NOT induce vomiting unless specifically instructed to do so.

Special Information

Patients with a history of constipation or hemorrhoids may choose magnesium hydroxide over other antacids because it can cause diarrhea. Diarrhea associated with magnesium hydroxide, unlike diarrhea brought on by other causes, does not necessarily cause stomach cramps or nocturnal bowel movements.

Because aluminum antacids may cause constipation, they are often taken with magnesium hydroxide to regulate bowel function.

Storage Instructions

The suspension form of magnesium hydroxide may be stored at room temperature, but to improve its taste, refrigerate it. Do not freeze it.

Special Populations

Pregnancy/Breast-feeding

Bulk-forming or emollient laxatives are the only laxatives recommended for pregnant women. Saline laxatives such as magnesium hydroxide can be absorbed into the mother's GI tract; both pregnant and nursing mothers should avoid using this product. Consider talking to your doctor about diet and mild exercise in the management of constipation.

Infants/Children

Laxative

Children age 2 and older may be given magnesium hydroxide as a laxative, in smaller doses than those taken by adults. For children under age 2, consult a doctor. In general, the use of laxatives should be avoided in children.

Antacid

The safety of antacid use in infants and children has not been established. Children under age 12 should not be given magnesium hydroxide as an antacid unless directed by a doctor.

Seniors

Laxative

Seniors commonly experience constipation, and consequently may become laxative-dependent. Be cautious of chronically turning to laxatives to ease constipation, and instead look to diet and increased fluid intake as therapeutic measures.

Saline laxatives such as magnesium hydroxide may not be the best choice for this group because they alter fluid and electrolyte balance, placing some seniors at risk for side effects. Bulk-forming laxatives are usually preferred for seniors.

Antacid

Seniors may safely take antacids. However, be advised that many older patients are at high risk for complications from ulcers, yet often do not show classic ulcer symptoms. Discuss with your pharmacist the possible causes of your gastric discomfort before self-medicating with an antacid and possibly delaying diagnosis of an ulcer. Be aware of possible interactions with other medications you may be taking.

Seniors may be more likely than younger adults to have diarrhea caused by magnesium hydroxide.

Generic Name

Magnesium Oxide

(mag-NEE-zee-um OKS-ide)

Definition

A form of the essential mineral magnesium used as an antacid and a mild laxative. It is often included in vitamin and mineral supplements as a source of magnesium.

Generic Name

Magnesium Salicylate

(mag-NEE-zee-um SAL-ih-SILL-ate)

Brand Names

Arthriten [S]
Backache From the Makers of Nuprin [C]
Doan's [C]
Momentum [C]
Mobigesic [S]
Pamprin Maximum Pain Relief [C]

Type of Drug

Analgesic (pain reliever) and antipyretic (fever reducer).

Used for

Temporary relief of mild to moderate pain and fever associated with the common cold, flu, viral infections, or other disorders (neuritis, neuralgia, bursitis, arthritis, rheumatism, simple headache, menstrual cramps, tooth and periodontic pain, sprains, and minor muscular aches). It may also be taken to relieve arthritis or inflammation of bones, joints, or body tissues.

General Information

Magnesium salicylate is a member of the group of drugs called salicylates. Other members of this group include aspirin, sodium salicylate, and choline salicylate. Magnesium salicylate reduces fever by causing the blood vessels in the skin to open, allowing heat to leave the body more rapidly. Magnesium salicylate's effects on pain and inflammation are thought to be related to its ability to prevent the manufacture of complex body hormones called prostaglandins.

Although magnesium salicylate has not been proven to be more effective than aspirin, it has some advantages that should be considered when choosing which pain reliever to take. Because aspirin has the greatest effect on prostaglandin production of the salicylates, it causes the strongest gastrointestinal effects; magnesium salicylate may be less irritating to the stomach. Magnesium salicylate can also be used by people who cannot tolerate the side effects associated with aspirin or who are allergic to aspirin. However, unlike aspirin, magnesium salicylate does not inhibit platelet aggregation and therefore cannot be substituted for aspirin in the prevention of heart attack or stroke. Magnesium salicylate is also more expensive than aspirin.

Magnesium salicylate is available by generic name and in combination brand-name products.

Cautions and Warnings

Do not take magnesium salicylate for more than 5 consecutive days or, in the presence of fever, 3 days, unless directed by your doctor. Notify your doctor if this product does not relieve your symptoms in that time.

Do not exceed the recommended daily dosage of magnesium salicylate.

Do not take magnesium salicylate if you have asthma.

People with chronically impaired kidney function should not use magnesium salicylate because of the risk of magnesium buildup in the body.

Stop taking this product and notify your doctor if you develop ringing in the ears or hearing loss.

Children with the flu or chicken pox who are given salicylates may develop Reye's syndrome, a life-threatening condition characterized by vomiting, progressive damage to the central nervous system, liver injury, and abnormally low blood sugar. Up to 30% of those who develop Reye's syndrome die and permanent brain damage is possible in those who survive. Because of the risk of Reye's syndrome, do not give salicylates to children under age 16. Acetaminophen can usually be substituted.

Possible Side Effects

- ▼ Most common: nausea, upset stomach, heartburn, loss of appetite, and appearance of small amounts of blood in the stool.
- ▼ Less common: hives, rashes, liver damage, fever, thirst, and difficulties with vision.

Drug Interactions

• Magnesium salicylate should not be used by individuals currently taking methotrexate, which is used to treat cancer, severe psoriasis, severe rheumatoid arthritis, and to induce abortion; or valproic acid, an anticonvulsant. It can increase the toxicity of these drugs.

• Magnesium salicylate should also not be taken with anticoagulant (blood-thinning) drugs, such as warfarin and dicumarol. It will exaggerate the effects of these drugs and increase the risk of abnormal bleeding.

• The possibility of stomach ulcer is increased if magnesium salicylate is taken together with an adrenal corticosteroid such as hydrocortisone; phenylbutazone, a nonsteroidal anti-inflammatory drug (NSAID); or alcoholic beverages.

• Magnesium salicylate will counteract the effects of the antigout medications probenicid and sulfinpyrazone and may counteract the effects of angiotensin-converting enzyme (ACE) inhibitors and beta blockers, which work to lower blood pressure.

• Magnesium salicylate can lower blood sugar, which can combine with the effects of oral sulfonylurea antidiabetes drugs, such as chlorpropamide or tolbutamide, and further suppress blood sugar levels in people with diabetes.

• Taking magnesium salicylate with an NSAID has no benefit and carries a greatly increased risk of side effects, especially stomach irritation.

Food Interactions

Take magnesium salicylate with food, milk, or water to reduce the chance of upset stomach or bleeding.

Usual Dose

Analgesic or Antipyretic

Adult (age 16 and over): initial dose 500 mg–1 g, followed by 500 mg every 4 hours, as needed. Do not take more than 3.5 g in 24 hours. Try to take the smallest possible dose that works for you.

Child (under age 16): not recommended because of the risk of Reye's syndrome (see "Cautions and Warnings").

Arthritis or Inflammation

Adult (age 16 and over): 545mg–1.2g, 3 or 4 times a day. Try to take the smallest possible dose that works for you.

Child (under age 16) : not recommended because of the risk of Reye's syndrome (see "Cautions and Warnings").

Overdosage

Do the following in case of accidental overdose: If the victim is unconscious or having convulsions, call for an ambulance immediately. If you take the victim to an emergency room, be sure to bring the bottle or container with you. If the victim is conscious, call your local poison control center or a health care professional. The poison control center may suggest inducing vomiting with ipecac syrup (available without a prescription at any pharmacy). DO NOT induce vomiting unless specifically instructed to do so.

Special Populations

Allergies

You may be able to take magnesium salicylate if you are allergic to aspirin, but check with your doctor first.

Pregnancy/Breast-feeding

Magnesium salicylate can cause bleeding problems in the developing fetus and can lead to a low-birth-weight infant; it can also cause bleeding problems in the mother before, during, or after pregnancy. Avoid magnesium salicylate if you are or might be pregnant.

Although magnesium salicylate passes into breast milk, no adverse effects have been shown to occur in the nursing infant if the drug is taken only occasionally, in low doses. Do not take magnesium salicylate on a regular basis unless it is approved by your physician. Acetaminophen may be a better choice if you are nursing.

Infants/Children

Magnesium salicylate is not recommended for use in children under age 16 because of the risk of Reye's syndrome.

Seniors

Seniors should exercise the same caution as younger adults when using magnesium salicylate.

Generic Name

Magnesium Sulfate

(mag-NEE-zee-um SULL-fate)

Brand Name

Epsom Salt
Metamucil Smooth Texture, Sugar-Free, Regular Flavor

Type of Drug

Laxative.

Used for

Relief of occasional constipation (irregularity).

General Information

The average, healthy individual defecates anywhere from 3 times a day to 3 times a week. Constipation is determined not necessarily by the frequency of bowel movements, but by the consistency of the stool, how difficult it is to eliminate, and other symptoms associated with constipation, such as dull headache, low back pain, and abdominal distention (swelling). Evaluate your condition carefully and discuss your symptoms and their possible causes with your pharmacist before taking a laxative. Laxatives are not always necessary, and when used improperly can either prevent the desired effect or result in laxative dependency. If you are indeed constipated, your condition may be best managed through proper diet, adequate fluid intake, and exercise. If you must use a laxative, choose the mildest effective product.

Laxatives may be classified by their mechanism of action: bulk forming, emollient (stool softeners), lubricant, saline, hyperosmotic, and stimulant. Magnesium sulfate is a saline laxative, which works by drawing water into the small intestine and increasing pressure and intestinal motility (ability to move spontaneously). Saline laxatives generally produce a bowel movement in 3 to 6 hours, or less. They are recommended for use when immediate and complete evacuation of the bowel is required; they are not recommended for the long-term management of constipation.

Magnesium sulfate is available by brand name in granule form.

Cautions and Warnings

Do not use magnesium sulfate for more than 7 days, unless directed by your doctor. Long-term use of laxatives has been linked with laxative dependence, chronic constipation, and loss of normal bowel function. Using laxatives too frequently can result in persistent diarrhea, hypokalemia (abnormally low potassium in the blood), loss of essential nutritional factors, and dehydration.

Do not exceed the recommended daily dosage of magnesium sulfate.

Do not take this product if you have abdominal pain, nausea, vomiting, or kidney disease, unless directed by your doctor.

If you notice a sudden change in bowel habits lasting for more than 2 weeks, do not take magnesium sulfate until you have spoken to your doctor. Also contact your doctor if there is blood in your stool, so that colon cancer or other significant disease can be ruled out before you begin self-medication with this product.

If you have had a disease or surgery affecting the gastrointestinal (GI) tract, using a laxative may affect your condition adversely.

If you have rectal bleeding after using magnesium sulfate, or if you do not have a bowel movement after several days of using the product, you may have a serious condition. Stop using the product and call your doctor.

Laxatives may decrease the absorption of other drugs that pass through the GI tract (see "Drug Interactions").

Because some of the magnesium is absorbed into the bloodstream and eliminated by the kidneys, people with impaired kidney function should not use magnesium sulfate. Such people are at high risk for magnesium toxicity, which can lead to muscle paralysis, severe hypotension (abnormally low blood pressure), respiratory depression, and other life-threatening complications.

Possible Side Effects

▼ Most common: abdominal cramping, diarrhea, nausea, vomiting, and dehydration.

Drug Interactions

• All laxatives potentially decrease the absorption of any oral drug taken at the same time. If you are currently taking an oral medication, talk to your pharmacist before taking magnesium sulfate.

Food Interactions

None known.

Usual Dose

Doses should be adjusted to individual usage. In general, saline laxatives should be taken at infrequent intervals. Do not exceed the recommended daily dosage.

Be sure to follow your dose with a full glass (8 oz.) of liquid.

Adult and Child (age 12 and over): 10–30 g once daily.

Child (age 6–11): 5–10 g once daily.

Child (age 2–5): 2.5–5 g once daily.

Child (under age 2): not recommended unless directed by a doctor.

Overdosage

Overdose with magnesium sulfate can cause hypermagnesemia (an accumulation of magnesium in the blood), which may be characterized by muscle weakness, sedation, and confusion. Overdose with this drug has been fatal in individuals with impaired kidney function.

Even if the victim is not displaying any of the symptoms listed above, do the following in case of accidental overdose: If the victim is unconscious or having convulsions, call for an ambulance immediately. If you take the victim to an emergency room, be sure to bring the bottle or container with you. If the victim is conscious, call your local poison control center or a health care professional. The poison control center may suggest inducing vomiting with ipecac syrup (available without a prescription at any pharmacy). DO NOT induce vomiting unless specifically instructed to do so.

Special Populations

Pregnancy/Breast-feeding

Saline laxatives such as magnesium sulfate can be absorbed into the mother's GI tract; both pregnant and nursing mothers should avoid using them. Toxicity with magnesium sulfate could cause diarrhea, drowsiness, or respiratory difficulty.

Only bulk-forming or emollient laxatives are recommended for pregnant women. Consider talking to your doctor about diet and mild exercise in the management of constipation.

Infants/Children

Observe your child carefully for patterns of bowel movements and the pain or difficulty with which the bowel movements are made before deciding whether the child is actually constipated. As with adults, "normal" bowel habits vary in children. If your child is indeed constipated, increasing fluid intake and adding fiber to his or her diet may be ways to manage the condition. In general, the use of laxatives should be avoided in children.

Do not give magnesium sulfate to a child under age 2 unless directed by a doctor

Seniors

Seniors commonly experience constipation, and consequently may become laxative-dependent. Be cautious of chronically turning to laxatives to ease constipation, and instead look to diet and increased fluid intake as therapeutic measures.

Saline laxatives such as magnesium sulfate may not be the best choice for this group because they alter fluid and electrolyte balance, placing some seniors at risk for side effects. They also should not be used by seniors with severe kidney impairment, which can affect the elimination of magnesium and lead to magnesium toxicity (see "Cautions and Warnings"). Bulk-forming laxatives are usually preferred for older individuals.

Generic Name

Magnesium Trisilicate

(mag-NEE-zee-um try-SILL-ih-kate)

Brand Name

†Gaviscon

†*Consult the OTC ingredient charts to determine whether different formulations in this brand-name group are alcohol-, caffeine-, or sugar-free.*

Type of Drug

Antacid.

Used for

Relief of heartburn, sour stomach, acid indigestion.

General Information

All antacids work in the same way, by neutralizing gastric acid. However, they differ in potency: Magnesium antacids such as magnesium trisilicate are more potent than aluminum antacids, but less potent than the antacids calcium carbonate and sodium bicarbonate. The higher the potency of an antacid, the less of it you will need to take to achieve the desired effect.

Antacids also vary according to adverse effects and drug interactions, as well as onset and duration of action. Magnesium antacids dissolve quickly in stomach acid and provide a rapid effect, unlike aluminum antacids, which dissolve more slowly in stomach acid and may take up to 30 minutes to begin working.

How long an antacid product works depends on how long it remains in the stomach. Magnesium antacids have a shorter duration of action than aluminum antacids and calcium carbonate. In general, an antacid taken on an empty stomach leaves the stomach rapidly, and works for only 20 to 40 minutes. However, when taken after a meal, it leaves the stomach more slowly. When taken 1 hour after a meal, an antacid can work for up to 3 hours.

Magnesium trisilicate is one of 4 types of magnesium antacids; the others are hydroxide, oxide, and carbonate.

Magnesium hydroxide is the most potent of the group. Magnesium trisilicate is the least effective.

Magnesium trisilicate is commercially available in combination with another antacid, aluminum hydroxide.

Cautions and Warnings

Do not take the maximum daily dosage of magnesium trisilicate for more than 2 weeks continuously except under a doctor's supervision. Antacids may relieve symptoms of a serious condition such as peptic ulcer disease. If you take an antacid for a prolonged period, you run the risk of unknowingly masking the symptoms of a serious gastrointestinal (GI) disease and delaying diagnosis.

Do not exceed the recommended daily dosage of magnesium trisilicate.

Call your doctor if you do not get relief from magnesium trisilicate, or if your stool is black or tarry, which indicates bleeding in the intestines or stomach. These may be signs of a serious GI disorder that cannot and should not be treated with an OTC product without your doctor's supervision.

Frequent use of magnesium trisilicate alone (as opposed to in combination with an aluminum antacid) can cause diarrhea, which may lead to fluid and electrolyte imbalances.

Because some of the magnesium is absorbed into the bloodstream and eliminated through the kidneys, people with impaired kidney function should not use magnesium trisilicate. Such people are at high risk for magnesium toxicity, which can lead to muscle paralysis, severe hypotension (abnormally low blood pressure), respiratory depression, and other life-threatening complications.

Prolonged use of magnesium trisilicate may result in the development of silicate kidney stones.

Possible Side Effect

▼ Most common: diarrhea.

Drug Interactions

• Magnesium trisilicate decreases the absorption of the following drugs, reducing their effect: tetracycline antibiotics; quinolone antibiotics, such as ciprofloxacin; isoniazid, used to treat tuberculosis; phenytoin, an anticonvulsant; dexamethasone, a corticosteroid; indomethacin, a nonsteroidal anti-inflammatory drug (NSAID); digoxin, used to treat congestive heart failure; and iron. If you are taking magnesium trisilicate at the same time as any of these drugs, separate your dose of each drug by at least 2 hours; with quinolone antibiotics, 4 to 6 hours is preferable.

• Magnesium trisilicate increases the absorption of the anticonvulsant valproic acid, creating the potential for valproic acid toxicity. If you are taking valproic acid, consult your doctor before taking magnesium trisilicate.

• Magnesium trisilicate decreases the elimination of the antiarrhythmic quinidine, raising the serum concentration of quinidine to potentially dangerous levels. If you are taking quinidine, consult your doctor before taking magnesium trisilicate.

• Concurrent use of magnesium trisilicate with sodium polystyrene sulfonate, a potassium remover, may be dangerous. Separate your dose of each drug by at least 2 hours.

Food Interactions

Magnesium trisilicate is best taken after meals (see "General Information").

Usual Dose

Adult and Child (age 12 and over): Take magnesium trisilicate as symptoms occur, but do not exceed the recommended daily dosage specified on the package.

Child (under age 12): not recommended.

Overdosage

Do the following in case of accidental overdose: If the victim is unconscious or having convulsions, call for an ambulance immediately. If you take the victim to an emergency room, be sure to bring the bottle or container with you. If the victim is conscious, call your local poison control center or a health care professional. The poison control center may suggest inducing vomiting with ipecac syrup (available without a prescription at any pharmacy). DO NOT induce vomiting unless specifically instructed to do so.

Special Information

Patients with a history of constipation or hemorrhoids may choose magnesium trisilicate over other antacids because it can cause diarrhea. Diarrhea associated with magnesium trisilicate, unlike diarrhea brought on by other causes, does not necessarily cause stomach cramps or nocturnal bowel movements.

Because aluminum antacids may cause constipation, they are often taken concurrently with magnesium trisilicate to regulate bowel function.

Special Populations

Pregnancy/Breast-feeding

Antacids can be safely taken in small doses for short periods of time during pregnancy and while breast-feeding. However, it is not generally recommended that pregnant women take any drugs, particularly during the first 3 months after conception. Check with your doctor before self-medicating with magnesium trisilicate if you are or might be pregnant, or if you are breast-feeding.

Infants/Children

The safety of antacid use in infants and children has not been established. Children under age 12 should not be given magnesium trisilicate unless directed by a doctor.

Seniors

Seniors may safely take antacids. However, be advised that many older patients are at high risk for complications from ulcers, yet often do not show classic ulcer symptoms. Discuss the possible causes of your gastric discomfort with your pharmacist before self-medicating with an antacid and possibly delaying diagnosis of an ulcer. Be aware of possible interactions with other medications you may be taking.

Seniors may be more likely than younger adults to have diarrhea caused by magnesium trisilicate. However, because constipation is a common complaint in this age group, magnesium trisilicate may be a good choice, as long as you don't have severe kidney impairment.

Generic Name

Meclizine Hydrochloride

(MEK-lih-zeen HYE-droe-KLOR-ide)

Brand Names

Bonine
Dramamine II Less Drowsy Formula

Type of Drug

Antihistamine used as an antiemetic.

Used for

The prevention and treatment of nausea, vomiting, and dizziness associated with motion sickness.

General Information

Nausea and emesis (vomiting) may be caused by various disorders, some minor, some serious. Various antiemetics are used to treat nausea and vomiting caused by motion sickness, pregnancy, mild infectious disease, radiation therapy, cancer chemotherapy, and metabolic, central nervous system (CNS), gastrointestinal (GI), and endocrine disorders.

Meclizine is only approved for the prevention and treatment of motion sickness, the nausea and vomiting associated with traveling, which is a relatively minor, temporary condition.

Meclizine is one of a group of drugs called antihistamines. Besides having many other uses, including the relief of allergy symptoms, antihistamines are the primary OTC antiemetic products. While it is not known precisely how meclizine works, certain antihistamines have a depressant effect on the overstimulated labyrinth (inner ear) function—which causes motion sickness. Meclizine is equal in effectiveness to the antihistamine/antiemetic dimenhydrinate, but causes drowsiness (a common side effect of antihistamines) less frequently.

As noted, meclizine is indicated for the prevention as well as the treatment of motion sickness. Motion sickness is much easier to prevent than to treat once it has already begun.

Meclizine begins working within 1 hour and continues to work for 8 to 24 hours. It has a longer duration of action than most other antihistamines, including dimenhydrinate.

Meclizine is available by brand and generic name in tablet and chewable tablet forms.

Cautions and Warnings

Do not use meclizine too frequently or for a prolonged period unless directed by a health care professional.

Do not exceed the maximum recommended daily dosage of meclizine.

Meclizine, like all antihistamines, may cause extreme drowsiness, which may be exacerbated by the concurrent use of alcoholic beverages, sedatives, hypnotics, or tranquilizers (see "Drug Interactions"). If you are taking meclizine, use caution when performing activities that require mental alertness or physical coordination, such as driving a motor vehicle or operating machinery.

Unless recommended by a doctor, meclizine should not be used by people who have a breathing problem, such as emphysema or chronic bronchitis, or by people with asthma.

Meclizine should be used with caution by people with glaucoma, an enlarged prostate, or an obstructive disease of the GI tract. If you have any of these conditions, consult your doctor before taking meclizine.

Nausea and vomiting associated with radiation therapy; cancer chemotherapy; and metabolic, CNS, GI, and endocrine disorders are serious conditions that should not be self-medicated with meclizine. Consult your doctor.

Meclizine should not be used for treating nausea and vomiting caused by pregnancy.

Possible Side Effects

▼ Most common: drowsiness, fatigue, dry mouth.

▼ Rare: blurred vision.

Drug Interactions

• Meclizine's effects can combine with those of other drugs that depress the CNS, including barbiturates, tranquilizers, sleeping medications, and alcohol (present in many OTC preparations). If you are taking other depressant drugs, check with your doctor before you take pheniramine or any other antihistamine. Avoid drinking alcohol if you are taking meclizine or any other antihistamine.

Food Interactions

None known.

Usual Dose

Adult and Child (age 12 and over): 25–50 mg once a day.

Child (under age 12): not recommended.

To prevent motion sickness, take meclizine 1 hour before departure for travel. Continue to take this product during travel.

Overdosage

Symptoms of antihistamine overdose in children include dilated pupils, flushed face, dry mouth, fever, excitability, hallucinations, loss of muscle coordination, and seizures.

In adults, severe overdose can cause drowsiness or coma, which may be followed by excitability or seizures. Eventually fluid can build up in the brain; the kidneys may fail, and the heart and lungs may stop working, resulting in death. Symptoms may develop within 30 minutes to 2 hours following an overdose, and death may occur within 18 hours.

Even if the victim is not displaying any of the symptoms listed above, do the following in case of accidental overdose: If the victim is unconscious or having convulsions, call for an ambulance immediately. If you take the victim to an emergency room, be sure to bring the bottle or container with you. If the victim is conscious, call your local poison control center or a health care professional. The poison control center may suggest inducing vomiting with ipecac syrup (available without a prescription at any pharmacy). DO NOT induce vomiting unless specifically instructed to do so.

Special Populations

Pregnancy/Breast-feeding

Meclizine has been known to cause fetal abnormalities; in general, antihistamines are not recommended for use during pregnancy unless directed by your doctor. Antihistamines are known to pass into the breast milk of nursing mothers and may cause side effects in infants. Check with your doctor before taking meclizine if you are or might be pregnant, or if you are breast-feeding.

Infants/Children

Because most studies involving antiemetics are conducted with adults, the use of antiemetics in children is controversial. Some clinicians question whether children suffering from a temporary, minor disorder, such as motion sickness, should be treated with meclizine.

An alternative to drug therapy in preventing motion sickness caused by automobile travel is to place the child in the car seat so he or she can see out the front window. Children may be more susceptible to the side effects of meclizine. They are also more susceptible to accidental antihistamine overdose. Do not give meclizine to a child under 12 unless directed by your doctor.

Seniors

Older persons may be more sensitive to the side effects of meclizine and may experience nervousness, irritability, and restlessness. Dizziness, sedation, and low blood pressure may also occur. Most mild reactions may be handled by either lowering your dose or trying another antihistamine.

Generic Name

Menthol (MEN-thol)

Brand Names

Absorbine Jr.
AllerMax
Arthricare
Arthritis Hot
Arthritis Rub
Babee Teething
Banalg
Ben-Gay
Betuline
Blistex
Cala-gel Clearly Calamine
Carmex
Celestial Seasonings Soothers
*Cepacol
Cepastat
ChapStick Medicated
Cold Sore Lotion
Cool Heat
Deep Down
Dencorub Cream
Dermamycin Spray

Dermarest Gel
Dermoplast
Dermtex Spray
Di-Delamine
*†Diabetic Tussin
Diphenylin Cough
Epiderm Balm
Eucalyptamint
First Aid Medicated Powder
†Fisherman's Friend
Flex-All
Gold Bond Medicated
Guaifed [A]
*GuiaCough
†Halls
Hayfebrol [A] [S]
Herbal-Menthol [S]
Icy Hot
Isodettes Lozenge
Koldets Cough Drops
†Luden's
Massengill Douche Powder
Medadyne
Menthacin
Mentholatum
Minit-Rub
Muscle Rub
Mycinettes Lozenge
N'Ice
Noxzema Original
Numol
Orabase Lip Cream [A]
Oragesic
Pain Doctor
Pain Gel Plus
Pain Patch
PainBreak
PMC Douche
Pramegel
Rhuli Gel
†Ricola
Rid-a-Pain Ointment
†Robitussin Cough Drops
Sarna
*†Scot-Tussin
Soltice Quick Rub
Sports Spray
Sucrets 4-Hour Cough Suppressant
Thera-Gesic
TheraPatch
*Therapeutic
Vaporizer in a Bottle Airwick Inhaler
Vaseline Lip Therapy
*†Vicks
Wonder Ice

**Not all products in this brand-name group contain menthol.*

†*Consult the OTC ingredient charts to determine whether different formulations in this brand-name group are alcohol-, caffeine-, or sugar-free.*

Type of Drug

Topical analgesic (pain reliever), topical anesthetic, and antitussive (cough suppressant).

Used for

Relief of soreness, stiffness, and pain in muscles, joints, and tendons; and suppression of dry, hacking, nonproductive cough.

General Information

Menthol can be extracted from peppermint oil or manufactured synthetically. When applied to the skin at concentrations of 1.25% to 16%, menthol produces the sensation of coolness and depresses the nerves that recognize pain; after a short time, the feelings of coolness give way to those of warmth. Used in this way, menthol is a counterirritant topical analgesic. A counterirritant works by producing a less severe pain to distract from a more intense pain. The smell or the feelings of warmth or coolness that counterirritant analgesics produce may also contribute to a placebo effect; that is, if you believe they will work to relieve your pain, they probably will.

Menthol's aromatic vapors work as an antitussive when this product is rubbed as an ointment on the throat or chest (in strengths of 2.6% to 2.8%). Menthol is commonly found in solutions for steam inhalation and cough drops or lozenges.

Menthol is also widely used to flavor candy, gum, cigarettes, toothpaste, and mouthwashes.

Cautions and Warnings

Do not use the maximum daily dosage of a menthol preparation for more than 10 days continuously except under a doctor's supervision.

Do not exceed the recommended daily dosage of a menthol preparation.

Topical menthol preparations should be used only on the skin. Don't apply them near your eyes or to mucous membranes (i.e., inside the mouth, nose, rectum, or vagina).

Don't use menthol on broken, irritated, or sunburned skin, or on an open wound.

If you wear contact lenses, don't take them out or put them in your eyes after you use a menthol preparation without first washing your hands.

Topical Analgesic

If your skin becomes irritated or red, or your pain gets worse or is constant and felt in any position, stop using this product and call your doctor.

Menthol preparations should not be used with a heating pad, hot water bottle, or any other heating device. You should also avoid sunlight and sunlamps after using these products.

Don't use menthol (or any other topical analgesic) after intense exercise, especially during hot and humid weather, when you will probably be flushed and warm. If you have a sore muscle from working out and want to use menthol to relieve the pain, wait until you cool down. You should also avoid applying this product before using a sauna or getting a professional massage.

To avoid the risk of irritation, redness, or blistering, don't use a tight bandage or dressing over the skin where you apply menthol or any other counterirritant analgesic.

Antitussive

To avoid the risk of serious burns when you are using menthol in a steam inhalation to treat a child's cough, never leave the child unsupervised.

Never expose menthol steam inhalation solution to flame or try to microwave it.

If your cough lasts longer than 7 days, is recurrent, or is accompanied by fever, rash, or persistent headache, call your doctor. A persistent cough may be a sign of a serious condition.

Possible Side Effects

▼ Rare: skin reactions such as itching, rashes, and contact dermatitis (inflammation). In at least one instance, a person with asthma experienced worsening of wheezing and shortness of breath that was linked to the use of peppermint-flavored toothpaste (peppermint oil contains 30% to 50% concentration of menthol). Rashes and blisters may be more likely to occur if menthol is applied to sensitive areas of the skin, such as behind your knees. If you develop any skin irritation or redness while using menthol, stop using it immediately.

Drug Interactions

None known.

Food Interactions

None known.

Usual Dose

Topical Analgesic

Adult and Child (age 2 and over): Gently massage a small amount over the area on the skin where pain is felt. Make sure to wash your hands thoroughly afterward. If you are treating pain in your hands, wait 30 minutes before washing. Reapply as needed, no more than 3–4 times a day.

Child (under age 2): not recommended unless directed by a doctor.

Topical Antitussive

Adult and Child (age 2 and over): Rub on the throat and chest in a thick layer. Repeat up to 3 times daily or as directed by your doctor.

Steam Inhalation

Adult and Child (age 6 and over): Add 1 tbs. of solution per quart of water directly to the water in a hot steam vaporizer, breathe in the vapors. Repeat up to 3 times daily or as directed by your doctor.

Child (under age 6): not recommended unless directed by your doctor.

Lozenge or Tablet

Adult and Child (age 2 and over): Allow the lozenge or tablet to dissolve slowly in your mouth. Repeat every hour, as needed, or as directed by your doctor.

Child (under age 2): not recommended unless directed by your doctor.

Overdosage

Do the following in case of accidental ingestion: If the victim is unconscious or having convulsions, call for an ambulance immediately. If you take the victim to an emergency room, be sure to bring the bottle or container with you. If the victim is conscious, call your local poison control center or a health care professional. The poison control center may suggest inducing vomiting with ipecac syrup (available without a prescription at any pharmacy). DO NOT induce vomiting unless specifically instructed to do so.

Special Information

Besides using a topical preparation, there are also physical methods of producing counterirritation, such as gently massaging the injured area. In fact, some of the benefit gained from using counterirritants may simply be due to the fact that they are applied by being rubbed and massaged into the skin. Another way to produce counterirritation is to apply heat to the skin with a hot water bottle or heating pad; in addition to reducing pain, heat helps the collagen in your skin regain its elasticity and lose its stiffness after a stretching injury. However, you should never use a counterirritant such as menthol with a heating device (see "Cautions and Warnings").

Special Populations

Pregnancy/Breast-feeding

It is not generally recommended that pregnant women take any drugs, particularly during the first 3 months after conception.

Check with your doctor before using menthol if you are or might be pregnant, or if you are breast-feeding.

Infants/Children

Menthol is not recommended as a steam inhalation in children under 6 or as a topical antitussive or a lozenge in children under 2 unless prescribed by a doctor.

Seniors

Seniors should exercise the same caution as younger adults when using these products.

Generic Name

Merbromin (mer-BROE-min)

Definition

An antiseptic ingredient used in OTC first-aid skin care products.

Generic Name

Methyl Nicotinate (METH-il NIK-oe-TIN-ate)

Definition

A counterirritant (a superficial irritation or inflammation in one area of the body that relieves irritation or inflammation in another part) used in OTC external analgesics to relieve pain from arthritis or muscle injury. It readily penetrates the skin, especially in gel formulations, and acts by dilating (widening) blood vessels. Available in concentrations from 0.25% to 10%, methyl nicotinate should not be applied more than 3 or 4 times a day. In some people, methyl nicotinate may cause a drop in blood pressure, decrease in pulse rate, and light-headedness when used over a large area. Methyl nicotinate should not be used on children under age 2.

Generic Name

Methyl Salicylate (METH-il SAL-ih-SILL-ate)

Brand Names

Arthricare Triple Medicated Rub
Arthritis Hot
Arthritis Rub
Banalg
*Ben-Gay
Betuline
Deep-Down
Dencorub Cream
Epiderm Balm
*Exocaine
First Aid Medicated
Flex-All
Gordogesic
Gold Bond
Heet
Icy Hot
*Mentholatum
Methagual
Minit-Rub
Muscle Rub
Numol
PainBreak
Pain Doctor
Sports Spray
Thera-Gesic
TheraPatch

**Not all products in this brand-name group contain methyl salicylate.*

Type of Drug

Topical analgesic (pain reliever).

Used for

Relief of soreness, stiffness, and pain in muscles, joints, and tendons.

General Information

Topical analgesics are one of the most popular types of OTC drugs, and the number of these drugs sold continues to increase year after year. Many of the people using these products are over age 50; in fact, 40% of individuals in this age group use topical analgesics on a regular basis. Younger people may use topical analgesics to relieve pain and soreness brought on by exercising or playing sports.

Methyl salicylate is a counterirritant topical analgesic. Counterirritation refers to the production of a less severe pain that distracts from a more intense pain. When a counterirritant medication is applied to the skin, it produces a feeling of warmth or cold that reduces the perception of more deep-seated pain in a muscle or joint. The smell or the feelings of warmth or coolness that counterirritant analgesics produce may also contribute to a placebo effect; that is, if you believe they will work to relieve your pain, they probably will.

Of the counterirritants, methyl salicylate is the most widely used. It is also used to flavor toothpaste, mouthwashes, and candy in much lower concentrations than those used in products meant to be applied to the skin. Methyl salicylate is also available in brand-name products in which it is combined with other counterirritants such as menthol or camphor.

Cautions and Warnings

If your symptoms persist or are not relieved by methyl salicylate after 7 days of continuous treatment, or if they stop but re-occur within several days, stop using the preparation and call your doctor.

Do not exceed the recommended daily dosage of a methyl salicylate preparation.

Topical preparations of methyl salicylate should be used only on the skin. Don't apply them near your eyes or to mucous membranes (i.e., inside the mouth, nose, rectum, or vagina).

Some people may overreact to the skin irritation caused by counterirritant medications such as methyl salicylate and develop rashes and blisters. This may be more likely to occur in sensitive areas of the skin, such as behind your knees. Counterirritants may also cause the skin to become oversensitive. If you develop any skin irritation or redness while using methyl salicylate, stop using it immediately and call your doctor.

If your pain gets worse or is constant and is not relieved by changing position, stop taking this product and call your doctor.

Methyl salicylate preparations should not be used with a heating pad, hot water bottle, or any other heating device. In at least one reported instance, this has caused greatly increased absorption of the agent, leading to death of skin and muscle cells and kidney inflammation. You should also avoid sunlight and sunlamps after using these products.

Don't use methyl salicylate (or any other topical analgesic) after intense exercise, especially during hot and humid weather, when you will probably be flushed and warm. If you have a sore muscle from working out and want to use methyl salicylate to relieve the pain, wait until you cool down. You should also avoid applying this product before using a sauna or getting a professional massage.

To avoid the risk of irritation, redness, or blistering, don't use a tight bandage or dressing over the skin where you apply methyl salicylate or any other counterirritant analgesic.

Don't use a methyl salicylate preparation on broken, irritated, or sunburned skin, or on an open wound.

If you wear contact lenses, don't take them out or put them in your eyes after you use a methyl salicylate preparation without first washing your hands.

Possible Side Effects

Methyl salicylate has been used for many years as a topical analgesic; when used in small doses, as recommended, preparations with this agent have been found to be very safe and effective. However, some people may overreact to the skin irritation caused by methyl salicylate (see "Cautions and Warnings").

Drug Interactions

- Some people taking the anticoagulant (blood-thinning) drug warfarin who also used a salicylate-containing topical analgesic have experienced an increase in the effect of warfarin. If you take warfarin, talk to your doctor or pharmacist before you self-medicate with methyl salicylate.

Usual Dose

Adult and Child (age 16 and over): Methyl salicylate is available in topical preparations in concentrations ranging from 10% to 60%. Gently massage a small amount over the area on the skin where pain is felt. Make sure to wash your hands thoroughly afterward. (If you are treating pain in your hands, wait 30 minutes before washing.) Reapply as needed, no more than 3 or 4 times a day.

Child (under age 16): not recommended because of the risk of Reye's syndrome (see "Special Populations").

Overdosage

Do the following in case of accidental ingestion: If the victim is unconscious or having convulsions, call for an ambulance immediately. If you take the victim to an emergency room, be sure to bring the bottle or container with you. If the victim is conscious, call your local poison control center or a health care professional. The poison control center may suggest inducing vomiting with ipecac syrup (available without a prescription at any pharmacy). DO NOT induce vomiting unless specifically instructed to do so.

Special Information

Besides using a topical preparation, there are also physical methods of producing counterirritation, such as gently massaging the injured area. In fact, some of the benefit gained from using counterirritants may simply be due to the fact that they are applied by being rubbed and massaged into the skin. Another way to produce counterirritation is to apply heat to the skin with a hot water bottle or heating pad; in addition to reducing pain, heat helps the collagen in your skin regain its elasticity and lose its stiffness after a stretching injury. However, you should never use a counterirritant such as methyl salicylate with a heating device (see "Cautions and Warnings").

Special Populations

Allergies

Individuals who are allergic to aspirin or who have nasal polyps or severe asthma should not use topical methyl salicylate preparations. In at least one reported incidence, a person allergic to aspirin experienced swelling and itching when exposed to methyl salicylate products.

Pregnancy/Breast-feeding
It is not generally recommended that pregnant women take any drugs, particularly during the first 3 months after conception. Check with your doctor if you are or might be pregnant, or if you are breast-feeding.

Infants/Children
Because methyl salicylate can be very dangerous if taken internally, even in small amounts, be sure to keep any methyl salicylate preparation out of the reach of children.

Reye's syndrome is a life-threatening condition characterized by vomiting, progressive damage to the central nervous system, liver injury, and abnormally low blood sugar. It is associated with the use of salicylates, although it has not been reported with the use of topical salicylates. However, considering the serious nature of this syndrome and the lack of documented benefits of salicylates, OTC products containing topical salicylates should not be given to children under 16 without first consulting your doctor.

Seniors
Seniors should exercise the same caution as younger adults when using methyl salicylate.

Generic Name

Methylbenzethonium Chloride

(METH-il-BEN-zuh-THOE-nee-uhm KLOR-ide)

Definition

See ***Benzethonium Chloride,*** *page 685*

Generic Name

Methylcellulose (METH-il-SELL-yew-loes)

Definition

See ***Carboxymethylcellulose Sodium,*** *page 745*

Generic Name

Methylparaben (METH-il-PARE-uh-buhn)

Definition

A bacterial preservative used in OTC eye care products, vaginal lubricants, and diaper rash medications. It is often used in conjunction with propylparaben, which is a fungal preservative. Some people have allergic reactions to eye products containing methylparaben.

Generic Name

Miconazole Nitrate
(mye-KON-uh-zole NYE-trate)

Brand Names

Absorbine Jr. Aerosol Spray Powder
Athlete's Foot Antifungal
Breezee Mist
*Desenex
Fungoid Tincture
*Lotrimin
Micatin
Monistat
Tetterine
Yeast-X
Zeasorb-AF

**Not all products in this brand-name group contain miconazole nitrate.*

Type of Drug

Topical and vaginal antifungal agent.

Used for

Topical Products
Curing tinea pedis (athlete's foot), tinea cruris (jock itch), and tinea corporis (ringworm), and relieving the itching, cracking, burning, and discomfort accompanying these conditions.

Vaginal Products
Treating vaginal yeast infection.

General Information

A fungus is an organism that obtains nutrients from other living organisms or from dead organic matter in order to survive. In doing so, fungi cause infections that only an antifungal agent can cure.

Miconazole nitrate is one of 4 antifungal agents known as imidazoles; 3 others in the group, clotrimazole, butoconazole, and tioconazole, are also available without a prescription. The imidazoles inhibit the growth of and kill fungi and also relieve the symptoms of the infection caused by the fungi.

Studies have shown that the 4 OTC imidazoles are equally effective in inhibiting the growth of and killing the fungus known as *Candida,* which causes yeast infections. They have an effectiveness rate of about 85% to 90%. Clotrimazole and miconazole must be taken for 7 days to cure a vaginal yeast infection, whereas butaconazole is effective after 3 days and tioconazole after 1 day.

Miconazole is equal in efficacy to clotrimazole in treating athlete's foot, and both are as effective as tolnaftate (Tinactin), the standard topical antifungal medication. Treatment of jock itch should be complete within 2 weeks; treatment of ringworm and athlete's foot, 4 weeks.

All 4 OTC imidazoles are well tolerated.

Miconazole topical products are available by generic name in cream form and by brand name in cream, ointment, powder, spray liquid, and spray powder forms. Sprays and powders may be less effective than creams and solutions because they are often not rubbed into the skin. However, sometimes a drying effect is desirable; powder products are the best choice in such cases.

Be aware that products of the same brand name in a different formulation do not necessarily contain the same active ingredient. For example, the active ingredient in Lotrimin AF spray powder is miconazole, but the active ingredient in Lotrimin AF cream is clotrimazole.

Miconazole vaginal products are available by brand name in cream and suppository form. The cream may be preferable if your vulva (outer genital tissue) has been significantly affected by the infection; it can be applied externally, to relieve itching, as well as internally.

Cautions and Warnings

Do not exceed the recommended daily dosage of miconazole nitrate.

Miconazole topical and vaginal products are for external use only. Avoid contact with your eyes. After applying one of the products, wash your hands with soap and water.

Topical Products

If there is no improvement in your athlete's foot or ringworm within 4 weeks or in your jock itch within 2 weeks or if your condition worsens in that time, stop using the product and call your doctor.

If irritation, itching, or swelling occurs, stop using the product and call your doctor.

Miconazole is not recommended for nail or scalp infections.

Apply miconazole with caution to areas of skin that are raw or oozing.

Miconazole spray liquids and powders are flammable. Do not use them while smoking or while near heat or flame, and do not puncture or incinerate the containers.

Although some antifungal agents have been shown to be effective in treating diaper rash caused by the *Candida* fungus, the FDA does not regard any OTC topical antifungal agent as safe and effective for the treatment and/or prevention of diaper rash. The agency maintains that diaper rash associated with fungal infection must be diagnosed and treated by a physician, and not self-medicated.

Vaginal Products

If you do not improve after 3 days of treatment with miconazole or if you do not get well in 7 days, you may have a condition other than a yeast infection. Call your doctor.

Self-medicate with a miconazole vaginal product only if you have had a doctor diagnose a vaginal yeast infection previously and you recognize the same symptoms now. If this is the first time you have had vaginal itch and discomfort, DO NOT SELF-MEDICATE WITH MICONAZOLE. Call your doctor, and have him or her determine whether what you have is truly a yeast infection and not another type of vaginal infection, such as one caused by bacteria, which can't be effectively treated with miconazole.

Do not use a miconazole vaginal product if you have abdominal pain, fever, or foul-smelling discharge. Call your doctor immediately.

Stop using the product and call your doctor if you develop abdominal cramping, headache, hives, or skin rash.

If your symptoms return within 2 months or if you have infections that do not clear up easily with treatment, call your physician. You could be pregnant, or there could be a serious underlying medical reason for your infections, such as diabetes or an impaired immune system (such as that associated with HIV infection).

You must use these products for 7 consecutive days for them to cure your fungal infection. Do not stop therapy before then even if your symptoms disappear right away, as often happens.

You may use miconazole vaginal products during your period, but do not use tampons. If your period begins after you have started your 7-day treatment, do not stop treatment.

It is recommended that you avoid sexual intercourse during your 7-day treatment. Be aware that miconazole can damage condoms, diaphragms, and cervical caps, thus increasing your risk of pregnancy.

Possible Side Effects

Miconazole topical and vaginal products are well tolerated.

Topical Products

▼ Rare: mild skin irritation, burning, and stinging.

Vaginal Products

Burning, itching, and irritation have been seen in a small percentage of individuals using miconazole vaginally. These effects usually occur after the first application.

▼ Rare: abdominal cramps, headache, and allergic reactions.

Drug Interactions

None known.

Usual Dose

Topical Products

Adult and Child (age 2 and over): Clean the affected area with soap and water, and dry thoroughly. Apply a thin layer of the product over the affected area twice daily (morning and night) or as directed by a doctor.

If you are treating athlete's foot, be sure to apply the cream, lotion, or solution to the spaces between the toes.

Athlete's foot almost always affects both feet. Be sure to treat both feet with equal thoroughness even if one foot looks worse than the other.

For best results, use miconazole for the length of time indicated on the package.

Child (under age 2): not recommended unless directed by a doctor.

Vaginal Products

Adult and Child (age 12 and over): Read the package carefully before using a miconazole vaginal product.

Wash your entire vaginal area with mild soap and water and dry thoroughly before applying the cream or suppository.

If you are using the cream, attach the applicator to the tube and squeeze the tube from the bottom to force the cream into the applicator. (The brand Monistat 7 is available in prefilled applicator form.) Once the applicator is full, remove it from the tube and insert it as far back into the vagina as possible.

If you are using the suppositories, unwrap 1 suppository, place it in the barrel of the applicator, and insert the applicator into your vagina. Press the plunger on the applicator until it deposits the suppository in your vagina.

Repeat either procedure daily for 7 consecutive days.

Be sure to wash the applicator in soap and water and air-dry it so that it is clean for use the next day.

It is best to use these products at bedtime to avoid the dripping or leaking that occurs when you are upright. There may still be some leakage; you may want to wear a sanitary pad but do not use a tampon to prevent leakage.

Child (under age 12): not recommended.

Overdosage

Do the following in case of accidental ingestion: If the victim is unconscious or having convulsions, call for an ambulance immediately. If you take the victim to an emergency room, be sure to bring the bottle or container with you. If the victim is conscious, call your local poison control center or a health care professional. The poison control center may suggest inducing vomiting with ipecac syrup (available without a prescription at any pharmacy). DO NOT induce vomiting unless specifically instructed to do so.

Special Information

Topical Products

When treating athlete's foot, certain measures can be taken, in addition to using an antifungal agent, to assist in curing the infection:

- Wash your feet with soap and water every day, and thoroughly dry them (but be careful not to scrub too hard between the toes and irritate the skin).
- Wear well-fitting, ventilated shoes and light socks.
- Change your shoes and socks at least once daily, and wash the socks thoroughly.
- Try not to wear canvas, leather, or rubber-soled shoes for too long.
- Keep your feet dry.
- Air your feet out as often as possible.

Storage Instructions

Do not expose miconazole spray liquid and powder products to temperatures above 120°F.

Special Populations

Pregnancy/Breast-feeding

Topical Products

It is not generally recommended that pregnant women take any drugs, particularly during the first 3 months after conception. Check with your doctor if you are or might be pregnant.

Vaginal Products

Do not use a miconazole vaginal product during pregnancy except under the advice and supervision of your doctor.

It is not known if miconazole passes into breast milk. Check with your doctor before using miconazole if you are breast-feeding.

Infants/Children

Topical Products

Do not use miconazole topical cream, powder, ointment, spray liquid, or spray powder on children under age 2 unless directed by a doctor. Supervise children under age 12 in the use of these products.

Vaginal Products

Miconazole vaginal cream and suppositories should not be used in children under 12.

Seniors

Seniors should exercise the same caution as younger adults when using miconazole products.

Generic Name

Mineral Oil (MIN-uhr-uhl)

Brand Names

Agoral	Kondremul
*†Fleet	Liqui-Doss [A]
Haley's M-O [A]	Milkinol

**Not all products in this brand-name group contain mineral oil.*

†Consult the OTC ingredient charts to determine whether different formulations in this brand-name group are alcohol-, caffeine-, or sugar-free.

Used for

Relief of occasional constipation (irregularity).

General Information

The average, healthy individual defecates anywhere from 3 times a day to 3 times a week. Constipation is determined not necessarily by the frequency of bowel movements, but by the consistency of the stool; how difficult it is to eliminate it; and other symptoms associated with constipation, such as dull headache, low back pain, and abdominal distention (swelling). Evaluate your condition carefully and discuss your symptoms and their possible causes with your pharmacist before using a laxative. Laxatives are not always necessary and, when used improperly, can either prevent the desired effect or result in laxative dependency. If you are indeed constipated, your condition may be best managed through proper diet, adequate fluid intake (6 to 8 glasses of water daily), and exercise. If you must use a laxative, choose the mildest effective product.

Laxatives may be classified by their mechanism of action: bulk forming, emollient (stool softeners), lubricant, saline, hyperosmotic, and stimulant. Mineral oil is a lubricant laxative. Lubricant laxatives work by coating fecal matter, thus helping it to retain water that might otherwise be absorbed by the intestinal tract. The increased water retention makes the feces softer and also increases its bulk, which speeds up evacuation. Mineral oil is recommended for people who have hard, dry stools or for people who should avoid straining during defecation (e.g., people with hernias).

Orally administered mineral oil generally produces a bowel movement in 6 to 8 hours.

Mineral oil is available by generic and brand name in oral liquid and enema forms. Emulsified oral mineral oil appears to be more effective than the nonemulsified oral product in softening feces, and also tastes better.

Cautions and Warnings

Do not use mineral oil for more than 1 week unless directed by your doctor. Long-term use of laxatives has been linked with laxative dependence, chronic constipation, and loss of normal bowel function. Using laxatives too frequently can result in persistent diarrhea, hypokalemia (abnormally low potassium in the blood), and fluid and electrolyte imbalance (dehydration and loss of essential nutritional factors). Symptoms of fluid and electrolyte imbalance include muscle cramps and dizziness. Prolonged use of mineral oil in particular may result in significant systemic absorption of the product and in malabsorption of certain vitamins (see "Possible Side Effects").

Do not exceed the recommended daily dosage of mineral oil. The higher the dose of mineral oil, the more likely you are to experience adverse effects.

Do not use mineral oil if you have abdominal pain, nausea, vomiting, or kidney disease unless directed by your doctor.

If you notice a sudden change in bowel habits lasting for more than 2 weeks, do not use mineral oil until you have spoken to your doctor. Also contact your doctor if there is blood in your stool so that colon cancer or other significant disease can be ruled out before you begin taking mineral oil.

If you have had a disease or surgery affecting the gastrointestinal (GI) tract, using a laxative may affect your condition adversely.

If you have rectal bleeding after using mineral oil or if you do not have a bowel movement after 1 week of using this medication, you may have a serious condition. Stop using the product and call your doctor.

Laxatives may decrease the absorption of other drugs that pass through the GI tract (see "Drug Interactions").

In rare cases, oral mineral oil may be aspirated (breathed into the lungs), resulting in pneumonia, especially in very young, very old, and bedridden and debilitated people. It should be used with caution in these people. Mineral oil should also not be taken by people with esophageal or gastric retention, dysphagia (difficulty swallowing), or hiatal hernia. It should generally not be used at bedtime.

If you are using a mineral oil enema product, be sure to follow the directions on the package carefully. An incorrectly administered enema can affect you adversely.

Possible Side Effects

Mineral oil has few adverse effects when used properly, the most common being seepage from the rectum. This may be minimized by reducing dosage or using mineral oil in emulsion.

In rare cases, chronic use of the product may cause impaired absorption of vitamins A, D, E, and K.

Drug Interactions

- All laxatives potentially decrease the absorption of any oral drug taken at the same time. If you are currently taking an oral medication, talk to your pharmacist before taking mineral oil.
- Mineral oil may interfere with the absorption of fat-soluble vitamins (A, D, E, and K); carotene; oral contraceptives;

and anticoagulant (blood-thinning) drugs, such as warfarin. It should not be taken at the same time as any of these products.

• Mineral oil may interfere with the antibacterial activity of nonabsorbable sulfonamides, such as phthalylsulfathiazole. They should not be taken at the same time.

• Mineral oil should not be taken at the same time as a stool softener (e.g., docusate potassium) as the amount of mineral oil absorbed may be increased. If you must take a stool softener wait for 2 hours before you take a dose of mineral oil.

Food Interactions

Take plain (nonemulsified) oral mineral oil on an empty stomach to minimize the malabsorption of vitamins. Oral mineral oil emulsions may be taken with meals.

Usual Dose

Doses should be adjusted to individual usage and taken with a full glass of water. Mineral oil should be used only occasionally. Do not exceed the recommended daily dosage.

Oral

Adult and Child (age 6 and over): Take plain (nonemulsified) mineral oil on an empty stomach.

Child (under age 6): not recommended.

Enema

Adult and Child (age 6 and over): Follow the directions on the package carefully. To administer an enema, lie on your side with your knees bent. Allow the solution to flow into the rectum *slowly.* Retain the solution until you feel stomach cramps.

Child (under age 6): not recommended.

Overdosage

Do the following in case of accidental overdose: If the victim is unconscious or having convulsions, call for an ambulance immediately. If you take the victim to an emergency room, be sure to bring the bottle or container with you. If the victim is conscious, call your local poison control center or a health care professional. The poison control center may suggest inducing vomiting with ipecac syrup (available without a prescription at any pharmacy). DO NOT induce vomiting unless specifically instructed to do so.

Special Populations

Pregnancy/Breast-feeding

It is not generally recommended that pregnant women take any drugs, particularly during the first 3 months after conception. Check with your doctor before using mineral oil if you are or might be pregnant, or if you are breast-feeding.

Chronic oral use of mineral oil by pregnant women can decrease the availability of vitamin K to the fetus, and has caused hypoprothrombinemia (decreased blood clotting) and hemorrhagic disease in newborns. Bulk-forming or emollient laxatives are generally recommended for pregnant women. Also, consider talking to your doctor about diet and mild exercise in the management of constipation.

Infants/Children

Observe your child carefully for patterns of bowel movements and the pain or difficulty with which the bowel movements are made before deciding whether the child is actually constipated. As with adults, "normal" bowel habits vary in children. If your child is indeed constipated, increasing fluid intake and adding fiber to his or her diet may be ways to manage the condition. In general, the use of laxatives should be avoided in children.

Very young children have been known to aspirate oral mineral oil (see "Cautions and Warnings"). Do not give oral mineral oil to children under 6 unless directed by a doctor.

Enemas are not generally recommended for children under 6.

Seniors

Seniors commonly experience constipation and, consequently, may become laxative-dependent. Be cautious of chronically turning to laxatives to ease constipation, and instead look to diet and increased fluid intake as therapeutic measures.

Seniors have been known to aspirate oral mineral oil (see "Cautions and Warnings"), and should not take it without contacting their physician or pharmacist. Bulk-forming laxatives are usually preferred for seniors.

Generic Name

Minoxidil (mih-NOKS-ih-dill)

Brand Name

Rogaine

Type of Drug

Topical hair growth stimulant.

Used for

Treatment of hereditary hair loss in men and women.

General Information

Hereditary hair loss is characterized by a progressive shrinking of the hair follicles, a shortened growth phase of the hair cycle, and a decrease in the size of the hair shaft. Also known as male-pattern hair loss, it occurs in both men and women.

Minoxidil is somewhat successful in stimulating hair growth in individuals experiencing hereditary hair loss or thinning. Studies in males ages 18 to 49 show that about 1/4 of the men noted moderate or better hair growth after using this product. Approximately 1/5 of women noted moderate hair growth.

It is not clear how minoxidil works, but it appears to involve direct stimulation of hair growth by affecting the hair follicle. It also appears to prolong the growth phase and enlarge existing follicles—although there is no evidence that it induces the growth of new follicles.

Minoxidil works best in men when they have thinning hair/hair loss on less than 1/4 of their scalp; in women, when less than 1/3 of the scalp is thinning. The longer the hair loss has occurred, the less likely treatment with minoxidil will be successful.

Minoxidil is not recommended for the treatment of patchy hair loss, sudden hair loss, or hair loss associated with childbirth. It is also not recommended for individuals without a family history of hair loss or individuals in whom the cause of hair loss is unknown.

Therapy with this product must be continuous—and undergone indefinitely—for hair regrowth to be maintained. It can take as long as 12 months to determine if minoxidil has been optimally effective. Some individuals may not respond at all.

Even if therapy with minoxidil is started soon after the onset of thinning and the product is used faithfully, individuals should realize that they may not have exactly the same head of hair they had before it began thinning. Some people achieve only minimal hair growth; i.e., hair is visible, but it does not cover thinning areas. Even with moderate regrowth, the hair in the treated area will be less dense than the hair on the rest of the head. Finally, not all of the hair grows back after treatment with minoxidil. On the plus side, the progressive loss of hair is usually slowed.

Minoxidil is available by generic or brand name in solution form.

Cautions and Warnings

Stop using minoxidil and call your doctor if you have detected no hair regrowth within 8 months if you are a woman or 12 months if you are a man.

Do not use more than the recommended daily dosage. Using minoxidil more than twice daily does not increase or expedite hair regrowth. In addition, it increases the risk of systemic absorption, which can cause adverse effects.

Stop using minoxidil and call your doctor if you experience any of the following systemic effects: chest pain, rapid heartbeat, faintness, dizziness, sudden unexplained weight gain, or swelling of the extremities.

Oral minoxidil (available by prescription only) is used to treat hypertension (high blood pressure). Although topical minoxidil is not absorbed to the extent that the oral medication is, individuals with heart problems should not use the topical product except under a doctor's supervision.

Do not use minoxidil if your scalp is inflamed, infected, irritated, or painful. Scalp psoriasis, severe sunburn, or scalp abrasions may increase absorption of minoxidil. If you have any of these conditions, talk to your doctor before using this product.

Minoxidil is for use on the scalp only. Do not apply it to other areas of your body.

Take care not to get any of the solution in your eyes; it can cause itching and burning. If you get the solution in your eyes, flush them with cool water.

Minoxidil is toxic if swallowed. Keep this product out of the reach of children.

Minoxidil must be taken continuously for an indefinite period. If therapy is interrupted, hair regrowth can be lost within 4 months or less, and hair loss will begin again.

Possible Side Effects

When minoxidil is used properly (i.e., the recommended daily dosage is not exceeded), the amount of the drug absorbed into the scalp is too small to cause serious, systemic side effects. The most common adverse effect is itching at the application site. Stop using the product and call your doctor if local irritation develops.

Drug Interactions

• Use minoxidil with caution if you are currently taking a corticosteroid or any other drug known to increase cutaneous (skin) absorption of drugs; you may increase the risk of systemic absorption of minoxidil. Consult your pharmacist.

• Do not use minoxidil without consulting a doctor if you are currently applying another topical drug preparation to your scalp.

Food Interactions

None Known.

Usual Dose

Adult (age 18 and over): Apply 1 ml of minoxidil to the scalp twice daily.

Keep the scalp dry for 4 hours after application. If you accidentally get your scalp wet during this time (e.g., from rain), dry your scalp and reapply the solution.

Wait to apply hair styling products (e.g., sprays, gels) until the medication has dried.

Child (under age 18): not recommended.

Overdosage

Although topical minoxidil is absorbed in a measurable amount, there are no known cases of overdosage. The risk of overdose is increased, however, if the product is used too much, applied too often, or applied to damaged or inflamed areas of the scalp, which can increase systemic absorption of the drug. Symptoms of overdose will likely be the systemic effects (see "Cautions and Warnings").

Accidental ingestion of topical minoxidil can cause cardiovascular effects, tachycardia (rapid heartbeat), and hypotension (abnormally low blood pressure).

Do the following in case of accidental ingestion: If the victim is unconscious or having convulsions, call for an ambulance immediately. If you take the victim to an emergency room, be sure to bring the bottle or container with you. If the victim is conscious, call your local poison control center or a health care professional. The poison control center may suggest inducing vomiting with ipecac syrup (available without a prescription at any pharmacy). DO NOT induce vomiting unless specifically instructed to do so.

Special Information

Cosmetic hair treatments (e.g., mousses and hair sprays, permanents, dyes) do not usually decrease the effectiveness of minoxidil.

Special Populations

Pregnancy/Breast-feeding
Do not use minoxidil if you are or might be pregnant. If you must use minoxidil, bottle-feed your baby with formula.

Infants/Children
Minoxidil should not be used in children under 18.

Minoxidil is toxic if swallowed. Keep this product out of the reach of children.

Seniors
Seniors should exercise the same caution as younger adults when using minoxidil.

Generic Name

Mustard Oil

Definition

A counterirritant (agent which causes a superficial irritation or inflammation in one area of the body that relieves irritation or inflammation in another part) used in OTC external analgesics in concentrations of 0.5% to 5.0%. The active ingredient in mustard oil and powder is allyl isothiocyanate, which is made from seeds of the mustard plant or synthetically. A poultice (a warm, moist bandage) containing mustard powder is often used as a home remedy to provide heat and pain relief. A poultice is made by mixing equal parts of mustard powder and flour, moistening with water to form a paste, and spreading the paste on a piece of clean cloth.

Allyl isothiocyanate is highly toxic. In preparing a poultice, avoid inhaling the fumes or tasting the substance. The poultice should remain on the skin for only a few minutes, or blisters may develop. It should be applied to the affected area no more than 3 times a day. Do not use on children under age 2.

Generic Name

Naphazoline Hydrochloride

(naff-AZE-oe-leen HYE-droe-KLOR-ide)

Brand Names

Allerest Eye Drops
Clear Eyes
Comfort Eye Drops
Degest 2
Estivin II
*4-Way
Naphcon A [A]
OcuHist
Opcon-A
Privine
Sensitive Eyes
20/20 Drops
Vasocon-A
Vaso Clear

**Not all products in this brand-name group contain naphazoline HCl.*

Type of Drug

Decongestant.

Used for

Relief of nasal congestion that may accompany allergies or colds; and relief of congestion, itching, and irritation of the eye.

General Information

Decongestants work by narrowing or constricting the blood vessels throughout the body, reducing the amount of blood supplied to the nose, and decreasing swelling in nasal mucous membranes that leads to the feeling of congestion. Decongestants are used to relieve the nasal stuffiness of colds and allergies. However, they cannot cure a cold or allergy. The best you can hope for is symptomatic relief. To effectively relieve allergy symptoms, decongestants are usually given in combination with an antihistamine.

Naphazoline, in either a spray form or drops, is administered directly into the nostril to relieve nasal congestion. For adults and adolescents, sprays are the easier to use and help to reduce the risk of swallowing the solution, which may lead to increased side effects. Drops are preferred for children. Naphazoline is also used in eyedrops to reduce redness and irritation by constricting the blood vessels in the eye. After administration into the nose or eye, the drug's effects last approximately 2 to 6 hours.

Naphazoline belongs to a group of drugs called imidazoles; the other imidazole decongestants are tetrahydrozoline and oxymetazoline. All 3 of these drugs are effective and have a low incidence of side effects, but naphazoline and tetrahydrozoline are less likely to cause rebound congestion (see "Cautions and Warnings").

Naphazoline is available by brand name in drops and spray form, both alone and in combination products.

Cautions and Warnings

In general, naphazoline nasal solutions should not be used for longer than 3 to 5 days; if your symptoms have not improved after this time, stop using the drug and call your doctor.

Naphazoline eyedrops should not be used for longer than 3 to 4 days unless directed by a doctor.

Do not exceed the recommended daily dosage of naphazoline products.

If you have hyperthyroidism, heart disease, high blood pressure, or diabetes, or difficulty urinating because of an enlarged prostate, you should use naphazoline only under the supervision of a health care professional because the drug can aggravate these conditions.

Do not use naphazoline eyedrops if you have glaucoma except under a doctor's supervision.

Naphazoline eyedrops may cause enlarged pupils; those with light-colored eyes may be more sensitive to this effect.

A problem common to all forms of topical decongestants, when used for a prolonged period of time, is rebound congestion; that is, you may still have a stuffy nose or red eyes even though you have been using naphazoline for several days. The lining of your nose may swell and turn red, or your eyes may become more inflamed each time you apply the drug. If this happens, stop using naphazoline and contact your doctor. The signs of rebound congestion will usually go away about a week after you stop using the drug.

If you experience eye pain or changes in your vision, continued redness or irritation, worsening or persistence of the condition for more than 48 hours, or signs of systemic absorption such as headache, nausea, or decreased body temperature while using naphazoline eyedrops, stop using the drug and call your doctor.

Naphazoline eyedrops should not be administered while contact lenses are being worn.

Always check the expiration date before using a naphazoline preparation. If the product is discolored or cloudy, do not use it.

To reduce the risk of spreading infection, droppers and spray bottles should not be used by more than 1 person. Do not let the dropper come into contact with any surface. Rinse dropper and bottle tips with hot water after use. Be careful not to let hot water into the bottle.

Possible Side Effects

Nasal Solutions

▼ Most common: Temporary burning, stinging, or dryness; sneezing, and rebound congestion (see "Cautions and Warnings").

Eyedrops

▼ Most common: blurred vision, mild temporary stinging and irritation, enlarged pupils, and increased or decreased pressure within the eye.

Possible Side Effects *(continued)*

Nasal Solutions or Eyedrops

▼ Less common: loss of sense of smell, headache, high blood pressure, heart irregularities, nervousness, nausea, dizziness, weakness, and sweating. If you develop any of these effects while using naphazoline, stop taking the drug immediately and contact your doctor.

Drug Interactions

• Naphazoline should not be used at the same time as a monoamine oxidase inhibitor (MAOI) or within 2 weeks of stopping treatment with an MAOI. MAOIs are used to treat depression, other psychiatric or emotional conditions, and Parkinson's disease. If you are not sure whether you are or have been taking an MAOI, check with your doctor or pharmacist before you use naphazoline.

• Naphazoline's effects may be increased if the drug is taken with a tricyclic antidepressant (such as imipramine or desipramine) or with the tetracyclic antidepressant maprotiline.

Usual Dose

Nasal Solutions

Adult and Child (age 12 and over): 0.05%–0.025% solution: 1–2 drops or sprays, no more than every 6 hours.

Child (age 6–11): 0.025% solution: 1–2 drops or sprays, not more often than every 6 hours. Do not use a 0.05% solution for children in this age group unless directed by a doctor.

Child (under age 6): not recommended except under the supervision of a doctor.

Eyedrops

Adult and Child (age 6 and over): Apply 1–3 drops of a 0.1% solution every 3–4 hours as needed, or 1–2 drops of a 0.01% to 0.03% solution up to 4 times daily, or as directed by a doctor.

Child (under age 6): not recommended except under the supervision of a doctor.

Overdosage

Overdose with naphazoline may produce drowsiness, lowered body temperature, slowed heartbeat, low blood pressure (giving the appearance of shock), and coma.

Even if the victim is not displaying any of the symptoms listed above, do the following in case of accidental ingestion: If the victim is unconscious or having convulsions, call for an ambulance immediately. If you take the victim to an emergency room, be sure to bring the bottle or container with you. If the victim is conscious, call your local poison control center or a health care professional. The poison control center may suggest inducing vomiting with ipecac syrup (available without a prescription at any pharmacy). DO NOT induce vomiting unless specifically instructed to do so.

Special Populations

Pregnancy/Breast-feeding

It is not generally recommended that pregnant women take any drugs, particularly during the first 3 months after conception. Check with your doctor if you are or might be pregnant.

It is not known whether naphazoline passes into breast milk. If you must take naphazoline, bottle-feed your baby with formula.

Infants/Children

The use of 0.1% naphazoline eyedrops in infants and children is not recommended because it may lead to central nervous system depression that may progress to abnormally low body temperature and coma.

Large doses of topical naphazoline can cause severe, noticeable sedation in children. If this happens, call your doctor.

Do not give naphazoline to a child under 6 unless directed by your doctor.

Seniors

Seniors should exercise the same caution as younger adults when using this product.

Generic Name

Neomycin Sulfate

(NEE-oe-MYE-sin SULL-fate)

Brand Names

Campho-phenique Triple Antibiotic
Clomycin
Lanabiotic
Medi-Quik Triple Antibiotic
Myciguent
Mycitracin
Neosporin
Tribiotic Plus

Type of Drug

Topical antibiotic.

Used for

Treatment of skin infections in minor cuts, scrapes, and burns.

General Information

Topical antibiotics are used to prevent or treat infections caused by bacteria that grow in wounds and cause inflammation, itching, and oozing. There are many types of antibiotics available, each effective against different forms of bacteria. Applied within 4 hours after an injury, antibiotics may reduce the risk of infection by killing any bacteria that have contaminated the wound. If infection is prevented, or minor infection contained, then the wound can heal more quickly. There are many types of antibiotics available, each effective against different forms of bacteria. Many OTC products combine different antibiotics so that they have a "broad spectrum" of effectiveness against a range of disease-causing bacteria.

Neomycin is used to treat or prevent wound infections caused by various bacteria, including staphylococcus germs. It works by interfering with the bacteria's ability to produce the proteins the organisms need in order to function. Neomycin is often combined with other antibiotics, such as polymyxin B sulfate and bacitracin zinc.

Neomycin is available by generic and brand name in cream and ointment forms, alone or in combination.

Cautions and Warnings

Overuse of antibiotics increases the risk that bacterial resistance will develop, making treatment ineffective. For this reason, neomycin and other antibiotics should be used only when needed and only as indicated, for short periods of time (no more than 7 days).

If there is no improvement in the infected area within 5 days, or if an allergic reaction develops, discontinue using the drug and contact your doctor.

Do not exceed the recommended daily dose of a neomycin product.

Neomycin is for external use on minor wounds only. In the case of deep puncture wounds or animal bites, contact your doctor immediately. These injuries generally require specific medical attention and should not be self-treated.

Some people who use neomycin may develop a hypersensitivity (allergic) reaction to the drug. Neomycin sometimes causes a secondary allergic reaction or rash during treatment. The rash may continue to be present even after the infection itself is cured.

Other inactive ingredients in antibiotic preparations, such as preservatives, may cause sensitivity reactions in some people. Read the ingredients on the label carefully.

Do not use neomycin over large areas of the body or in large quantities; this poses a risk that too much of the drug will be absorbed, which can lead to kidney toxicity and other dangerous reactions (see "Possible Side Effects").

Do not use first aid products containing neomycin sulfate in the eyes.

By destroying a bacterial infection, neomycin use sometimes allows a fungal infection to develop in its place. If this problem (known as a superinfection) occurs, discontinue use of the drug and ask a health care professional for advice.

Possible Side Effects

- ▼ Common: allergic reaction, itching, or rash in the infected area during use.
- ▼ Rare: Hearing loss, kidney toxicity, and problems with nerves and muscles can occur if too much of the drug is absorbed systemically.

Drug Interactions

• Using hydrocortisone, a topical corticosteroid for treatment of inflammation, at the same time as neomycin can disguise the presence of an infection. It also makes it hard to notice if the antibiotic is causing an allergic reaction. Do not use hydrocortisone along with topical antibiotics except under advice from a health care professional.

Usual Dose

Adult and Child (age 2 and over): Apply a thin layer to the wound after the area has been cleaned with soap and water and patted dry. Do not apply more than 3 times a day. The affected area should be covered with a sterile bandage for the maximum effect.

Child (under age 2): Consult your doctor.

Overdosage

Do the following in case of accidental ingestion: If the victim is unconscious or having convulsions, call for an ambulance immediately. If you take the victim to an emergency room, be sure to bring the bottle or container with you. If the victim is conscious, call your local poison control center or a health care professional. The poison control center may suggest inducing vomiting with ipecac syrup (available without a prescription at any pharmacy). DO NOT induce vomiting unless specifically instructed to do so.

Special Populations

Pregnancy/Breast-feeding

It is not generally recommended that pregnant women take any drugs, particularly during the first 3 months after conception. Check with your doctor if you are or might be pregnant, or if you are breast-feeding.

Infants/Children

This drug should not be used on diaper rash in infants unless approved by your doctor. Using this antibiotic on such a large area of the child's body poses an increased risk that too much of the drug will be absorbed, causing allergic reactions and possibly serious internal complications.

Seniors

Neomycin should not be used on incontinence rash in older individuals. Using this antibiotic on such a large area of the body poses an increased risk of serious internal complications, especially in people with kidney disorders.

Generic Name

Nonoxynol-9 (noe-NOKS-ih-nole)

Brand Names

Advantage 24
Conceptrol
Delfen
Emko
Encare
Gynol II
K-Y Plus
Koromex
Ortho-Creme
Ortho-Gynol
Ramses Personal Spermicidal Lubricant
Semicid Inserts
Shur-Seal
VCF

Type of Drug

Contraceptive.

Used for

Prevention of pregnancy.

General Information

Vaginal spermicides are available in a variety of forms, including jellies, creams, foams, suppositories, and film. They prevent pregnancy by killing sperm before it can fertilize an egg. Nonoxynol-9 is the most widely used spermicidal agent; octoxynol-9 is another spermicide available in the U.S.

In addition to their contraceptive use, nonoxynol-9 and other spermicides have come under growing scrutiny for their ability to protect against sexually transmitted diseases (STDs), including human immunodeficiency virus (HIV), the virus that causes AIDS. However, although nonoxynol-9 has been shown to inactivate HIV in laboratory studies, it has not been proven to decrease the risk of HIV infection in women who use spermicides containing this ingredient. Spermicides have been shown to possibly have a protective effect against other STDs such as chlamydia and gonorrhea.

Cautions and Warnings

Do not exceed the recommended daily dosage of nonoxynol-9.

To get the maximum effectiveness from any nonoxynol-9 product, it is very important to read the directions for use and ask your pharmacist, doctor, or other health care professional if you are unsure about how to use the product correctly. Nonoxynol-9 used alone has a high failure rate. Of women who use nonoxynol-9 or other spermicides, 21% will have an unintended pregnancy in the first year of use. If used with a barrier method such as a diaphragm, cervical cap, or condom, the failure rate improves to varying degrees, from 18% for the diaphragm and cervical cap (the figure for cap use is for women who have not previously had children) to 12% for the condom. These figures are for the "average user"; the rate of accidental pregnancy with spermicides is reduced to 6% for the "perfect user", who uses spermicides both consistently (i.e., every time intercourse occurs) and correctly.

Nonoxynol-9's effectiveness also varies according to the dosage form used. Foams are generally thought to be the most effective when used alone, but they may not provide enough lubrication for women who experience vaginal dryness. Vaginal suppositories are the least effective method. If you decide to use a spermicidal product without a barrier method, make sure you choose one with a higher concentration of nonoxynol-9.

To give nonoxynol-9 the time it needs to work, you should wait at least 8 hours after use before douching.

Possible Side Effects

Both sexual partners may experience allergic reactions to products containing nonoxynol-9, although these happen rarely.

The tissue lining the vagina and cervix may become irritated or damaged if a product with a high concentration of nonoxynol-9 is used, especially if it is used frequently.

Foams may irritate the vagina or penis and may cause pain, itching, or a sensation of heat.

Regular use of spermicides and diaphragms may increase a woman's risk of developing urinary tract infections.

Drug Interactions

None known.

Usual Dose

Vaginal Cream or Jelly

If used alone, insert a full applicator as high into the vagina as possible and push the plunger. Although cream or jelly may be applied 30–60 minutes before intercourse, it is advisable to apply it as short a time as possible before intercourse (under 15 minutes). You must insert another full applicator before each time you have intercourse, or if more than 60 minutes goes by before intercourse occurs.

If used with a diaphragm or cervical cap, fill 1/3 of the diaphragm or cap with cream or jelly before insertion. Diaphragms should be left in place for at least 6 hours after intercourse; after 6 hours, the diaphragm can be removed and washed and reinserted with a new application of cream or jelly before intercourse takes place again. If you have intercourse again before the 6 hours are up, a full applicator of additional cream or jelly must be inserted into the vagina. The diaphragm should NOT be removed.

Cervical caps can remain in place for up to 48 hours. They do not need to be removed if intercourse reoccurs, but it's a good idea to apply more cream or jelly using an applicator.

Vaginal Foam

If the foam is in a can, shake the can about 20 times to make sure that the spermicide is well mixed (it tends to settle in the bottom). Insert a full applicator as high into the vagina as possible and push the plunger. Remove the applicator *without pulling on the plunger.* Because some brands of foam need 2 full applicators to work, be sure to read the directions for the particular product you are using. Although foam may be applied 30–60 minutes before intercourse, it is advisable to apply it as short a time as possible before intercourse (under 15 minutes). You must insert another full applicator each time you have intercourse or if more than 60 minutes goes by before intercourse occurs.

Carefully follow the directions for use of any nonoxynol-9 product to ensure maximum effectiveness.

Vaginal Suppositories
Unwrap 1 suppository and insert it high into the vagina at least 10–15 minutes before intercourse. Another suppository should be used before each additional act of intercourse or if more than 60 minutes goes by before intercourse occurs.

Contraceptive Film
With dry hands, place one 2-inch sheet of film on the tip of your finger and insert the film high up in the vagina, either on your cervix or as close to the cervix as possible. The film should be allowed to dissolve for at least 5 minutes but no longer than 15 minutes before intercourse. If intercourse reoccurs or does not take place for more than 60 minutes, another sheet of film must be applied.

Overdosage

Do the following in case of accidental ingestion: If the victim is unconscious or having convulsions, call for an ambulance immediately. If you take the victim to an emergency room, be sure to bring the bottle or container with you. If the victim is conscious, call your local poison control center or a health care professional. The poison control center may suggest inducing vomiting with ipecac syrup (available without a prescription at any pharmacy). DO NOT induce vomiting unless specifically instructed to do so.

Special Information

You may want to apply nonoxynol-9 *after* oral sex (but *before* intercourse) to avoid the unpleasant taste of these products.

Special Populations

Pregnancy/Breast-feeding
It is not generally recommended that pregnant women use any drug, particularly during the first 3 months after conception. Check with your doctor if you are or might be pregnant, or if you are breast-feeding.

Seniors
Seniors should exercise the same caution as younger adults when using nonoxynol-9.

Generic Name

Oat bran

Definition

A form of dietary fiber that may have some significant health benefits. The actual form of fiber is the product known as beta glucan. Oat bran is thought to be effective in reducing the level of cholesterol in the blood, which may decrease incidence of heart disease. The FDA is considering allowing manufacturers of products containing 20 gm of oatmeal, 13 gm of oatbran, or 1 gm of beta glucan per serving to make health benefit claims.

Generic Name

Oatmeal

Definition

A product containing oat bran.

Generic Name

Oxymetazoline Hydrochloride

(OKS-ee-met-AZE-oh-leen HYE-droe-KLOR-ide)

Brand Name

Afrin
Allerest
Benzedrex 12 HR
Cheracolz
Chlorphed-LA
Dristan 12-Hour
Duramist Plus
Duration
4-Way Long Lasting
*Neo-Synephrine 12-Hour
Nostrilla
NTZ
Oxymeta
Sinarest
Twice-A-Day
Vicks Sinex 12-Hour Ultra Fine Mist

**Not all products in this brand-name group contain oxymetazoline HCl.*

Type of Drug

Decongestant.

Used for

Clearing up the stuffy nose that may accompany allergies or colds; relieving congestion and itching and reducing irritation of the eye.

General Information

Decongestants work by narrowing or constricting the blood vessels, which in turn reduces the blood supplied to the nose, which then decreases the swelling in mucous membranes. They are used to treat the nasal stuffiness of both colds and allergies. However, because decongestants do not work against histamine or any other substance released during allergic reactions, they are usually given in combination with an antihistamine to treat allergies.

Oxymetazoline, in either a spray form or drops, is applied topically to the nose to relieve nasal congestion. Oxymetazoline is also used in eye drops to reduce redness and irritation. After administration, the drug's effects last for about 5 to 6 hours.

Cautions and Warnings

When used topically, in recommended doses, oxymetazoline is generally safe in most individuals. Do not use oxymetazoline if you have angle-closure glaucoma, or if you are taking monoamine oxidase inhibitors, unless recommended by a doctor.

A problem common to all forms of topical decongestants is rebound congestion; that is, you may still have a stuffy nose or red eyes even though you have been using oxymetazoline for several days. The lining of your nose may swell and turn red, giving you the appearance of allergic rhinitis, or your eyes may become more inflamed each time you apply the drug. If this happens, stop using oxymetazoline and contact your doctor. The signs of rebound congestion will usually go away about a week after you stop using the drug.

In children, oxymetazoline in excessive dosage, or if ingested, can cause severe depression of the central nervous system if large doses are given. If this happens, call your doctor.

In general, oxymetazoline nasal solutions should not be used for longer than 3 days; if your symptoms have not improved after this time, stop using the drug and call your doctor.

Possible Side Effects

Oxymetazoline, like other topical decongestants, is minimally absorbed by the body and has a low incidence of side effects.

▼ Most common: when used in the nose, temporary burning, stinging, or dryness; sneezing, and rebound congestion (see Cautions and Warnings).

▼ Less common: high blood pressure, nervousness, nausea, dizziness, headache, insomnia, heart palpitation, or slow heartbeat. If you develop any of these effects while using oxymetazoline, stop taking the drug immediately and contact your doctor.

Drug Interactions

• Oxymetazoline should not be used at the same time as a monoamine oxidase inhibitor (MAOI) or within 2 weeks of stopping treatment with an MAOI. MAOIs are used to treat depression, other psychiatric or emotional conditions, and Parkinson's disease. If you are not sure whether you are or have been taking an MAOI, check with your doctor or pharmacist before you use oxymetazoline.

• Oxymetazoline's effects may be increased if the drug is taken with a tricyclic antidepressant (such as imipramine or desipramine) or with the tetracyclic antidepressant maprotiline.

Food Interactions

None known.

Usual Dose

Nasal Solutions

Adult and Child (over age 12): 0.05–0.025 percent solutions, 2–3 drops or sprays twice a day in the morning and evening.

Child (ages 6–11): 0.05–0.025 percent solutions, 2–3 drops or sprays twice a day in the morning and evening. Do not use a 0.05 percent solution for children in this age group unless prescribed by a doctor.

Child (under age 6): not recommended unless prescribed by a doctor.

Eyedrops

Adult and Child (age 6 and over): Apply 1–2 drops every 6 hours as needed, or as directed by a doctor.

Child (under age 6): not recommended unless prescribed by a doctor.

Overdosage

Overdose with oxymetazoline may produce depression of the central nervous system, low blood pressure (giving the appearance of shock), and coma.

Even if the victim is not displaying any of the symptoms listed above, do the following in case of accidental overdose: If the victim is unconscious or having convulsions, call for an ambulance immediately. If you take the victim to an emergency room, be sure to bring the bottle or container with you. If the victim is conscious, call your local poison control center or a health care professional. The poison control center may suggest inducing vomiting with ipecac syrup (available without a prescription at any pharmacy). DO NOT induce vomiting unless specifically instructed to do so.

Special Information

Remember that oxymetazoline (or any other decongestant) cannot cure a cold or allergy. The best you can hope for is symptom relief.

For adults and adolescents, sprays are the easiest dosage method to use, and help to reduce the risk of swallowing the solution, since they are applied with the head upright. Drops are preferred for children. Follow the manufacturer's instructions for use.

Always check the expiration date before using an oxymetazoline preparation. If the product is discolored or cloudy, do not use it.

To reduce the risk of spreading infection, droppers and spray bottles should not be used by more than 1 person. Do not let the dropper come into contact with any surface. Rinse dropper and bottle tips with hot water after use. Be careful not to let hot water into the bottles.

Colds will usually go away in 1 to 2 weeks whether they are treated or not. There are other ways to temporarily treat congestion caused by colds, including taking tea with lemon and honey, chicken soup, and hot broths.

Special Populations

Pregnancy/Breast-feeding

It is not generally recommended that pregnant women take any drugs, particularly during the first 3 months after conception. Check with your doctor if you are or might be pregnant.

It is not known whether oxymetazoline passes into breast milk. If you must take oxymetazoline, bottle-feed your baby with formula.

Infants/Children

Children may be more susceptible to the effects caused by oxymetazoline. Do not give oxymetazoline to a child under age 6 except on the advice of a doctor.

Seniors

Seniors should exercise the same caution as younger adults when using oxymetazoline.

Generic Name

Oxyquinoline (OKS-ee-KWIN-oe-leen)

Definition

An antimicrobial agent used in OTC ointments and aerosols to prevent infection from minor burns and sunburn. Oxyquinoline sulfate, another form of oxyquinoline, is used as an anti-infective ingredient in feminine hygiene products.

Generic Name

Pamabrom (PAM-uh-brom)

Definition

A mild diuretic, related to caffeine and theophylline, that helps remove excess water from the body. Pamabrom, along with analgesics and antihistamines, is contained in

OTC combination products used to treat premenstrual syndrome (PMS), the symptoms of which include cramps, bloating, water-weight gain, headaches, and backache. The usual dosage is 50 mg, taken up to 4 times a day. Daily doses should not exceed 200 mg.

Generic Name

Peppermint Oil

Definition

A colorless or pale yellow liquid distilled from the flowering peppermint plant, used as a flavoring agent (e.g., in candy and chewing gum), carminative (helps expel gas from alimentary canal), antiseptic, and local anesthetic. It is often included in cough and cold preparations as an antitussive (cough suppressant), but it has not been proven to be effective for this purpose.

Generic Name

Permethrin (per-METH-rin)

Brand Name

A-200 Lice Killing Shampoo
Nix

Type of Drug

Pediculicide (antiparasite).

Used for

Treatment of head lice.

General Information

Lice are 8-legged wingless parasites that live on the human body. Their front legs are well suited for holding tightly to human skin. Lice feed on the blood of their host, and their bites cause an irritating itch. Head lice appear on the scalp.

Lice do not jump or fly. Instead, the infestation is transmitted by direct contact or by sharing personal items such as combs, brushes, or headwear. Lice infestation is common among children in schools and day care centers.

Lice infestation is an annoying and stubborn problem, but it can be treated effectively with OTC products that contain permethrin. Pyrethrins is the other commonly available OTC pediculicide. Medications containing pediculicides paralyze the parasites, thus preventing them from reproducing and eventually killing them.

Permethrin cures 99% of head lice infestations with a single application. In a few cases, a second application is needed 5 to 7 days later to destroy any remaining lice that may have hatched since the first treatment.

Permethrin is available by brand name in shampoo form.

Cautions and Warnings

Do not use more than 2 doses of permethrin. If infestation is still present after 2 doses spaced by 5 to 7 days, contact your doctor.

Do not exceed the recommended dosage of permethrin.

NOTE: Some OTC products for lice treatment, such as household spray, are intended for use on animals or inanimate objects only, not on humans. Read labels carefully.

Permethrin products are for external use only.

If the infestation involves the eyebrows or eyelashes, do not use a lice treatment containing permethrin, because the drug can cause serious complications if it comes in contact with eye tissues. Instead, contact your doctor for recommendations of an alternate treatment. Meanwhile, applying petroleum jelly for 10 days can be effective in the treatment of eyelash and eyebrow infestations.

Permethrin shampoos must be left on the scalp for about 10 minutes. Keep eyes closed tightly while the product is working. If the shampoo comes in contact with your eyes, flush them immediately with cool water.

The fumes from permethrin products can be harmful, especially to people with asthma or chronic bronchitis. Use the medication in a well-ventilated area, and stay there until it is time to rinse off the medication.

If one person in the family develops a head lice infestation, all household members should be treated to reduce the risk of the infestation spreading and reinfestation.

After treatment, examine the affected area very carefully, especially the nape of the neck and behind the ears. Use a specially-designed comb to remove lice bodies and eggs (nits).

Wash all infected bedding and clothing in hot water, and dry at high temperatures for at least 20 minutes to prevent reinfestation. Items that can't be washed may be sealed in a plastic bag for 2 weeks.

Possible Side Effects

Permethrin products may cause temporary stinging, itching, burning, or irritation in the area being treated. These effects are not long-lasting and usually stop within 20 minutes after removal of the product.

Drug Interactions

None known.

Usual Dose

Adult and Child (age 2 months and over): Wash the affected area with a mild soap or shampoo and water; rinse and dry thoroughly. Apply the product in a sufficient amount to saturate the hair and scalp. Allow it to remain on the scalp for 10 minutes, but no longer. Rinse thoroughly, and dry the area with a towel. Afterward, inspect the area carefully, and use a special nit comb to remove the lice bodies and eggs (nits).

Do not exceed 2 applications in 24 hours. Repeat procedure in 5–7 days to kill any newly hatched lice.

Child (under age 2 months): not recommended unless directed by a doctor.

Overdosage

Do the following in case of accidental ingestion: If the victim is unconscious or having convulsions, call for an ambulance immediately. If you take the victim to an emergency room, be sure to bring the bottle or container with you. If the victim is conscious, call your local poison control center or a health care professional. The poison control center may suggest inducing vomiting with ipecac syrup (available without a prescription at any pharmacy). DO NOT induce vomiting unless specifically instructed to do so.

Special Populations

Pregnancy/Breast-feeding
It is not generally recommended that pregnant women use any drugs, particularly during the first 3 months after conception. Check with your doctor if you are or might be pregnant, or if you are breast-feeding.

Infants/Children
Do not use these products in children under 2 months of age unless directed by a doctor.

Seniors
Seniors should exercise the same caution as younger adults when using permethrin.

Generic Name

Petrolatum (PET-roe-LAY-tum)

Brand Names

*A and D
Akwa Tears Ointment
Caldesene Medicated Ointment
Care-Creme Cream
*Desitin
Diaper Guard
DML Lotion
Duolube
DuraTears Naturale
Dyprotex
Flanders Buttocks
*Hemorid for Women
Hem-Prep
Hydropel
Hydrosal Hemorrhoidal
Hypotears
Johnson's Baby Diaper Rash Ointment
Lacri-Lube
Little Bottoms
Lobana Peri-Gard
Medicone
Pazo
Plexolan Lanolin
*Preparation H
Protective Barrier
Refresh P.M.
Stye Sterile Lubricant
Tears Renewed Ointment
Triple Paste
Vaseline Pure Petroleum Jelly

**Not all products in this brand-name group contain petrolatum.*

Type of Drug

Topical protectant and lubricant.

Used for

Protective skin barrier and lubricant.

General Information

Petrolatum (also known as mineral jelly or petroleum jelly), which is derived from petroleum, is commonly used in hemorrhoidal, artificial tears, diaper rash, and prickly heat products. It soothes the skin surface, protects it against outside irritants, and prevents the evaporation of moisture. It is more easily removed from the skin than protectants such as zinc oxide and calamine.

Petrolatum (sometimes called "yellow petrolatum") has a yellowish tinge; white petrolatum is petrolatum that has had this coloring removed so the product is clearer and more cosmetically pleasing.

Petrolatum is generally used in OTC products to ensure prolonged contact with the affected area. It should make up at least 50% to 60% of the product to be effective.

Products containing petrolatum have many uses, including:

- protecting hemorrhoids from exposure to fecal matter, thus reducing irritation, itching, burning, and discomfort
- protecting an infant's genital area from the irritating effects of urine and fecal matter, thus relieving diaper rash
- aiding in the removal of lice infestations in the eyelashes and eyebrows
- prolonging the time that eye medications remain on the eye's surface, allowing them the time they need to take effect
- protecting and moisturizing tissues to relieve pain from cold sores and other sources of discomfort and allow them to heal more quickly
- maintaining moisture in the skin and promoting health by assisting the skin's natural defenses against infection
- easing the symptoms of skin conditions such as dermatitis (skin inflammation)
- acting as a mild sunscreen by absorbing ultraviolet radiation

Petrolatum is available by brand name in combination with other ingredients in the following forms: creams, effervescent tablets, ointments, sticks, and suppositories.

Cautions and Warnings

Hemorrhoidal Products

Do not use hemorrhoidal products containing petrolatum for more than 7 days without consulting your doctor. If your condition worsens or fails to improve within that time, or if there is bleeding, consult your doctor.

Artificial Tears

Do not use artificial tears containing petrolatum for more than 3 days without consulting your doctor.

Diaper Rash or Prickly Heat Products

Do not use diaper rash or prickly heat products containing petrolatum for more than 7 days without consulting your doctor. If your condition or that of your child worsens or fails to improve within that time, consult your doctor.

Do not exceed the recommended daily dosage of petrolatum products.

These products are for external use only.

Products containing petrolatum have been shown to impair the natural healing process of superficial burns, which need exposure to oxygen. Consult your doctor before using petrolatum products on burns.

If your condition does not improve or worsens with the use of any of these products, discontinue use and contact your doctor.

Possible Side Effects

White petrolatum may irritate the skin. When petrolatum products are used as directed, there are no other known side effects. However, you may have a reaction to other ingredients in products containing petrolatum. Read the ingredients on the label carefully.

Drug Interactions

None known.

Usual Dose

Application instructions will vary, depending on the condition for which you are using the product. Always read the instructions carefully.

When appropriate, protect the product from accidental removal before it has had time to work, by using bandages or other dressings.

Hemorrhoidal Products

Adult and Child (age 12 and over): If using an ointment or cream, apply up to 4 times a day, particularly at night, in the morning, or after bowel movements. Suppositories may be used up to 6 times a day.

Child (under age 12): Consult your doctor.

Artificial Tears

Adult and Child: Use 1–2 drops, 3–4 times a day.

Diaper Rash

Apply ointment liberally with each diaper change and after baths, especially at night to prevent long exposure to moisture.

Prickly Heat

Adult and Child (age 2 and over): Apply 3–4 times a day as needed, or as directed by a doctor.

Child (under age 2): Consult your doctor.

Overdosage

Do the following in case of accidental ingestion: If the victim is unconscious or having convulsions, call for an ambulance immediately. If you take the victim to an emergency room, be sure to bring the bottle or container with you. If the victim is conscious, call your local poison control center or a health care professional. The poison control center may suggest inducing vomiting with ipecac syrup (available without a prescription at any pharmacy). DO NOT induce vomiting unless specifically instructed to do so.

Special Populations

Pregnancy/Breast-feeding

It is not generally recommended that pregnant women take any drugs, particularly during the first 3 months after con-

ception. Check with your doctor if you are or might be pregnant, or if you are breast-feeding.

Infants/Children

Special care should be taken to ensure that a diaper rash product containing petrolatum is not accidentally removed before it has time to work.

Seniors

Seniors should exercise the same caution as younger adults when using petrolatum products.

Generic Name

Phenazopyridine Hydrochloride

(FEN-ah-zoe-PEER-ih-deen HYE-droe-KLOR-ide)

Brand Names

Azo-Dine
Azo-Standard
Baridium [C]
Uristat

Type of Drug

Analgesic (pain reliever).

Used for

Symptomatic relief of pain, burning, urgency and frequency of urination, and other discomfort caused by irritation of the lower urinary tract, often associated with a urinary tract (bladder) infection.

General Information

Phenazopyridine is used only to relieve the pain and discomfort associated with a bladder infection. Phenazopyridine does not kill the bacteria that cause infection, and thus cannot eradicate a bladder infection.

Phenazopyridine is available by brand and generic name in tablet form.

Cautions and Warnings

Do not use phenazopyridine for longer than 2 days.

Do not exceed the recommended daily dosage of phenazopyridine.

If your symptoms last for more than 2 days or if you have fever, chills, back pain, or bloody urine, stop taking phenazopyridine and call your doctor.

People with kidney or liver disorders such as glomerulonephritis, severe hepatitis, uremia, pyelonephritis during pregnancy, or impaired kidney function should not take phenazopyridine. If your skin or the whites of your eyes turn a yellowish color while you are taking phenazopyridine, stop taking it immediately and call your doctor.

Phenazopyridine should not be used as a substitute for surgery or antimicrobial therapy. It relieves symptoms, but does not treat the underlying problem.

Possible Side Effects

- ▼ Most common: headache, dizziness, rash, itching, and mild stomach upset or cramps.
- ▼ Less common: methemoglobinemia [a blood disorder resulting in headache, dizziness, fatigue, nausea, vomiting, drowsiness, stupor, coma, and (rarely) death], hemolytic anemia, skin pigmentation, and transient acute kidney failure. These reactions have usually occurred with high doses, overdose, or prolonged therapy, or with usual doses in people with impaired kidney function.
- ▼ Rare: jaundice, hepatitis, a shocklike reaction, and kidney stones.

Drug Interactions

- Because it discolors urine, phenazopyridine can interfere with the results of urine tests based on spectrometry or color reactions. If you are diabetic, phenazopyridine may interfere with testing your urine for sugar. Other urine tests that may be affected include those for bilirubin, ketones, protein, steroids, and urobilinogen, and spectrophotofluorimetric screening tests and assays for porphyrins.

Food Interactions

None known.

Usual Dose

Adult (age 12 and over): 200 mg, taken 3 times a day after meals.

Child (under age 12): Consult your doctor.

Overdosage

Skin discoloration and deep staining of vomit and urine are some of the more obvious signs of phenazopyridine overdose.

Even if the victim is not displaying any of the symptoms listed above, do the following in case of accidental overdose: If the victim is unconscious or having convulsions, call for an ambulance immediately. If you take the victim to an emergency room, be sure to bring the bottle or container with you. If the victim is conscious, call your local poison control center or a health care professional. The poison control center may suggest inducing vomiting with ipecac syrup (available without a prescription at any pharmacy). DO NOT induce vomiting unless specifically instructed to do so.

Special Information

Phenazopyridine produces an orange-to-red color in the urine that may stain fabric. The stains can be removed by soaking the fabric in a 0.25% solution of sodium dithionate or sodium hydrosulfite. Staining of soft contact lenses has also occurred in people taking this drug.

Special Populations

Pregnancy/Breast-feeding

It is not generally recommended that pregnant women take any drugs, particularly during the first 3 months after conception. Check with your doctor if you are or might be pregnant, or if you are breast-feeding.

Infants/Children

Phenazopyridine is not recommended in children under age 12 unless directed by a doctor.

Seniors

Seniors should exercise the same caution as younger adults when using phenazopyridine.

Generic Name

Phenindamine Tartrate

(fen-IN-dah-meen TAHR-trate)

Definition

An antihistamine used in OTC cough, cold, and allergy products.

Generic Name

Pheniramine Maleate

(fen-EER-ah-meen MAL-ee-ate)

Brand Name

Scot-Tussin Original [A] [S]

Type of Drug

Antihistamine.

Used for

Temporary relief of runny nose, sneezing, itchy eyes, scratchy throat, and other symptoms associated with cold and allergy.

General Information

Histamine is one of the substances released by the body tissues during an allergic reaction. When it is released, the body reacts with a variety of symptoms, including itching and sneezing. Antihistamines work by competitively inhibiting the pharmacological action of histamine, which makes them very effective for relieving the symptoms of allergic reactions. Antihistamines may also help relieve a runny nose. However, because antihistamines do not work against the other substances released by the body during an allergic reaction, they can reduce only about 40% to 60% of allergic symptoms. They are also not effective in clearing up a stuffy nose.

If you have seasonal allergies, antihistamines work best if you take them before your allergy season begins. Those who suffer from allergies regardless of the season may need to take antihistamines all year.

Antihistamines will not cure or prevent allergies, viral infections (colds), or bacterial infections. The best you can hope for is symptomatic relief.

Pheniramine maleate is classified as an alkylamine antihistamine. Others in this group include chlorpheniramine and brompheniramine. Of the antihistamines available without a prescription, these are the least likely to make you sleepy. However, drowsiness is still a significant side effect of pheniramine. Newer antihistamines do not have the common antihistamine side effect of drowsiness, but they are currently available only by prescription.

In cold and allergy products, pheniramine is often combined with a nasal decongestant, such as phenylpropanolamine or pseudoephedrine. In combination with the decongestant naphazoline, pheniramine is available in eyedrop form to temporarily relieve red and itchy eyes due to allergies or irritants.

Pheniramine is available by brand name in combination products, in liquid or eyedrop form.

Cautions and Warnings

In eyedrop form, pheniramine should not be used longer than 3 to 4 days continuously, unless directed by your doctor.

Do not exceed the recommended daily dosage of pheniramine.

Unless recommended by a doctor, pheniramine and other antihistamines should not be used by people who have a breathing problem, such as emphysema or chronic bronchitis, or by individuals with asthma. Antihistamines dry the mucous membranes, which can inhibit the ability of the lungs to move or get rid of the excess secretions that these conditions produce.

Pheniramine and other antihistamines should be used with caution by people with glaucoma, hyperthyroidism, heart disease, high blood pressure, or an enlarged prostate. If you have any of these conditions, take pheniramine only on the advice of your doctor.

Pheniramine's effects on the central nervous system (CNS) can make you feel sleepy or reduce your concentration. Your ability to perform activities that require your full alertness and coordination, such as driving a motor vehicle or operating machinery, may be affected. Drinking alcohol while you are taking pheniramine can add to these effects.

Possible Side Effects

Oral Formulation

▼ Most common: restlessness, nervousness, sleeplessness or drowsiness, sedation, excitability, dizziness, poor coordination, and upset stomach.

▼ Less common: dry eyes, nose, and mouth; blurred vision; difficulty urinating; irritability (at high doses); increased or irregular heart rate; and heart palpitations.

Eyedrops

▼ Most common: blurred vision, mild temporary stinging and irritation, enlarged pupils, increased or decreased pressure within the eye.

▼ Less common: loss of sense of smell, headache, high blood pressure, heart irregularities, nervousness, nausea, dizziness, weakness, and sweating. If you develop any of these effects, stop taking the eyedrops immediately and contact your doctor.

Drug Interactions

• Pheniramine's effects can combine with those of other drugs that depress the CNS, including barbiturates, tranquilizers, sleeping medications, and alcohol (present in many OTC preparations). If you are taking other depressant drugs, check with your doctor before you take pheniramine or any other antihistamine. Avoid drinking alcohol if you are taking pheniramine or any other antihistamine.

• Pheniramine should not be used at the same time as a monoamine oxidase inhibitor (MAOI) or within 2 weeks of stopping treatment with an MAOI. MAOIs are used to treat depression, other psychiatric or emotional conditions, and Parkinson's disease. If you are not sure whether you are or have been taking an MAOI, check with your doctor or pharmacist before you use pheniramine.

• Antihistamines can affect the results of skin and blood tests. Notify your health care professional before scheduling these tests if you are taking pheniramine.

Food Interactions

None known.

Usual Dose

Because histamine is released nearly continuously, it is best to take antihistamines on a schedule rather than as needed.

Oral Formulation

Adult and Child (age 12 and over): 12.5 to 25 mg every 4 to 6 hours. Do not take more than 150 mg in 24 hours.

Child (age 6-11): 6.25 to 12.5 mg every 4 to 6 hours. Do not give more than 75 mg in 24 hours.

Child (under age 6): Consult your doctor.

Eyedrops

Adult and Child (age 6 and over): Apply 1 or 2 drops to each eye 3 or 4 times daily.

Child (under age 6): Consult your doctor.

The inconvenience of the sedating effects of pheniramine may be minimized by either taking a full dose at bedtime or using the smallest recommended doses, combined with a decongestant, during the day. Another alternative is to start with the lowest dose when you begin taking the drug and gradually increase the dosage over several days.

If you forget to take a dose of pheniramine, do so as soon as you remember. If it is almost time for your next dose, skip the one you forgot and continue with your regular schedule. Do not take a double dose.

Overdosage

Symptoms of antihistamine overdose in children include dilated pupils, flushed face, dry mouth, fever, excitability, hallucinations, loss of muscle coordination, and seizures.

In adults, severe overdose can cause drowsiness or coma, which may be followed by excitability or seizures. Eventually fluid can build up in the brain; the kidneys may fail, and the heart and lungs may stop working, resulting in death. Symptoms may develop within 30 minutes to 2 hours following an overdose, and death may occur within 18 hours.

Even if the victim is not displaying any of the symptoms listed above, do the following in case of accidental ingestion or overdose: If the victim is unconscious or having convulsions, call for an ambulance immediately. If you take the victim to an emergency room, be sure to bring the bottle or container with you. If the victim is conscious, call your local poison control center or a health care professional. The poison control center may suggest inducing vomiting with ipecac syrup (available without a prescription at any pharmacy). DO NOT induce vomiting unless specifically instructed to do so.

Special Populations

Pregnancy/Breast-feeding

Antihistamines are not recommended for use during pregnancy unless directed by your doctor. Antihistamines are known to pass into the breast milk of nursing mothers and may cause side effects in infants. Check with your doctor before using pheniramine if you are or might be pregnant, or if you are breast-feeding.

Infants/Children

Children may be more susceptible to the side effects of pheniramine. They are also more susceptible to accidental antihistamine overdose. Do not give pheniramine to a child under 6 unless directed by your doctor.

Seniors

Older persons may be more sensitive to the side effects of pheniramine and other antihistamines and may experience nervousness, irritability, and restlessness. Dizziness, sedation, and low blood pressure may also occur. Most mild reactions may be handled by either lowering your dose or trying another antihistamine.

Generic Name

Phenol (FEE-nol)

Definition

A powerful counterirritant (agent which causes a superficial irritation or inflammation in one area of the body that relieves irritation or inflammation in another part) related to menthol and derived from plants or coal tar; or manufactured synthetically. Phenol dissolved in a concentrated (90%) liquid form is carbolic acid, a powerful irritant and disinfectant with a pungent, distinctive odor. Phenol is a component in OTC antimicrobial drugs, throat sprays, lozenges, douche products, mouthwashes, teething pain relievers, and first aid treatments for minor burns and insect bites or stings. Used in mouth rinses, phenol acts as a local anesthetic, antiseptic, and bactericidal agent that penetrates plaque. Phenol is safe and effective for topical anesthesia in adults and children over age 2 when applied no more than 3 or 4 times a day in concentrations of 0.5% to 1.5%. Do not use teething pain preparations containing more than 0.5% phenol in a water base. These products may be applied up to 6 times daily, but they should not be used on infants under age 4 months.

Because phenol is such a powerful substance, its use in recent years has been called into question. While it is an ingredient in douche products, its effectiveness in these has not been substantiated. In the past, phenol has been used for treatment of pain caused by ear disorders, but it is no longer recommended because there is a risk that it might perforate (puncture) the eardrum or cause other tissue damage. Similarly, the American Dental Association does not recommend phenol to treat canker sores because overuse may cause tissue damage and systemic toxicity.

Generic Name

Phenolphthalein (FEE-nol-THAL-een)

Brand Names

Agoral
Alophen
Caroid
Dialose Plus
Docusate Calcium and Yellow Phenolphthalein
Doxidan
Espotabs
Evac-U-Gen
Evac-Q-Kwik
*Ex-Lax
Femilax
Fletcher's Children's
Lax-Pills
Medilax
*Modane
Phillips' Gelcap
Prulet
Unilax [S]
Woman's Gentle Laxative

**Not all products in this brand-name group contain phenolphthalein.*

Type of Drug

Laxative.

Used for

Relief of occasional constipation (irregularity).

General Information

The average, healthy individual defecates anywhere from 3 times a day to 3 times a week. Constipation is determined not necessarily by the frequency of bowel movements, but by the consistency of the stool, how difficult it is to eliminate, and symptoms such as dull headache, low back pain, and abdominal distention (swelling). Evaluate your condition carefully and discuss your symptoms and their possible causes with your pharmacist before taking a laxative. Laxatives are not always necessary, and when used improperly can either prevent the desired effect or result in laxative dependency. If you are indeed constipated, it may be best managed through proper diet, adequate fluid intake (6 to 8 glasses a day), and exercise. If you must use a laxative, choose the mildest effective product.

Laxatives may be classified by their mechanism of action: bulk-forming, emollient (stool softeners), lubricant, saline, hyperosmotic, and stimulant. Phenolphthalein is a stimulant laxative. According to different studies, stimulant laxatives work by either increasing the propulsive activity of the intestine or stimulating the secretion of water and electrolytes in the intestine, thus leading to evacuation of the colon. Phenolphthalein increases activity of the small intestine. Phenolphthalein is specifically a diphenylmethane laxative, which produces a more intense effect than other stimulant laxatives, such as the anthraquinone stimulant senna.

The intensity of action of stimulant laxatives is dose-proportional. Phenolphthalein is effective in small doses. It generally produces a bowel movement in 6 to 8 hours.

Phenolphthalein is available by generic name in powder form and by brand name in the following forms: tablets, chewable tablets, gelcaps, capsules, emulsion, and suspension.

Cautions and Warnings

Do not use for more than 7 days, unless directed by your doctor. Long-term use of laxatives has been linked with laxative dependence, chronic constipation, loss of normal bowel function, and, in severe cases, nerve, muscle, and tissue damage to the intestines. Using laxatives too frequently can result in persistent diarrhea, hypokalemia (abnormally low potassium in blood), loss of essential nutrients, and dehydration.

Do not exceed the recommended daily dosage of phenolphthalein. The higher the dose, the more likely you are to experience adverse effects.

Of all the types of laxatives, stimulant laxatives such as phenolphthalein are particularly habit-forming and with longterm use are the most likely to cause adverse effects such as diarrhea, gastrointestinal (GI) irritation, and fluid and electrolyte depletion.

Phenolphthalein may continue its laxative effect for several days after it has been taken.

Overuse of phenolphthalein can impair the absorption of vitamin D and calcium. This can cause osteomalacia (softening of the bones), which is characterized by pain, tenderness, muscular weakness, loss of appetite, and weight loss.

Do not take phenolphthalein if you have abdominal pain, nausea, vomiting, or kidney disease, unless directed by your doctor.

If you notice a marked change in bowel habits lasting for more than 2 weeks, do not take phenolphthalein until you have spoken to your doctor. Also contact your doctor if there is blood in your stool, so that colon cancer or other significant disease can be ruled out before you begin taking phenolphthalein.

If you have had a disease or surgery affecting the GI tract, using a laxative may affect your condition adversely.

If you have rectal bleeding after using phenolphthalein, or if you do not have a bowel movement after 7 days of using this medication, you may have a serious condition. Stop using phenolphthalein and call your doctor.

Phenolphthalein can cause 2 types of allergic reactions in susceptible people. One is a pink or purple skin rash. The other, associated with large doses, causes diarrhea, colic, cardiac and respiratory distress, or circulatory collapse. If you experience any of these reactions, stop using phenolphthalein and call your doctor or pharmacist.

Laxatives may decrease the absorption of other drugs that pass through the GI tract.

Possible Side Effects

Stimulant laxatives like phenolphthalein are more likely to cause cramping than other types.

▼ Most common: abdominal discomfort, faintness, nausea, cramps, pinching and spasmodic pain in the bowels, colic, and increased mucus secretion.

▼ Less common (associated with chronic use of phenolphthalein): metabolic acidosis or alkalosis (imbalances of acid and base in body fluids); hypocalcemia (too little calcium in blood); tetany (characterized by foot spasms, muscular twitching, and cramps); electrolyte and fluid deficiencies (characterized by vomiting and muscle weakness); impaired intestinal absorption of nutrients; burning sensation in the rectum (suppository only); cathartic colon (weak or dilated colon).

Drug Interactions

• All laxatives potentially decrease the absorption of any oral drug taken at the same time. If you are currently taking an oral medication, talk to your pharmacist before self-medicating with phenolphthalein.

Food Interactions

None known.

Usual Dose

Doses should be adjusted to individual usage.

Chewable Tablets

Adult and Child (age 12 and over): 1–2 tablets a day.

Child (under age 12): not recommended.

Suspension

Adult and Child (age 12 and over): 2–4 tsp. a day.

Child (under age 12): not recommended.

Gelcaps

Adult and Child (age 12 and over): 1–2 gelcaps a day taken with a glass (8 oz.) of water.

Child (under age 12): not recommended.

Overdosage

Symptoms of overdosage include persistent diarrhea and dehydration.

Even if the victim is not displaying any of the symptoms listed above, do the following in case of accidental overdose: If the victim is unconscious or having convulsions, call for an ambulance immediately. If you take the victim to an emergency room, be sure to bring the bottle or container with you. If the victim is conscious, call your local poison control center or a health care professional. The poison control center may suggest inducing vomiting with ipecac syrup (available without a prescription at any pharmacy). DO NOT induce vomiting unless specifically instructed to do so.

Special Information

Phenolphthalein may cause your urine or feces to appear pink or red. This is not a cause for alarm.

Special Populations

Allergies

Phenolphthalein has been known to cause 2 types of allergic reactions in susceptible people (see "Cautions and Warnings"). Do not take phenolphthalein if you have ever had an unusual or allergic reaction to this product.

Pregnancy/Breast-feeding

Stimulant laxatives such as phenolphthalein should be avoided during pregnancy. Only bulk-forming or emollient laxatives are recommended for pregnant women. Consider talking to your doctor about diet and mild exercise in the management of constipation.

It is not known whether phenolphthalein passes into breast milk. Check with your doctor before using phenolphthalein if you are breast-feeding.

Infants/Children

Observe your child carefully for patterns of bowel movements and the pain or difficulty with which the bowel movements are made before deciding whether the child is actually constipated. As with adults, "normal" bowel habits vary in children. If your child is indeed constipated, increasing fluid intake and adding fiber to his or her diet may help to manage the condition. In general, the use of laxatives should be avoided in children.

Do not give phenolphthalein to children under 12 unless directed by a doctor.

Seniors

Seniors commonly experience constipation, and consequently may become laxative-dependent. Be cautious of chronically turning to laxatives to ease constipation, and instead look to diet and increased fluid intake as therapeutic measures.

Stimulant laxatives such as phenolphthalein may not be the best choice for this age group because they alter fluid and electrolyte balance, placing some seniors at risk for side effects. Bulk-forming laxatives are usually preferred for seniors.

Generic Name

Phenylephrine Hydrochloride

(FEN-il-EFF-rin HYE-droe-KLOR-ide)

Brand Names

AK-Nefrin
Alconefrin
Anusert
Cerose-DM
*Codimal [A]
Coldonyl
Dallergy-D [A]
Dristan Nasal Spray
Dristan Cold Multi-Symptom
Emagrin Forte
Fendol
*4-Way
Gendecon
Hemorid for Women
Hem-Prep
Histatab Plus
Isopto-Frin
Little Noses Decongestant
Medicone
ND-Gesic
*Neo-Synephrine
Novahistine
Prefrin Liquifilm
Preparation H
Quelidrine Cough
Relief
Rhinall
Scot-Tussin Original [A] [S]
Spec-T Sore Throat Decongestant
Vicks Sinex Ultra Fine Mist
Zincfrin

**Not all products in this brand-name group contain phenylephrine HCl.*

Type of Drug

Decongestant.

Used for

Relief of nasal congestion that may accompany allergies or colds.

General Information

Decongestants work by narrowing or constricting the blood vessels throughout the body, reducing the blood supplied to the nose, which then decreases the swelling in mucous membranes. They are used to treat both colds and allergies. However, because decongestants do not work against histamine or any other substance that works in allergic reactions, they are formulated in combination with an antihistamine to treat allergies.

In OTC products, oral phenylephrine hydrochloride is used in combination with other drugs to relieve nasal congestion associated with colds and allergies. Phenylephrine is often used as a topical decongestant. Phenylephrine, in either spray form or drops, is applied directly in the nose to relieve nasal congestion. It is also used in eye drops to clear up redness and reduce irritation and in hemorrhoid medications to reduce swelling and itching.

Phenylephrine is available by generic name as sprays and drops, and by brand name in the following forms: sprays, drops, liquids, tablets, lozenges, creams, ointments, and suppositories.

Cautions and Warnings

Oral Decongestant

Unless directed by your doctor, do not use oral phenylephrine for longer than 7 consecutive days, or 3 consecutive days in the presence of fever.

Phenylephrine should be used with caution by people with hyperthyroidism, heart disease, high blood pressure, diabetes, or difficulty urinating because of an enlarged prostate because the drug can aggravate these conditions. If you have any of these conditions, ask your doctor before using phenylephrine.

Eyedrops or Nasal Products

Topical phenylephrine (nasal drops or sprays, and eyedrops) should not be used for longer than 3 consecutive days. If your symptoms have not improved after this time, stop using the drug and call your doctor.

A problem common to all forms of topical decongestants is rebound congestion; that is, you may still have a stuffy nose or red eyes even though you have been using phenylephrine for several days. The lining of your nose may swell and turn red, giving the appearance of allergic rhinitis, or your eyes may become more inflamed each time you use the drug. If this happens, stop using phenylephrine and contact your doctor. The signs of rebound congestion will usually go away in about a week after you stop using the drug.

If you experience visual disturbances, pain, or increased redness while using phenylephrine eye drops, or if your condition worsens over a 3-day period, stop using the drug and contact your doctor.

Phenylephrine eye drops should not be used by people with glaucoma or other eye diseases except under a doctor's supervision.

Hemorrhoids

Do not use phenylephrine hemorrhoidal preparations for longer than 7 days. If symptoms have not improved in this time, call your doctor.

If you are using a phenylephrine preparation to treat hemorrhoids, discontinue use and call your doctor immediately if bleeding from the rectal area occurs. Anorectal bleeding can be a sign of a more serious underlying condition.

Do not exceed the recommended daily dosage of phenylephrine.

Excessive use of phenylephrine should be avoided, especially in children (see "Special Populations").

Possible Side Effects

Oral Decongestant

▼ Less common: heart palpitations, increased or irregular heartbeat, headache, pallor or blanching, trembling or tremors, increased perspiration, nausea, insomnia, weakness, dizziness, and high blood pressure. If you develop any of these effects while using phenylephrine, stop taking the drug immediately and contact your doctor.

Possible Side Effects ***(continued)***

Eyedrops or Nasal Products

▼ Most common: temporary burning or stinging, dryness of the mucosa, rebound congestion (see "Cautions and Warnings").

Drug Interactions

• Phenylephrine should not be used at the same time as a monoamine oxidase inhibitor (MAOI) or within 3 weeks of stopping an MAOI. MAOIs are used to treat depression, other psychiatric or emotional conditions, and Parkinson's disease. If you are not sure whether you are or or have been taking an MAOI, check with your doctor or pharmacist before you use phenylephrine.

• Phenylephrine's effects may be increased if the drug is taken with a tricyclic antidepressant (such as imipramine or desipramine).

• Taking oral phenylephrine along with another decongestant can increase the risk of adverse effects and toxicity. If you are taking another decongestant, do not use phenylephrine without first asking your doctor.

• The effects of oral phenylephrine may combine with those of caffeine, a CNS stimulant found in many prescription and OTC drugs. This combination can cause disorientation, delirium, and other side effects.

Food Interactions

When taken orally, phenylephrine interacts adversely with caffeine (see "Drug Interactions"), which is found in many popular beverages, including coffee, tea, and cola, and in chocolate.

Usual Dose

Oral Decongestant

Adult and Child (age 12 and over): 10 mg every 4 hours.
Child (under age 12): Consult your doctor.

Eyedrops

Adult and Child (age 12 and over): 0.08–0.25% solution, 1–2 drops every 3–4 hours. Do not exceed 4 doses in a

24-hour period.

Child (under age 12): Consult your doctor.

Nasal Products

Adult and Child (over age 12): 0.25%–1% solutions, 2–3 drops or sprays no more often than every 4 hours. In case of extreme congestion in adults, a 1% solution may be used initially.

Child (under age 12): Consult your doctor.

Hemorrhoids

Adult and Child (age 12 and over): Read package instructions carefully. Apply externally or intrarectally as directed. Do not exceed 4 doses in a 24-hour period.

Overdosage

Do the following in case of accidental ingestion or overdose: If the victim is unconscious or having convulsions, call for an ambulance immediately. If you take the victim to an emergency room, be sure to bring the bottle or container with you. If the victim is conscious, call your local poison control center or a health care professional. The poison control center may suggest inducing vomiting with ipecac syrup (available without a prescription at any pharmacy). DO NOT induce vomiting unless specifically instructed to do so.

Special Information

Remember that phenylephrine (or any other decongestant) cannot cure a cold or allergy. The best you can hope for is symptomatic relief. Colds will usually go away in 1-2 weeks whether they are treated or not. There are other ways to temporarily treat congestion caused by colds, including drinking tea with lemon and honey, and eating chicken soup and hot broths.

For adults and adolescents, sprays are the easiest method and help to reduce the risk of swallowing the solution since they are applied with the head upright. Drops are preferred for younger children. Follow the manufacturer's instructions for use.

Always check the expiration date before using a phenylephrine preparation. If the product is brown or otherwise discolored, do not use it.

To reduce the risk of spreading infection, droppers and spray bottles should not be used by more than one person. Rinse dropper and bottle tips with hot water after use. Be careful not to let hot water into the bottles.

Special Populations

Allergies

Some formulations of phenylephrine contain sulfites, which may cause allergic-type reactions, including anaphylaxis and life-threatening or less severe asthmatic episodes, in some people. Individuals with asthma are more likely to be sensitive to sulfites.

Pregnancy/Breast-feeding

It is not generally recommended that pregnant women take any drugs, particularly during the first 3 months after conception. Check with your doctor before using phenylephrine if you are or might be pregnant.

It is not known whether phenylephrine passes into breast milk. If you must take phenylephrine, bottle-feed your baby with formula.

Infants/Children

Excessive use of phenylephrine in children can cause systemic (whole-body) complications, including increased blood pressure. Consult your doctor for the appropriate dose for children under age 12. To ensure proper administration, adult supervision is recommended.

Do not use phenylephrine in children under age 6 unless supervised by your doctor.

Seniors

Older people may be more susceptible to the side effects of phenylephrine. Individuals with an enlarged prostate or a history of cardiovascular disease should ask their doctor before using phenylephrine.

In some older individuals, the use of phenylephrine eyedrops, especially in high concentrations, may cause tiny fragments of the iris (colored portion of the eye) to become detached. If this happens, call your doctor.

Generic Name

Phenylpropanolamine

(FEN-il-PROE-pah-NOLE-ah-meen)

Brand Names

A.R.M.
Acutrim
*Alka-Seltzer Plus
Amfed T.D.
BC
Bromatapp
Bromotap
Cheracol Plus
*†Chlor-Trimeton
Comtrex
*Contac
Coricidin D
†Demazin
Dexatrim
Dieutrim
*†Dimetapp
Duadacin
GuiaCough CF
Ipsatol [A]
Kophane [A]
Mini Slims
*Naldecon [A]
Pediacon [A]
Permathene
Prominicol Cough
Propagest [S]
Protrim
Pyrroxate
Robitussin CF [A]
Sinapils
Sinulin [S]
Spec-T Sore Throat Decongestant
Super Odrinex
Tavist-D
Teldrin
Thinz
Tri-Nefrin
*Triaminic [A]
Triaminicin
Triaminicol [A]
*Tricodene [A]
*†Vicks

**Not all products in this brand-name group contain phenylpropanolamine.*

†Consult the OTC ingredient charts to determine whether different formulations in this brand-name group are alcohol-, caffeine-, or sugar-free.

Type of Drug

Decongestant and appetite suppressant.

Used for

Temporary relief of nasal congestion (stuffy nose) that may accompany allergies and colds.

General Information

Decongestants relieve nasal congestion by narrowing or constricting blood vessels in the nose. This action reduces the blood supplied to the nose and decreases the swelling of nasal mucous membranes. Unlike topical decongestants (decongestant nasal sprays), which act on local blood vessels, oral decongestants may constrict blood vessels throughout the body.

Decongestants are used to treat the nasal stuffiness of both colds and allergies. However, they cannot cure a cold or allergy. The best you can hope for is symptomatic relief. To effectively relieve allergy symptoms, decongestants are usually given in combination with an antihistamine, which works against histamine, a chemical substance released by the body during an allergic reaction.

Phenylpropanolamine hydrochloride, an oral decongestant, is available by generic and brand name, both alone and in combination with other drugs used to treat allergy or cold symptoms. It starts to work withing 15 to 30 minutes after it is taken and its decongestant effects last for about 3 hours. There have been no well-controlled clinical studies performed with phenylpropanolamine and some doctors have questioned whether it is an effective decongestant. Phenylpropanolamine is also an ingredient in OTC appetite suppressants.

Cautions and Warnings

Do not exceed the recommended daily dosage of phenylpropanolamine.

If you have hyperthyroidism, heart disease, high blood pressure, diabetes, or an enlarged prostate gland, you should take phenylpropanolamine only under the supervision of a doctor, because it can aggravate these conditions. People with high blood pressure should be especially cautious about taking this drug because it may increase blood pressure and, in large doses, may increase stimulation of the heart or alter its rhythm. When used in individuals with diabetes, phenylpropanolamine hydrochloride may increase blood sugar.

Possible Side Effects

Phenylpropanolamine has a low incidence of side effects in people taking recommended doses. Most side effects that are seen are related to phenylpropanolamine's effect on the central nervous system. If you develop any of the following side effects, stop taking phenylpropanolamine. Call your doctor if you experience any of the effects listed as "less common" or "rare."

▼ Most common: nervousness, restlessness, insomnia, dizziness, and headache. Nausea may also occur.

▼ Less common: increased blood pressure, increased or irregular heart rate, and heart palpitations.

▼ Rare: severe headache, feelings of tightness in the chest, greatly elevated blood pressure, rapid heartbeat, and heart contractions.

Drug Interactions

• Phenylpropanolamine should not be used at the same time as a monoamine oxidase inhibitor (MAOI) drug or within 2 weeks of stopping treatment with an MAOI. MAOIs are used to treat depression, other psychiatric or emotional conditions, and Parkinson's disease. If you are not sure whether you are or have been taking an MAOI, check with your doctor or pharmacist before you use phenylpropanolamine.

• Do not use with other nasal decongestants (i.e., pseudoephedrine) or with other combination products containing phenylpropanolamine.

• Phenylpropanolamine's actions may combine with those of caffeine, which also affects the central nervous system, to cause disorientation, delirium, and other side effects. Be aware that in addition to being found in coffee, tea, colas, and chocolate, caffeine is also an ingredient in many prescription and OTC drugs.

Food Interactions

Avoid foods and beverages containing caffeine if you are taking phenylpropanolamine hydrochloride (see "Drug Interactions").

Usual Dose

Decongestant

Adult and Child (age 12 and over): 20–5 mg every 4 hours. Do not take more than 150 mg in 24 hours. As an alternative, one 75-mg extended-release capsule can be taken every 12 hours.

Child (age 6–11): 10–12.5 mg every 4 hours. Do not give more than 75 mg in 24 hours.

Child (age 2–5): 6.25 mg every 4 hours. Do not give more than 37.5 mg in 24 hours.

These guidelines do not take the weight of the child into consideration; if your child is large or small for his or her age, check with your doctor about the appropriate dose.

Appetite Suppressant

Adult and Child (age 12 and over): 25 mg 3 times a day, or 37.5 mg twice a day, taken 30 minutes before meals, with a full glass of water. As an alternative, one 50-mg or 75-mg extended-release capsule or tablet can be taken once a day (in the mid-morning) with a full glass of water.

Child (under age 12): not recommended.

Do not divide, crush, chew, or dissolve extended release product—swallow whole. Use of these products should not exceed 3 months.

Overdosage

Do the following in case of accidental overdose: If the victim is unconscious or having convulsions, call for an ambulance immediately. If you take the victim to an emergency room, be sure to bring the bottle or container with you. If the victim is conscious, call your local poison control center or a health care professional. The poison control center may suggest inducing vomiting with ipecac syrup (available without a prescription at any pharmacy). DO NOT induce vomiting unless specifically instructed to do so.

Special Information

Colds will usually go away in 1 to 2 weeks whether they are treated or not. There are other ways to temporarily relieve congestion caused by colds, including taking tea with lemon and honey, or eating chicken soup or hot broth.

Special Populations

Allergies

Some phenylpropanolamine products contain the dye tartrazine, which may cause allergic reactions (including bronchial asthma) in some people. People who are allergic to aspirin are more likely to react to tartrazine.

Pregnancy/Breast-feeding

It is not generally recommended that pregnant women take any drugs, particularly during the first 3 months after conception. Studies of phenylpropanolamine in animals have revealed adverse effects in the fetus, but there are no controlled studies of this drug in pregnant women. Do not take phenylpropanolamine if you are or might be pregnant without first checking with your doctor.

Small amounts of decongestants such as phenylpropanolamine have been shown to pass into breast milk. If you must take phenylpropanolamine hydrochloride, bottle-feed your baby with formula.

Infants/Children

Phenylpropanolamine should not be used as a decongestant in children younger than 2 or as an appetite suppressant in children younger than age 12.

Seniors

Seniors taking phenylpropanolamine should be especially cautious about the amount of caffeine they ingest because they may be more susceptible to this combination's effect on the central nervous system (see "Drug Interactions").

Generic Name

Phenyltoloxamine Citrate

(FEN-il-tol-OKS-uh-meen SYE-trate)

Definition

An antihistamine that is sometimes combined with pain relievers such as acetaminophen to enhance the effectiveness of OTC analgesics.

Generic Name

Phosphorated Carbohydrate Solution

(FOSS-foe-RATE-ed KAR-boe-HYE-drate)

Brand Names

Emecheck
Naus-A-Way
Especol [A]
Nausetrol

Type of Drug

Antiemetic (relieves nausea and vomiting).

Used for

Prevention and treatment of nausea and vomiting associated with upset stomach caused by intestinal flu, overeating, or emotional upset.

General Information

Nausea and emesis (vomiting) may be caused by various disorders: some minor, some serious. Various antiemetics are used to treat nausea and vomiting caused by motion sickness; pregnancy; mild infectious disease; radiation therapy; cancer chemotherapy; and metabolic, central nervous system (CNS), gastrointestinal (GI), and endocrine disorders. Phosphorated carbohydrate solution is approved only for the treatment of a relatively minor, transient condition: nausea and vomiting associated with upset stomach.

Phosphorated carbohydrate solution is a mixture of the simple sugars fructose and glucose, and phosphoric acid, an antiemetic that is also commercially available alone under the brand names Cola (a syrup) and Emetrol (a liquid).

Phosphorated carbohydrate solution in theory has the potential to inhibit gastric emptying and reduce gastric tone. It is taken at 15-minute intervals until vomiting ceases.

Phosphorated carbohydrate solution is available by brand name in solution form.

Cautions and Warnings

Do not take more than 5 doses of phosphorated carbohydrate solution in 1 hour. Do not consume other fluids for

15 minutes after taking a dose. Call your doctor if vomiting does not stop after 5 doses.

Do not exceed the recommended daily dosage of phosphorated carbohydrate solution.

Because of the product's high glucose content, individuals with diabetes should use phosphorated carbohydrate solution with caution.

Nausea and vomiting associated with radiation therapy; cancer chemotherapy; and metabolic, CNS, GI, and endocrine disorders are serious conditions that should not be self-medicated with phosphorated carbohydrate solution. Consult your doctor.

This product should probably not be used to treat nausea and vomiting associated with pregnancy (see "Special Populations").

Possible Side Effects

Large doses of fructose, one of the ingredients in phosphorated carbohydrate solution, may cause abdominal pain and diarrhea.

Drug Interactions

None known.

Food Interactions

None known.

Usual Dose

Adult and Child (age 12 and over): 15–30 ml (1–2 tbs.) at 15-minute intervals until vomiting stops. Do not exceed 5 doses in 1 hour or take for more than 1 hour.

Child (under age 12): 5–10 ml (1–2 tsp.) at 15-minute intervals until vomiting stops. Do not exceed 5 doses in 1 hour or take for more than 1 hour.

Do not dilute the solution.

Do not consume other liquids for 15 minutes after taking a dose.

Overdosage

Do the following in case of accidental overdose: If the victim is unconscious or having convulsions, call for an ambulance immediately. If you take the victim to an emergency room, be sure to bring the bottle or container with you. If the victim is conscious, call your local poison control center or a health care professional. The poison control center may suggest inducing vomiting with ipecac syrup (available without a prescription at any pharmacy). DO NOT induce vomiting unless specifically instructed to do so.

Special Populations

Allergies

Individuals with fructose intolerance should not take phosphorated carbohydrate solution.

Pregnancy/Breast-feeding

Phosphorated carbohydrate solution has been used to treat nausea and vomiting associated with pregnancy, but has not been proven to be particularly effective. Currently, OTC antiemetics approved by the FDA are not indicated for this purpose.

It is not generally recommended that pregnant women take any drugs, particularly during the first 3 months after conception. Check with your doctor before self-medicating with phosphorated carbohydrate solution if you are or might be pregnant, or if you are breast-feeding.

Infants/Children

Because most studies involving antiemetics are conducted with adults, the use of antiemetics in children is controversial. Some clinicians question whether children suffering from an acute, temporary disorder such as upset stomach due to intestinal flu should be treated with any antiemetic, including phosphorated carbohydrate solution.

If you choose to give this product to your child, exercise the same caution as you would with an adult (see "Cautions and Warnings").

Seniors

Seniors should generally exercise the same caution as younger adults when using phosphorated carbohydrate solution.

Generic Name

Phosphoric Acid (foss-FOR-ik ASS-id)

Definition

An ingredient used in OTC products for the prevention of nausea and vomiting associated with an intestinal virus, indigestion, or an emotional upset. Phosphoric acid is mixed with the sugars fructose and glucose to create phosphorated carbohydrate solution.

Generic Name

Pine Tar Oil

Definition

A blackish-brown liquid derived from the wood of pine trees. It is used externally as a mild irritant and local antibacterial agent in OTC products to treat chronic skin diseases such as eczema, psoriasis, and dandruff.

Generic Name

Piperonyl Butoxide
(PYE-per-ON-il bew-TOKS-ide)

Definition

A chemical used in pediculicides (lice treatments) to enhance the killing power of the main active ingredient, pyrethrins.

Generic Name

Polycarbophil (POLL-ee-KAR-boe-fill)

Definition

A synthetic resin used in OTC products to treat diarrhea. By absorbing water, polycarbophil helps decrease the looseness of stool.

Generic Name

Polyethylene Glycol

(POLL-ee-ETH-ih-leen GLYE-kol)

Definition

A substance used as a vehicle (carrier) for the active drug in various OTC products. Because it dissolves in water, polyethylene glycol releases the active drug more readily in certain tissues, such as the anal region (for treatment of hemorrhoids) and the feet (for treatment of fungal infections), than does an oil-based vehicle. However, in other areas, such as the hands, a polyethylene glycol base can draw moisture out of the tissue, causing dryness and reducing the ability of the active drug to penetrate the skin. Polyethylene glycol is also used as a moisturizing agent in eyedrops and is combined with electrolytes (salts) for bowel preparations and enemas.

Generic Name

Polymyxin B Sulfate

(POLL-ee-MIKS-in BEE SULL-fate)

Brand Names

Betadine First Aid Antibiotic Plus Moisturizer
Campho-phenique Triple Antibiotic
Clomycin
Lanabiotic
Medi-Quik Triple Antibiotic
Mycitracin
Neosporin
Polysporin
Tribiotic Plus

Type of Drug

Topical antibiotic.

Used for

Treatment of ear, eye, and skin infections.

General Information

Topical OTC antibiotics are used to prevent microscopic organisms, such as bacteria, from growing in wounds and causing inflammation, itching, and oozing. There are many types of antibiotics available, each effective against different forms of bacteria. Many OTC products combine different antibiotics so that they have what is called a broad spectrum of effectiveness against a range of disease-causing germs.

Applied within 4 hours after an injury—before the bacteria have a chance to grow—topical antibiotics reduce the risk of wound infection by preventing tissue breakdown, relieving pain, removing dead skin cells (which can delay healing), and helping the wound to close.

Often, bacteria develop resistance to antibiotics. This means that they evolve quickly and develop new ways to defend themselves against the antibiotic, making it useless.

Many physicians believe that, to reduce the problem of resistance, topical antibiotics should be used only to prevent skin infection, not to treat an infection after it develops. Also, antibiotics should be used only when needed and only as indicated, for short periods of time.

Polymyxin B sulfate works by weakening the cell walls of the bacteria, causing the walls to leak and the bacteria eventually to die.

Polymyxin B is not effective against fungal infections.

Polymyxin B is available by itself and in combination with other antibiotics, such as bacitracin and neomycin, so that it has a better chance of being effective against germs. However, overuse of these combination antibiotics increases the risk that bacterial resistance will develop, making treatment ineffective.

Polymyxin B is also available by prescription, alone or in combination with other antibiotics, for treating superficial infections of the eye, such as some forms of conjunctivitis. More serious eye infections require treatment with antibiotics taken by mouth or injection. Combined with other antibiotics, prescription forms of polymyxin B can be used to treat superficial infections of the outer ear.

Cautions and Warnings

Do not use polymyxin B for more than 7 consecutive days. Overuse of antibiotics can lead to bacterial resistance. If there is no improvement in the infected area within 7 days, discontinue using the drug and contact your doctor.

Do not exceed the recommended daily dosage of polymyxin B.

Do not use polymyxin B products over large areas of injured skin or in large quantities.

OTC products containing polymyxin B are for external use only.

By itself, polymyxin B rarely causes an allergic reaction. But this drug is often teamed with other antibiotics, such as neomycin, in "triple-strength" formulations. These other ingredients are more likely to cause a secondary rash or inflammation. If you develop an allergic reaction to any polymyxin product, stop using it and call your doctor.

Do not use first-aid skin care products containing polymyxin B in or near the eyes.

In the case of deep puncture wounds or animal bites, contact your doctor immediately. These injuries generally require specific medical attention.

By destroying bacteria, polymyxin B sometimes allows a fungal infection to develop in its place. If this problem (known as a superinfection) occurs, discontinue use of the drug and ask a health care professional for advice.

Possible Side Effects

Polymyxin alone carries little risk of a sensitivity reaction. When used in combination with neomycin, there can be adverse effects due to the combination. If you experience itching, diarrhea, nausea, hearing loss, dizziness, ringing in the ears, or a rash, discontinue the medication and contact your doctor.

Other ingredients in antibiotic preparations, such as preservatives, may cause sensitivity reactions in some people.

Drug Interactions

- Using hydrocortisone, a topical corticosteroid for treatment of inflammation, at the same time as polymyxin B can disguise the presence of a secondary infection. It also makes it hard to notice whether the antibiotic is causing an allergic reaction. Do not use hydrocortisone along with topical antibiotics except under the advice of a health care professional.

Usual Dose

Adult and Child (age 2 and over): Apply a thin layer to the wound after the area has been cleaned with soap and water and patted dry. Do not apply more than 3 times a day. The affected area may be covered with a sterile bandage. Wash hands prior to and after administering these products.

Child (under age 2): Consult a doctor.

Overdosage

The risk for overdose with polymyxin is quite low. However, if you use polymyxin in combination with neomycin products, you should be concerned if you experience itching, diarrhea, nausea, hearing loss, dizziness, ringing in the ears, or a rash. If you have these symptoms, discontinue use of the drug and contact your doctor.

Even if the victim is not displaying any of the symptoms listed above, do the following in case of accidental ingestion: If the victim is unconscious or having convulsions, call for an ambulance immediately. If you take the victim to an emergency room, be sure to bring the bottle or container with you. If the victim is conscious, call your local poison control center or a health care professional. The poison control center may suggest inducing vomiting with ipecac syrup (available without a prescription at any pharmacy). DO NOT induce vomiting unless specifically instructed to do so.

Special Populations

Pregnancy/Breast-feeding

There is no indication that using topical polymyxin B for superficial skin infections poses a risk to pregnant women, nursing mothers, or their infants. However, it is not generally recommended that pregnant women take any drugs, particularly during the first 3 months after conception. Check with your doctor if you are or might be pregnant, or if you are breast-feeding.

Infants/Children

Antibiotics, including polymyxin B, should not be used for treatment of diaper rash. This is especially true of combination products that contain neomycin. Using antibiotics on such a large area of the child's body poses an increased risk that too much of the drug will be absorbed, causing allergic reactions and possibly serious internal complications.

Polymyxin B is not recommended in children under age 2 unless directed by a doctor.

Seniors

Combination medications containing polymyxin B sulfate may also contain neomycin, which should never be used on incontinence rash in older individuals. The possibility of allergic reaction to the neomycin and the large area of skin requiring treatment can lead to serious internal complications.

Generic Name

Polyparaben (POLL-ee-PARE-uh-ben)

Definition

A preservative used in OTC eye care products, vaginal lubricants, and diaper rash medications.

Generic Name

Polyquaternium #5

(POLL-ee-KWA-ter-nee-um)

Definition

A preservative used in OTC vaginal lubricants.

Generic Name

Polyvinyl Alcohol (PVA)

(POLL-ee-VYE-nil AL-kuh-hall)

Definition

An ingredient used to enhance viscosity (the ability of the product to remain on the tissue and thus provide moisture) in OTC artificial tear products. PVA also aids healing of scratches on the cornea (outer surface of the eye). In artificial tear preparations, PVA is usually present in a 1.4% concentration.

Generic Name

Potassium Salicylate

(poe-TASS-ee-uhm SAL-ih-SILL-ate)

Definition

A pain-relieving ingredient used in OTC products for relief of menstrual symptoms, especially combination products that also include a diuretic.

Generic Name

Potassium Sorbate (poe-TASS-ee-um SOR-bate)

Definition

A preservative used in OTC vaginal lubricants and other products. It is also used in contact lens wetting products. It is considered less irritating to the eyes than mercury-based preservatives such as thimerosal. However, potassium sorbate may increase the yellowing of certain contact lenses, especially those made with a methacrylic acid.

Generic Name

Povidone (POE-vih-doan)

Definition

*see **Povidone-Iodine** below*

Generic Name

Povidone-Iodine (POE-vih-doan EYE-oe-dine)

Brand Names

Aerodine
Betadine
Isodine Antiseptic
Massengill Medicated Disposable Douche
Minidyne
Polydine
Summer's Eve Douche
Vaginex Douche
*Yeast-Guard

**Not all products in this brand-name group contain povidone-iodine.*

Type of Drug

Topical anti-infective agent.

Used for

Preventing infection in minor scrapes, cuts, and burns; relieving symptoms of minor itching and irritation associated with vaginitis due to certain types of fungal, protozoan, and bacterial infection; treating fungal skin infections.

Although povidone-iodine can be effective for treating minor bacterial infections of the skin and vagina, there are better OTC products available for this purpose. For minor bacterial infection of the skin, triple antibiotic ointment is preferable, and for vaginal fungal infections, athlete's foot and jock itch, clotrimazole-containing products are recommended.

General Information

Iodine is a germicide effective against bacteria, fungi, and protozoa. Povidone-iodine is a complex produced by reacting iodine with the chemical compound povidone, which slowly releases iodine. It contains 0.5% to 1% available iodine.

Solutions of iodine alone stain skin and may be irritating to tissue; povidone-iodine is less irritating to the skin and mucous membranes.

Povidone-iodine has many different uses, according to formulation. It is 1 of only 7 OTC antifungal drug products regarded as safe and effective by the FDA, and it is also regarded by the agency as a safe and effective first aid antiseptic. For these topical uses, povidone-iodine is available by generic name in ointment and solution forms and by brand name in spray, gel, ointment, cream, and solution forms. Sprays are less effective than the other forms because they are often not rubbed into the skin.

Reduced concentrations of povidone-iodine are used in medicated douche products, available by brand name in solution form, for mixing the douche yourself, or ready-mixed in disposable form. Although douching is quite common, the benefits of this practice, for either therapeutic or hygienic reasons, are questionable, and there exist several risks (see "Cautions and Warnings").

Cautions and Warnings

Do not exceed the recommended daily dosage of povidone-iodine.

These products are for external use only. Avoid contact with your eyes.

Topical Products

Do not use iodine skin preparations for more than 3 or 4 days continuously except under a doctor's supervision.

In general, first aid antiseptics are best used to disinfect the intact skin around a wound rather than the wound itself. Antiseptics have been shown to kill white blood cells, which promote healing, when applied to open wounds, resulting in increased inflammation. However, reduced concentrations of povidone-iodine (0.001%) are less toxic to white blood cells than to bacteria. Be sure to read the label of your povidone-iodine preparation.

Povidone-iodine should be used with caution when treating large wounds or severe burns. In such cases, the iodine is absorbed through the skin, which can result in excess iodine concentrations. If kidney function is normal, the iodine is rapidly eliminated from the body; but if kidney function is impaired, temporary thyroid dysfunction or hyperthyroidism (marked by palpitations, nervousness and tremors, excessive sweating, and other symptoms) can occur.

If you are using povidone-iodine to treat a fungal skin infection and you do not see substantial improvement in 7 days, call your doctor. Recurring skin infections may be a sign of an underlying serious disease, such as diabetes or immune system dysfunction.

Vaginal Products

If symptoms persist after 7 days or if redness, swelling, or pain develops, call your doctor.

An association has been reported between douching and pelvic inflammation disease (PID— a serious infection of the reproductive system that can lead to sterility and ectopic pregnancy). The most common symptom of PID is pain and/or tenderness in the lower abdomen and pelvis. Other symptoms include vaginal discharge, vaginal bleeding, nausea, and fever. If you are using a povidone-iodine douche and suspect that you have PID, stop using the product and call your doctor.

Certain sexually transmitted diseases (STDs) have symptoms similar to those of PID, as well as additional symptoms. Do not use a povidone-iodine douche if you are experiencing unusual vaginal discharge, vaginal bleeding, painful and/or frequent urination, lower abdominal/pelvis pain, or if you or your partner has genital sores or ulcers. Call your doctor.

Douching may alter the chemical environment in the vagina, leading to an increased risk for cervical cancer or for acquiring an STD.

Do not use povidone-iodine douche to self-treat a PID or STD.

Do not use a medicated douche for routine cleansing.

While povidone-iodine douches reduce total bacteria, they may also conversely allow some species to multiply, thus actually increasing the risk of vaginal infection.

Povidone-iodine may be systemically absorbed. Do not use any of these products if you have an iodine sensitivity or allergy.

Use povidone-iodine douche for the full 7-day regimen even if your symptoms are relieved earlier.

If vaginal dryness or irritation occurs, stop using the product.

Do not use forceful pressure when douching.

If you are not using a disposable product, be sure to keep your douche equipment clean and to use lukewarm water to mix the douche. If you are using a douche bag, do not use the rectal tip (used for enemas) to douche; this can lead to vaginal infections.

Douching does not prevent pregnancy.

Do not douche until at least 8 hours after intercourse if a diaphragm, cervical cap, or contraceptive jelly, cream, or foam was used.

Do not douche in the 24 to 48 hour period before a gynecological exam.

Possible Side Effects

Topical Products

Povidone-iodine is usually nonirritating, but take care when treating large wounds or when applying the medication to the wound itself (see "Cautions and Warnings").

Possible Side Effects ***(continued)***

Vaginal Products

Few allergic reactions have been seen with these products, but povidone-iodine taken intravaginally may be systemically absorbed; individuals with iodine sensitivity should not use povidone-iodine douches.

Vaginal dryness and irritation have been reported.

Douching has been associated with PID (see "Cautions and Warnings").

Drug Interactions

None known.

Usual Dose

Topical Products

Use as needed, but do not exceed the recommended daily dose.

Vaginal Products

Use once a day for 7 consecutive days. Be sure to complete the full 7-day regimen. Read the package instructions carefully.

Overdosage

Do the following in case of accidental ingestion: If the victim is unconscious or having convulsions, call for an ambulance immediately. If you take the victim to an emergency room, be sure to bring the bottle or container with you. If the victim is conscious, call your local poison control center or a health care professional. The poison control center may suggest inducing vomiting with ipecac syrup (available without a prescription at any pharmacy). DO NOT induce vomiting unless specifically instructed to do so.

Special Populations

Allergies

Do not use any povidone-iodine product if you are allergic to iodine.

Pregnancy/Breast-feeding

Topical Products

It is not generally recommended that pregnant women take any drugs, particularly during the first 3 months after conception. Check with your doctor before using povidone-iodine if you are or might be pregnant, or if you are breast-feeding.

Vaginal Products

Do not douche during pregnancy or while breast-feeding unless directed by a doctor. Povidone-iodine douche presents a particular risk; because it is absorbed, it can result in iodine-induced goiter and deficient thyroid activity in the fetus.

Infants/Children

Topical Products

Children should not use povidone-iodine products without supervision to prevent accidental ingestion.

Vaginal Products

Consult your doctor before allowing a child or adolescent to use a medicated douche.

Seniors

Seniors should exercise the same caution as younger adults when using povidone-iodine products.

Generic Name

Pramoxine Hydrochloride

(prah-MOKS-een HYE-dro-KLOR-ide)

Brand Names

Anti-Itch
Anusol Ointment
Aveeno Anti-Itch
Caladryl
Calamycin
Curasore
Fleet Pain-Relief
*Hemorid for Women
Itch-X
Pramegel
Prax
Procto Foam
Tronothane Hydrochloride
Sooth-It Plus
Tronolane cream

**Not all products in this brand-name group contain pramoxine HCl.*

Type of Drug

Topical anesthetic.

Used for

Temporary relief of pain and itching from minor cuts and burns; insect bites; hemorrhoids; poison ivy, oak, and sumac; and minor skin and mouth irritations.

General Information

Topical anesthetics work by blocking pain signals in the skin and keeping them from traveling along the nerves to the brain. The duration of pain relief from OTC anesthetics for skin conditions is often short, lasting only 15 to 45 minutes. However, these medications should be applied only 3 or 4 times a day. Consequently, they will not provide around-the-clock relief.

Pramoxine and a related compound, pramoxine hydrochloride, are found in a variety of OTC products, including burn and sunburn treatments, hemorrhoid treatments, and products for treatment of poison ivy, poison oak, and insect bites and stings.

Pramoxine is available in concentrations ranging from 0.5% to 1%. Higher concentrations are used for conditions in which the skin is intact, while lower concentrations are appropriate if the skin has been broken.

Pramoxine is one of the few topical anesthetics that is not derived from lidocaine. It therefore is not likely to cause the same sensitivity or allergic reactions that people often experience from products made with lidocaine or procaine. People who are sensitive to benzocaine, for example, may experience relief from pramoxine for their skin complaints.

Pramoxine is available by brand name in the following forms: ointments, creams, lotions, liquids, gels, foams, medicated pads, and sprays.

Cautions and Warnings

Do not use pramoxine for longer than 7 consecutive days. If your symptoms persist, return, or worsen within 7 days or if redness, irritation, swelling, or pain occurs, discontinue using the drug and contact your doctor.

Do not exceed the recommended dosage of pramoxine.

While there is a very low risk for systemic (whole-body) complications with topical anesthetics, using the product more often than recommended increases the risk of developing an allergic reaction or internal side effects.

To avoid systemic toxicity, do not use pramoxine in large quantities, especially on scraped or blistered skin. If a wound is sufficiently large or painful to require a large amount of the drug, do not self-medicate. See your doctor.

Pramoxine preparations are for external use only.

Topical anesthetics should not be used for serious burns, animal bites, or puncture wounds, which need appropriate medical attention.

Pramoxine should not be used near the eyes or nose or applied to large areas of the body.

There is a risk that use of topical anesthetics can hide the symptoms of a more serious condition, which may require different or stronger medical treatment from your doctor.

If the product is being used for hemorrhoid treatment and increased pain or bleeding occurs, discontinue use of the product and contact your doctor.

Topical anesthetics for hemorrhoid treatment should be used only in the external anal area. Do not insert the product into the rectum, because there is a risk that too much of the drug can be absorbed and can cause toxicity.

Do not use products containing pramoxine if you are allergic to any ingredient the formulation contains.

Possible Side Effects

Reactions to pramoxine are rare. However, some people may experience rash, hives, and localized swelling. Should these symptoms develop, wash the area thoroughly with soap and water and discontinue use of the medication.

Topical application of anesthetics can cause temporary burning or stinging in sensitive individuals.

In rare cases, anaphylactic shock might develop, resulting in difficulty breathing, low blood pressure, swelling of the tongue or throat, and diarrhea.

Drug Interactions

None known.

Usual Dose

Pain Relief

Adult and Child (age 2 and over): Apply 3–4 times a day or as directed by your doctor. The affected area should be cleansed and dried thoroughly before application of the medication. Apply a thin layer to extend to the edges of the inflammation. Pain relief should be felt within a few minutes.

Child (under age 2): Consult your doctor.

Hemorrhoids

Adult and Child (age 12 and over): Apply up to 5 times a day or after each bowel movement. Follow package directions for the specific product you are using.

Child (under age 12): Consult your doctor.

Overdosage

Do the following in case of accidental ingestion: If the victim is unconscious or having convulsions, call for an ambulance immediately. If you take the victim to an emergency room, be sure to bring the bottle or container with you. If the victim is conscious, call your local poison control center or a health care professional. The poison control center may suggest inducing vomiting with ipecac syrup (available without a prescription at any pharmacy). DO NOT induce vomiting unless specifically instructed to do so.

Special Populations

Pregnancy/Breast-feeding

It is not generally recommended that pregnant women take any drug, particularly during the first 3 months after conception. Check with your doctor before using pramoxine if you are or might be pregnant, or if you are breast-feeding.

If you experience dry, sore, or cracked nipple tissues while breast-feeding, do not use an OTC anesthetic except on advice from a physician. Your baby could ingest the medication during feeding.

Infants/Children

Children under 2 should not use pramoxine except under your doctor's supervision. Children under 12 should not be given pramoxine hemorrhoidal preparations unless directed by your doctor.

To avoid accidental ingestion, children treated with pramoxine should be instructed not to put the affected area in the mouth.

Seniors

Seniors should exercise the same caution as younger adults when using pramoxine products.

Generic Name

Propylene Glycol (PROP-uh-leen GLYE-kol)

Definition

A substance used as a preservative in OTC vaginal lubricants and as a wetting agent in artificial tear products. In OTC ear preparations, it is a vehicle (carrier) of the active drug, and adheres to tissues, thus increasing the amount of time the active drug remains in contact with the affected area. When combined with acetic acid, propylene glycol helps fight infection. However, with long-term use, propylene glycol can cause dermatitis (skin inflammation).

Generic Name

Propylparaben (PROE-pull-PAH-ruh-ben)

Definition

A substance used as a fungal preservative in eye care products, vaginal lubricants, and other OTC products. It is often used in conjunction with methylparaben, which is a bacterial preservative. Some people have allergic reactions to eye products containing propylparaben.

Generic Name

Pseudoephedrine (SOO-doe-eh-FED-rin)

Brand Names

Actifed
Advil Cold & Sinus
*Alka-Seltzer Plus
Allerest
Bayer Select Aspirin-Free Sinus Pain Relief
*†Benadryl
Benylin Multi-Symptom Formula [A] [S]
Bromfed [A]
†Cenafed
*†Chlor-Trimeton
*†Codimal
*Comtrex
Congestac
Congestion Relief
*Contac
*Creomulsion [A]
DayGel
Dimacol
*†Dimetapp
Disophrol Chronotabs
Dorcol Children's Cough [A]
*Dristan Cold & Cough
*Drixoral
Dynafed
Efidac/24
Excedrin Sinus
Fedahist
Flu-Relief
GuiaCough PE
Guaifed [A]
Hayfebrol [A] [S]
Kodet SE
*†Kolephrin
Mini Thin Pseudo
Napril
Nasal-D [S]
NiteGel
*Novahistine
Oranyl
Ornex
P.C. Nasal Decongestant
PediaCare [A]
*†Robitussin
Sinarest
Sine-Aid
Sine-Off
Singlet
Sinutab
Sinutol Maximum Strength
†Sudafed
Sudanyl
Tetrahist
TheraFlu
Tri-Fed
*Triaminic [A]
†Tussar
*†Tylenol
*†Vicks

**Not all products in this brand-name group contain pseudoephedrine.*

†Consult the OTC ingredient charts to determine whether different formulations in this brand-name group are alcohol-, caffeine-, or sugar-free.

Type of Drug

Decongestant.

Used for

Temporary relief of nasal congestion (stuffy nose) that may accompany allergies and colds.

General Information

Decongestants relieve nasal congestion by narrowing or constricting blood vessels in the nose. This action reduces the blood supplied to the nose and decreases the swelling of nasal mucous membranes. Unlike topical decongestants (decongestant nasal sprays), which act on local blood vessels, oral decongestants may constrict blood vessels throughout the body.

Decongestants are used to treat the nasal stuffiness of colds and allergies. However, they cannot cure a cold or allergy. The best you can hope for is symptomatic relief. To effectively relieve allergy symptoms, decongestants are usually given in combination with an antihistamine, which works against histamine, a chemical substance released by the body during an allergic reaction.

Pseudoephedrine, an oral decongestant, is available by generic and brand name, either alone as pseudoephedrine hydrochloride or in combination products as pseudoephedrine sulfate. It is manufactured in many forms, including caplets, tablets, drops, gelcaps, liqui-caps, and liquids. At its usual dose of 60 mg, pseudoephedrine begins to work within 30 minutes after it is taken, and its effect lasts for up to 8 hours.

Cautions and Warnings

Do not take pseudoephedrine for more than 7 days continuously except under a doctor's supervision.

Do not exceed the recommended daily dosage of pseudoephedrine.

If you have hyperthyroidism, heart disease, high blood pressure, diabetes, or an enlarged prostate, you should take pseudoephedrine only under the supervision of a doctor, because it can aggravate these conditions. People with high blood pressure should be especially cautious about taking this drug because it may increase blood pressure and, in large doses, may increase stimulation of the heart or alter its rhythm. When used in individuals with diabetes, pseudoephedrine may increase blood sugar.

Possible Side Effects

Pseudoephedrine has a low incidence of side effects in people taking recommended doses. Most of the side effects seen are related to the drug's effect on the central nervous system. If you develop any of the following side effects, stop taking pseudoephedrine. Call your doctor if you experience any of the effects listed as "less common" or "rare."

- ▼ Most common: nervousness, restlessness, excitability, insomnia, dizziness, and weakness. Headache and drowsiness may also occur.
- ▼ Less common: increased blood pressure, increased or irregular heart rate, and heart palpitations.
- ▼ Rare: fear, anxiety, tenseness, tremor, hallucinations, seizures, pallor, breathing difficulty, difficulty or pain when urinating, and cardiovascular collapse.

Drug Interactions

• Pseudoephedrine should not be used at the same time as a monoamine oxidase inhibitor (MAOI) drug or within 2 weeks of stopping treatment with an MAOI. MAOI drugs are used to treat depression, other psychiatric or emotional conditions, and Parkinson's disease. If you are not sure whether you are taking or have taken an MAOI, check with your doctor or pharmacist before you use pseudoephedrine.

• Taking pseudoephedrine along with another decongestant can increase the risk of adverse effects and toxicity. If you are taking another decongestant, do not take pseudoephedrine without first asking your doctor.

• Pseudoephedrine's actions may combine with those of caffeine, which also affects the central nervous system, and cause disorientation, delirium, and other side effects. Be aware that caffeine is an ingredient in many prescription and OTC drugs.

Food Interactions

Pseudoephedrine interacts with caffeine, which is found in many popular beverages, including coffee, tea, and cola, and in chocolate. (see "Drug Interactions").

Usual Dose

Adult and Child (age 12 and over): 60 mg every 4–6 hours. Do not take more than 240 mg in 24 hours.

Child (age 6–11): 30 mg every 4–6 hours. Do not give more than 120 mg in 24 hours.

Child (age 2–5): 15 mg every 4–6 hours. Do not give more than 60 mg in 24 hours. As an alternative, some pediatricians recommend 4 mg/kg daily, given in 4 divided doses.

Child (under age 2): Consult a doctor.

Extended-release

Some preparations of pseudoephedrine are available with an extended-release core and an immediate-release outer coating. These should be taken as 1 tablet every 24 hours and should be swallowed whole with fluid—never chewed, crushed, or dissolved.

Extended-release preparations of pseudoephedrine hydrochloride or sulfate should not be used in children under age 12.

Overdosage

Do the following in case of accidental overdose: If the victim is unconscious or having convulsions, call for an ambulance immediately. If you take the victim to an emergency room, be sure to bring the bottle or container with you. If the victim is conscious, call your local poison control center or a health care professional. The poison control center may suggest inducing vomiting with ipecac syrup (available without a prescription at any pharmacy). DO NOT induce vomiting unless specifically instructed to do so.

Special Information

Colds will usually go away in 1 to 2 weeks whether they are treated or not. There are other ways to temporarily treat congestion caused by colds, including taking tea with lemon and honey or eating chicken soup or hot broth.

Special Populations

Pregnancy/Breast-feeding

It is not generally recommended that pregnant women take any drugs, particularly during the first 3 months after conception. Do not take pseudoephedrine if you are or might be pregnant without first checking with your doctor.

Small amounts of decongestants such as pseudoephedrine have been shown to pass into breast milk. Check with your doctor before self-medicating with pseudoephedrine if you are breast-feeding.

Infants/Children

Children under age 2 should not take pseudoephedrine unless directed by a physician. Children under age 12 should not take extended-release preparations of pseudoephedrine.

Seniors

Seniors taking pseudoephedrine should be especially cautious about the amount of caffeine they ingest (see "Drug Interactions"). They may also be especially sensitive to the side effects of pseudoephedrine. They may experience nervousness, irritability, restlessness, dizziness, sedation, hallucinations, seizures, and low blood pressure. Most mild reactions may be handled by lowering your dose. Seniors should not take extended-release preparations of pseudoephedrine unless they have first taken a short-acting version and experienced no adverse effects.

Generic Name

Psyllium Hydrophilic Mucilloid

(SILL-ee-um HYE-droe-FILL-ik MEW-sih-loid)

Brand Names

*Fiberall
Garfields Tea
Hydrocil Instant (psyllium)
Innerclean Herbal (psyllium seed husks-buckthorn bark)
*Konsyl
Metamucil
Modane Bulk Powder
Natural Bulk
Perdiem (psyllium)
Serutan
Swiss Kriss [S] (psyllium seed husks)
V-Lax

**Not all products in this brand-name group contain psyllium hydrophilic mucilloid.*

Type of Drug

Laxative.

Used for

Relief of occasional constipation (irregularity). Also used to increase the bulk of stools in people with chronic, watery diarrhea.

General Information

The average, healthy individual defecates anywhere from 3 times a day to 3 times a week. Constipation is determined not necessarily by the frequency of bowel movements, but by the consistency of the stool, how difficult it is to eliminate it, and symptoms such as dull headache, low back pain, and abdominal distention (swelling). Evaluate your condition carefully and discuss your symptoms and their possible causes with your pharmacist before taking a laxative. Laxatives are not always necessary, and when used improperly can either prevent the desired effect or result in laxative dependency. If you are indeed constipated, it may be best managed through proper diet, adequate fluid intake (6 to 8 glasses a day), and exercise. If you must use a laxative, choose the mildest effective product.

Laxatives may be classified by their mechanism of action: bulk-forming, emollient (stool softeners), lubricant, saline, hyperosmotic, and stimulant. Psyllium hydrophilic mucilloid is a bulk-forming laxative. Bulk-forming laxatives work by dissolving or swelling in water to form an emollient gel. The increased bulk of the fecal material helps the intestine to contract in waves, forcing the feces out. Of all laxatives, bulk-forming products most closely approximate the natural, physiologic mechanism of defecation. Consequently, they are considered by most doctors to be the best initial therapy for simple constipation, which is generally caused by a low-fiber and/or low-fluid diet.

Bulk-forming laxatives are recommended for people with colostomies and irritable bowel syndrome, and for people who should avoid straining during defecation (e.g., individuals with hernias). However, they are not recommended for treating constipation associated with hard, dry stools. They are also not the best choice when a prompt or complete emptying of the bowel is desired.

Bulk-forming laxatives generally begin to work within 12 to 24 hours, but the full effect may not be achieved for 2 to 3 days.

Psyllium is available by generic name in powder form and by brand-name in tablet, powder, granule, and wafer form.

Cautions and Warnings

Do not use for more than 7 days unless directed by your doctor.

Do not exceed the maximum daily dosage of psyllium. The higher the dose, the more likely you are to experience adverse effects.

Long-term use of laxatives has been linked with laxative dependence, chronic constipation, loss of normal bowel function, and, in severe cases, nerve, muscle, and tissue damage to the intestines. Using laxatives too frequently can result in persistent diarrhea, hypokalemia (abnormally low potassium in blood), loss of essential nutrients, and dehydration.

Do not take psyllium if you have abdominal pain, nausea, vomiting, or kidney disease, unless directed by your doctor.

If you notice a marked change in bowel habits lasting for more than 2 weeks, do not take psyllium until you have spoken to your doctor. Also contact your doctor if there is blood in your stool, so that colon cancer or other significant disease can be ruled out before you begin self-medication with psyllium.

If you have had a disease or surgery affecting the gastrointestinal (GI) tract, using a laxative may affect your condition adversely.

If you have rectal bleeding after using psyllium, or if you do not have a bowel movement after 7 days of using this medication, you may have a serious condition. Stop using psyllium and call your doctor.

Psyllium should not be used by people with partial bowel obstruction.

Two special populations should note the inactive ingredients in their psyllium product. People with diabetes should be aware that some psyllium preparations contain large amounts of sugar. Individuals with phenylketonuria should avoid sugar-free preparations, which contain aspartame. Read the label carefully.

Take care not to inhale psyllium dust particles, in case of an allergic reaction (see "Special Populations: Allergies").

Each dose of psyllium must be taken with at least 8 oz. of water or other fluid. If you do not drink enough with your bulk-laxative dose, a semisolid mass can form, resulting in bowel and/or esophageal obstruction, swelling or blockage of the throat, choking, or asphyxiation. Psyllium should not be used by people with throat problems or who have difficulty swallowing. Call your doctor if, after taking this product, you have chest pain or pressure, you regurgitate or vomit, or you have difficulty swallowing or breathing.

Possible Side Effects

When used properly, psyllium rarely causes adverse effects. However, a dose of psyllium taken without enough fluid (8 oz.) can result in bowel and/or esophageal obstruction, swelling or blockage of the throat, choking, or asphyxiation (see "Cautions and Warnings").

▼ Less common: diarrhea, abdominal discomfort, flatulence (gas), and excessive loss of fluid.

Drug Interactions

• All laxatives potentially decrease the absorption of any oral drug taken at the same time. If you are currently taking an oral medication, talk to your doctor or pharmacist before self-medicating with a psyllium product.

• If you are taking the heart medication digitalis, the urinary anti-infective nitrofurantoin, or a salicylate such as aspirin, consult your doctor or pharmacist before beginning self-medication with psyllium. Some physicians recommend separating doses by at least 3 hours if you take psyllium concurrently with any of the above drugs.

Food Interactions

None known.

Usual Dose

Doses should be adjusted to individual usage.

Each dose of psyllium must be taken with at least 8 oz. of water or other fluid (see "Cautions and Warnings").

To mask the grittiness of the powder, mix it with a pleasant-tasting fluid such as fruit juice or a sugar-free fruit drink.

Tablets

Adult and Child (over age 12): 2 tablets, 1–4 times a day.

Child (age 6–12): 1 tablet, 1–3 times a day.

Child (under age 6): Consult your doctor.

Powder

Adult and Child (over age 12): 1 tsp., 1–3 times a day. Put 1 tsp. of powder in a closed container with 8 oz. of water or juice. Shake for 3–5 seconds (do not stir) and then drink immediately.

Child (age 6–12): 1/2 tsp., 1–3 times a day. Follow the instructions above, using 8 oz. of water or juice.

Child (under age 6): Consult your doctor.

Wafers

Adult and Child (over age 12): 2 wafers, 1–3 times a day.

Child (age 6–12): 1/2 tsp., 1 wafer, 1–3 times a day.

Child (under age 6): Consult your doctor.

If you are taking the maximum daily dosage of psyllium, take it in divided doses.

Overdosage

Do the following in case of accidental overdose: If the victim is unconscious or having convulsions, call for an ambulance immediately. If you take the victim to an emergency room, be sure to bring the bottle or container with you. If the victim is conscious, call your local poison control center or a health care professional. The poison control center may suggest inducing vomiting with ipecac syrup (available without a prescription at any pharmacy). DO NOT induce vomiting unless specifically instructed to do so.

Special Populations

Allergies

Susceptible individuals (e.g., those with psyllium sensitivity or suffering from respiratory disorders) who have accidentally inhaled dry psyllium particles have experienced potentially severe hypersensitivity reactions, including bronchospasm. To avoid possible allergic reaction to airborne powdered psyllium, use a spoon to add the powder to your glass rather than pouring it directly from the container.

Pregnancy/Breast-feeding

It is not generally recommended that pregnant women take any drugs, particularly during the first 3 months after conception. However, emollient and bulk-forming laxatives such as psyllium are the only laxatives recommended for use by pregnant women.

Check with your doctor before self-medicating with psyllium if you are or might be pregnant, or if you are breastfeeding. Also, consider talking to your doctor about diet and mild exercise in the management of constipation.

Infants/Children

Observe your child carefully for patterns of bowel movements and the pain or difficulty with which the bowel movements are made before deciding whether the child is actually constipated. As with adults, "normal" bowel habits vary in children. If your child is indeed constipated, increasing fluid intake and adding fiber to his or her diet may help to manage the condition.

In general, the use of laxatives should be avoided in children.

Consult your doctor before giving psyllium to a child under 6 years of age.

Seniors

Seniors commonly experience constipation, and consequently may become laxative-dependent. Avoid chronically turning to laxatives to ease constipation, and instead look to diet and increased fluid intake as therapeutic measures.

Although esophageal obstruction has occurred in seniors taking bulk-forming laxatives, these products are usually the preferred choice for seniors.

Generic Name

Pyrantel Pamoate (pih-RAN-tel PAM-oe-ate)

Definition

A tasteless and odorless powder, used in liquid, suspension, or caplet form to treat infection with roundworms, hookworms, and pinworms.

Generic Name

Pyrethrins (pye-RETH-rinz)

Brand Names

Barc
End-Lice
Licetrol
Licide
Pronto Lice Killing
R&C
Tisit

Type of Drug

Pediculicide (antilice medication).

Used for

Treatment of lice infestation.

General Information

Lice are 8-legged, wingless parasites that live on the human body. Their front legs are well suited for holding tightly to human skin. Lice feed on the blood of their host, and their bites cause an irritating itch. Head lice appear on the scalp, pubic lice (also known as crab lice or crabs) appear in the groin area, and body lice occupy seams and folds of clothing and feed on various parts of the body.

Lice do not jump or fly. Instead, the infestation is transmitted by direct contact or by sharing personal items such as combs, brushes, or headwear. Lice infestation is common among children in schools and day care centers. Among adults, pubic lice can be transmitted during sexual intercourse.

Lice infestation is an annoying and stubborn problem, but it can be treated effectively with OTC products that contain pyrethrins. Permethrin is the other commonly available OTC pediculicide. Medications containing pediculicides paralyze the parasites, thus preventing them from reproducing and eventually killing them. Pyrethrins is effective at killing all kinds of lice and their nits (eggs).

Most pediculicides with pyrethrins also contain piperonyl butoxide. This chemical does not work against lice directly, but it enhances the effect of pyrethrins.

Pyrethrins is available by brand name in gel, liquid, and shampoo form.

Cautions and Warnings

Do not use more than 2 doses of pyrethrins. If infestation is still present after 2 doses spaced by 7 to 10 days, contact your doctor.

Do not exceed the recommended daily dosage of pyrethrins products.

Some OTC products for lice treatment, such as household sprays, are intended for use on animals or inanimate objects only, not on humans. Read labels carefully.

Pyrethrins products are for external use only.

If the infestation involves the eyebrows or eyelashes, do not use a lice treatment containing pyrethrins, because the drug can cause serious complications if it comes in contact with eye tissues. Instead, contact your doctor for recommendations of an alternate treatment. Meanwhile, applying petroleum jelly for 10 days can be effective in the treatment of eyelash and eyebrow infestations.

Pyrethrins-containing shampoo must be left on the scalp or body for about 10 minutes. Keep eyes closed tightly while the product is working. If the shampoo comes in contact with your eyes, flush them immediately with cool water.

The fumes from pyrethrins products can be harmful, especially to people with asthma or chronic bronchitis. Use the medication in a well-ventilated area, and stay there until it is time to rinse off the medication.

If one person in the family develops a lice infestation, all other household members should be treated to reduce the risk of the infestation spreading and reinfestation.

Wash all infected bedding and clothing in hot water and dry at high temperatures for at least 20 minutes to prevent reinfestation. Items that can't be washed may be sealed in a plastic bag for 2 weeks.

Possible Side Effects

Pyrethrins products may cause temporary stinging, itching, burning, or irritation in the area being treated. These effects are not long-lasting and usually stop within 20 minutes after removal of the product.

Drug Interactions

None known.

Usual Dose

Adult and Child (age 2 months and over): Wash the affected area with a mild soap or shampoo and water; rinse and dry thoroughly. Apply the product in a sufficient amount to saturate the hair and skin. Allow it to remain on the scalp for 10 minutes, but no longer. Rinse thoroughly and dry the area with a towel. Afterward, inspect the area carefully and use a special nit comb to remove the lice bodies and eggs (nits).

Do not exceed 2 applications in 24 hours. Repeat procedure in 7–10 days to kill any newly hatched lice.

Child (under age 2 months): not recommended unless prescribed by a doctor.

Overdosage

Very little pyrethrins is absorbed into the skin, so the risk of toxicity is low.

Do the following in case of accidental ingestion: If the victim is unconscious or having convulsions, call for an ambulance immediately. If you take the victim to an emergency room, be sure to bring the bottle or container with you. If the victim is conscious, call your local poison control center or a health care professional. The poison control center may suggest inducing vomiting with ipecac syrup (available without a prescription at any pharmacy). DO NOT induce vomiting unless specifically instructed to do so.

Special Populations

Allergies

Pyrethrins is derived from a chrysanthemumlike plant. Products containing pyrethrins should not be used by individuals who have an allergic reaction to ragweed or chrysanthemums.

Pregnancy/Breast-feeding

It is not generally recommended that pregnant women take any drugs, particularly during the first 3 months after conception. However, due to the low absorption rate of pyrethrins with piperonyl butoxide, use of this product is preferred over other pediculicides for pregnant women.

Check with your doctor before using pyrethrins if you are or might be pregnant, or if you are breast-feeding.

Infants/Children

Do not use a pyrethrins product on a child under 2 months (see "Usual Dosage") without first consulting your doctor.

Seniors

Seniors should exercise the same caution as younger adults when using pyrethrins.

Generic Name

Pyrethrum Extract (pye-RETH-rum)

Definition

A substance obtained from pyrethrum flowers (chrysanthemums), used as a treatment for lice infestations.

Generic Name

Pyrilamine Maleate

(peer-ILL-uh-meen MAL-ee-ate)

Brand Names

†*Codimal	ND-Gesic [A]
*4-Way Fast Acting Nasal Spray	Robitussin Night Relief [A]
	Tricodene No. 1 [A]

** Not all products in this brand-name group contain pyrilamine maleate.*

† Consult the OTC ingredient charts to determine whether different formulations in this brand-name group are alcohol-, caffeine-, or sugar-free.

Type of Drug

Antihistamine.

Used for

Temporary relief of itchy eyes or throat, runny nose, sneezing, and inflammation associated with cold and allergy.

General Information

Antihistamines block the release of histamine in the body, relieving the sneezing and itching that often occur with colds and allergies. They can also aid in stopping a runny nose by reducing the secretions caused by histamine release. (Generally, though, a decongestant is included for that purpose in combination products with antihistamines.)

Since histamine is only one of several substances released by the body during an allergic reaction, antihistamines can only reduce about 40% to 60% of allergic symptoms.

If you have seasonal allergies, antihistamines work best if you begin treatment before the allergy season starts. Once these allergies begin, the body releases histamine continuously. Thus the best method of controlling histamine release is to keep taking antihistamines on a continuous schedule once you start. This helps the antihistamine keep up with the constant release of histamine. People who experience allergies year-round (e.g., allergies to pet hair or dust mites) may need to take antihistamines throughout the year.

Pyrilamine maleate is one of the few antihistamines approved by the U.S. Olympic Committee for use by athletes with asthma.

Antihistamines such as pyrilamine will not cure or prevent allergies or colds. The best you can hope for is symptomatic relief.

Pyrilamine is available by generic and brand name in tablet and liquid form, both alone and in combination products.

Cautions and Warnings

Do not take the maximum daily dosage of pyrilamine for

more than 3 days continuously except under a doctor's supervision.

Do not exceed the recommended daily dosage of pyrilamine.

Pyrilamine and other antihistamines should be used with caution if you have a condition that causes breathing problems, such as emphysema, chronic bronchitis, or asthma. Antihistamines dry out the mucous membranes. This in turn can inhibit the ability of the lungs to move or get rid of the excess secretions that these diseases produce.

Antihistamines should be used with caution by people with glaucoma, hyperthyroidism, heart disease, high blood pressure, or difficulty in urinating due to an enlarged prostate. If you have any of these conditions, consult your doctor before taking pyrilamine.

Antihistamines act as a depressant on the central nervous system (CNS), which can cause sleepiness or grogginess and can interfere with the ability to concentrate. Your ability to perform activities that require your full alertness and coordination, such as driving a motor vehicle or operating machinery, may be affected. Refrain from drinking alcohol while you are taking pyrilamine because alcohol aggravates these effects.

Possible Side Effects

▼ Most common: restlessness, nervousness, sleeplessness or drowsiness, dizziness, excitability, poor muscle coordination, headache, and upset stomach.

▼ Less common: blurred vision, difficulty urinating, irritability (at high doses), increased blood pressure, increased or irregular heart rate, heart palpitations, and dry eyes, nose, and mouth.

Drug Interactions

• Antihistamines can enhance the effect of other CNS depressants, such as barbiturates, tranquilizers, sleeping medications, and alcohol (present in many OTC preparations). If you are taking other depressant drugs, check with your doctor before using pyrilamine or any other antihistamine. Avoid drinking alcohol if you are taking pyrilamine.

• Antihistamines should not be used at the same time as a monoamine oxidase inhibitor (MAOI) or within 2 weeks of stopping treatment with an MAOI. MAOIs are used to treat depression, other psychiatric or emotional conditions, and Parkinson's disease. If you are not sure whether you are or have been taking an MAOI, check with your doctor or pharmacist before you use pyrilamine.

• Antihistamines can affect the results of skin and blood tests. Notify your health care professional before scheduling these tests if you are taking pyrilamine.

Food Interactions

None known.

Usual Dose

Because histamine is released nearly continuously, it is best to take pyrilamine on a schedule rather than as needed.

Adult and Child (age 12 and over): 25–50 mg every 6–8 hours. Do not exceed 200 mg in 24 hours.

Child (age 6–11): 12.5–25 mg every 6–8 hours. Do not exceed 100 mg in 24 hours.

Child (under age 6): Consult your doctor.

You may minimize the inconvenience of the sedative effects of antihistamines by taking a full dose at bedtime and using the smallest recommended doses combined with a decongestant during the day. You can establish the lowest dose necessary for effective relief by starting with the lowest dose when you begin taking the drug, and gradually increasing the dosage over several days as needed.

If you forget to take a dose of pyrilamine, do so as soon as you rememeber. If it is almost time for your next dose, skip the one you forgot and continue with your regular schedule. Do not take a double dose.

Overdosage

Symptoms of antihistamine overdose in children include dilated pupils, flushed face, dry mouth, fever, excitability, hallucinations, loss of muscle coordination, and seizures.

In adults, severe overdose can cause drowsiness or coma, which may be followed by excitability or seizures. Eventually fluid can build up in the brain; the kidneys may fail, and the heart and lungs may stop working, resulting in death. Symptoms may develop within 30 minutes to 2 hours following an overdose, and death may occur within 18 hours.

Even if the victim is not displaying any of the symptoms listed above, do the following in case of accidental overdose: If the victim is unconscious or having convulsions, call for an ambulance immediately. If you take the victim to an emergency room, be sure to bring the bottle or container with you. If the victim is conscious, call your local poison control center or a health care professional. The poison control center may suggest inducing vomiting with ipecac syrup (available without a prescription at any pharmacy). DO NOT induce vomiting unless specifically instructed to do so.

Special Populations

Pregnancy/Breast-feeding
Antihistamines are not recommended for use during pregnancy unless directed by your doctor. Antihistamines are known to pass into the breast milk of nursing mothers and may cause side effects in infants. Check with your doctor before taking pyrilamine if you are or might be pregnant, or if you are breast-feeding.

Infants/Children
Children may be more susceptible to the side effects of pyrilamine. They are also more susceptible to accidental antihistamine overdose. Do not give pyrilamine to a child under age 6 unless directed by your doctor.

Seniors
Seniors may be more sensitive to the side effects of antihistamines. They may experience nervousness, irritability, restlessness, dizziness, sedation, hallucinations, seizures, and low blood pressure. Most mild reactions may be handled by either lowering the dose or switching to another product.

Generic Name

Pyrithione Zinc (pih-RITH-ee-own zink)

Brand Names

Brylcreem Anti-Dandruff
DHS Zinc
*Head & Shoulders
Sebulon
*X-Seb
Zincon
ZNP Bar

**Not all products in this brand-name group contain pyrithione zinc.*

Type of Drug

Antiseborrheic.

Used for

Treatment and control of dandruff and seborrhea (seborrheic dermatitis).

General Information

Pyrithione zinc is a cytostatic agent. It works by slowing down the rate at which cells grow and multiply. This action can reduce or even eliminate the excessive amount of skin cells produced in flaking scalp conditions such as dandruff and seborrhea (seborrheic dermatitis).

Pyrithione zinc is one of two cytostatic chemicals that have been approved by the FDA for use in OTC shampoo preparations; the other is selenium sulfide. Pyrithione zinc may take longer to work than selenium sulfide, because its absorption increases the longer it is used. It is also available in a bar soap to control seborrheic dermatitis of the body.

Pyrithione zinc adheres to the scalp surface and the hair, building up over a period of weeks.

Pyrithione zinc is available by brand name in shampoo form.

Cautions and Warnings

Do not exceed the recommended daily dosage of pyrithione zinc.

These products are for external use only. Care should be taken to avoid contact with the eyes. If this occurs, flush the eyes well with water.

If the condition persists or worsens with regular use as directed, stop using the product and consult your doctor.

There are no indications that long-term use of these products is associated with a toxic reaction. Pyrithione zinc is not readily absorbed into the deeper layers of the skin, and systemic (whole-body) overdose is highly unlikely. However, to minimize the risk of a skin reaction, do not use these products on broken skin.

Many experts advise switching from a medicated dandruff shampoo to regular shampoo on alternate days or using dandruff shampoos no more than twice a week.

Possible Side Effects

There is a risk that products used for the treatment of dandruff and seborrhea can cause excessive dryness of the skin, scalp, or hair. Using these products more often than directed can cause scalp or skin irritation and the development of inflamed hair follicles.

Pyrithione zinc products must be rinsed thoroughly from the hair and scalp, or discoloration may result, especially in blond, gray, or dyed hair.

Frequent use of a pyrithione zinc product can cause a residual odor and may leave an oily coating on the scalp.

Drug Interactions

None known.

Usual Dose

Adult and Child (age 2 and over): Before using a pyrithione zinc product, first wash hair with a nonmedicated, nonresidue shampoo and rinse well to remove any dirt, oil, or loose scales. Next, apply a lotion shampoo product with a 1%–2% pyrithione zinc concentration to the scalp, massage it in thoroughly, and leave it on for 5 minutes before rinsing.

Child (under age 2): Consult your doctor.

Overdosage

Do the following in case of accidental ingestion: If the victim is unconscious or having convulsions, call for an ambulance immediately. If you take the victim to an emergency room, be sure to bring the bottle or container with you. If the victim is conscious, call your local poison control center or a health care professional. The poison control center may suggest inducing vomiting with ipecac syrup (available without a prescription at any pharmacy). DO NOT induce vomiting unless specifically instructed to do so.

Special Populations

Pregnancy/Breast-feeding

It is not generally recommended that pregnant women take any drug, particularly during the first 3 months after conception. Check with your doctor if you are or might be pregnant, or if you are breast-feeding.

Infants/Children

Pyrithione zinc preparations available over the counter are not recommended for children under 2 unless under the supervision of a doctor.

Seniors

Seniors should exercise the same caution as younger adults when using pyrithione zinc.

Generic Name

Resmethrin (rez-METH-rin)

Definition

A lice-killing ingredient, similar to permethrin, used in OTC products for treating lice infestations.

Generic Name

Resorcinol (ruh-SOR-sih-nol)

Brand Names

*Acne Treatment
Acnomel
Acnotex
Rezamid Acne Lotion
Sulforcin
Bicozene External Analgesic Creme
Rid-Itch
Resinol Medicated
Vagisil

**Not all products in this brand-name group contain resorcinol.*

Type of Drug

Topical anti-infective, keratolytic (skin-cell remover), and antipruritic (anti-itch agent).

Used for

Treatment of acne (in combination with sulfur); temporary relief of pain and itching associated with minor burns, sunburn, minor cuts, scrapes, insect bites and stings, and minor skin irritations.

General Information

Resorcinol performs several functions. As an anti-infective, it kills both bacteria and fungi. As a keratolytic, it softens and dissolves or peels off the top layer of the skin. As an antipruritic, it relieves and prevents itching. Resorcinol is not available as a single-ingredient product, but is used in combination with several other medications.

Resorcinol is combined with sulfur in several acne products. Resorcinol alone is regarded by the FDA as safe but not effective as an acne remedy, but the combination with sulfur, another keratolytic, is safe and effective in resolving acne lesions.

Resorcinol is also combined with benzocaine in preparations that are used for temporary relief of pain and itching associated with minor burns, sunburn, scrapes, insect bites and stings, and minor cuts and skin irritations.

Resorcinol is combined with the astringents zinc oxide and calamine in products used to treat poison ivy, oak, and sumac.

Resorcinol is combined with the anesthetic benzocaine in OTC products used to treat vaginal yeast infections. However, OTCs that contain an antifungal such as clotrimazole, miconazole, or butoconazole, are much more effective in the treatment of yeast infections.

Resorcinol is combined with benzoic acid and chlorothymol in a preparation marketed as an athlete's foot treatment, however none of these 3 ingredients is regarded by the FDA as a safe and effective topical antifungal drug.

Cautions and Warnings

Do not use resorcinol for pain and itching for longer than 7 days consecutively. If your symptoms persist for more than 7 days, or clear up and recur within a few days, stop using the product and call your doctor.

Do not exceed the recommended daily dosage of resorcinol products.

Do not apply resorcinol preparations to large areas of the body.

Do not cover the affected area with a compress or bandage.

Stop using resorcinol preparations and call your doctor if a rash or irritation develops.

Resorcinol products are for external use only. Avoid contact with your eyes. Be aware of manufacturer's cautions and warnings listed on the label.

Resorcinol/sulfur acne products have a distinct odor and color, due to the sulfur. You may want to use your product at bedtime or use a tinted product during the day. Resorcinol may produce a dark brown scale on some darker-skinned individuals. This goes away once the medication is stopped.

Possible Side Effects

- ▼ Common: rash, irritation.
- ▼ Less common: temporary, dark brown scale on those with darker skin.

Drug Interactions

None known.

Usual Dose

Skin Products

Adult and Child (age 2 and over): Apply to the affected area not more than 3 or 4 times daily.

Child (under age 2): Do not use unless advised by a physician.

Acne Products

Adult and Child (age 12 and over): Apply in a thin film to the affected area once or twice daily.

Child (under age 12): Consult your doctor.

Overdosage

Do the following in case of accidental ingestion: If the victim is unconscious or having convulsions, call for an ambulance immediately. If you take the victim to an emergency room, be sure to bring the bottle or container with you. If the victim is conscious, call your local poison control center or a health care professional. The poison control center may suggest inducing vomiting with ipecac syrup (available without a prescription at any pharmacy). DO NOT induce vomiting unless specifically instructed to do so.

Special Populations

Pregnancy/Breast-feeding

It is not generally recommended that pregnant women take any drugs, particularly during the first 3 months after conception. Check with your doctor before using resorcinol preparations if you are or might be pregnant, or if you are breast-feeding.

Infants/Children

Do not give resorcinol skin products to children under age 2 except under the advice and supervision of a doctor. Resorcinol acne preparations should not be used by children under 12 unless directed by a doctor.

Resorcinol may be absorbed through the skin and should not be used on large areas of the bodies of infants and children, because of the risk of systemic (whole-body) toxicity. Resorcinol should not be used on wounds in infants and children because of the risk of the blood disease methemoglobinemia.

Seniors

Seniors should exercise the same caution as younger adults when using resorcinol products.

Generic Name

Salicylamide (SAL-ih-SILL-am-ide)

Brand Names

Anodynos
Diurex Water Pills
Emagrin
Fendol

Type of Drug

Analgesic (pain reliever).

Used for

Temporary relief of mild to moderate aches and pains associated with the common cold, flu, viral infections, or other disorders (neuritis, neuralgia, bursitis, arthritis, rheumatism, simple headache, menstrual cramps, tooth and periodontic pain, sprains, and minor muscular aches).

General Information

Salicylamide is structurally and pharmacologically related to the salicylates (aspirin, sodium salicylate, magnesium salicylate, and choline salicylate) and is theorized to have the same pain-reducing effects as these agents. However, salicylamide is rapidly broken down into inactive metabolites after it is taken and does not consistently produce these effects. Because salicylamide has not been proven to work, especially at its usually prescribed dose, some physicians have recommended that this drug no longer be used.

Salicylamide is available by brand name in tablet and powder form combined with analgesics and antipyretics (fever reducers) such as aspirin and acetaminophen, as well as antihistamines, antitussives (cough suppressants), caffeine, decongestants, and expectorants (used to clear the respiratory tract).

Cautions and Warnings

Do not use salicylamide for more than 10 consecutive days unless directed by your physician.

Do not exceed the recommended daily dosage of salicylamide.

Because salicylamide is related to the salicylates, people who cannot take salicylates such as aspirin should also avoid salicylamide. However, salicylamide is not associated with the same risk of gastrointestinal bleeding as aspirin.

Children with the flu or chicken pox who are given salicylates may develop Reye's syndrome, a life-threatening condition characterized by vomiting, progressive damage to the central nervous system, liver injury, and abnormally low blood sugar. Up to 30% of those who develop Reye's syndrome can die, and permanent brain damage is possible in those who survive. Because salicylamide is related to the salicylates which carry a risk of Reye's syndrome, do not give salicylamide to children under age 16. Acetaminophen can usually be substituted.

Possible Side Effects

▼ Most common: nausea, vomiting, heartburn, loss of appetite, diarrhea, dizziness, drowsiness, light-headedness, faintness, headache, flushing, hyperventilation, sweating, dry mouth, and rash. These effects may be more likely to occur with higher doses.

Drug Interactions

- Taking salicylamide with aspirin may result in increased concentrations of both drugs in the blood. This effect may also occur if salicylamide is taken with acetaminophen.

• The drug interactions usually seen with salicylates have not been reported to occur with salicylamide.

Food Interactions

Take salicylamide with food, milk, or water to reduce the chance of upset stomach.

Usual Dose

Adult (age 16 and over): 325–650 mg 3–4 times a day, as needed.

Child (under age 16): not recommended, because of the risk of Reye's Syndrome (see "Cautions and Warnings").

Overdosage

Do the following in case of accidental overdose: If the victim is unconscious or having convulsions, call for an ambulance immediately. If you take the victim to an emergency room, be sure to bring the bottle or container with you. If the victim is conscious, call your local poison control center or a health care professional. The poison control center may suggest inducing vomiting with ipecac syrup (available without a prescription at any pharmacy). DO NOT induce vomiting unless specifically instructed to do so.

Special Populations

Pregnancy/Breast-feeding

It is not generally recommended that pregnant women take any drugs, particularly during the first 3 months after conception. If you are pregnant or nursing a baby, check with a doctor before using salicylamide.

Infants/Children

Salicylamide has not been proven to be safe or effective in infants or children and should not be taken by children younger than age 16 unless directed by a doctor, due to the risk of Reye's Syndrome (see "Cautions and Warnings").

Seniors

Seniors should exercise the same caution as younger adults when using salicylamide.

Generic Name

Salicylic Acid (SAL-ih-SILL-ik ASS-id)

Brand Names

Acne Treatment Cleanser
Acno
AMBI 10 Acne Pads
Aveeno Medicated Cleanser
Cantharone Plus
Carmex
*Clean & Clear
*Clearasil
Clear Away
Compound W Wart Remover
Corn Fix
Creamy Dandruff Shampoo
Dandruff Shampoo Maximum Strength
Dandruff Wash, Medicated
DHS Sal
Dr. Scholl's
Drytex
DuoFilm
Duoplant Plantar Wart Remover
ExACT Pore Treatment
*Fostex
Freezone Corn and Callus Remover
Fung-O
Gets-It
Glover's Medicated For Dandruff
Gordofilm
Ionax Astringent Skin Cleanser
*Ionil
Meted
MG217 for Psoriasis Sal-Acid
Mosco Corn & Callus Remover
*Neutrogena
Occlusal HP
OFF-Ezy
*Oxy
P&S
Pernox
Poslam Psoriasis
Propa pH
Psor-A-Set
SalAc Cleanser
Salicylic Acid and Sulfur Soap
Sal-Acid Wart Remover
Salactic Film
Sal-Plant
Scalpicin Maximum Strength
Sebasorb Liquid
Sebucare
Sebulex
Sebutone
Stri-Dex
Therac
Trans-Ver-Sal
Verrex
Verrusol
Verukan-20
Wart Fix
Wart-Off

**Not all products in this brand-name group contain salicylic acid.*

Type of Drug

Topical keratolytic (skin-cell remover) and antiseptic.

Used for

Treatment and control of skin disorders, such as dandruff, seborrhea, psoriasis, common warts (rough, cauliflower-like appearance) and plantar warts (bottom of foot), calluses, corns, and acne. It is also used as an antiseptic in some insect bite medications.

General Information

Salicylic acid works by lowering the pH (increasing the acidity) of the skin and attracting fluid to the area. This action causes the skin to swell, soften, and slough (shed) off the surface cells more rapidly than normal, which promotes healing of the underlying condition.

Depending on the condition to be treated, some products with salicylic acid also contain sulfur, another keratolytic agent. Sulfur causes minor inflammation of the skin surface and dissolves the chemical that binds skin cells together.

Recent studies have shown that acne pads containing salicylic acid are superior to pads containing benzoyl peroxide in the treatment and prevention of acne. It is suggested that the increased fluid in the affected area can enhance the performance of other chemical agents in these products.

Salicylic acid, on its own or combined with other ingredients, is available by brand name in the following forms: lip balm, shampoo, liquid, pad, soap, cream, mask, disc, gel, solution, patch, and plaster. It is available generically in soap form.

Cautions and Warnings

Acne or Warts

If your condition worsens or persists for more than 12 weeks of regular use as directed, stop using the product and consult your doctor.

Do not exceed the recommended daily dosage of salicylic acid products.

Dandruff, Psoriasis, or Seborrhea

Salicylic acid products may be used indefinitely as long as the manufacturer's directions are followed. If the condition worsens discontinue treatment and call your doctor.

These products are for external use only. Avoid contact with the eyes. If the drug gets into the eyes, rinse thoroughly with water.

Products containing salicylic acid should not be used over large areas of the body or on broken, infected, or inflamed skin.

Diabetics and people with poor circulation should not use OTC corn, callus, or plantar wart medications. Because of their poor circulation problems, such people may experience serious and even life-threatening complications with foot injury or infection. If you have diabetes, and the corns, calluses, or warts on your foot become bothersome, consult your doctor.

Care should be taken to avoid getting hair products containing salicylic acid in the ears. This chemical can act as an irritant to delicate ear tissues.

Many experts advise switching from dandruff shampoo to regular shampoo on alternate days or using dandruff shampoos no more than twice a week.

Salicylic acid products used to treat psoriasis should not be used at the onset of psoriasis, as they may irritate and prolong the flare-up. After the condition has subsided and the usual scales appear, these products may then be used to help remove the scaly skin. Also, these products should not be used to treat psoriasis in the genital and underarm areas, because these areas are susceptible to irritation. Treatment with a cream containing hydrocortisone is usually more appropriate.

When used for foot care, products containing salicylic acid should be used to treat common and plantar warts only. Facial warts, growths around the nail beds, and genital warts should be treated by your doctor to avoid complications.

Possible Side Effects

Using a salicylic acid product more often than directed can cause excessive dryness of the skin or scalp. The stimulation salicylic acid provides can also cause skin cells to overmultiply, creating patches of thick, hard skin.

Drug Interactions

• Using salicylic acid acne products at the same time as other acne medications poses a risk of excess skin irritation or inflammation.

Usual Dose

Acne

Adult and Child (age 2 and over): Wash the skin thoroughly and pat dry. Apply a thin layer 1–3 times per day, depending on the severity of the problem, or as directed by a doctor. To avoid excessive dryness, start with 1 application daily and increase gradually. Follow package directions and doctor recommendations.

Child (under age 2): not recommended unless directed by your doctor.

Dandruff and Seborrhea

Adult and Child (age 2 and over): Use a lotion shampoo product with a 1.8%–3.0% salicylic acid concentration. Apply a small amount to the scalp, massage it in thoroughly, rinse, and repeat the application. Use this shampoo no more than twice weekly.

Child (under age 2): not recommended unless directed by your doctor.

Psoriasis

Adult and Child (under age 2): Use a product with a 2%–10% salicylic acid concentration for mild to moderate cases. For more severe, thicker-scaled outbreaks, a concentration of 5% salicylic acid in combination with 20% juniper tar and 10% sulfur may be more effective. Apply a thin layer to the affected skin surface.

Child (under age 2): not recommended unless directed by your doctor.

Warts

Adult and Child (age 2 and over): Use a product containing a 5%–17% salicylic acid concentration. Prior to application, the wart should be cleansed and soaked in warm water for 5 minutes. Application of the product should be restricted to the wart only; circling the wart with petroleum jelly may help you avoid contact between the medication and healthy skin. When using a solution, apply one drop at a time and allow to dry so the solution does not run on to healthy skin. Repeat this process once or twice daily for up to 12 weeks, or until the wart is removed (wart treatment typically takes up to 12 weeks). To avoid the spread of warts thoroughly wash hands after treatment.

Child (under age 2): not recommended unless directed by your doctor.

Corns or Calluses

Adult and Child (age 2 and over): Product concentrations of salicylic acid vary, from 12%–17.6% in liquid applications, and from 12%–40% in adherent pads or disks. Prior to application, the affected area should be washed and soaked in warm water for 15–30 minutes. Application of the product should be restricted to the affected area only; circling the corn or callus with petroleum jelly may help you avoid contact between the medication and healthy skin. Repeat the liquid procedure once daily for 7 days (treatment often needed for 2 weeks), or until the corn or callus is flattened. Pads or disks, which are cut to cover only the corn or callus, remain in place for 48 hours and are then removed. Following removal, the foot should be soaked in warm water for 15–30 minutes and softened tissue may be removed by gently rubbing with a washcloth, callus file, or pumice stone.

Child (under age 2): should not be treated with salicylic acid products unless directed by a physician.

Overdosage

Do the following in case of accidental ingestion: If the victim is unconscious or having convulsions, call for an ambulance immediately. If you take the victim to an emergency room, be sure to bring the bottle or container with you. If the victim is conscious, call your local poison control center or a health care professional. The poison control center may suggest inducing vomiting with ipecac syrup (available without a prescription at any pharmacy). DO NOT induce vomiting unless specifically instructed to do so.

Special Information

In the process of attracting moisture to the affected area, salicylic acid can affect the cellular structure of the hair and can cause a difference in texture and appearance. Changing products may reduce this problem.

Special Populations

Pregnancy/Breast-feeding

It is not generally recommended that pregnant women take any drugs, particularly during the first 3 months of pregnancy. Check with your doctor if you are or might be pregnant, or if you are breast-feeding.

Infants/Children

Do not use a salicylic acid product on a child under age 2 unless directed by a doctor.

Seniors

Seniors should exercise the same caution as younger adults when using salicylic acid.

Generic Name

Selenium Sulfide (seh-LEH-nee-um SULL-fide)

Brand Names

Head & Shoulders Intensive Treatment
Selsun

Type of Drug

Antiseborrheic.

Used for

Treatment and control of dandruff and seborrhea (seborrheic dermatitis).

General Information

Selenium sulfide is a cytostatic agent. It works by slowing down the rate at which cells grow and multiply. This action can reduce or even eliminate the excessive amount of skin cells produced in flaking scalp conditions such as dandruff and seborrhea.

Selenium is 1 of 2 cytostatic chemicals that have been approved by the FDA for use in OTC shampoo preparations; the other is pyrithione zinc. Pyrithione zinc appears to be the more effective, but may take longer to produce results than selenium.

Selenium adheres to the scalp surface and the hair, building up over a period of weeks.

For OTC products that are intended to be applied and washed off after a brief exposure, the recommended concentration of selenium is 1.0% for the treatment of dandruff and seborrhea. A higher concentration is available by prescription for cases that prove resistant to OTC treatment.

Selenium is available by generic and brand name in shampoo form.

Cautions and Warnings

There are no indications that long-term use of selenium is associated with a toxic reaction. Selenium is not readily absorbed into the deeper layers of the skin, and systemic (whole-body) overdose is highly unlikely. However, to minimize the risk of a skin reaction, do not use these products on broken or abraded skin.

Do not exceed the recommended daily dosage of selenium products.

Selenium is for external use only. Care should be taken to avoid contact with the eyes. If this occurs, flush the eyes well with water.

If dandruff or seborrhea persists or worsens with regular use of selenium as directed, stop using selenium and consult your doctor.

Many experts advise switching from medicated dandruff shampoo to regular shampoo on alternate days or using dandruff shampoos no more than twice a week.

Possible Side Effects

There is a risk that products used for the treatment of dandruff and seborrhea can cause excessive dryness of the skin, scalp, and hair.

Selenium sulfide products must be rinsed thoroughly from the hair and scalp, or discoloration may result, especially in blond, gray, and dyed hair.

Frequent use of selenium can cause a residual odor and may leave an oily coating on the scalp.

Drug Interactions

None known.

Usual Dose

Adult and Child (age 2 and over): Before using a selenium product, first wash your hair with a nonmedicated, non-residue shampoo to remove any dirt, oil, or loose scales. Next, apply a shampoo with a 1% selenium concentration to the scalp, massage it in thoroughly, and leave it on for 5 minutes before rinsing. Repeat twice weekly for 2 weeks, then once every 1–4 weeks as needed.

Child (under age 2). Consult your doctor.

Overdosage

Do the following in case of accidental ingestion: If the victim is unconscious or having convulsions, call for an ambulance immediately. If you take the victim to an emergency room, be sure to bring the bottle or container with you. If the victim is conscious, call your local poison control center or a health care professional. The poison control center may suggest inducing vomiting with ipecac syrup (available without a prescription at any pharmacy). DO NOT induce vomiting unless specifically instructed to do so.

Special Populations

Pregnancy/Breast-feeding

It is not generally recommended that pregnant women take any drugs, particularly during the first 3 months after conception. Check with your doctor if you are or might be pregnant, or if you are breast-feeding.

Infants/Children

Selenium preparations available over the counter are not recommended for children under 2 unless under the supervision of a doctor.

Seniors

Seniors should exercise the same caution as younger adults when using selenium.

Generic Name

Senna (SEN-uh)

Brand Names

Correctol Herbal Tea
Dr. Caldwell Senna
Ex-Lax Gentle Nature Natural
Fletcher's Castoria
Garfields Tea
Gentlax S
Innerclean Herbal
Perdiem Granule
†Senokot
Senolax
Swiss Kriss [S]

† *Consult the OTC ingredient charts to determine whether different formulations in this brand-name group are alcohol-, caffeine-, or sugar-free.*

Type of Drug

Laxative.

Used for

Relief of occasional constipation (irregularity).

General Information

The average, healthy individual defecates anywhere from 3 times a day to 3 times a week. Constipation is determined not necessarily by the frequency of bowel movements, but by the consistency of the stool; how difficult it is to eliminate it; and symptoms such as dull headache, low back pain, and abdominal distention (swelling). Evaluate your condition carefully and discuss your symptoms and their possible causes with your pharmacist before self-medicating with a laxative. Laxatives are not always necessary and, when used improperly, can either prevent the desired effect or result in laxative dependency. If you are indeed constipated, your condition may be best managed through proper diet, adequate fluid intake, and exercise. If you must use a laxative, choose the mildest effective product.

Laxatives may be classified by their mechanism of action: bulk forming, emollient (stool softeners), lubricant, saline, hyperosmotic, and stimulant. Senna is a stimulant laxative. According to different studies, stimulant laxatives work by either increasing the propulsive activity of the intestine or stimulating the secretion of water and electrolytes in the intestine, thus leading to evacuation of the colon.

Senna, made from the dried leaflet of *Cassia acutifolia* or *Cassia angustifolia,* is specifically an anthraquinone laxative. It is milder than other stimulant laxatives, such as the diphenylmethane stimulant phenolphthalein. Senna is more potent and more likely to cause abdominal cramps than another commonly used anthraquinone, cascara sagrada. Senna is also found in a form called sennosides (also known as sennosides A and B), which is the primary active laxative component of senna. Sennosides is prepared as calcium salts from the same herbs as senna.

Oral senna generally produces a bowel movement in 6 to 12 hours, but may take as long as 24 hours.

Senna is available by brand name, as either senna leaf, standardized senna concentrate, or sennosides, in tablet, suppository, liquid, granule, and tea forms. It is also available in several combination products containing other laxatives.

Cautions and Warnings

Do not use senna for more than 7 days unless directed by your doctor. Long-term use of laxatives has been linked with laxative dependence, chronic constipation, and loss of normal bowel function. Using laxatives too frequently can result in persistent diarrhea, hypokalemia (abnormally low potassium in the blood), loss of essential nutritional factors, and dehydration.

Of all the types of laxatives, stimulant laxatives, such as senna, are particularly habit-forming and are the most likely to cause adverse effects, such as diarrhea, gastrointestinal (GI) irritation, and fluid and electrolyte depletion, with long-term use.

Do not exceed the recommended daily dosage of senna. The higher the dose of senna, the more likely you are to experience adverse effects.

Do not take senna if you have abdominal pain, nausea, vomiting, or kidney disease unless directed by your doctor.

If you notice a sudden change in bowel habits lasting for more than 2 weeks, do not take senna until you have spoken to your doctor. Also contact your doctor if there is blood in your stool so that colon cancer or other significant disease can be ruled out before you begin self-medication with senna.

If you have had a disease or surgery affecting the GI tract, using a laxative may affect your condition adversely.

If you have rectal bleeding after using senna or if you do not have a bowel movement after 7 days of using this medication, you may have a serious condition. Stop using the product and call your doctor.

Laxatives may decrease the absorption of other drugs that pass through the GI tract (see "Drug Interactions").

Possible Side Effects

▼ Most common: abdominal discomfort, faintness, nausea, cramps, pinching and spasmodic pain in the bowels, colic, increased mucus secretion.

▼ Less common (chronic use of product only): metabolic acidosis or alkalosis (imbalances of acid and base in body fluids), hypocalcemia (too little calcium in the blood), tetany (characterized by foot spasms, muscular twitching, and cramps), electrolyte and fluid deficiencies (characterized by vomiting and muscle weakness), impaired intestinal absorption of nutrients, burning sensation in the rectum (suppository only), "cathartic colon" (weak or dilated colon).

Drug Interactions

• All laxatives potentially decrease the absorption of any oral drug taken at the same time. If you are currently taking an oral medication, talk to your pharmacist before self-medicating with senna.

Food Interactions

None known.

Usual Dose

Doses should be adjusted to individual usage. Take senna as needed, but do not exceed the recommended daily dosage.

Suppository
Administer the suppository at the time a bowel movement is desired. Lie on your side, and with pointed end up, push the suppository high into the rectum. Hold it there for as long as possible. If you feel the suppository slipping out, push it higher into the rectum.

Overdosage

Symptoms of overdosage include persistent diarrhea and dehydration. In the event of an accidental overdose, call your doctor or local poison control center immediately.

Special Information

Senna may cause your urine to appear pink, red, brown, or black. This is not a cause for alarm.

Storage Instructions

Store liquid senna at room temperature in a light-resistant container.

Special Populations

Pregnancy/Breast-feeding
Stimulant laxatives, such as senna, should generally be avoided during pregnancy. Only bulk-forming or emollient laxatives are recommended for pregnant women. Also, consider talking to your doctor about diet and mild exercise in the management of constipation.

Senna passes into breast milk. A brown discoloration of breast milk has been reported in nursing infants of mothers who have taken senna. One study of breast-feeding mothers taking senna reported diarrhea in 17% of the nursing infants. If you choose to take this product while breast-feeding, watch for diarrhea in your baby.

It is not generally recommended that pregnant women take any drugs, particularly during the first 3 months after conception. Check with your doctor before self-medicating with senna if you are or might be pregnant or if you are breast-feeding.

Infants/Children
Observe your child carefully for patterns of bowel movements and the pain or difficulty with which the bowel move-

ments are made before deciding whether the child is actually constipated. As with adults, "normal" bowel habits vary in children. If your child is indeed constipated, increasing fluid intake and adding fiber to his or her diet may be ways to manage the condition. In general, the use of laxatives should be avoided in children.

Do not give senna to children under age 6 unless directed by a doctor.

Seniors

Seniors commonly experience constipation and, consequently, may become laxative-dependent. Be cautious of chronically turning to laxatives to ease constipation, and instead look to diet and increased fluid intake as therapeutic measures.

Stimulant laxatives, such as senna, may not be the best choice for this age group because they alter fluid and electrolyte balance, placing some seniors at risk for side effects. Bulk-forming laxatives are usually preferred for seniors.

Generic Name

Shark Liver Oil

Definition

An oil obtained from the liver of the shark with high concentrations of vitamins A and D. Shark liver oil is used topically in OTC creams and ointments as a skin protectant and emollient (skin softener/soothing agent) for the treatment of minor skin conditions including diaper rash, abrasions, and minor burns.

Generic Name

Silicone (SILL-ih-kone)

Definition

An ingredient used in OTC diaper rash products as a skin protectant. Silicone oil is a lubricant found in vaginal moisturizers. Injected silicone is being tested as a possible treatment for corns, since it can cushion skin and reduce pain.

Generic Name

Simethicone (sih-METH-ih-kone)

Brand Names

Alka-Seltzer Anti-Gas
Di-Gel
†Gas-X
Gelusil
Kudrox
Little Tummy's Infant Gas Relief S
Losopan Plus
*Maalox
*Mylanta
Mylicon, Infant's
Phazyme
Riopan
Simaal
Tempo Drops
Titralac Plus
Tums

**Not all products in this brand-name group contain simethicone.*

†Consult the OTC ingredient charts to determine whether different formulations in this brand-name group are alcohol-, caffeine-, or sugar-free.

Type of Drug

Antiflatulent.

Used for

Alleviating or relieving the pain and pressure symptoms of excess gas in the digestive tract.

General Information

Stomach gas is frequently caused by excessive swallowing of air or by eating foods that disagree with you. The retention of gas may also be a problem in conditions such as postoperative gaseous distention, peptic ulcer, spastic or irritable colon, and diverticulosis. Excess gas is often accompanied by complaints of bloating, distention, fullness, pressure, pain, cramps, and excess flatulence.

Simethicone works by preventing the formation of gas pockets in the gastrointestinal (GI) tract and relieving gas entrapment in both the stomach and the intestines. The freed gas is then eliminated through belching or passing flatus (gas).

Simethicone is regarded by the FDA and clinicians as a safe and effective antiflatulent, but there is no conclusive evidence that it relieves the symptoms of immediate post-prandial upper abdominal distress, which occurs within 30 minutes after a meal and is characterized by GI bloating, distention, fullness, or pressure with abdominal discomfort; or of intestinal distress, which is abdominal discomfort not accompanied by constipation or diarrhea. While both of these conditions are commonly thought to be caused by excess gas, this has not been proven in either case.

Simethicone does not work as an antacid, but it is paired with various antacids in several brand name combination products. However, the efficacy of these combinations has not been well studied.

Simethicone is regarded as a particularly safe medication because it is not absorbed from the GI tract, and thus has no known systemic side effects.

Generic simethicone is available in chewable tablet form and as drops; brand name products are available in chewable tablet and capsule forms, and as drops.

Cautions and Warnings

Do not exceed the recommended daily dosage of simethicone.

If your condition persists, consult your doctor.

Possible Side Effects

None known.

Drug Interactions

None known.

Food Interactions

None known.

Usual Dose

Adult and Child (age 12 and over): The usual dose schedule for all forms of simethicone is 40–80 mg 4 times a day, after meals and at bedtime. Do not exceed the maximum daily dosage (500 mg). Be sure to chew the tablets thoroughly.

Child (under age 12): Consult your doctor.

Overdosage

Do the following in case of accidental overdose: If the victim is unconscious or having convulsions, call for an ambulance immediately. If you take the victim to an emergency room, be sure to bring the bottle or container with you. If the victim is conscious, call your local poison control center or a health care professional. The poison control center may suggest inducing vomiting with ipecac syrup (available without a prescription at any pharmacy). DO NOT induce vomiting unless specifically instructed to do so.

Special Populations

Pregnancy/Breast-feeding

It is not generally recommended that pregnant women take any drugs, particularly during the first 3 months after conception.

Check with your doctor before taking simethicone if you are or might be pregnant, or if you are breast-feeding.

Infants/Children

There is limited information on the safety of simethicone use in children and infants, although this product is apparently nontoxic. Simethicone was once thought to be effective in the treatment of infant colic, but recent trials have shown it to be no more effective than a placebo.

The dosage for children under 12 should be determined by a doctor, based on the severity of the condition and the child's size.

For children under 2 years, the drops may be added to liquids.

Seniors

Seniors should exercise the same caution as younger adults when using simethicone. However, you should be advised that many older patients are at high risk for complications from ulcers, yet often do not show classic ulcer symptoms. You may want to discuss with your pharmacist the possible causes of your gastric discomfort before self-medicating with simethicone and possibly delaying diagnosis of an ulcer.

Generic Name

Sodium Benzoate (SOE-dee-um BEN-zoe-ate)

Definition

A preservative used in OTC vaginal lubricants. Some mouth rinses also contain this ingredient, which may help remove plaque from the teeth.

Generic Name

Sodium Bicarbonate
(SOE-dee-um bye-KAR-buh-nate)

Brand Names

*Alka-Seltzer
Arm & Hammer Pure Baking Soda
Bell/ans
Bromo-Seltzer
Citrocarbonate
*Gaviscon
Ceo-Two
Massengill with Baking Soda

**Not all products in this brand-name group contain sodium bicarbonate.*

Type of Drug

Antacid.

Used for

Relief of heartburn, sour stomach, and acid indigestion.

General Information

All antacids work in the same way, by neutralizing stomach acid. However, they differ in potency: Sodium bicarbonate, commonly known as baking soda, is less potent than the antacid calcium carbonate, more potent than magnesium and aluminum antacids. The higher the potency of an antacid, the less of it you will need to take to achieve the desired effect.

Antacids also vary in their adverse effects and in their interactions with other drugs, as well as in their speed of onset and duration of action. Sodium bicarbonate dissolves quickly in stomach acid and provides a rapid effect, unlike aluminum antacids, which dissolve more slowly in stomach acid and may take up to 30 minutes to begin working.

How long an antacid product works depends on how long it remains in the stomach. Sodium bicarbonate has the shortest duration of action of these products. In general, an antacid taken on an empty stomach leaves the stomach rapidly, and works for only 20 to 40 minutes. However, when taken after a meal, it leaves the stomach more slowly. When taken 1 hour after a meal, an antacid can work for up to 3 hours.

Sodium bicarbornate is also used in OTC laxative suppositories, and in vaginal douches.

Sodium bicarbonate is available by generic and brand name in powder and chewable tablet forms. It is also available in combination products containing the antacids aluminum hydroxide and magnesium carbonate or trisilicate.

Cautions and Warnings

Do not take the maximum daily dosage of sodium bicarbonate for more than 2 weeks continuously except under a doctor's supervision. Antacids may relieve symptoms of a serious condition such as peptic ulcer disease. If you take an antacid for a prolonged period, you run the risk of unknowingly masking the symptoms of a serious gastrointestinal (GI) disease and delaying diagnosis.

Do not exceed the recommended daily dosage of sodium bicarbonate.

Call your doctor if you have severe stomach pains after taking sodium bicarbonate.

Call your doctor if you do not get relief from sodium bicarbonate, or if your stool is black or tarry or looks like coffee grounds, which indicates bleeding in the intestines or stomach. These may be signs of a serious GI disorder that cannot and should not be treated with an OTC product without your doctor's supervision.

Unlike other antacids, sodium bicarbonate is completely absorbed into the blood stream. When taken in large doses or by people with impaired kidney function, it can cause systemic metabolic alkalosis (a condition in which the blood becomes low in acidity, affecting the kidney, blood, and salt balance).

Large doses of sodium bicarbonate, when combined with milk or calcium, can cause milk-alkali syndrome, which occurs when there is a high intake of calcium combined with anything producing alkalosis (imbalance of acid and base in body fluids). Symptoms include headache, nausea, irritability, vertigo (dizziness), and vomiting. Left unchecked, the syndrome can cause irreversible kidney damage.

Do not use this product if you are on a sodium-restricted diet, or if you have hypertension (abnormally high blood pressure), edema (fluid retention), congestive heart failure, kidney failure, or cirrhosis.

To avoid serious stomach injury, do not take sodium bicarbonate powder until it is completely dissolved.

Do not take sodium bicarbonate if you are overfull from eating or drinking.

Possible Side Effects

▼ Most common: gastric distension (swelling), flatulence (gas).

▼ Less common: fluid retention, weight gain.

Drug Interactions

• Sodium bicarbonate decreases the absorption of iron and ketoconazole, an antifungal agent, reducing their effects. If you are taking sodium bicarbonate at the same time as either of these, separate your dose of each by at least 2 hours.

• Sodium bicarbonate decreases the elimination of amphetamine, used to treat narcolepsy and obesity; and quinidine, an antiarrhythmic, leading to possible retention of these drugs and intoxication. Do not use sodium bicarbonate at the same time as either of these products.

Food Interactions

Sodium bicarbonate is best taken after meals (see "General Information").

Usual Dose

Adult and Child (age 5 and over): Take sodium bicarbonate as symptoms occur, but do not exceed the recommended daily dosage specified on the package.

Child (under age 5): not recommended.

Overdosage

Do the following in case of accidental overdose: If the victim is unconscious or having convulsions, call for an ambulance immediately. If you take the victim to an emergency room, be sure to bring the bottle or container with you. If the victim is conscious, call your local poison control center or a health care professional. The poison control center may suggest inducing vomiting with ipecac syrup (available without a prescription at any pharmacy). DO NOT induce vomiting unless specifically instructed to do so.

Special Populations

Pregnancy/Breast-feeding

It is not generally recommended that pregnant women take any drugs, especially during the first 3 months after conception. However, antacids can be safely taken in small doses for short periods of time during pregnancy and while breast-feeding. Pregnant women who increase their milk or calcium intake should be especially aware of the risk of milk-alkali syndrome (see "Cautions and Warnings") before choosing sodium bicarbonate as an antacid.

Check with your doctor before self-medicating with sodium bicarbonate if you are or might be pregnant, or if you are breast-feeding.

Infants/Children

The safety of antacid use in infants and children has not been established. Children under age 5 should not be given sodium bicarbonate unless directed by a doctor.

Seniors

Seniors may safely take antacids. However, be advised that many older patients are at high risk for complications from ulcers, yet often do not show classic ulcer symptoms. Discuss the possible causes of your gastric discomfort with your pharmacist before self-medicating with an antacid and possibly delaying diagnosis of an ulcer. Be aware of possible interactions with other medications you may be taking.

Many seniors are on low-salt diets because of high blood pressure or congestive heart failure. Do not take sodium bicarbonate if you should restrict your salt intake.

Generic Name

Sodium Chloride (SOE-dee-um KLOR-ide)

Definition

An essential nutrient for the body; also known as table salt. When sodium chloride is dissolved in water in a concentration of 0.9%, it is known as normal saline solution. Normal saline solution is used in many nasal mist drops or sprays for relief of dryness and irritation. Sodium chloride solution can be mixed with inhaled bronchodilator medications to relieve inflamed breathing passages during an asthma attack.

Generic Name

Sodium Diacetate
(SOE-dee-um dye-ASS-eh-tate)

Definition

An antiseptic found in OTC first-aid skin care products.

Generic Name

Sodium Hypochlorite
(SOE-dee-um HYE-poe-KLOR-ite)

Definition

An antiseptic used in OTC first-aid skin care products. In concentrations of 5% or more, sodium hypochlorite is used as a bleach and should not be used topically.

Generic Name

Sodium Iodide (SOE-dee-um EYE-oe-dide)

Definition

An antiseptic found in OTC first-aid skin care products.

Generic Name

Sodium Lauryl Sulfate

(SOE-dee-um LAW-ril SULL-fate)

Definition

An ingredient that contributes to the moisturizing ability of various OTC products and that works as a mild detergent. Used in vaginal lubricant products and some douches, it helps moisture to spread across the surface of the vagina and penetrate the membrane tissue. In toothpastes and mouth rinses, sodium lauryl sulfate through its detergent action helps remove plaque and bacteria. In shampoos, this ingredient can break up dandruff flakes into smaller pieces to make them easier to remove.

Generic Name

Sodium Peroxyborate Monohydrate

(SOE-dee-um per-OKS-ee-BOR-ate MON-oe-HYE-drate)

Definition

A cleansing agent used in OTC products that relieve minor oral discomfort.

Generic Names

Sodium Phosphate, Monobasic and Dibasic

(SOE-dee-um FOSS-fate, MON-oe-BAY-sik, dye-BAY-sik)

Brand Names

*Fleet Ready-to-Use Enema
Phospho-Soda Buffered Saline

Type of Drug

Laxative.

Used for

Relief of occasional constipation (irregularity).

General Information

The average, healthy individual defecates anywhere from 3 times a day to 3 times a week. Constipation is determined not necessarily by the frequency of bowel movements, but by the consistency of the stool, how difficult it is to eliminate, and symptoms such as dull headache, low back pain, and abdominal distention (swelling). Evaluate your condition carefully and discuss your symptoms and their possible causes with your pharmacist before self-medicating with a laxative. Laxatives are not always necessary, and when used improperly can either prevent the desired effect or result in laxative dependency. If you are indeed constipated, your condition may be best managed through proper diet, adequate fluid intake (6 to 8 glasses a day), and exercise. If you must use a laxative, choose the mildest effective product.

Laxatives may be classified by their mechanism of action: bulk-forming, emollient (stool softeners), lubricant, saline, hyperosmotic, and stimulant. Monobasic sodium phosphate and dibasic sodium phosphate, 2 substances that are used in combination, are saline laxatives, which work by drawing water into the small intestine, thus increasing pressure and intestinal motility (ability to move spontaneously). Oral doses of monobasic and dibasic sodium phosphate generally produce a bowel movement in 3 to 6 hours or less. Enemas cause evacuation in 2 to 5 minutes. Saline laxatives are recommended for use when immediate and complete evacuation of the bowel is required; they are not recommended for the long-term management of constipation.

The sodium phosphates are also used in OTC opthalmic decongestants, irrigants, and hyperosmotics as buffers.

The sodium phosphates are available by brand name in the following forms: liquids, suppositories, and tablets.

Cautions and Warnings

Do not use sodium phosphate laxatives for more than 7 days unless directed by your doctor. Long-term use of laxatives has been linked with laxative dependence, chronic constipation, loss of normal bowel function, and, in severe cases, nerve, muscle, and tissue damage to the intestines. Using laxatives too frequently can result in persistent diarrhea, hypokalemia (abnormally low potassium in the blood), loss of essential nutrients, and dehydration. Long-term use of a sodium phosphate laxative in particular can cause serious, life-threatening dehydration. It can also cause phosphate poisoning, which reduces calcium concentrations in the blood.

Do not exceed the recommended daily dosage of a sodium phosphate preparation.

Do not take a sodium phosphate product if you have abdominal pain, nausea, vomiting, or kidney disease, unless directed by your doctor.

If you notice a marked change in bowel habits lasting for more than 2 weeks, do not take a sodium phosphate preparation until you have spoken to your doctor. Also contact your doctor if there is blood in your stool, so that colon cancer or other significant disease can be ruled out before you begin self-medication with this product.

If you have had a disease or surgery affecting the gastrointestinal (GI) tract, using a laxative may affect your condition adversely.

If you have rectal bleeding after using a sodium phosphate preparation, or if you do not have a bowel movement after 7 days of using this medication, you may have a serious condition. Stop using sodium phosphate and call your doctor.

Laxatives may decrease the absorption of other drugs that pass through the GI tract (see "Drug Interactions").

People with impaired kidney function should use sodium phosphate preparations only under the supervision of a doctor. Such people are at high risk for sodium overload. In children with kidney disease, tetany (a condition characterized by spasms, muscular twitching, and cramps) has occurred after administration of 1 sodium phosphate enema.

Sodium phosphate products should be used with caution by individuals on low-sodium diets. They should not be used by people with cardiac disease, edema, or cirrhosis. Indiscriminate use of saline laxatives containing sodium has lead to congestive heart failure.

Sodium phosphate preparations should be used with caution by individuals currently taking a diuretic or another medication that might affect electrolyte concentrations.

Be sure to read the label carefully before purchasing a sodium phosphate product. These preparations are available in several volumes, including adult and pediatric. Selecting the age-appropriate product reduces the risk of potential overdose.

If you are using a sodium phosphate enema product, be sure to follow the directions on the package carefully. An enema that is incorrectly administered can have adverse effects.

Possible Side Effects

Serious side effects such as dehydration, hyperphosphatemia (high phosphate levels in the blood), hypocalcemia (low calcium in the blood), and renal (kidney) failure may occur with prolonged use of sodium phosphates or overdose. Nausea, vomiting, and diarrhea can also occur.

Drug Interactions

- All laxatives potentially decrease the absorption of any oral drug taken at the same time. If you are currently taking an oral medication, talk to your doctor or pharmacist before self-medicating with a sodium phosphate product.

Food Interactions

None known.

Usual Dose

Doses should be adjusted to individual usage. In general, saline laxatives should be taken at infrequent intervals.

Oral solutions of sodium phosphate laxatives should be diluted with water before administration. Follow your dose with a glass (8 oz.) of water.

Laxative

Adult and Child (age 12 and over): 3.4–7.6 g a day as a single dose (dibasic). 9.1–20.2 g a day as a single dose (monobasic).

Child (age 10–11): 1.7–3.8 g a day as a single dose (dibasic). 4.5–10 g a day as a single dose (monobasic).

Child (age 5–9): 860–1900 mg a day as a single dose (dibasic). 2200–5100 mg a day as a single dose (monobasic).

Child (under age 5): Consult your doctor.

Enema

If you are using the enema product, follow the directions on the package carefully. To administer an enema, lie on your side with your knees bent. Allow the solution to flow into the rectum *slowly.* Retain the solution until you feel stomach cramps.

Adult and Child (age 12 and over): 6.8–7.6 g a day as a single dose (dibasic). 18–20 g a day as a single dose (monobasic).

Child (age 2-11): 3.4–3.8 g a day as a single dose (dibasic). 9.1–10 g a day as a single dose (monobasic).

Child (under age 2): not recommended.

Overdosage

Overdose with sodium phosphate laxatives can cause serious, life-threatening dehydration. It may also cause phosphate poisoning, which reduces calcium concentrations in the blood.

Even if the victim is not displaying any of the symptoms listed above, do the following in case of accidental ingestion or overdose: If the victim is unconscious or having convulsions, call for an ambulance immediately. If you take the victim to an emergency room, be sure to bring the bottle or container with you. If the victim is conscious, call your local poison control center or a health care professional. The poison control center may suggest inducing vomiting with ipecac syrup (available without a prescription at any pharmacy). DO NOT induce vomiting unless specifically instructed to do so.

Special Populations

Pregnancy/Breast-feeding

Sodium phosphate laxatives should be avoided during pregnancy. Only bulk-forming and emollient laxatives are recommended for pregnant women. Consider talking to your doctor about diet and mild exercise in the management of constipation.

It is not known whether sodium phosphate passes into breast milk. Check with your doctor before using the sodium phosphates if you are breast-feeding.

Infants/Children

Observe your child carefully for patterns of bowel movements and the pain or difficulty with which the bowel movements are made before deciding whether the child is actually constipated. As with adults, "normal" bowel habits vary in children. If your child is indeed constipated, increasing fluid intake and adding fiber to his or her diet may help to manage the condition. In general, the use of laxatives should be avoided in children.

Children age 5 and over may be given sodium phosphate preparations orally, in smaller doses than those taken by adults. For children under age 5, consult a doctor.

Children age 2 and over may be given sodium phosphate products rectally, in smaller doses than those taken by adults. Enemas are not generally recommended for children under this age.

Do not give a sodium phosphate preparation to a child under age 2 without consulting a doctor. Sodium phosphates can cause dehydration, loss of calcium, tetany, and phosphate accumulation in children under age 2.

Seniors

Seniors commonly experience constipation, and consequently may become laxative dependent. Avoid chronically turning to laxatives to ease constipation, and instead look to diet and increased fluid intake as therapeutic measures.

Sodium phosphate laxatives may not be the best choice for this group because they alter fluid and electrolyte balance, placing some seniors at risk for side effects. They also should not be used by seniors with severe kidney impairment or cardiac disease (see "Cautions and Warnings"). Bulk-forming laxatives are usually preferred for seniors.

Generic Name

Sodium Salicylate

(SOE-dee-um SAL-ih-SILL-ate)

Brand Names

Cystex

Scot-Tussin Original [A] [S]

Type of Drug

Analgesic (pain reliever); antipyretic (fever reducer); anti-inflammatory.

Used for

Sodium salicylate is used to treat mild to moderate pain and fever associated with the common cold, flu, and viral infections. It is useful in treating mild-to-moderate pain associated with a variety of disorders, including neuritis, neuralgia, bursitis, arthritis, rheumatism, simple headache, menstrual cramps, tooth and periodontic pain, sprains, and minor muscular aches. It may also be taken to relieve inflammation of bones, joints, or other body tissues.

General Information

Sodium salicylate is a member of the group of drugs called salicylates. Other members of this group include aspirin, choline salicylate, and magnesium salicylate. Sodium salicylate reduces fever by causing the blood vessels in the skin to dilate, allowing heat to leave the body more rapidly. Its effects on pain and inflammation are thought to be related to its ability to prevent the manufacture of complex body hormones called prostaglandins, which sensitize pain receptors and stimulate the inflammatory response.

Sodium salicylate is absorbed more quickly from the stomach than aspirin, but it is not as effective as an equivalent dose of aspirin in reducing pain or fever. However, when used in the treatment of rheumatoid arthritis, the two drugs (in enteric-coated form) have been proven equally effective in relieving pain, reducing joint tenderness and swelling, and increasing grip strength. There are also other differences between these pain relievers that should be considered when choosing one agent over another. Of all the salicylates, aspirin has the greatest effect on prostaglandin production and, therefore, causes the strongest gastrointestinal effects. Sodium salicylate may be less irritating to the stomach and can be used by people who cannot tolerate the side effects associated with aspirin or who are allergic to aspirin. However, sodium salicylate is more expensive than aspirin.

Sodium salicylate is available by generic and brand name in tablet form. It is also available in a combination product with phenylephrine, a decongestant; pheniramine, an antihistamine; and sodium citrate, an expectorant, to relieve aches associated with coughs, colds, and allergies.

Cautions and Warnings

Do not take sodium salicylate for more than 10 consecutive days or, in the presence of fever, for more than 3 days, unless directed by your doctor.

Do not exceed the recommended daily dosage of sodium salicylate.

Do not take sodium salicylate if you have gout.

Notify your doctor if you develop ringing in the ears or hearing loss while taking sodium salicylate.

Because of its high sodium content, sodium salicylate should not be used by people with congestive heart failure, hypertension (high blood pressure), or other conditions in which sodium intake is restricted.

Children with the flu or chicken pox who are given salicylates may develop Reye's syndrome, a life-threatening condition characterized by vomiting, progressive damage to the central nervous system, liver injury, and abnormally low blood sugar. Up to 30% of those who develop Reye's syndrome die, and permanent brain damage is possible in those who survive. Because of the risk of Reye's syndrome, do not give salicylates to children under age 16. Acetaminophen can usually be substituted.

Possible Side Effects

- ▼ Common: nausea, upset stomach, heartburn, loss of appetite, and loss of small amounts of blood in the stool.
- ▼ Rare: hives, rashes, liver damage, fever, thirst, and difficulties with vision.

Drug Interactions

- Sodium salicylate should not be used by individuals currently taking methotrexate (used to treat cancer, severe psoriasis, severe rheumatoid arthritis and to induce abortion) or valproic acid, an anticonvulsant. It can increase the toxicity of these drugs.

• Sodium salicylate should not be taken with anticoagulant (blood-thinning) drugs such as warfarin and dicumarol. It will exaggerate the effects of these drugs and increase the risk of abnormal bleeding.

• The possibility of stomach ulcer is increased if sodium salicylate is taken together with an adrenal corticosteroid such as hydrocortisone; phenylbutazone, a nonsteroidal anti-inflammatory drug (NSAID); or alcoholic beverages.

• Sodium salicylate will counteract the effects of the antigout medications probenecid and sulfinpyrazone and may counteract the effects of angiotensin-converting enzyme (ACE) inhibitors and beta blockers, which work to lower blood pressure.

• Taking sodium salicylate with an NSAID has no benefit and carries a greatly increased risk of side effects, especially stomach irritation.

Food Interactions

Take sodium salicylate with food, milk, or water to reduce the risk of stomach irritation.

Usual Dose

Pain and Fever Relief

Adult (age 16 and over): 325–650 mg every 4 hours, as needed.

Anti-inflammatory

Adult (age 16 and over): 325 to 650 mg every 4 hours; 325 to 500 mg every 3 hours; or 650 mg to 1 gram every 6 hours. Do not take more than 4 grams (4000 mg) in 24 hours. Try to take the smallest possible dose that is effective for you.

Pain and Fever Relief or Anti-inflammatory

Child (under age 16): not recommended because of the risk of Reye's syndrome (see "Cautions and Warnings").

Overdosage

Symptoms of mild overdosage include rapid and deep breathing, nausea, vomiting, dizziness, ringing or buzzing in the ears, flushing, sweating, thirst, headache, drowsiness, diarrhea, and rapid heartbeat. Severe overdose may cause fever, excitability, confusion, convulsions, liver or kidney failure, coma, or bleeding.

Even if the victim is not displaying any of the symptoms listed above, do the following in case of accidental overdose: If the victim is unconscious or having convulsions, call for an ambulance immediately. If you take the victim to an emergency room, be sure to bring the bottle or container with you. If the victim is conscious, call your local poison control center or a health care professional. The poison control center may suggest inducing vomiting with ipecac syrup (available without a prescription at any pharmacy). DO NOT induce vomiting unless specifically instructed to do so.

Special Populations

Allergies

You may be able to take sodium salicylate if you are allergic to aspirin, but check with your doctor first.

Pregnancy/Breast-feeding

Sodium salicylate can cause bleeding problems in the developing fetus and can lead to a low-birth-weight infant; it can also cause bleeding problems in the mother before, during, or after pregnancy. Avoid sodium salicylate if you are pregnant.

Although sodium salicylate passes into breast milk, no adverse effects have been proven to occur in the nursing infant. However, acetaminophen may be a better choice if you are nursing.

Infants/Children

Sodium salicylate should not be used in children younger than age 16 because of Reye's syndrome (see "Cautions and Warnings").

Seniors

Seniors should exercise the same caution as younger adults when using this drug.

Generic Name

Sorbic Acid (SOR-bik ASS-id)

Definition

A preservative used in OTC vaginal lubricants.

Generic Name

Sorbitol (SOR-bih-tol)

Definition

A sweetening agent included in a range of OTC products, including mouthwashes and tooth care products. It is added to activated charcoal, a poison antidote, to make it easier to drink. In dry skin products, sorbitol helps to allow moisture to penetrate cells. Sorbitol in higher concentrations (20% to 70%) is used as a laxative.

Generic Name

Starch

Definition

A fine powder made from corn, wheat, or potatoes, used as a dusting powder for its ability to absorb moisture and as a filler, binder, or disintegrant (an agent that causes tablets to disintegrate and release medicine on contact with moisture) in various OTC products.

Generic Name

Stearic Acid (STEER-ik ASS-id)

Definition

A fatty substance that promotes moisturization, used in OTC vaginal lubricants.

Generic Name

Stearyl Alcohol (STEER-il AL-kuh-hall)

Definition

An astringent (drying agent) used in OTC products for treatment of dermatitis (skin inflammation) and relief of poison ivy.

Generic Name

Sulfur (SULL-fer)

Brand Names

Acne Treatment
Acno
Acnomel
Acnotex
Bensulfoid
Creamy Dandruff Shampoo
Cuticura Ointment
Dandruff Shampoo Maximum Strength
Dandruff Wash, Medicated
Fostril
*Glover's
Liquimat
Meted
Novacet Lotion
Pernox
Poslam Psoriasis
Rezamid Acne Lotion
Salicylic Acid & Sulfur Soap
SAStid
Seales Lotion-Modified
Sebex-T
Sebulex
Sebutone
Sulfacet-R
Sulfoam Medicated Antidandruff
Sulforcin
Sulfoxyl
Sulmasque
Sulpho-Lac
Sulray
Therac
Thylox Acne Treatment

**Not all products in this brand-name group contain sulfur.*

Type of Drug

Topical keratolytic (skin-cell removing) agent.

Used for

Treatment and control of skin disorders, such as dandruff, seborrhea, psoriasis, scabies, and acne.

General Information

Sulfur (sometimes spelled *sulphur*) is an element that plays a number of important roles in the body. It is needed for production of vitamin B1; amino acids; and collagen, which is an important component of skin, bones, and connective tissues. Sulfur is also found in keratin, a component of skin, hair, and nails.

This chemical is found in a number of prescription medications used to treat a variety of conditions, including gout, arthritis, inflammatory bowel disease, and bronchitis.

In OTC ointments, creams, and skin preparations, sulfur is indicated for treatment of acne, dandruff, psoriasis, scabies, diaper rash, and minor fungal infections.

Sulfur works as a mild irritant. It causes minor inflammation of the skin surface and dissolves the substance that binds skin cells together. These actions increase the sloughing (removal) of dead cells, which promotes healing of the underlying condition.

Products containing sulfur in concentrations between 2% and 5% are effective for the treatment of the majority of skin disorders. Acne medications usually have higher concentrations, ranging from 3% to 10%.

When used to treat acne, sulfur appears to work by removing the surface skin that traps dirt, oil, and debris and causes acne blemishes (pimples and blackheads). The dead skin, dirt, and oil can then be removed with gentle scrubbing, promoting healing of the blemish.

Acne products that combine sulfur and another acne medication, benzoyl peroxide, may be more effective than products that contain only one of these ingredients. People who are sensitive to benzoyl peroxide may experience more severe reactions if they use products that also contain sulfur. Some products contain combinations of sulfur and resorcinol, an antiseptic.

Sulfur works to relieve mild cases of dandruff by loosening flakes of skin on the scalp and breaking them into smaller pieces so they can be rinsed away more easily. Many dandruff-control products also contain salicylic acid to enhance sulfur's efficacy.

Some sulfur products work against seborrheic dermatitis, a skin condition resulting from excess skin growth and production of a waxy substance called sebum.

Scabies—a skin infection caused by mites—can also be treated with sulfur-containing ointments. However, these products tend to be messy and smelly. Other treatments, such as permethrin, are easier and more pleasant to use.

Sulfur also has mild antifungal and antibiotic effects, but other products that are specifically designed to fight fungal and bacterial infections are generally more effective for this purpose.

Cautions and Warnings

Do not use sulfur-containing products for more than 7 days unless under the supervision of a doctor.

Do not exceed the recommended daily dosage of sulfur.

Sulfur-containing products have a noticeable color and odor.

Using these products more often than directed can cause excessive dryness of skin or scalp. The stimulation sulfur provides can cause skin cells to overmultiply, creating patches of thick, hard skin.

These products are for external use only. Avoid contact with the eyes. If the drug gets into the eyes, rinse thoroughly with water.

If the condition persists or worsens with regular use as directed, stop using the product and consult your doctor.

Products containing sulfur and resorcinol should not be used over large areas of the body or on broken or already inflamed skin.

Do not use a sulfur ointment to treat an infant with scabies (see "Special Populations").

Possible Side Effects

There is a risk that sulfur can cause excessive dryness of the skin, scalp, or hair. Also, products containing sulfur might cause irritation and dermatitis, resulting in a hardening of the skin surface or mild scabbing. Allergic reactions are rare.

Drug Interactions

- Do not use a sulfur-containing acne product at the same time as other acne medications. This poses a risk of excess skin irritation or inflammation.

Usual Dose

Acne

Adult and Child (age 2 and over): Generally, these products are applied after skin has been washed and dried.

Apply a thin layer 1–3 times per day, depending on the severity of the problem, or as directed by a doctor. To avoid excessive dryness, start with 1 application daily and increase gradually. Follow package directions and physician's recommendations.

Child (under age 2): not recommended unless directed by your doctor.

Dandruff

Adult and Child (age 2 and over): Use a lotion shampoo product with 2%–5% sulfur concentration. Apply an amount to the scalp, massage it in thoroughly, rinse, and repeat the application. Many experts advise switching from dandruff shampoo to regular shampoo on alternate days or using sulfur shampoos no more than twice a week.

Child (under age 2): not recommended unless directed by your doctor.

Scabies

Adult and Child (age 2 and over): Apply a thin layer of sulfur ointment to the entire skin surface from the neck to the soles of the feet. Repeat the application every 2–3 days. Bathe prior to application and after the last application. Adults will need approximately 30 g of ointment to cover the body. Children will need smaller amounts.

Child (under age 2): not recommended unless directed by your doctor.

Overdosage

Do the following in case of accidental ingestion: If the victim is unconscious or having convulsions, call for an ambulance immediately. If you take the victim to an emergency room, be sure to bring the bottle or container with you. If the victim is conscious, call your local poison control center or a health care professional. The poison control center may suggest inducing vomiting with ipecac syrup (available without a prescription at any pharmacy). DO NOT induce vomiting unless specifically instructed to do so.

Special Information

Sulfur dissolves the substance that holds skin cells together. This can affect the cellular structure of the hair and can cause a difference in texture and appearance. Changing dandruff products may relieve this effect.

Special Populations

Pregnancy/Breast-feeding

It is not generally recommended that pregnant women take any drug, particularly during the first 3 months after conception. Check with your doctor if you are or might be pregnant, or if you are breast-feeding.

Infants/Children

Sulfur products should not be used on children under age 2 unless directed by a doctor.

Sulfur ointments should not be used for treating infants with scabies, because there is a risk of serious toxicity and even death.

Seniors

Residents of long-term nursing facilities are at higher risk of scabies infection. Because the infection can be easily passed to others, and because reinfestation is likely, intensive treatment is needed. Generally in such conditions, scabies is more effectively treated with products other than sulfur ointments, such as benzyl benzoate lotion, gamma benzene hexachloride cream or lotion, or crotamiton cream or lotion, all available by prescription only.

Generic Name

Talc

Definition

A powdered form of magnesium silicate used in OTC diaper rash and skin care products. Talc relieves irritation, prevents chafing, and absorbs moisture. In some foot-care products, talc is used as a vehicle (carrier) for the active ingredient (such as an antifungal drug) and as an absorbent to dry moisture from an oozing infection.

Generic Name

Tetrahydrozoline Hydrochloride

(TET-rah-hye-DROZ-oe-leen HYE-droe-KLOR-ide)

Brand Names

Collyrium Fresh
Eye-Sed
Eye Sine
Murine Plus Lubricant Eye Redness Reliever
Optigene
Soothe
Tyzine
*Visine

**Not all products in this brand-name group contain tetrahydrozoline HCL.*

Type of Drug

Decongestant.

Used for

Relief of congestion, itching, and irritation of the eye.

General Information

Decongestants relieve congestion by narrowing or constricting the blood vessels. Tetrahydrozoline hydrochloride is classified as an imidazole; other decongestants in this family are naphazoline and oxymetazoline. Administered as eyedrops, these chemicals are considered effective in relieving the surface discomfort of itchy, red eyes, without unduly affecting the underlying blood vessels of the eye structure. After administration, tetrahydrozoline starts to work within a few minutes; its effects can last from 1 to 4 hours.

Tetrahydrozoline is available both generically and in brand-name form.

Cautions and Warnings

Tetrahydrozoline eyedrops should not be used for longer than 3 to 4 days continuously unless directed by a doctor.

Do not exceed the recommended daily dosage of tetrahydrozoline.

Excessive use of tetrahydrozoline should be avoided, especially in children (see "Special Populations").

Tetrahydrozoline is less likely to cause the pupils to alter in size than other ophthalmic decongestants. This prevents the symptom of light sensitivity during use of a product containing tetrahydrozoline. However, some individuals may experience a mild, temporary stinging sensation immediately after using one of these products.

These products are not to be taken internally.

If you have hyperthyroidism, heart disease, high blood pressure, or diabetes, you should consult your doctor before using one of these products, because there is a slight risk that it could aggravate these conditions. People with high blood pressure should be cautious about taking tetrahydrozoline since it may also increase the irritability of the heart or alter its rhythm, especially if taken in large doses.

Discontinue use of tetrahydrozoline if you experience visual disturbances, pain, or increased redness. If your condition worsens over a 72-hour period, discontinue use and contact your doctor.

A problem common to all forms of topical decongestants is rebound congestion; that is, you may still have a stuffy nose or red eyes even though you have been using tetrahydrozoline for several days. The lining of your nose may swell and turn red, giving you the appearance of allergic rhinitis, or your eyes may become more inflamed each time you apply the drug. If this happens, stop using tetrahydrozoline and contact your doctor. The signs of rebound congestion will usually go away about a week after you stop using the drug.

These medications should not be used by people with glaucoma or other serious eye diseases except under a doctor's supervision.

To reduce the risk of spreading infection, eye drops should not be used by more than one person. Rinse dropper and bottle tips with hot water after use. Be careful not to let hot water into the bottle. Do not let the bottle tip come into contact with any surface.

Possible Side Effects

Used as directed, there are very few adverse reactions with tetrahydrozoline. However, excessive use of these drugs can irritate tissues.

Upon application, some people may experience temporary burning, stinging, and a feeling of surface dryness. Blurred vision and dilation of the pupils may occur.

Drug Interactions

None known.

Food Interactions

None known.

Usual Dose

Adult and Child (age 12 and over): 1–2 drops of a 0.05%–0.01% concentration solution up to 4 times daily.

Child (age 2–11): Consult your doctor for the appropriate dose for children in this age group. Do not overuse (see "Special Populations").

Child (under age 2): not recommended.

Overdosage

Overuse of tetrahydrozoline can cause central nervous system depression, drowsiness, lowered body temperature, slowed heartbeat, lowered blood pressure, shortness of breath, and eventually, coma.

Even if the victim is not displaying any of the symptoms listed above, do the following in case of accidental ingestion: If the victim is unconscious or having convulsions, call for an ambulance immediately. If you take the victim to an emergency room, be sure to bring the bottle or container with you. If the victim is conscious, call your local poison control center or a health care professional. The poison control center may suggest inducing vomiting with ipecac syrup (available without a prescription at any pharmacy). DO NOT induce vomiting unless specifically instructed to do so.

Special Populations

Pregnancy/Breast-feeding

It is not generally recommended that pregnant women take any drugs, particularly during the first 3 months after conception. There have been no studies regarding the effects of tetrahydrozoline on the developing fetus. Check with your doctor if you are or might be pregnant before using tetrahydrozoline.

It is not known if tetrahydrozoline passes into breast milk. If you must take tetrahydrozoline, bottle-feed your baby with formula.

Infants/Children

Do not use tetrahydrozoline in children under age 2. Excessive use of tetrahydrozoline in children can cause systemic complications, including severe drowsiness and profuse sweating. Consult your doctor for the appropriate dose in children under age 12.

Seniors

In some older individuals, use of tetrahydrozoline, especially in high doses, may cause tiny fragments of the iris (colored portion of the eye) to become detached. If this happens, call your doctor.

Generic Name

Thimerosal (thye-MER-oe-sal)

Definition

A mercury-based chemical used in OTC nasal saline solutions and decongestants as a preservative, and in first aid skin care products as an antiseptic. Some artificial tear preparations also contain thimerosal. In some people, thimerosal can cause allergic reactions.

Generic Name

Thymol (THYE-mol)

Definition

A chemical obtained from thyme oil, used as an antifungal and antibacterial ingredient in vaginal douches and mouthwashes.

Generic Name

Tolnaftate (tol-NAFF-tate)

Brand Names

*Absorbine Jr.	FungiCure
Aftate	Johnson's Odor-Eaters
Blis-To-Sol	NP-27
Desenex Antifungal Spray Liquid	Odor-Eaters Antifungal
Dr. Scholl's Athletes Foot	Tinactin
	Ting Antifungal

**Not all products in this brand-name group contain tolnaftate.*

Type of Drug

Topical antifungal agent.

Used for

Cure of tinea pedis (athlete's foot), tinea cruris (jock itch), and tinea corporis (ringworm), and relief of the itching, cracking, burning, and discomfort accompanying these conditions; prevention of the recurrence of athlete's foot.

General Information

A fungus is an organism that obtains nutrients from other living organisms or from dead organic matter in order to survive. In doing so, fungi cause infections that only an antifungal agent can cure.

Tolnaftate has been commercially available since 1965, and has become the standard topical antifungal medication. It is the only OTC drug approved for both the treatment and prevention of athlete's foot.

Tolnaftate is effective in inhibiting the growth of and killing many types of fungus. It is ineffective, however, against *Candida,* the fungus that causes yeast infection.

Tolnaftate is most effective against the dry, scaly type of athlete's foot. It is not as effective against the soggy type of athlete's foot often associated with bacterial infection.

Tolnaftate relieves itching, burning, and soreness within 24 to 72 hours of beginning therapy. Treatment of jock itch should be complete within 2 weeks; treatment of ringworm and athlete's foot, 4 weeks. However, it may take up to 6 weeks to treat some cases of athlete's foot; for example, when lesions are between the toes or when the skin has thickened.

To help prevent recurrence of infection, treatment should be continued for 2 weeks after the disappearance of all symptoms.

Tolnaftate is available by brand name in powder, cream, solution, gel, liquid, spray liquid, and spray powder form. Sprays and powders may be less effective than creams and solutions because they are often not rubbed into the skin. The solution may be more effective than the cream. An advantage of the powder is that it retains water; it is important in the treatment of athlete's foot that the foot be kept dry.

Be aware that products of the same brand name do not necessarily contain the same active ingredient. For example, the active ingredient in Desenex spray liquid is tolnaftate, but the active ingredient in Desenex powder is a different antifungal medication, undecylenic acid-zinc undecylenate. (To add to the potential confusion, the active ingredient in Desenex AF spray liquid is yet another antifungal agent, miconazole; and in Desenex AF cream, it is the antifungal clotrimazole.)

Cautions and Warnings

Do not take the maximum daily dosage of tolnaftate continuously for more than 2 weeks for jock itch, or 4 weeks continuously for athlete's foot.

Do not exceed the recommended daily dosage of tolnaftate.

Tolnaftate is for external use only. Avoid contact with your eyes. After applying the medication, wash your hands with soap and water.

If there is no improvement in your athlete's foot, jock itch, or ringworm within 10 days, or if your condition worsens in that time, stop using the product and call your doctor.

If irritation or hypersensitivity occurs, stop using the product and call your doctor.

If oozing lesions are present, treat them with a wet compress before applying the tolnaftate (see "Special Information").

Tolnaftate creams and solutions are not recommended for nail or scalp infections, and the powders and spray powders are not recommended for use on the scalp.

Tolnaftate spray liquids and powders are flammable. Do not use them while smoking or while near heat or flame, and do not puncture or incinerate the containers. Avoid inhaling.

Possible Side Effects

Most people don't experience side effects while using tolnaftate, but it may sting slightly when applied. Slight local irritation may occur when it is applied to broken skin.

Drug Interactions

None known.

Usual Dose

Adult and Child (age 2 and over): Clean the affected area with soap and water and dry thoroughly. Apply a thin layer of the product over the affected area twice daily (morning and night), or as directed by a doctor.

Child (under age 2): Consult your doctor.

If you are treating athlete's foot, be sure to apply the medication to the spaces between the toes.

Athlete's foot almost always affects both feet. Be sure to treat both feet equally, even if one foot looks worse than the other.

For best results, use tolnaftate for the length of time indicated on the package.

For prevention of athlete's foot, apply a thin layer of tolnaftate to the feet once or twice daily (morning and/or night).

Overdosage

Do the following in case of accidental ingestion: If the victim is unconscious or having convulsions, call for an ambulance immediately. If you take the victim to an emergency room, be sure to bring the bottle or container with you. If the victim is conscious, call your local poison control center or a health care professional. The poison control center may suggest inducing vomiting with ipecac syrup (available without a prescription at any pharmacy). DO NOT induce vomiting unless specifically instructed to do so.

Special Information

When treating athlete's foot, certain measures can be taken, in addition to using an antifungal agent, to assist in curing the infection:

- Wash your feet with soap and water every day, and thoroughly dry them (but be careful not to scrub too hard between the toes and irritate the skin).
- Wear well-fitting, ventilated shoes and light socks.
- Change your shoes and socks at least once daily, and wash the socks thoroughly.
- Try not to wear canvas, leather, or rubber-soled shoes for too long.
- Keep your feet dry.
- Air your feet out as often as possible.

When treating pressure areas of the foot, you may use a keratolytic agent (a substance that facilitates the removal of the thickened layer of the skin) such as Whitfield's ointment along with the tolnaftate. You may also use a wet compress—e.g., an aluminum acetate solution—to help heal oozing lesions. Neither interacts adversely with tolnaftate.

Storage Instructions

Do not expose the spray liquid and powder products to temperatures above 120°F. Tolnaftate solutions solidify when exposed to the cold, but return to liquid form, with no loss of potency, when they return to room temperature.

Special Populations

Pregnancy/Breast-feeding

It is not generally recommended that pregnant women take any drugs, particularly during the first 3 months after conception. Check with your doctor before self-medicating with tolnaftate if you are or might be pregnant, or if you are breast-feeding.

Infants/Children

Do not use any tolnaftate product on a child under age 2 unless directed by a doctor. Supervise children under age 12 in the use of these products.

Seniors

Older individuals should exercise the same caution as younger adults when using tolnaftate.

Generic Name

Triclosan (TRYE-kloe-san)

Definition

An antimicrobial agent found in OTC products for treatment of acne and in antibacterial bar soaps. Some diaper rash products also contain triclosan, but further research is needed to prove that this ingredient is effective in fighting infections that cause diaper rash. Triclosan is being tested as a possible antibacterial additive for mouthwashes and other oral care products.

Generic Name

Tripelennamine (TRYE-puhl-LEN-ah-min)

Definition

A topical antihistamine that reduces pain and itching and is used in OTC products for treatment of poison ivy and minor burns. Tripelennamine in concentrations of 0.5% to 2% is safe when applied no more than 3 or 4 times a day.

Generic Name

Triprolidine Hydrochloride

(trye-PROL-uh-deen HYE-droe-KLOR-ide)

Brand Names

*Actifed
Cenafed Plus
Tri-Fed

**Not all products in this brand-name group contain triprolidine HCl.*

Type of Drug

Antihistamine.

Used for

Temporary relief of sneezing, itchy eyes, runny nose, scratchy throat, and other symptoms (skin rash, itching, or hives) caused by seasonal allergy.

General Information

Histamine is one of the substances released by the body tissues during an allergic reaction. When it is released, the body reacts with a variety of symptoms, including itching and sneezing. Antihistamines work by competitively inhibiting the pharmacological action of histamine, which makes them very effective for relieving the symptoms of allergic reactions. Antihistamines may also help relieve a runny nose. However, because antihistamines do not work against the other substances released by the body during an allergic reaction, they can reduce only about 40% to 60% of allergic symptoms. They are also not effective in clearing up a stuffy nose.

If you have seasonal allergies, antihistamines work best if you begin treatment before the allergy season starts. Those who suffer from allergies regardless of the season may need to take antihistamines all year.

Antihistamines will not cure or prevent allergies, viral infections (colds), or bacterial infection. The best you can hope for is symptomatic relief.

Triprolidine hydrochloride is classified as an alkylamine antihistamine. Others in this group include chlorpheniramine and pheniramine. Of the antihistamines available without a prescription, these are the least likely to make you sleepy. Newer antihistamines do not have the common antihistamine side effect of drowsiness, but they are currently available only by prescription.

In cold and allergy products, triprolidine is often combined with the nasal decongestant pseudoephedrine.

Triprolidine is one of the few antihistamines that is considered generally safe for children even under age 2. However, always check with your doctor before giving triprolidine to children under age 6.

Triprolidine starts to work within 15 to 30 minutes after it is taken, and its effects last for 3 to 6 hours.

Triprolidine is available by brand name in tablet and liquid form.

Cautions and Warnings

Do not exceed the recommended daily dosage of triprolidine.

Triprolidine and other antihistamines should be used with caution if you have breathing problems, such as emphysema, chronic bronchitis, or asthma. These drugs dry the mucous membranes, which can inhibit the ability of the lungs to move or get rid of the excess secretions that these conditions produce.

Triprolidine and other antihistamines should be used with caution by people with glaucoma, hyperthyroidism, heart disease, high blood pressure or an enlarged prostate. If you have any of these conditions, take triprolidine only on the advice of your doctor.

Antihistamines act as a depressant on the central nervous system (CNS), which can cause sleepiness or grogginess and can interfere with the ability to concentrate. Your ability to perform activities that require your full alertness and coordination, such as driving a motor vehicle or operating machinery, may be affected. Refrain from drinking alcohol while you are taking triprolidine because alcohol aggravates these effects.

Possible Side Effects

▼ Most common: restlessness, nervousness, sleeplessness or dizziness, excitability, poor muscle coordination, headache, and upset stomach.

▼ Less common: dry eyes, nose, and mouth; blurred vision; difficulty urinating; irritability (at high doses); increased blood pressure; increased or irregular heart rate; and heart palpitations.

Drug Interactions

• Triprolidine can enhance the effect of other drugs that depress the CNS, such as barbiturates, tranquilizers, sleeping medications, and alcohol (present in many OTC preparations). If you are taking other depressant drugs, check with your doctor before using triprolidine or any other antihistamine. Avoid drinking alcohol if you are taking triprolidine.

• Triprolidine should not be used at the same time as a monoamine oxidase inhibitor (MAOI) or within 2 weeks of stopping treatment with an MAOI. MAOIs are used to treat depression, other psychiatric or emotional conditions, and Parkinson's disease. If you are not sure whether you are or have been taking an MAOI, check with your doctor or pharmacist before you use triprolidine.

• Antihistamines can affect the results of skin and blood tests. Notify your health care professional before scheduling these tests if you are taking triprolidine.

Usual Dose

Because histamine is released nearly continuously, it is best to take antihistamines on a schedule rather than as needed.

Adult and Child (age 12 and over): 2.5 mg every 4–6 hours. Do not exceed 10 mg in a 24-hour period.

Child (age 6–11): 1.25 mg every 4–6 hours. Do not exceed 5 mg in a 24-hour period.

Child (under age 6): Consult your doctor.

The inconvenience of the sedating effects of triprolidine may be minimized by either taking a full dose at bedtime or using the smallest recommended doses, combined with a decongestant, during the day. Another alternative is to start with the lowest dose when you begin taking the drug and gradually increase the dosage over several days.

If you forget to take a dose of triprolidine hydrochloride, do so as soon as you remember. If it is almost time for your next dose, skip the one you forgot and continue with your regular schedule. Do not take a double dose.

Overdosage

Symptoms of antihistamine overdose in children include dilated pupils, flushed face, dry mouth, fever, excitability, hallucinations, loss of muscle coordination, and seizures.

In adults, severe overdose can cause drowsiness or coma, which may be followed by excitability or seizures. Eventually fluid can build up in the brain; the kidneys may fail, and the heart and lungs may stop working, resulting in death. Symptoms may develop within 30 minutes to 2 hours following an overdose, and death may occur within 18 hours.

Even if the victim is not displaying any of the symptoms listed above, do the following in case of accidental overdose: If the victim is unconscious or having convulsions, call for an ambulance immediately. If you take the victim to an emergency room, be sure to bring the bottle or container with you. If the victim is conscious, call your local poison

control center or a health care professional. The poison control center may suggest inducing vomiting with ipecac syrup (available without a prescription at any pharmacy). DO NOT induce vomiting unless specifically instructed to do so.

Special Populations

Pregnancy/Breast-feeding

Antihistamines are not recommended for use during pregnancy unless directed by your doctor. Antihistamines are known to pass into the breast milk of nursing mothers and may cause side effects in infants. Check with your doctor before taking triprolidine if you are or might be pregnant, or if you are breast-feeding.

Infants/Children

Children may be be more susceptible to the side effects of triprolidine. They are also more susceptible to accidental antihistamine overdose. Unlike other antihistamines, triprolidine is considered safe for use in children as young as 4 months, but only with a doctor's supervision. Do not give triprolidine to a child under age 6 unless directed by your doctor.

Seniors

Older individuals may be more sensitive to the side effects of triprolidine and other antihistamines. They may experience nervousness, irritability, restlessness, dizziness, sedation, hallucinations, seizures, and low blood pressure. Most mild reactions may be handled by either lowering your dose or by trying another antihistamine.

Generic Name

Trolamine Salicylate

(TROE-luh-meen SAL-ih-SILL-ate)

Brand Names

Aspercreme
Mobisyl
Myoflex
Sportscreme

Type of Drug

Topical analgesic (pain reliever).

Used for

Relief of soreness, stiffness, and pain in muscles, joints, and tendons.

General Information

Topical analgesics are one of the most popular types of OTC drugs, and the number of these drugs sold continues to increase year after year. Many of the people using these products are over age 50; in fact, 40% of individuals in this age group use topical analgesics on a regular basis. Younger people may use topical analgesics to relieve pain and soreness brought on by exercising or playing sports.

Salicylates (e.g., aspirin, sodium salicylate, magnesium salicylate) are thought to relieve pain by affecting the body's production of complex hormones known as prostaglandins. However, it has not been proven that trolamine salicylate, a topical member of the group, works in this way when applied to the skin, nor does it work as a counterirritant to relieve pain, as does methyl salicylate, another topical analgesic. There have been some published reports indicating that trolamine salicylate may be effective in relieving pain and soreness caused by exercise and weight training; however, the FDA does not recognize trolamine salicylate as an effective OTC analgesic.

Trolamine salicylate is available in brand-name products as a single ingredient and in combination with other topical analgesics.

Cautions and Warnings

Trolamine salicylate should not be used for longer than 10 consecutive days. If your pain persists for more than 7 days, stop using the preparation and call your doctor.

Do not exceed the recommended daily dosage of a trolamine salicylate preparation.

Trolamine salicylate should be used only on the skin. Don't apply it near your eyes or to mucous membranes (i.e., inside the mouth, nose, rectum, or vagina).

Don't use trolamine salicylate on red or irritated skin. Stop using it if irritation develops, and call your doctor.

To avoid the risk of irritation, redness, or blistering, don't use a tight bandage or dressing over the skin where you apply trolamine salicylate.

Don't use a trolamine salicylate preparation on broken, irritated, or sunburned skin, or on an open wound.

If you wear contact lenses, don't take them out or put them in your eyes after you use a trolamine salicylate preparation without first washing your hands.

Drug Interactions

Some people taking the anticoagulant (blood-thinning) drug warfarin who also used a salicylate-containing topical analgesic have experienced an increase in the effect of warfarin. If you take warfarin, talk to your doctor or pharmacist before you self-medicate with trolamine salicylate.

Possible Side Effects

None known

Usual Dose

Adult and Child (age 12 and over): Massage a generous amount into the painful area until it is thoroughly absorbed into the skin. Repeat as needed. Don't apply more than 4 times in 24 hours. Be sure to wash your hands thoroughly afterward. If you are treating pain in your hands, wait 30 minutes before washing.

Child (under age 12): not recommended.

Overdosage

Do the following in case of accidental ingestion: If the victim is unconscious or having convulsions, call for an ambulance immediately. If you take the victim to an emergency room, be sure to bring the bottle or container with you. If the victim is conscious, call your local poison control center or a health care professional. The poison control center may suggest inducing vomiting with ipecac syrup (available without a prescription at any pharmacy). DO NOT induce vomiting unless specifically instructed to do so.

Special Information

Besides using a topical preparation, there are also physical methods of easing the pain of an overworked muscle, such as by gently massaging the injured area. In fact, some of the benefit gained from using topical medications may simply be due to the fact that they are applied by being rubbed and massaged into the skin. Another way to ease pain is to apply heat to the skin with a hot water bottle or heating pad; in addition to reducing pain, heat helps the collagen in your skin regain its elasticity and lose its stiffness after a stretching injury.

Special Populations

Allergies
If you are allergic to aspirin or to other salicylates, check with your doctor before using trolamine salicylate.

Pregnancy/Breast-feeding
It is not generally recommended that pregnant women take any drugs, particularly during the first 3 months after conception.

Check with your doctor before using trolamine salicylate if you are or might be pregnant or if you are breast-feeding.

Infants/Children
Trolamine salicylate should not be taken by children under age 12 unless prescribed by a doctor.

Seniors
Seniors should exercise the same caution as younger adults when using trolamine salicylate.

Generic Name

Undecylenic Acid (UN-des-uhl-EN-ik)

Brand Names

Blis-To-Sol
*Cruex
*Desenex
FungiCure
Undelenic

**Not all products in this brand-name group contain undecylenic acid.*

Type of Drug

Antifungal agent.

Used for

Curing tinea pedis (athlete's foot), tinea cruris (jock itch), and tinea corporis (ringworm), and relieving the itching, cracking, burning, and discomfort accompanying these conditions.

General Information

A fungus is an organism that obtains nutrients from other living organisms or from dead organic matter in order to survive. In doing so, they cause infections that only an antifungal agent can cure.

Undecylenic acid and its salts—calcium undecylenate, copper undecylenate, and zinc undecylenate—are topical antifungal medications. Undecylenic acid inhibits the growth of fungi. To be effective, it requires extended exposure at relatively high concentrations.

Undecylenic acid is most often used in combination with its zinc salt, with the combination labeled as a "total undecylenate." Zinc undecylenate is thought to free undecylenic acid on contact with perspiration. The zinc salt also has astringent activity, which lessens irritation and inflammation associated with the fungal infection.

Sprays and powders may be less effective than creams and solutions because they are often not rubbed into the skin. However, when a drying effect is desirable, powder products are the best choice.

Treatment of jock itch should be complete within 2 weeks; treatment of ringworm and athlete's foot, within 4 weeks.

The combination undecylenic acid-zinc undecylenate is available by brand name in cream, ointment, powder, and spray powder form. Undecylenic acid alone is available by brand name as a liquid and a tincture. Zinc undecylenate alone is available by brand name as a powder.

Cautions and Warnings

If there is no improvement in your condition within 2 weeks for jock itch or 4 weeks for ringworm or athlete's foot, or if it worsens in that time, stop using an undecylenic preparation and call your doctor.

Do not exceed the recommended daily dosage of an undecylenic preparation.

These undecylenic preparations are for external use only. Avoid contact with your eyes. After applying the medication, wash your hands with soap and water. Be careful not to inhale the powder.

If irritation or hypersensitivity occurs, stop using an undecylenic preparation and call your doctor.

Undecylenic preparations are not recommended for nail or scalp infections.

People with impaired circulation, including diabetics, should not use an undecylenic preparation without their doctor's supervision.

The spray powder is flammable. Do not use it while smoking or while near heat or flame, and do not puncture or incinerate the container.

Although at least 1 brand name product containing calcium undecylenate is promoted as a treatment for diaper rash, the FDA does not regard any OTC topical antifungal product as safe and effective for the treatment and/or prevention of diaper rash. The agency maintains that diaper rash associated with fungal infection must be diagnosed and treated by a physician.

Possible Side Effects

Undecylenic acid-zinc undecylenate is relatively nonirritating and rarely causes hypersensitivity reactions.

The high alcohol content of the undecylenic acid tincture or liquid may cause stinging if the product is applied to broken skin.

Drug Interactions

None known.

Usual Dose

Adult and Child (age 2 and over):

Clean the affected area with soap and water and dry thoroughly. Apply a thin layer of the product over the affected area twice daily (morning and night), or as directed by a doctor.

If you are treating athlete's foot, be sure to apply the medication to the spaces between the toes.

For best results, use undecylenic preparations for the length of time indicated on the package.

Child (under age 2): not recommended unless directed by your doctor.

Overdosage

Do the following in case of accidental ingestion: If the victim is unconscious or having convulsions, call for an ambulance immediately. If you take the victim to an emergency room, be sure to bring the bottle or container with you. If the victim is conscious, call your local poison control center or a health care professional. The poison control center may suggest inducing vomiting with ipecac syrup (available without a prescription at any pharmacy). DO NOT induce vomiting unless specifically instructed to do so.

Special Information

When treating athlete's foot, certain measures can be taken, in addition to using an antifungal agent, to assist in curing the infection:

- Wash your feet with soap and water every day, and thoroughly dry them (but be careful not to scrub too hard between the toes and irritate the skin).
- Wear well-fitting, ventilated shoes and light socks.
- Change your shoes and socks at least once daily, and wash the socks thoroughly.
- Try not to wear canvas, leather, or rubber-soled shoes for too long.
- Keep your feet dry.
- Air your feet out as often as possible.

Storage Instructions

Do not expose the aerosol spray powder to temperatures above 120°F.

Special Populations

Pregnancy/Breast-feeding

It is not generally recommended that pregnant women take

any drugs, particularly during the first 3 months after conception. Check with your doctor before self-medicating with an undecylenic preparation if you are or might be pregnant, or if you are breast-feeding.

Infants/Children

Do not use any undecylenic product on a child under 2 years of age unless directed by a doctor. Supervise older children under the age of 12 in the use of these products.

Do not use an undecylenic preparation to treat your child's diaper rash unless directed by your doctor (see "Cautions and Warnings").

Seniors

Older individuals should exercise the same caution as younger adults when using any of these products.

Generic Name

White Petrolatum

(PET-roe-LAY-tum)

Definition

See ***Petrolatum, page 955***

Generic Name

Witch Hazel

Definition

An astringent (drying agent) commonly used to relieve minor skin irritations; also known as hamamelis water. It is also sometimes used to stop bleeding from small wounds. Witch hazel is extracted from the twigs and leaves of a shrub, *Hamamelis virginiana,* native to the forests of North America. The product is included in rectal pads and wipes for treatment of hemorrhoids and in liquid preparations for relief of poison ivy.

Generic Name

Xylometazoline Hydrochloride

(zye-loe-met-AZE-oh-leen HYE-droe-KLOR-ide)

Brand Name

Otrivin

Type of Drug

Decongestant.

Used for

Temporary relief of nasal congestion (stuffy nose) that may accompany allergies or colds.

General Information

Decongestants relieve nasal congestion by narrowing or constricting the blood vessels in the nose. This action reduces the blood supplied to the nose and decreases the swelling in mucous membranes.

Decongestants are used to treat the nasal stuffiness of colds and allergies. However, they cannot cure a cold or allergy. The best you can hope for is symptomatic relief. To effectively relieve allergy symptoms, decongestants are usually given in combination with an antihistamine, which works against histamine, a chemical substance released by the body during an allergic reaction.

Xylometazoline hydrochloride, in either a spray form or drops, is applied topically to the nose to relieve nasal congestion. Sprays are easier to use and help to reduce the risk of swallowing the solution, since they are applied with the head upright. Drops are preferred for children. After administration, the drug's effects last for about 5 to 6 hours.

Cautions and Warnings

Xylometazoline should not be used for longer than 3 days continuously; if your symptoms have not improved after this time, stop using the drug and call your doctor.

Do not exceed the recommended daily dosage of xylometazoline.

Do not use xylometazoline if you have angle-closure glaucoma, unless recommended by your doctor.

A problem common to all forms of topical decongestants is rebound congestion; that is, you may still have a stuffy nose even though you have been using xylometazoline for several days. The lining of your nose may swell and turn red, giving you the appearance of allergic rhinitis. If this happens, stop using xylometazoline and contact your doctor. The signs of rebound congestion will usually go away in about a week after you stop using the drug.

Always check the expiration date before using a xylometazoline preparation. If the product is discolored or cloudy, do not use it.

To reduce the risk of spreading infection, droppers and spray bottles should not be used by more than one person. Rinse dropper and bottle tips with hot water after use. Be careful not to let hot water into the bottle. Do not let the bottle tip come into contact with any surface.

Possible Side Effects

▼ Most common: temporary burning, stinging, or dryness; sneezing; and rebound congestion (see "Cautions and Warnings").

▼ Less common: high blood pressure, nervousness, nausea, dizziness, headache, sleeplessness, heart palpitations, and fast or irregular heartbeat. If you develop any of these effects while using xylometazoline, stop taking the drug immediately and contact your doctor.

Drug Interactions

• Xylometazoline should not be used at the same time as a monoamine oxidase inhibitor (MAOI) or within 2 weeks of stopping treatment with an MAOI. MAOIs are used to treat depression, other psychiatric or emotional conditions, and Parkinson's disease. If you are not sure whether you are or have been taking an MAOI, check with your doctor or pharmacist before you use xylometazoline.

• If you are taking a tricyclic antidepressant (such as imipramine or desipramine), you should not use xylometazoline.

Food Interactions

None known.

Usual Dose

Adult and Child (age 12 and over): 0.1% solution, 2–3 drops or sprays every 8–10 hours.

Child (age 2–12): 0.05% solution, 2–3 drops or sprays every 8–10 hours. Do not use a 0.1% solution for children in this age group unless directed by a doctor.

Child (under age 2): not recommended except under the supervision of a doctor.

Overdosage

Even if the victim is not displaying any of the symptoms listed above, do the following in case of accidental ingestion: If the victim is unconscious or having convulsions, call for an ambulance immediately. If you take the victim to an emergency room, be sure to bring the bottle or container with you. If the victim is conscious, call your local poison control center or a health care professional. The poison control center may suggest inducing vomiting with ipecac syrup (available without a prescription at any pharmacy). DO NOT induce vomiting unless specifically instructed to do so.

Special Information

Colds will usually go away in 1 to 2 weeks whether they are treated or not. There are other ways to temporarily treat congestion caused by colds, including taking tea with lemon and honey or eating chicken soup or hot broth.

Special Populations

Pregnancy/Breast-feeding

It is not generally recommended that pregnant women take any drug, particularly during the first 3 months after conception. It is not known whether topically applied xylometazoline can harm the developing fetus if taken during pregnancy. Check with your doctor if you are or might be pregnant before taking xylometazoline.

It is not known whether xylometazoline passes into breast milk. If you must take xylometazoline, bottle-feed your baby with formula.

Infants/Children
Xylometazoline is not recommended in children under 2 unless directed by a doctor.

Seniors
Seniors should exercise the same caution as younger adults when using xylometazoline.

Generic Name

Zinc Acetate (ZINK ASS-eh-tate)

Definition

A skin protectant used in OTC products for treatment of diaper rash, minor burns, and sunburn. There is some evidence that this chemical may not be as effective as other available protectants, such as petrolatum and cocoa butter. The FDA recommends that products with zinc acetate not be used on children under age 2.

Generic Name

Zinc Oxide (ZINK OKS-ide)

Brand Names

*A and D
Ammens
Anusol Ointment
Balmex
Caldesene Medicated Ointment
Desitin
Diaperene Diaper Rash
Diaper Guard
Diaper Rash Ointment
Dyprotex
First Aid Medicated Powder
Flanders Buttocks
Gold Bond
Hem-Prep
Hemorid for Women Suppository
Hydrosal
*Johnson's
Little Bottoms
Mexsana Medicated
Nupercainal
Nutra Soothe
Ostiderm
Pazo
Plexolan Lanolin
Resinol
Schamberg's Anti-Itch
Triple Paste
Tronolane

**Not all products in this brand-name group contain zinc oxide.*

Type of Drug

Topical astringent; antiseptic; skin protectant.

Used for

Protecting the skin from harmful irritants and aiding healing.

General Information

Zinc oxide is used to shield the skin surface from chemical irritants and harmful sun overexposure. It provides a protective coating that does not dissolve in water or alcohol.

It promotes healing by attracting protein to the affected area and thus encouraging new tissue growth. It also helps to dry the skin by hastening removal of skin-surface moisture, which further promotes healing.

In addition to its role as a sunscreen to block out ultraviolet rays, this drug is used for relief of a number of common skin conditions, such as diaper rash; poison ivy, oak, and sumac exposure; external hemorrhoids; and insect bites.

Zinc oxide is also used in a number of skin care products to thicken lotions and creams and make them easier to apply.

Cautions and Warnings

If there is no improvement in the infected area within 7 days or an allergic reaction develops, discontinue using the drug and contact your doctor.

Do not exceed the recommended daily dosage of a zinc oxide product.

Zinc oxide is for external use only.

Zinc oxide is often used in combination products containing lanolin. While zinc oxide itself has no tendency to cause allergic reactions, some individuals may become sensitized to the lanolin and develop a rash. Should this occur, discontinue using the product and contact your doctor.

People who are sensitive to any ingredient in a zinc oxide preparation should avoid using the product.

Do not apply zinc oxide ointments to deep or puncture wounds, areas of broken skin, or cuts.

When using baby powders containing zinc oxide, keep the powder away from the child's face to prevent accidental inhalation.

Possible Side Effects

The thickness and consistency of zinc oxide prevents it from being absorbed into the skin. Consequently, topical or systemic side effects or allergic reactions, even with long-term use, are rare.

Hemorrhoid ointments containing zinc oxide may cause a burning sensation in some people, especially if the skin in the affected area is not intact.

Drug Interactions

None known.

Usual Dose

Sunscreen

Adult and Child (age 6 and over): Apply to exposed areas before going out in the sun. Repeat as needed.

Child (under age 6): Consult your doctor.

Poison Ivy, Itching, Insect Bites

Adult and Child (age 6 and over): Apply to the affected area no more than 3–4 times per day.

Child (under age 6): Consult your doctor.

Diaper rash

Remove soiled diaper promptly. Wash the genital and anal area thoroughly with water; pat dry. Apply ointment liberally with each diaper change and after baths, especially at night to prevent long exposure to moisture.

Hemorrhoids

Adult and Child (age 12 and over): Clean the area with mild soap and warm water; rinse thoroughly; gently pat dry. Apply a layer of the product to the area up to 5 times per day or after each bowel movement.

Suppositories containing zinc oxide may be used up to 6 times a day.

Child (under age 12): Consult your doctor.

Prickly Heat, Chafing

Adult and Child (age 2 and over): Apply 3–4 times a day as needed, or as directed by a doctor.

Child (under age 2): Consult a doctor.

Overdosage

Because zinc oxide is so dense, it is not readily absorbed through the pores of the skin. The risk of overdose is very low.

Do the following in case of accidental ingestion: If the victim is unconscious or having convulsions, call for an ambulance immediately. If you take the victim to an emergency room, be sure to bring the bottle or container with you. If the victim is conscious, call your local poison control center or a health care professional. The poison control center may suggest inducing vomiting with ipecac syrup (available without a prescription at any pharmacy). DO NOT induce vomiting unless specifically instructed to do so.

Special Populations

Pregnancy/Breast-feeding

Since zinc oxide is not absorbed into the skin, there is little risk to either pregnant women or nursing mothers and their babies. However, it is not generally recommended that pregnant women take any drugs, particularly during the first 3 months after conception. Check with your doctor if you are or might be pregnant, or if you are breast-feeding.

Infants/Children

Zinc oxide products are generally safe when used as directed for diaper rash (see "Cautions and Warnings"). However, hemorrhoid products should not be used in children younger than 12, and skin products should not be used in children younger than 6, without first consulting a doctor.

Seniors

Seniors should exercise the same caution as younger adults when using a zinc oxide product.

Generic Name

Zinc Stearate (ZINK STEER-ate)

Definition

A skin protectant used in OTC diaper rash products.

Generic Name

Zinc Undecylenate (ZINK UN-des-UHL-en-ate)

Definition

*see **Undecylenic Acid,** page 1081*

Index

The entries listed in bold refer to brand-name products.

ABOUT THE EDITORS

Robert P. Rapp, Pharm. D., is Professor and Director of the Division of Pharmacy Practice and Science at the University of Kentucky College of Pharmacy and is the Associate Director of the Department of Pharmacy at the University of Kentucky Hospital. He is also Professor of Surgery in the Department of Surgery, College of Medicine, University of Kentucky. He is a member of the United States Pharmacopeia Subcommittee on Surgical Drugs and Devices.

Aimee R. Gelhot, Pharm. D., is Ambulatory Care Clinical Specialist at the University of Kentucky Medical Center and Assistant Professor in both the Department of Medicine and the Division of Pharmacy Practice and Science, Colleges of Medicine and Pharmacy, University of Kentucky.

Mary Lea Gora-Harper, Pharm. D., directs the Drug Information Center at the University of Kentucky Hospital and is Assistant Professor in the Division of Pharmacy Practice and Science, College of Pharmacy, University of Kentucky. She is a member of the Consortium for Medical Information, Policy, and Research, and an editorial advisory board member and reviewer for several professional publications in the area of drug information and pharmacoeconomics.

Angela Hoth, Pharm. D., is Family Practice Clinical Pharmacy Specialist at the University of Kentucky Medical Center and Assistant Professor in both the Department of Family Practice and the Division of Pharmacy Practice and Science, Colleges of Medicine and Pharmacy, University of Kentucky.

Michael B. Jacobs, M.D., is Professor of Medicine and section head of Primary Care Internal Medicine at Stanford University School of Medicine. He also directs teaching programs there and practices primary care medicine at Stanford Medical Group.